MANUAL OF
CLINICAL PROBLEMS
IN NEPHROLOGY

MANUAL OF CLINICAL PROBLEMS IN NEPHROLOGY

Burton David Rose, M.D.

Associate Professor of Medicine, Harvard Medical School and Harvard Center for the Study of Kidney Diseases; Director of Clinical Nephrology, Brigham and Women's Hospital, Boston, Massachusetts

Robert Mark Black, M.D.

Assistant Professor of Medicine, University of Massachusetts Medical School; Director of Nephrology, The Fallon Clinic, Worcester, Massachusetts

Little, Brown and Company
Boston/Toronto

Library of Congress Catalog Card No. 88-
81597

ISBN 0-316-75637-7

Printed in the United States of America

DON

For our children,
Amy, Rebecca, Emily, Anne, and Daniel

CONTENTS

PREFACE

The purpose of this manual is to provide medical students, house officers, and practicing physicians with basic concepts of clinical nephrology and hypertension in a concise format. Each chapter is devoted to a single disorder and generally contains brief reviews of pathology (when appropriate), pathophysiology, clinical manifestations, diagnosis, and therapy. Bibliographies of pertinent and current references are also included.

The book is divided into several major sections: acid-base and electrolyte disorders, hypertension, acute renal failure, glomerular diseases, vascular and tubulointerstitial diseases, and chronic renal failure (including dialysis and renal transplantation). Each of these sections is subdivided into chapters covering those conditions that are most commonly seen in the clinical setting. The section on acid-base and electrolyte disorders, for example, has separate chapters on hyponatremia and hypernatremia, metabolic acidosis and alkalosis, and disorders of potassium balance. There are also separate chapters devoted to new concepts in lactic acidosis, ketoacidosis, renal tubular acidosis, polyuria (including diabetes insipidus), and the clinical use of diuretics.

Information is also presented on more general issues that the clinician should, in our opinion, possess. Included, therefore, are discussions on the use and misuse of the plasma creatinine concentration and creatinine clearance as estimates of the glomerular filtration rate, the diagnostic approach to the patient with renal disease, the evaluation and management of renal calculi, and possible therapies to prevent progressive renal failure.

This book could not have been completed without the help of many people. We would particularly like to thank Drs. Diego Garcia and William Crooks as well as the many students and residents at the University of Massachusetts Medical School and Harvard Medical School and the St. Vincent Hospital and Brigham and Women's Hospital who reviewed parts of the text, and Susan Pioli at Little, Brown for her continued encouragement.

B.D.R.
R.M.B.

I. ACID-BASE AND ELECTROLYTE DISORDERS

1. HYPONATREMIA

Basic Physiology

An understanding of the meaning of the plasma sodium concentration is essential in the approach to the patient with hyponatremia. In particular, it is important to appreciate that hyponatremia represents a *disorder of water balance*; this is in contrast to true volume depletion (due to gastrointestinal or renal losses) or to edematous states, which are *disorders of sodium balance*.

This distinction can be illustrated by a review of the difference between osmoregulation and volume regulation (Table 1-1). The former involves maintenance of the *plasma osmolality*, which is usually composed primarily of sodium salts. Changes in the plasma osmolality are, therefore, sensed as changes in the plasma sodium concentration by osmoreceptors in the hypothalamus [1]. These receptors affect both water intake and water excretion by influencing thirst and the release of antidiuretic hormone (ADH), respectively. The latter increases the urine osmolality and causes water retention by enhancing the permeability of the collecting tubules to water.

Volume regulation, on the other hand, attempts to maintain *tissue perfusion*. Different sensors and effectors are involved in this process, including the sympathetic nervous system, the renin-angiotensin-aldosterone system, intrarenal hemodynamics, and possibly atrial natriuretic peptide [2]. These mediators regulate volume balance by affecting urinary sodium excretion* rather than the urine osmolality. ADH does play a small role since its release is enhanced by hypovolemia, acting via the aortic and perhaps the atrial baroreceptors [1]. The associated increase in water reabsorption will tend to cause some extracellular volume expansion, although about two-thirds of the water will enter the cells.

A few simple examples can highlight the clinical significance of the difference between osmoregulation and volume regulation. Ingestion of a water load lowers the plasma osmolality and plasma sodium concentration. This leads to a reduction in ADH release, a fall in urine osmolality (to below 100 mosmol/kg in some cases), and rapid excretion of the excess water. This process is so efficient that volume-maintaining mechanisms are usually not affected. A normal subject, for example, can excrete more than 10 liters of water per day. This has important implications for the development of hyponatremia; since water excretion is so efficient (normally keeping the plasma osmolality within a 1–2 % range), *water retention leading to hyponatremia* occurs in only two settings: when water excretion is impaired due primarily to an inability to shut off ADH; and rarely when there is a marked increase in water intake to overwhelm excretory capacity.

An infusion of isotonic saline, on the other hand, elicits a different set of responses. The extracellular volume is increased in this setting without an alteration in the plasma osmolality. As a result, there is no change in ADH release. However, the secretion of renin is reduced, resulting in decreased formation of angiotensin II and aldosterone. These hormonal changes promote the excretion of the excess sodium and water.

The lack of correlation between the plasma sodium concentration and the extracellular volume can also be illustrated by the response induced by exercising in hot weather. The loss of water (as sweat, which usually has a sodium concentration under 50 meq/L) produces both a *rise* in the plasma sodium concentration and a *fall* in volume. As a result, there will be activation of both the osmoregulatory and volume regulatory systems. If, however, the sweat losses are replaced entirely by free water, marked hyponatremia may ensue. This sequence has been described in ultramarathon runners who have massive sweat losses that are replaced by dilute juices and colas [3].

Etiology

With the understanding that hyponatremia and hypoosmolality usually represent the retention of ingested water, the causes of this problem can be divided into those disorders in which water excretion is abnormal and those in which water excretion is normal

---

*In addition to their renal effects, the sympathetic nervous system and angiotensin II also help to maintain the systemic blood pressure (by arteriolar constriction) and cardiac output (via β-adrenergic effects on the heart) in hypovolemic states.

Table 1-1. Difference between osmoregulation and volume regulation

	Osmoregulation	Volume regulation
What is being sensed	Plasma osmolality	Effective circulating volume
Sensors	Hypothalamic osmoreceptors	Carotid sinus Afferent arteriole Atria
Effectors	Antidiuretic hormone Thirst	Sympathetic nervous system Renin-angiotensin-aldosterone system Atrial natriuretic peptide Intrarenal hemodynamics Antidiuretic hormone
What is affected	Urine osmolality and, via thirst, water intake	Urinary sodium excretion

but intake is dramatically enhanced (called primary polydipsia) (Table 1-2) [4]. In both hypovolemic states and the syndrome of inappropriate ADH secretion (SIADH), for example, ADH release is enhanced, thereby impairing the excretion of ingested or administered water [1]. It is important to remember that, in addition to true volume depletion induced by fluid losses, advanced congestive heart failure and hepatic cirrhosis also lead to decreased tissue perfusion due to diminished cardiac function and splanchnic and peritoneal pooling, respectively. Thus, ADH release (as well as that of the other hypovolemic hormones, renin and norepinephrine) is enhanced in these disorders [5–7].

Although hyponatremia is almost always due to water retention, it can, in theory, also occur when effective solute (sodium plus potassium*) is lost in excess of water. There is only one setting, however, in which this is likely to occur: patients treated with a thiazide diuretic who have a large initial diuresis. In this setting, the diuretic increases sodium and potassium loss and the hypovolemia-induced release of ADH minimizes the loss of water. As an example, some patients with marked hyponatremia (plasma sodium concentration averaging 105 meq/L) have urinary sodium plus potassium losses that can exceed 150 meq/L [9]. These losses will directly lower the plasma sodium concentration, a problem that will be exacerbated by any associated water intake.

It might be assumed that loop diuretics can initiate the same sequence. However, *almost all reported cases of diuretic-induced hyponatremia have been caused by the thiazides* [9,10]. The decrease in susceptibility with the loop diuretics is probably related to their site of action; by impairing sodium reabsorption in the ascending limb of the loop of Henle, these agents also impair production of the medullary osmotic gradient that is required for countercurrent multiplication and the production of a hyperosmotic interstitium. Consequently, the ability of ADH to promote water retention and the development of hyponatremia is reduced. This effect of the loop diuretics can actually be used to *treat hyponatremia* in the SIADH (see *SIADH*). The thiazides, in comparison, act in the distal tubule in the cortex and do not interfere with concentrating ability [11].

One other diagnostic consideration is *pseudohyponatremia* in which hyponatremia is associated with a plasma osmolality that is normal or even elevated, rather than reduced (Table 1-2). The most common causes of this problem are hyperglycemia and hyperlipidemia [4]. Hyperglycemia directly raises the plasma osmolality; this creates an osmotic gradient that favors the movement of water out of the cells, lowering the plasma sodium concentration by dilution. In general, the plasma sodium concentration falls by 1 meq/L for every 62 mg/dl rise in the plasma glucose concentration. Therapy must be aimed at correcting the hyperosmolar state with insulin and fluids, not at raising the plasma sodium concentration.

---

*The effect of potassium must be included since it is the primary intracellular solute and is as osmotically active as sodium [8].

Table 1-2. Major causes of hyponatremia[a]

Disorder	Causes
IMPAIRED WATER EXCRETION	
Hypovolemic states	True volume depletion due to gastrointestinal or renal losses
	Diuretics—particularly the thiazides
	Heart failure
	Hepatic cirrhosis
SIADH	Neuropsychiatric disorders
	Drugs—most common with chlorpropamide or high-dose intravenous cyclophosphamide[b]
	Malignancy—especially oat-cell carcinoma
	Pulmonary infections or acute diseases
	Postoperative patient
Advanced renal failure	
Endocrine abnormality	Hypothyroidism
	Hypoadrenalism—cortisol deficiency more important for hyponatremia; aldosterone deficiency can contribute and causes hyperkalemia
Reset osmostat	Normal pregnancy (plasma sodium falls about 5 meq/L)
	Some cases of SIADH
	Severe malnutrition
NORMAL WATER EXCRETION (URINE OSMOLALITY BELOW 100 MOSMOL/KG)	
Primary polydipsia	Psychiatric diseases—particularly if dry mouth due to phenothiazines
	Hypothalamic disorders
PSEUDOHYPONATREMIA	
Normal plasma osmolality	Severe hyperlipidemia or hyperproteinemia
	Glycine irrigation in urologic surgery
Elevated plasma osmolality	Hyperglycemia
	Hypertonic mannitol in renal failure

[a]A more complete list is presented in ref. 4.
[b]Intravenous cyclophosphamide may be particularly dangerous because it is often given with water loading to prevent hemorrhagic cystitis. This combination can lead to severe and potentially fatal hyponatremia.

In contrast, the plasma osmolality is normal with hyperlipidemia. The hyponatremia in this setting is a laboratory artifact. The space taken up by the extra lipids means that each liter of plasma contains less water and therefore less sodium. The standard flame photometer measures the concentration of sodium per liter of plasma; although this value is decreased, the physiologically important plasma sodium concentration *per liter of plasma water* is actually normal.

The use of large volumes of isotonic glycine irrigation fluids during transurethral resection of the prostate or bladder can also lead to pseudohyponatremia as some of this solution is absorbed [12]. The net effect is a dilutional fall in the plasma sodium concentration (occasionally to below 115 meq/L) but maintenance of a normal plasma osmolality. Neurologic symptoms can occur but it is unclear whether they are due to the low sodium concentration or possibly to glycine toxicity [12].

Symptoms
The symptoms directly attributable to hyponatremia are primarily neurologic. Nausea and malaise are the earliest findings, with possible progression to headache, lethargy,

Table 1-3. Major steps in initial evaluation of hyponatremia

Plasma osmolality
Low: true hyponatremia
Normal or elevated: pseudohyponatremia or renal failure
Urine osmolality
< 100 mosmol/kg: primary polydipsia with normal water excretion
> 100 mosmol/kg: other causes of true hyponatremia in which water excretion is impaired
Urine sodium concentration
< 15 meq/L: effective volume depletion
> 20 meq/L: other causes in which normovolemia or renal salt wasting is present

obtundation, seizures, coma, and death or irreversible neurologic deficits in severe cases (plasma sodium concentration usually below 110–115 meq/L) [9,13,14].

The likelihood of developing these changes is related *both to the severity of the hyponatremia and to the rapidity with which the plasma sodium concentration falls* [13,14]. The reduction in the plasma osmolality creates an osmolar gradient that favors the movement of water from the extracellular fluid into the brain (as well as other cells). This cerebral overhydration appears to be the major factor leading to neurologic dysfunction. In one recently reported series, for example, 15 previously healthy young women with postoperative SIADH were given a relatively large quantity of intravenous water. As a result, there was a mean reduction in the plasma sodium concentration from 138 to 108 meq/L, occurring over a 48-hour period [14]. Four of the women died and the remainder had severe permanent neurologic deficits.

In comparison, more slowly developing hyponatremia results in a lesser degree of cerebral edema and generally fewer neurologic symptoms [13]. The return of brain volume toward normal appears to be due to a specific adaptive response of the brain that leads to the net loss of effective osmoles (such as sodium, potassium, and perhaps amino acids) from the brain cells [15]. How this occurs is not known.

Diagnosis

Hyponatremia is most often due to the SIADH, one of the hypovolemic states, or marked hyperglycemia [16]. The history and physical examination are often helpful in identifying, for example, the presence of heart failure, hepatic cirrhosis, or a possibly offending drug. Three simple laboratory tests are also diagnostically important: *the plasma osmolality, the urine osmolality, and the urine sodium concentration* (Table 1-3)[4]. The plasma osmolality (normal 275–290 mosmol/kg) is reduced in true hyponatremia but is normal or elevated with pseudohyponatremia, which generally does not require therapy aimed at raising the plasma sodium concentration. When evaluating the plasma osmolality, it is essential to subtract the osmotic contribution of urea (estimated from the blood urea nitrogen [BUN] concentration divided by 2.8) from the measured plasma osmolality; urea readily crosses cell membranes and is therefore an ineffective osmole that, unlike glucose, does not affect the plasma sodium concentration. Patients with advanced renal failure, for example, are susceptible to developing hyponatremia due to an impaired ability to excrete free water. The measured plasma osmolality is often elevated in this setting because of the high BUN. This does not, however, represent pseudohyponatremia since the effective plasma osmolality is actually reduced.

Determination of the urine osmolality is used to estimate water excretory ability. True hyponatremia with hypoosmolality should *completely suppress* ADH release (see Fig. 2-1), resulting in a urine osmolality below 100 mosmol/kg (or specific gravity ≤ 1.003). A higher value is usually found, indicating impaired water excretion, most often due to elevated ADH levels. In comparison, the finding of a maximally dilute urine suggests that primary polydipsia is the major problem. In this setting, the urine osmolality should remain low until the plasma sodium concentration returns to normal, a response that occurs rapidly once water intake is diminished [4,17].

The urine sodium concentration is used to distinguish between volume depletion and the SIADH. This parameter should be less than 15 meq/L with hypovolemia (unless there is salt wasting due to diuretic therapy, hypoaldosteronism, or underlying renal disease) but is generally above 20 meq/L in the SIADH, since water retention leads to initial volume expansion. The response to the administration of sodium chloride is often helpful in nonedematous patients if a borderline value is obtained. The urine sodium concentration should remain low initially with true volume depletion as sodium is retained to replete the extracellular volume. In comparison, the extra sodium is rapidly and appropriately excreted in the SIADH, resulting in a marked rise in the urine sodium concentration that can exceed 100 meq/L.

If the above laboratory evaluation suggests the SIADH (low plasma osmolality, high urine osmolality, and high urine sodium concentration), it is then important to identify the cause (Table 1-2) [4]. If no cause is apparent, hypothyroidism and adrenal insufficiency should be excluded. Idiopathic SIADH does occur, but many of these patients have an underlying occult malignancy (particularly oat-cell carcinoma of the lung) [18,19].

Concurrent acid-base or potassium disturbances also may be helpful in selected patients. Hypokalemia and metabolic alkalosis suggest vomiting or diuretic therapy whereas hyperkalemia suggests decreased potassium excretion due to renal failure, marked volume depletion, or adrenal insufficiency with hypoaldosteronism.

Treatment
Elevating the plasma sodium toward normal in patients with true hyponatremia is most often achieved by administering sodium or by restricting water intake. As will be seen, the proper regimen varies with the underlying cause. Before addressing these issues, however, it is important to review the controversy surrounding the *rate* at which the plasma sodium concentration should be corrected.

Rate of Correction
Clearly, patients with severe hyponatremia (plasma sodium concentration below 110–115 meq/L) are at risk of developing severe and potentially irreversible neurologic damage [9,13,14,20]. On the other hand, both experimental and clinical studies suggest that overly rapid correction also may be dangerous, possibly leading to central pontine myelinolysis, a severe neurologic disorder characterized by paraparesis or quadriparesis, dysarthria, and dysphagia [21,22].

A definitive recommendation for the treatment of severe hyponatremia cannot be made at this time, but it is probably adviseable to *raise the plasma sodium concentration by 0.5 to 1.0 meq/liter/hour until a level of 120 to 125 meq/L* is reached, a concentration at which the patient should be out of danger [20,23]. The plasma sodium concentration can then be slowly normalized over a period of days. Central demyelinating lesions are most likely to occur with more rapid correction, particularly if the plasma sodium concentration is raised within the first 48 hours by more than 25 meq/L or to above 140 meq/L [20,24].

True Volume Depletion
Asymptomatic patients with hyponatremia and true volume depletion are treated with isotonic saline, usually given at an empiric rate of 50 to 100 ml/hour. In this setting, correction of the hyponatremia will occur in two stages: the plasma sodium concentration will initially rise slowly since the administered fluid has a higher sodium concentration than the plasma; once volume repletion occurs, however, ADH release will be suppressed, leading to rapid excretion of the excess water and normalization of the plasma sodium concentration. Oral sodium chloride, given in the diet or in tablet form, is a safe alternative in patients who are able to eat.

In contrast, hypertonic saline should be administered to patients with symptomatic or severe hyponatremia (plasma sodium concentration ≤ 110 meq/L). The quantity given can be estimated from calculation of the sodium deficit:

Na deficit = volume of distribution of plasma sodium × deficit per liter

Although sodium is restricted to the extracellular space, changes in the plasma sodium concentration are distributed through the total body water (TBW) since water will equilibrate between the extracellular and intracellular compartments. The TBW is approximately 60 and 50 percent of lean body weight in men and women, respectively. If, for example, a 60-kg woman has a plasma sodium concentration of 105 meq/L, and the initial aim of therapy is to reach 120 meq/L, then:

$$Na\ deficit\ =\ 0.5\ \times\ 60\ \times\ (120\ -\ 105)\ =\ 450\ meq$$

Each liter of hypertonic saline contains 513 meq of sodium. Thus, 900 ml should be given over 15 hours to raise the plasma sodium concentration at a safe rate of 1.0 meq/liter/hour [20,23]. It must be emphasized that this formula is only an estimate and serial monitoring of the plasma sodium concentration is required to ascertain that the desired effect is achieved.

Edematous States

Therapy is different in the edematous states (heart failure, hepatic cirrhosis, or renal failure) since administering sodium will worsen the fluid overload. Restricting water intake to less than urine output is usually sufficient in patients with mild-to-moderate hyponatremia. In emergent cases, the plasma sodium concentration can be raised more quickly by the use of loop diuretics in combination with hypertonic saline. Sodium and water are lost with the diuretic, and only the sodium (as estimated from the urine volume and the urine sodium concentration) is replaced. The net effect is pure water loss and correction of the hyponatremia.

Therapy should also be aimed at the underlying disorder. Although this cannot be easily achieved with hepatic cirrhosis, the administration of a converting enzyme inhibitor to decrease afterload may be effective in raising the plasma sodium concentration toward normal in patients with severe congestive heart failure [25-27]. An increase in cardiac output leading to a reduction in ADH release may play an important role in this effect [26]. In addition, converting enzyme inhibition may, via local prostaglandin release, diminish the response to ADH [28], producing an increase in water excretion not seen with other unloading agents [27]. Concurrent administration of a loop diuretic may have a synergistic effect in this setting, perhaps by diminishing the urine osmolality and allowing more free water to be excreted [25].

SIADH

Treatment of the SIADH is potentially more complicated. Water restriction alone is often effective in mild cases. If, however, fluid is to be given, the sodium content is extremely important. The SIADH differs from volume depletion in that *sodium handling is normal,* since ADH only affects water balance. This distinction can be appreciated by the response to isotonic saline in a patient with the SIADH, a plasma sodium concentration of 116 meq/L, and a urine osmolality that is relatively fixed at 616 mosmol/kg [8]. Each liter of isotonic saline contains 308 mosmol (154 meq each of sodium and chloride). This fluid will initially raise the plasma sodium concentration because it is more concentrated than the plasma. In the steady state, however, all of the salt will be excreted (since salt balance is normal) but in only 500 ml of urine due to the high urine osmolality (308 mosmol in 500 ml equals 616 mosmol/kg). The net effect, therefore, is water retention and a *further reduction in the plasma sodium concentration.*

Thus, correction of the hyponatremia requires that the *osmolality of the administered fluid exceeds that of the urine* [8]. If, for example, a liter of hypertonic saline is given (containing 1026 mosmol of sodium chloride), all of the salt will again be excreted but now in about 1.7 liters of urine (1026 mosmol in 1.7 liters equals 616 mosmol/kg); the net effect is the loss of 700 ml of water and only a small rise in the plasma sodium concentration. (The plasma sodium concentration will at first rise quickly because of the highly concentrated solution and then fall back toward the baseline level as the sodium is excreted; the urine sodium concentration can exceed 100–200 meq/L at this time.)

These findings indicate that even hypertonic saline is relatively ineffective when the urine osmolality is very high. In this setting, optimal therapy requires that the urine osmolality be lowered. This can be most easily achieved with a loop diuretic that interferes with urinary concentrating ability by impairing sodium chloride reabsorption in the ascending limb of the loop of Henle [11]. If, for example, the urine osmolality is reduced to 300 mosmol/kg, the 1026 mosmol of salt in 1 liter of hypertonic saline will now be excreted in 3.4 liters; this loss of 2.4 liters of water will raise the plasma sodium concentration by up to 10 meq/L.

The calculations described above to estimate the sodium deficit and the rate at which it should be corrected can also be used in the SIADH. Although the SIADH is initially a water overload syndrome, the ensuing volume expansion promotes sodium and water loss in the urine. The net effect is that both water excess and sodium loss contribute to the fall in the plasma sodium concentration [29]. Thus, administering sodium is physiologically appropriate in this setting.

Similar considerations apply to the outpatient treatment of the chronic SIADH (as might occur with an oat-cell carcinoma). Restricting the intake of water and encouraging the intake of sodium will control the plasma sodium concentration in most patients. If compliance is poor or the urine osmolality is high, then therapy to diminish concentrating ability may be required. This can be achieved with low doses of a loop diuretic (such as 20 mg twice daily of furosemide, with a high-salt diet to prevent volume depletion) or with demeclocycline (a tetracycline derivative) or lithium, agents that directly antagonize the renal effect of ADH [4,30]. Demeclocycline has also been used successfully to raise the plasma sodium concentration in heart failure or hepatic cirrhosis; in these disorders, however, the decrease in hepatic function frequently results in impaired drug metabolism and subsequent nephrotoxicity [31].

Other Disorders

Treatment of the other causes of hyponatremia is variable. Hormone replacement is clearly indicated in patients with hypothyroidism or adrenal insufficiency. On the other hand, restricting water intake will rapidly normalize the plasma sodium concentration in patients with primary polydipsia in whom water excretory capacity is normal. It may also be helpful to alter the drug regimen when phenothiazines stimulate water intake by causing the sensation of a dry mouth.

Therapy aimed at raising the plasma sodium concentration is not required in pseudohyponatremia since the effective plasma osmolality is not reduced. The one exception may occur with the use of glycine irrigation solutions during transurethral urologic surgery. In this setting, the acute and marked reduction in the plasma sodium concentration may produce symptoms even in the absence of hypoosmolality [12].

References

1. Robertson, GL. Thirst and vasopressin function in normal and disordered states of water balance. *J Lab Clin Med* 101:351, 1983.
2. Rose, BD. *Clinical Physiology of Acid-Base and Electrolyte Disorders* (2nd ed.). New York: McGraw-Hill, 1987. Pp. 171-186.
3. Frizzell, RT, Lang, GH, Lowance, DC, Lathan, SR. Hyponatremia and ultramarathon running. *J Am Med Assoc* 255:772, 1985.
4. Rose, BD. *Clinical Physiology of Acid-Base and Electrolyte Disorders* (2nd ed.). New York: McGraw-Hill, 1984. Pp. 482-508.
5. Dzau, VJ, Packer, M, Lilly, LS, Swartz, SL, Hollenberg, NK, Williams, GH. Prostaglandins in severe congestive heart failure. *N Engl J. Med* 310:347, 1984.
6. Bichet, DG, Kortas, C, Mettauer, B, Manzini, C, Marc-Aurèle, J, Rouleau, JL, Schrier, RW. Modulation of plasma and platelet vasopressin by cardiac function in patients with heart failure. *Kidney Int* 29:1188, 1986.
7. Perez-Ayuso, RM, Arroyo, V, Campos, J, Rimola, A, Gaya, J, Costa, J, Rivera, F,

Rodes, J. Evidence that renal prostaglandins are involved in renal water metabolism in cirrhosis. *Kidney Int* 26:72, 1984.

8. Rose, BD. New approach to disturbances in the plasma sodium concentration. *Am J Med* 81:1033, 1986

9. Ashraf, N, Locksley, R, Arieff, AI. Thiazide-induced hyponatremia associated with death or neurologic damage in outpatients. *Am J Med* 70:1163, 1981.

10. Ashouri, OS. Severe diuretic-induced hyponatremia in the elderly. *Arch Intern Med* 146:1355, 1986.

11. Szatalowicz, VL, Miller, PD, Lacher, JW, Gordon, JA, Schrier, RW. Comparative effect of diuretics on renal water excretion in hyponatremic oedematous states. *Clin Sci* 62:235, 1982.

12. Sunderrajan, S, Bauer, JH, Vopat, RL, Wanner-Barjenbruch, P, Hayes, A. Posttransurethral prostatic resection hyponatremic syndrome: Case report and review of the literature. *Am J Kid Dis* 4:80, 1984.

13. Arieff, AI, Llach, F, Massry, SG. Neurological manifestations and morbidity of hyponatremia: Correlation with brain water and electrolytes. *Medicine* 55:121, 1976.

14. Arieff, AI. Hyponatremia, convulsions, respiratory arrest, and permanent brain damage after elective surgery in healthy women. *N Engl J Med* 314:1529, 1986.

15. Melton, JE, Patlak, CS, Pettigrew, KD, Cserr, HF. Volume regulatory loss of Na, Cl, and K from rat brain during acute hyponatremia. *Am J Physiol* 252:F661, 1987.

16. Anderson, RJ, Chung, H-M, Kluge, R, Schrier, RW. Hyponatremia: A prospective analysis of its epidemiology and the pathogenetic role of vasopressin. *Ann Intern Med* 102:164, 1985.

17. Gillum, DM, Linas, SL. Water intoxication in a psychotic patient with normal water excretion. *Am J Med* 77:773, 1986.

18. Martinez-Maldonado, M. Inappropriate antidiuretic hormone secretion of unknown origin. *Kidney Int* 17:554, 1980.

19. Cullen, MJ, Cusack, DA, O'Briain, S, Devlin, JB, Kehely, A, Lyons, TA. Neurosecretion of arginine vasopressin by an olfactory neuroblastoma causing reversible syndrome of antidiuresis. *Am J Med* 81:911, 1986.

20. Ayus, JC, Krothapalli, RK, Arieff, AI. Treatment of symptomatic hyponatremia and its relation to brain damage: A prospective study. *N Engl J Med* 317:1190, 1987.

21. Laureno, R. Central pontine myelinolysis following rapid correction of hyponatremia. *Ann Neurol* 13:232, 1983.

22. Sterns, RH, Riggs, JE, Schochet, SS, Jr. Osmotic demyelination syndrome following correction of hyponatremia. *N Engl J Med* 314:1535, 1986.

23. Narins, RG. Therapy of hyponatremia. Does haste make waste? *N Engl J Med* 314:1573, 1986.

24. Ayus, JC, Krothapalli, RK, Armstrong, DL. Rapid correction of severe hyponatremia: Histopathological changes in the brain. *Am J Physiol* 248:F711, 1985.

25. Dzau, VJ, Hollenberg, NK. Renal response to captopril in severe heart failure: Role of furosemide in natriuresis and reversal of hyponatremia. *Ann Intern Med* 100:777, 1984.

26. Riegger, GA, Kochsiek, K. Vasopressin, renin and norepinephrine levels before and after captopril administration in patients with congestive heart failure due to idiopathic dilated cardiomyopathy. *Am J Cardiol* 58:300, 1986.

27. Packer, M. Medina, N, Yushak, M. Correction of dilutional hyponatremia in severe chronic heart failure by converting-enzyme inhibition. *Ann Intern Med* 100:782, 1984.

28. Rouse, D, Dalmeida, W, Williamson, FC, Suki, WN. Captopril inhibits the hydroosmotic effect of ADH in the cortical collecting tubule. *Kidney Int* 32:845, 1987.

29. Verbalis, JG. An experimental model of syndrome of inappropriate antidiuretic hormone secretion in the rat. *Am J Physiol* 247:E540, 1984.

30. Forrest, JN, Jr, Cox, M, Hong, C, Morrison, G, Bia, M, Singer, I. Superiority of demeclocycline over lithium in the treatment of chronic syndrome of inappropriate secretion of antidiuretic hormone. *N Engl J Med* 298:173, 1978.

31. Miller, PD, Linas, SL, Schrier, RW. Plasma demeclocycline levels and nephrotoxicity: Correlation in hyponatremic cirrhotic patients. *J Am Med Assoc* 243:2513, 1980.

2. HYPERNATREMIA

The introductory basic physiology section of the preceding chapter, which reviewed the meaning of the plasma sodium concentration and the manner in which it is normally regulated, should be read before proceeding with this discussion.

Protective Mechanisms

Hypernatremia always represents hyperosmolality, since sodium salts are the main determinants of the plasma osmolality. The major protective mechanisms against this problem are depicted in Fig. 2-1: increased release of antidiuretic hormone (ADH) and enhanced thirst [1]. The former decreases water loss by increasing water reabsorption in the collecting tubules, and the latter augments water intake. The net effect is water retention and return of the plasma sodium concentration toward normal. This homeostatic mechanism demonstrates that the plasma sodium concentration is regulated by changes in water intake and excretion and, as a corollary, that hypernatremia is, with the unusual exception of sodium loading, a *disorder of water balance*.

Osmoregulation is normally so effective that the plasma osmolality and the plasma sodium concentration are maintained within a range of 1 to 2 percent, despite wide variations in sodium and water intake. Although ADH clearly plays an important role, it is *thirst that provides the ultimate protection against hypernatremia*. This can be illustrated by patients with central diabetes insipidus (DI) who secrete little or no ADH. As a result, renal water reabsorption falls and the urine output can exceed 10 to 15 liters/day. These patients, however, do not become hypernatremic because water intake is augmented to match output [2]. Conversely, even with maximum ADH secretion, the kidney may be unable to retain enough water to offset insensible losses from the skin and respiratory tract in a patient with hypodipsia (diminished thirst) [3]. Thus, *hypernatremia primarily occurs in patients with hypodipsia or, much more commonly, in infants and comatose patients who may have an intact thirst mechanism but are unable to ask for water*. Elderly patients may be at greater risk because of a decline in the efficacy of the thirst mechanism with age [4]. On the other hand, a plasma sodium concentration above 150 meq/L is virtually never seen in an alert patient with intact thirst and access to water.

Etiology

The major causes of hypernatremia, which also require decreased thirst or access to water to be present, are listed in Table 2-1. As can be seen, the plasma sodium concentration can rise if water is lost in excess of solute or if hypertonic sodium solutions are administered or ingested. The latter can occur after the use of sodium bicarbonate to treat lactic acidosis, the administration of hypertonic saline to induce a therapeutic abortion, or high-sodium feedings in infants or elderly patients [5-8]. As an extreme example, the inadvertent administration of only 1 tablespoon of sodium chloride to a newborn can raise the plasma sodium concentration by as much as 70 meq/L [7].

Much more commonly, however, hypernatremia results from water loss. A classic example is an elderly nursing home patient who develops a urinary tract infection and stops eating and drinking. In this setting, insensible losses from the skin and respiratory tract are not replaced, and the plasma sodium concentration rises.

Water loss in excess of effective solute can also occur from the kidney and gastrointestinal tract. Central and nephrogenic diabetes insipidus are conditions in which either ADH secretion or its renal effect is impaired. Although these disorders can produce hypernatremia, they will be discussed in the following chapter since patients with these conditions are usually alert and complain primarily of polyuria and polydipsia. An osmotic diuresis is a unique form of nephrogenic DI in which enhanced water loss is induced by the presence of large amounts of nonreabsorbed solute in the tubular lumen. Glucosuria in uncontrolled diabetes mellitus is the most common cause of an osmotic

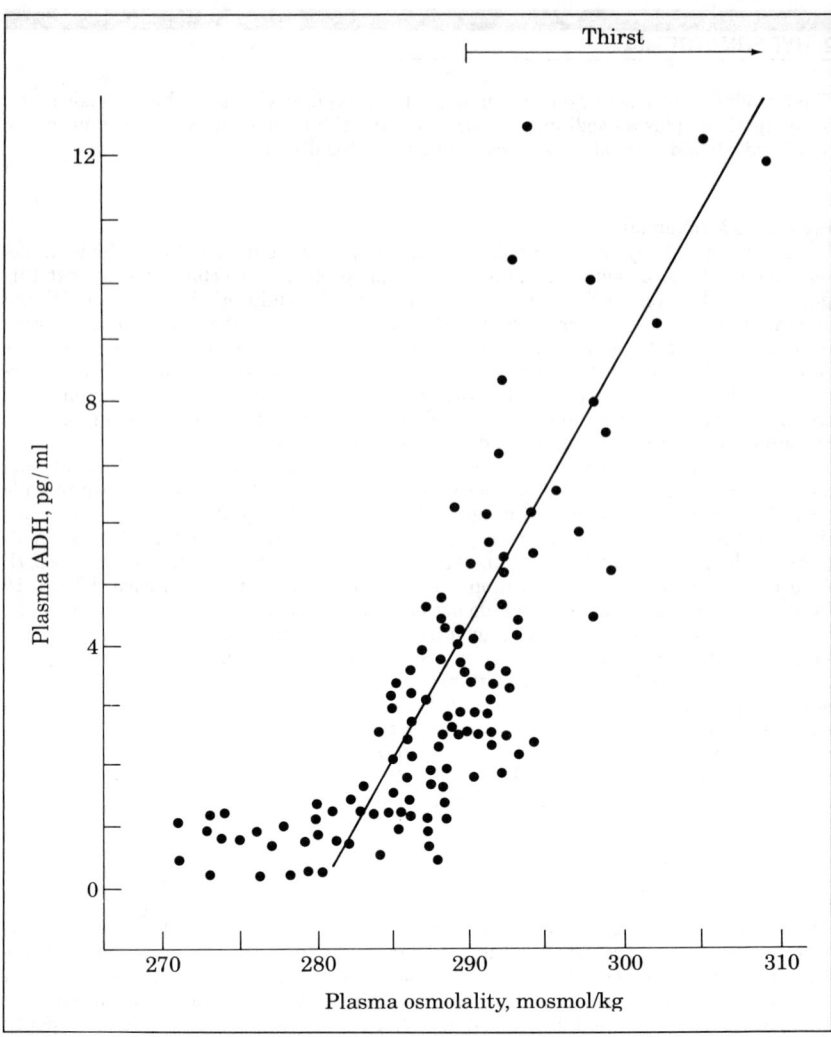

Fig. 2-1. Relationship of plasma ADH concentration to plasma osmolality in normal humans in whom the latter was varied by changing the state of hydration. Notice that the osmotic threshold for thirst appears to be 5 to 10 mosmol/kg higher than that for the release of ADH. (From Robertson, GL, Aycinena, P, Zerbe, RL. *Am J Med* 72:339, 1982.)

Table 2-1. Major causes of hypernatremia

WATER LOSS
Insensible losses
    Increased sweating—fever, exposure to high temperature
    Respiratory infections
    Burns
Renal losses
    Central diabetes insipidus
    Nephrogenic diabetes insipidus
    Osmotic diuresis—glucose, urea, mannitol
Gastrointestinal losses
    Osmotic diarrhea—infectious, lactulose
Hypothalamic disorders
    Hypodipsia
    Resetting of osmostat due to primary mineralocorticoid excess
Water loss into cells
    Seizures, severe exercise, rhabdomyolysis

SODIUM RETENTION
Administration of hypertonic NaCl or NaHCO$_3$
Ingestion of sodium

diuresis*, but a similar problem can occur with high-protein tube feedings (resulting in excess urea production and excretion) and with prolonged infusions of hypertonic mannitol [5,11].

Osmotic water loss can also occur from the gastrointestinal tract. Lactulose-induced diarrhea is a common example [12], but malabsorption and some infectious diarrheas can produce a similar effect [13]. In comparison, the fluid lost in a secretory diarrhea (such as cholera or that seen with a vasoactive intestinal peptide-producing tumor) is an isosmotic solution composed almost entirely of sodium and potassium salts [13]. Volume depletion will ensue, but there will be no direct change in the plasma sodium concentration since effective solute and water are lost in proportion.

Primary hypothalamic lesions are rare caues of hypernatremia. Hypodipsia must be present in this setting and is usually but not always accompanied by a defect in ADH release [1,3,14]. Osmoreceptor function is typically abnormal in many of these patients. In some cases, however, it has been proposed that there is true resetting of the osmostat in which a high plasma sodium concentration is recognized as normal. This possibility has been confirmed only in states of primary mineralocorticoid excess such as primary hyperaldosteronism [1]. In this condition, the chronic mild hypervolemia induced by the mineralocorticoid retards ADH secretion, shifting the osmotic threshold for its release (which normally occurs at a plasma osmolality of 280–285 mosmol/kg) upward by 5 to 10 mosmol/kg. As a result, the plasma sodium concentration tends to be 145 to 147 meq/L. Normal osmoregulation can be restored by removing the source of hormone secretion or by lowering the effective circulating volume with diuretics [1].

A final rare form of transient hypernatremia may occur during seizures, severe exercise, or rhabdomyolysis [5,15]. In these conditions, it is presumed that the breakdown of cellular macromolecules into smaller compounds (as with the conversion of glycogen into lactate with seizures or intense exercise) raises the cell osmolality, promoting water movement into the cells.

*Hyperglycemia directly lowers the plasma sodium concentration by dilution as the increase in plasma osmolality pulls water out of the cells. In general, the plasma sodium concentration should fall by 1 meq/L for every 62 mg/dl rise in the plasma glucose concentration [9]. With the water loss induced by the osmotic diuresis, however, the plasma sodium concentration is often higher than predicted from this correction and occasionally reaches hypernatremic levels [10].

Table 2-2. Urine osmolality and response to ADH in hypernatremia

Urine osmolality	Response to ADH
< 300 mosmol/kg	
Central DI	+
Nephrogenic DI	−
300–800 mosmol/kg	
Volume depletion in central DI	+
Partial central DI	+
Partial nephrogenic DI	−
Osmotic diuresis	−
> 800 mosmol/kg	
Sodium overload	−
Insensible water loss	−
Primary hypodipsia	−

Diagnosis

Several factors are helpful in establishing the cause of hypernatremia. A hypothalamic lesion affecting thirst is almost certainly present if the patient is alert and has access to water. Although the history may be helpful (polyuria, polydipsia, decreased intake, diabetes mellitus?), the amount of past information that can be obtained is often limited because most patients have impaired mental status due to underlying neurologic disease or hypernatremia itself. In this setting, *measurement of the urine osmolality and its response to ADH* may be extremely important. As shown in Fig. 2-1, ADH release and, therefore, the urine osmolality should be very high in hypernatremic states, exceeding 800 mosmol/kg (specific gravity usually > 1.022) if ADH release and renal function are intact [2]. It is also important to note that the maximum ADH effect on the kidney is reached at a plasma osmolality of 295 to 300 mosmol/kg, a value that is exceeded in hypernatremic patients with a plasma sodium concentration above 150 meq/L [2]. Thus, the administration of exogenous ADH (given as 5 units of aqueous vasopressin subcutaneously or 10 μg of dDAVP by nasal insufflation) should produce no increment in the urine osmolality *unless endogenous release is impaired.*

The following responses should be seen in hypernatremia (Table 2-2). Concentrating ability should be normal in patients with sodium overload, enhanced insensible losses, or pure hypodipsia without DI. Thus, the initial urine osmolality should exceed 800 mosmol/kg and there should be no response to ADH administration. In comparison, either severe central or nephrogenic DI is present if the urine is dilute to plasma. These disorders can be differentiated by the response to ADH: there should be at least a 50 percent rise in urine osmolality and a marked fall in urine volume in central DI but no effect in nephrogenic DI, since this disorder is characterized by ADH resistance.

Many patients fall in an intermediate area with the urine osmolality ranging from 300 to 800 mosmol/kg. This can reflect volume depletion in central DI (as the slow flow in the tubules allows relatively more water reabsorption in the medullary collecting duct even in the absence of ADH) [16], partial central or nephrogenic DI, or an osmotic diuresis. The first two conditions will respond to ADH, and an osmotic diuresis can be diagnosed by the presence of glucosuria or by a history of high-protein feedings and confirmation that most of the urinary solute is urea (by measuring the urine urea nitrogen).

Partial nephrogenic DI is a more difficult problem to interpret. Many elderly patients, who are most at risk of developing hypernatremia due to impaired mental status, have a decline in concentrating ability due in large part to a fall in the glomerular filtration rate (GFR) [17]. This defect is generally mild and can cause some nocturia; polyuria, however, does not occur. Thus, the common sequence of decreased intake leading to unreplaced insensible losses is often associated with an inadequately concentrated urine. Although this does represent nephrogenic DI, the small amount of extra water

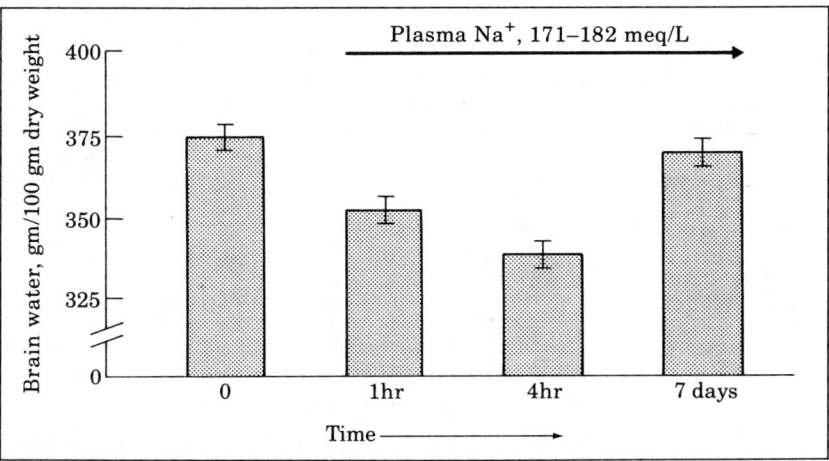

Fig. 2-2. Effect of sustained hypernatremia on brain-water content in rabbits. Brain water is substantially reduced by 1 to 4 hours but returns to normal within 1 week. (From Pollock, AS, Arieff, AI. *Am J Physiol* 239:F195, 1980.)

lost in the urine in this setting does not importantly contribute to the development of hypernatremia.

Other Causes of Hyperosmolality
In addition to hypernatremia, hyperosmolality can be seen in a variety of other conditions including hyperglycemia, renal failure (in which urea and other organic solutes accumulate), and the ingestion of ethanol, methanol, or ethylene glycol [18]. With the exception of hyperglycemia or the administration of hypertonic mannitol, however, the other solutes are able to cross cell membranes and do not cause osmotic water shifts or the symptoms of hyperosmolality.

Symptoms and Treatment
The symptoms of hypernatremia are primarily neurologic. Lethargy, weakness, and irritability are the earliest findings, which can progress to twitching, seizures, coma, and death or irreversible neurologic damage. These problems are related less to the absolute level of the plasma sodium concentration than to the movement of water out of the brain cells down an osmotic gradient created by the rise in effective plasma osmolality [19]. This acute decrease in brain volume causes rupture of the cerebral veins, resulting in focal intracerebral and subarachnoid hemorrhages.

As depicted in Fig. 2-2, however, this cerebral dehydration is transient [19]. Within 24 hours the brain begins to adapt to the hyperosmolal state with an increase in brain cell osmolality, resulting in water movement back into the brain and the return of brain volume toward normal. This adaptive response may be mediated by the uptake of sodium and potassium and by the generation of osmolytes, such as betaine glycine (a derivative of choline) [19,20]. Osmolytes, in comparison to sodium and potassium, may be less likely to interfere with the activity of cell proteins. Thus, changing the concentration of osmolytes, which occurs in many different species of animals and plants, has the important advantage of allowing cell volume to be maintained without interfering with cell function [20].

The normalization of brain water content has two important clinical consequences. First, chronic hypernatremia is often well tolerated, with a plasma sodium concentration as high as 170 meq/L frequently producing mild or even no symptoms [21]. Thus, the severity of neurologic dysfunction[1] is more importantly related to the *rate of development of hypernatremia* than to the absolute level of the plasma sodium concentration [19].

Second, overly rapid correction of the plasma sodium concentration can now lead to cerebral overhydration, potentially producing seizures and permanent neurologic damage [19]. As a result, it has been suggested that the *plasma sodium concentration be gradually normalized over a 48-hour period*. This can be achieved by appropriate water replacement and serial monitoring of the plasma sodium concentration in patients in whom the hypernatremia is due to water loss. Estimation of the free water deficit[2] is a helpful guide in determining the rate at which fluid repletion should be initiated [5]:

$$\text{Water deficit} = \text{total body water} \times ([P_{Na}/140] - 1)$$

The approximate total body water is normally about 60 and 50 percent of lean body weight in men and women, respectively. However, it is probably more accurate to use values 10 percent lower (50 and 40%) in hypernatremic patients who are water depleted. In a 70-kg man with a plasma sodium concentration of 168 meq/L, for example:

$$\text{Water deficit} = 0.5 \times 70 \times ([168/140] - 1) = 7 \text{ liters}$$

Giving 150 ml/hour of free water will correct this deficit over 48 hours. Since the aim is to induce positive water balance, however, estimated insensible losses (usually 30–40 ml/hour) and dilute urine losses in DI should also be replaced.

It must be emphasized that the above formula is based on assumptions of the total body water that may not be correct. For example, the total body water may be substantially lower than estimated in an elderly cachectic patient with little muscle mass. In this setting, the calculated water deficit will be inappropriately high, leading to a more rapid reduction in the plasma sodium concentration than is desired. Thus, careful monitoring of the plasma sodium concentration is an essential adjunct to fluid repletion.

Although it may seem risky to give this much fluid to an elderly patient with possible underlying cardiac disease, it should be remembered that two-thirds of the water will enter the cells, resulting in a much lesser degree of extracellular volume expansion. Going slower leads to a longer period of hypernatremia, with possible neurologic damage if the plasma sodium concentration remains above 160 meq/L.

The type of fluid administered is variable, depending on the patient's clinical state and the cause of the hypernatremia:

1. Free water can be given orally or intravenously (as D/W) in patients with pure water loss. In some patients, the administration of more than 300 ml/hour as 5 % D/W can lead to marked hyperglycemia since the quantity of glucose given can exceed the maximum rate of utilization [22]. Thus, the plasma glucose concentration should be monitored in this setting and insulin given if necesary.

2. An infusion of quarter-isotonic saline is preferable if sodium depletion is also present. Since this solution is only three-quarters free water, 200 ml must be given per hour to supply 150 ml of free water.

3. Isotonic saline should be used initially if the patient is hypotensive. Restoration of tissue perfusion is of primary importance in this setting. Furthermore, this solution can lower the plasma sodium concentration since it is still hypoosmotic to the hypernatremic patient.

4. The contribution of any added potassium, which is as osmotically active as sodium, must be taken into account when calculating the tonicity of the fluid that is to be given. For example, quarter-isotonic saline (sodium concentration equals 37 meq/L) to which

---

[1]It should be emphasized that underlying neurologic disease, particularly associated with decreased mentation and thirst, frequently precedes the development of hypernatremia. It may be difficult, therefore, to ascertain the relative roles of hyperosmolality and the underlying disease until the plasma sodium concentration has been normalized.

[2]This formula calculates the amount of free water that must be added to return the plasma sodium concentration to 140 meq/L. It does not include any isosmotic fluid deficit that is also frequently present when both sodium and water have been lost, as with an osmotic diuresis.

40 meq of potassium chloride is added is osmotically equivalent to half-isotonic saline and, therefore, has less free water. On the other hand, the contribution of dextrose usually can be ignored since it is rapidly metabolized to carbon dioxide and water.

Some patients require therapy in addition to water replacement. In central DI, for example, raising the urine osmolality with an ADH preparation or with drugs that increase ADH release or its renal effect can dramatically reduce the urine volume and eliminate the complaints of polyuria and polydipsia (see Chap. 3). Patients with hypodipsia, on the other hand, should be put on a chronic regimen of fixed water intake to prevent water depletion. If ADH is also given because of concurrent DI, careful observation is required to prevent water retention and hyponatremia [14].

Finally, water administration may not be safe in patients with primary sodium overload who are already volume expanded. Therefore, therapy is best aimed at removing the excess sodium. This is easy to achieve when renal function is normal, since the sodium load will be rapidly excreted in the urine. Net sodium removal can be facilitated, if necessary, by inducing sodium and water loss with a diuretic and then replacing the urine output with free water. Careful monitoring of the plasma sodium concentration is again essential to prevent overly rapid correction of the hypernatremia.

References

1. Robertson, GL, Aycinena, P, Zerbe, RL. Neurogenic disorders of osmoregulation. *Am J Med* 72:339, 1982.
2. Miller, M, Kalkos, T, Moses, AM, Fellerman, H, Streeten, D. Recognition of partial defects in antidiuretic hormone secretion. *Ann Intern Med* 73:721, 1970.
3. Hammond, DN, Moll, GW, Robertson, GL, Chelmicka-Schorr, E. Hypodipsic hypernatremia with normal osmoregulation of vasopressin. *N Engl J Med* 315:433, 1986.
4. Phillips, PA, Rolls, BJ, Ledingham, JGG, Forsling, ML, Morton, JJ, Crowe, MJ, Wollner, L. Reduced thirst after water deprivation in healthy elderly men. *N Engl J Med* 311:753, 1984.
5. Rose, BD. *Clinical Physiology of Acid-Base and Electrolyte Disorders* (2nd ed.). New York: McGraw-Hill, 1984. Pp. 515-542.
6. Mattar, JA, Weil, MH, Shubin, H, Stein, L. Cardiac arrest in the critically ill. II. Hyperosmolal states following cardiac arrest. *Am J Med* 56:162, 1974.
7. Miller, NL, Finberg, L. Peritoneal dialysis for salt poisoning. *N Engl J Med* 263:1347, 1960.
8. Addleman, M, Pollard, A, Grossman, RF. Survival after severe hypernatremia due to salt ingestion by an adult. *Am J Med* 78:176, 1985.
9. Katz, M. Hyperglycemia-induced hyponatremia: Calculation of expected serum sodium depression. *N Engl J Med* 289:843, 1973.
10. Arieff, AI, Carroll, HJ. Nonketotic hyperosmolar coma with hyperglycemia: Clinical features, pathophysiology, renal function, acid-base balance, plasma-cerebrospinal fluid equilibria and the effects of therapy in 37 cases. *Medicine* 51:73, 1972.
11. Gault, MH, Dixon, ME, Doyle, M, Cohen, WM. Hypernatremia, azotemia, and dehydration due to high-protein tube feeding. *Ann Intern Med* 68:778, 1968.
12. Nelson, DC, McGrew, WRG, Hoyumpa, AM. Hypernatremia and lactulose therapy. *J Am Med Assoc* 249:1295, 1983.
13. Shiau, Y-F, Feldman, GM, Resnick, MA, Coff, PM. Stool electrolyte and osmolality measurements in the evaluation of diarrheal disorders. *Ann Intern Med* 102:773, 1985.
14. Robertson, GL. Abnormalities of thirst regulation. *Kidney Int.* 25:460, 1984.
15. Felig, P, Johnson, C. Levitt, M, Cunningham, J, Keefe, F, Boglioli, B. Hypernatremia induced by maximal exercise *J Am Med Assoc* 248:1209, 1982.
16. Valtin, H, Edwards, BR. GFR and the concentration of urine in the absence of vasopressin. Berliner-Davidson re-explored. *Kidney Int* 31:634, 1987.
17. Sporn, IN, Lancestremere, RG, Papper, S. Differential diagnosis of oliguria in aged patients. *N Engl J Med* 267:130, 1962.
18. DiNubile, MJ. Serum osmolality (letter). *N Engl J Med* 310:1609, 1984.

19. Pollock, AS, Arieff, AI. Abnormalities of cell volume regulation and their functional consequences. *Am J Physiol* 239:F195, 1980.
20. Somero, GN. Protons, osmolytes, and fitness of internal milieu for protein function. *Am J Physiol* 251:R197, 1986.
21. Kastin, AJ, Lipsett, MB, Ommaya, AK, Moser, JM, Jr. Asymptomatic hypernatremia *Am J Med* 38:306, 1965.
22. Freidenberg, GR, Kosnik, EJ, Sotos, JF. Hyperglycemic coma after suprasellar surgery. *N Engl J Med* 303:863, 1980.

3. EVALUATION OF THE POLYURIC PATIENT

Polyuria is a relatively common clinical complaint. It is characterized by an absolute rise in urine output and should be differentiated from urinary frequency in which multiple small voidings are typically present with no increase in total output.

Diagnosis
It is useful to begin the evaluation of the polyuric patient by asking two questions:

1. Does the polyuria reflect a solute or a water diuresis?
2. Is the diuresis appropriate or inappropriate?

The latter question is important because *polyuria is often an appropriate response to an increase in intake,* rather than a manifestation of an underlying disease process.

Solute versus Water Diuresis
Polyuria represents an increase in urine volume due to reduced tubular water reabsorption. Renal water transport occurs by two passive mechanisms: it follows the reabsorption of sodium in the proximal tubule and loop of Henle*; and, in the presence of antidiuretic hormone (ADH), it is reabsorbed down a favorable osmotic gradient in the cortical and medullary collecting tubules. Thus, polyuria can occur during a solute diuresis when net sodium reabsorption is reduced or during a pure-water diuresis when there is decreased activity of ADH (Table 3-1). This discussion will not include those drugs expressly given to enhance the urine output such as diuretics and mannitol.

If polyuria is arbitrarily defined as a urine output exceeding 3 liters/day, then a solute diuresis can usually be differentiated from a water diuresis simply by measuring the urine osmolality. A dilute urine with an osmolality below 250 mosmol/kg indicates a water diuresis (unless sodium excretion is also very high as with the infusion of half-isotonic saline). In this setting, the differential diagnosis is central or nephrogenic diabetes insipidus (DI) (due to deficient secretion and renal resistance to ADH, respectively) or primary polydipsia in which there is a primary increase in water intake that *appropriately* suppresses ADH release by lowering the plasma osmolality.

In contrast, a urine osmolality above 300 mosmol/kg is generally indicative of a solute diuresis. Although partial central or nephrogenic DI can also result in a similar urine osmolality, *these disorders will not lead to polyuria if solute excretion is normal.* This can be appreciated from a few simple calculations. The normal range of solute excretion (composed predominantly of sodium and potassium salts and urea) is 600 to 900 mosmol per day. If the urine osmolality is 300 mosmol/kg, then the maximum daily urine output is 2 to 3 liters. A higher output can be achieved only if solute excretion (equal to the urine osmolality times volume) is increased or the urine osmolality is further reduced.

SOLUTE DIURESIS.   The most common cause of a solute diuresis is the osmotic diuresis seen in uncontrolled diabetes mellitus. In this disorder, the presence of a nonreabsorbed

---

*Although the ascending limb of the loop of Henle is impermeable to water, sodium chloride reabsorption in this segment increases medullary interstitial osmolality, thereby promoting water reabsorption out of the water-permeable *descending* limb.

Table 3-1. Causes of polyuria

	Appropriate	Inappropriate
Water diuresis (U_{osm} < 250 mosmol/kg)	Primary polydipsia	Central diabetes insipidus Nephrogenic diabetes insipidus
Solute diuresis (U_{osm} > 300 mosmol/kg)	Postobstructive diuresis Saline loading	Hyperglycemia High-protein tube feedings Sodium-wasting nephropathy

solute such as glucose in the tubular lumen results in obligatory sodium and water losses. These losses play a central role in the frequently associated problems of volume depletion and hyperosmolality [1]. This diagnosis can be easily established by documenting the presence of both hyperglycemia and marked glucosuria. Restoration of normoglycemia with insulin returns the urine output to the normal range.

An inappropriate solute diuresis can also occur with high-protein tube feedings. In this setting, urea production and subsequent urinary excretion are enhanced, resulting in an elevation in the urine output [2].

Increased sodium excretion (in which sodium rather than glucose or urea is the major urinary solute) can also lead to polyuria. True sodium wasting does occur in some renal diseases [3-5], particularly tubulointerstitial disorders such as acute tubular necrosis and medullary cystic kidney disease in which predominant tubular damage impairs sodium reabsorption both directly and indirectly by reducing the responsiveness to aldosterone [5]. However, the degree of sodium loss is generally mild and the obligatory urine output is typically less than 2 liters/day. Thus, patients may complain of nocturia but usually not polyuria.

Although tubular damage and the osmotic diuresis induced by increased urea excretion in the remaining functioning nephrons may contribute, the sodium wasting in many chronic renal diseases appears to be due to an inability to acutely shut off natriuretic forces. If sodium intake is normal in a patient with a reduced number of functioning nephrons, then sodium excretion per nephron must increase if balance is to be maintained. This requires a fall in sodium reabsorption that may be mediated at least in part by chronic hypersecretion of a natriuretic hormone (atrial natriuretic peptide being one possibility). Thus, the obligatory sodium wasting that occurs when sodium intake is abruptly lowered could be mediated by persistent hormone release and, if so, could initially be equal to the previous level of intake (which may exceed 200 meq/day) [4]. Consistent with this hypothesis is the observation that apparent sodium wasters can maintain sodium balance on an intake of only 5 meq/day if intake is reduced slowly over a period of weeks, presumably the time required for regression of the hyperplastic hormone secretory apparatus [4].

A *post obstructive diuresis* after the release of bilateral urinary tract obstruction is often cited as an example of polyuria (which can acutely exceed 500 ml/hour) due to a marked sodium-wasting state. In the great majority of patients, however, the diuresis represents an *appropriate* attempt to excrete the fluid that was retained during the period of obstruction [6,7]. As a result, complete replacement of urinary losses is both unnecessary and, by perpetuating the hypervolemic state, can lead to persistent polyuria in which the urine output can exceed 10 liters/day. Standard replacement therapy, such as 50 to 75 ml/hour of half-isotonic saline, is usually sufficient during the acute diuresis, which will cease spontaneously when the excess fluid is excreted. (Management of a postobstructive diuresis is reviewed in Chap. 55).

A similar sequence of persistent hypervolemia leading to marked polyuria can also occur if a euvolemic patient is initially given an infusion of 1 to 2 liters of saline, followed by orders to "avoid volume depletion" by replacing the urine output with an equivalent volume of saline. This example again illustrates that polyuria due to a sodium diuresis may well be *appropriate* and should be treated by limiting intake and allowing the excess fluid to be excreted. Inappropriate losses should be suspected only if the patient develops hypotension, reduced skin turgor, or an acute decline in renal function.

WATER DIURESIS.   Patients with polyuria due to a water diuresis (in which large volumes of dilute urine are excreted) typically present with a normal plasma sodium concentration because thirst prevents the development of negative water balance. The three causes of this problem, central DI, nephrogenic DI, and primary polydipsia (in which the polyuria is appropriate) can be distinguished by history, the plasma sodium concentration, and the response to a water restriction test.

Patients with central DI frequently have a predilection for very cold or iced water, a finding that does not appear to be present in the other two disorders. In addition, central DI usually begins abruptly as the patient can date the exact onset of the disease. A more gradual onset suggests nephrogenic DI or primary polydipsia.

Measurement of the plasma sodium concentration also may be helpful in selected cases. Patients with primary polydipsia tend to be somewhat water overloaded. As a result, the plasma sodium concentration may be low-normal (135–138 meq/L) or rarely reduced if intake is extraordinarily high [8]. In comparison, patients with primary renal water loss due to either form of DI may have a plasma sodium concentration in the high-normal range (143–145 meq/L) [8,9]. More commonly, however, a clearly normal value is obtained [9].

Routine history and laboratory testing also may identify the 3 major causes of nephrogenic DI in adults: *lithium toxicity, hypercalcemia, and hypokalemia*. Although there are many other disorders that can impair urinary concentrating ability, they are usually not severe enough to produce true polyuria (see *Determinants of Polyuria* below). As described earlier, a fall in maximum urine osmolality from the normal of 800 to 1200 mosmol/kg to any value above 300 mosmol/kg will not produce a urine output above 3 liters/day unless solute excretion is also enhanced. These patients may, however, complain of nocturia since it is overnight, when there is no water intake, that the urine nomally becomes most concentrated.

The definitive diagnosis can be established by raising the plasma osmolality with complete water restriction, thereby stimulating endogenous ADH release (Fig. 3-1). ADH should then increase the urine osmolality and reduce the urine volume [9]. The urine volume, urine osmolality, and body weight are measured hourly, and the plasma osmolality is measured every 2 to 4 hours. Water restriction is continued until the urine osmolality reaches a plateau (defined as < a 30-mosmol/kg increment in two consecutive hourly specimens) or the plasma osmolality reaches 295 mosmol/kg, the level at which *maximum endogenous ADH effect on the kidney* should be present.* At this point, exogenous ADH is given (5 units of aqueous vasopressin subcutaneously or 10 μg of dDAVP by nasal insufflation) and the hourly measurements continued. Several different patterns of response may be seen (Fig. 3-2):

1. The urine becomes highly concentrated (urine osmolality above 800 mosmol/kg) and the urine volume falls to less than 0.5 ml/min in normal subjects; the administration of ADH is without effect since endogenous activity on the kidney is maximal.

2. The urine osmolality usually stays below 300 mosmol/kg in severe central or nephrogenic DI. A positive response to ADH with at least a 50 percent rise in urine osmolality and fall in urine volume is seen in central DI since ADH secretion is deficient; there is no response to ADH in nephrogenic DI. Patients with milder, partial forms of either of these disorders achieve a higher urine osmolality following water restriction.

3. Patients with primary polydipsia might be expected to respond in a similar fashion to normals. However, the prolonged suppression of ADH release due to chronic water loading leads to washout of the medullary interstitial osmotic gradient and therefore a reduction in the maximum urine osmolality. Thus, primary polydipsia is often a reversible form of nephrogenic DI. It can be differentiated from nephrogenic DI by the history

---

*A similar rise in plasma osmolality can be achieved by the intravenous infusion of hypertonic (5 %) saline. This solution, which has a sodium concentration of 855 meq/L, is infused at the rate of 0.05 ml/kg/min for no more than 2 hours. This method has the advantage of shortening the duration of water restriction but can produce circulatory overload in susceptible patients.

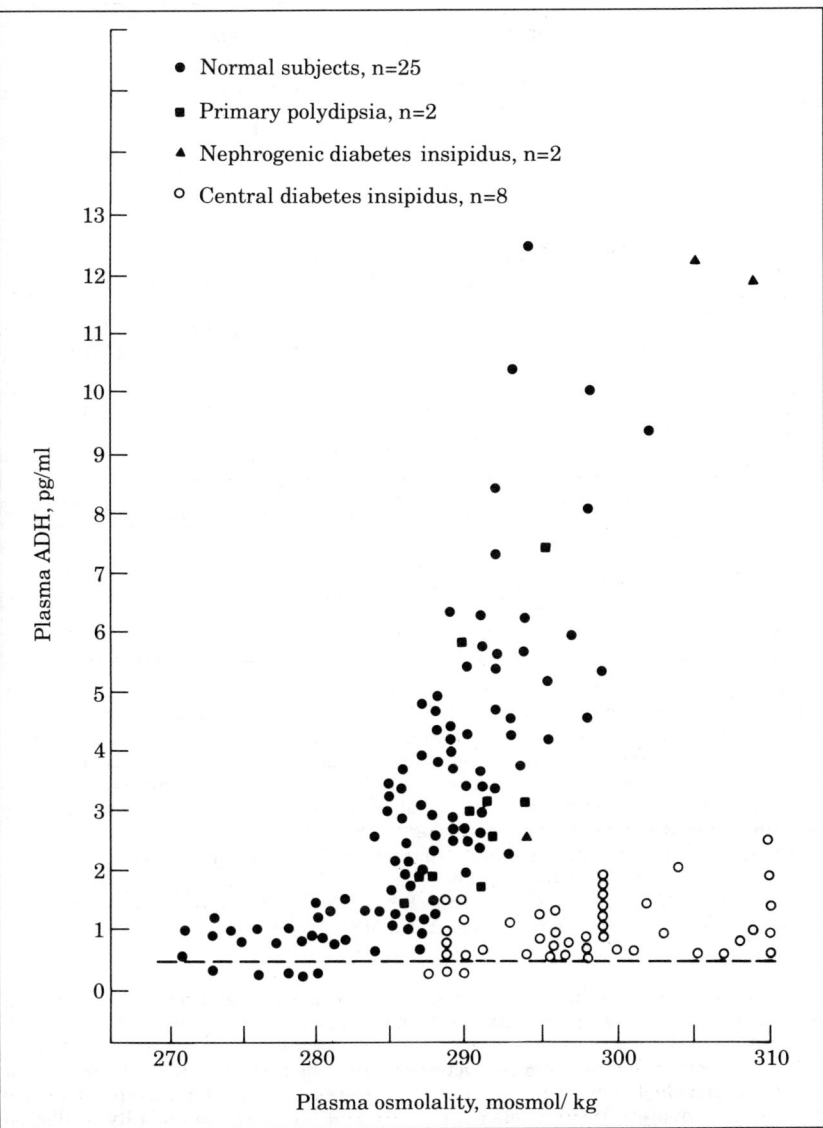

Fig. 3-1. Relationship between plasma ADH levels and plasma osmolality in normal subjects and patients with polyuria of diverse etiologies. ADH secretion is reduced only in central diabetes insipidus. (From Robertson, GL, Mahr, EA, Atkar, S, Sinka, T. *J Clin Invest* 52:2340, 1973, by copyright permission of the American Society for Clinical Investigation.)

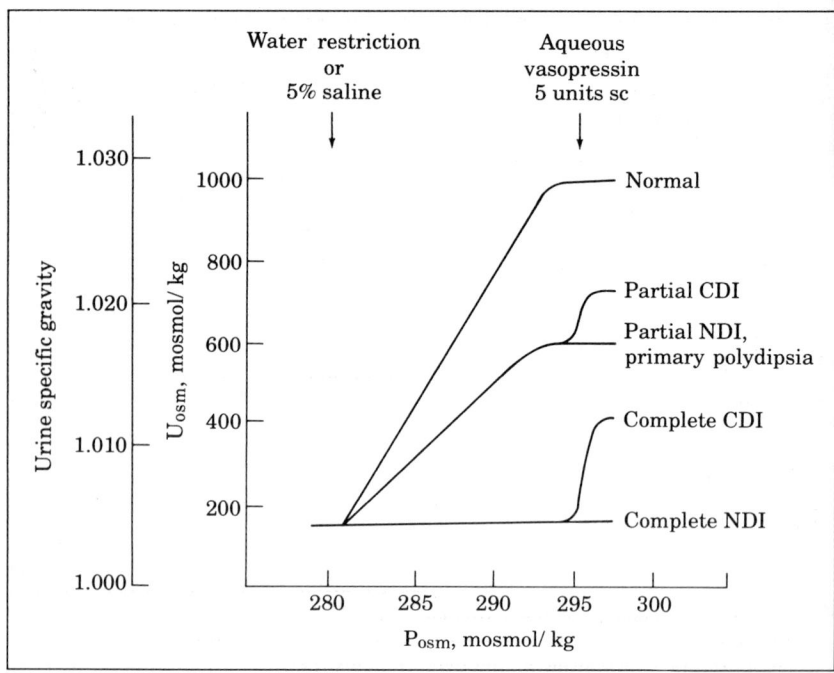

Fig. 3-2. Effect of a rise in plasma osmolality (P_{osm}), induced by either water restriction or hypertonic saline, on the urine osmolality or specific gravity. In normal subjects, there is maximum ADH effect on the kidney as the plasma osmolality reaches 290 to 295 mosmol/kg, resulting in a urine osmolality exceeding 800 mosmol/kg and no further increment after exogenous vasopressin. In comparison, the urine remains hypoosmotic to plasma with complete central or nephrogenic DI; vasopressin will raise the urine osmolality only in central DI where ADH secretion is impaired. Patients with partial DI show an intermediate response; those with primary polydipsia may behave similar to normal or to partial nephrogenic DI since chronic polyuria washes out the medullary osmotic gradient. (From Rose, BD. *Clinical Physiology of Acid-Base and Electrolyte Disorders* (2nd ed.). New York: McGraw-Hill, 1984.)

and laboratory data (? lithium, hypercalcemia, hypokalemia) and by rapid reversal of the polyuria by limiting water intake to the normal range.

Patients undergoing the water restriction test must be monitored carefully to prevent marked volume depletion. Some patients with severe central DI can excrete 700 to 800 ml/hour and symptomatic hypovolemia may ensue if the plasma osmolality is allowed to rise above 295 mosmol/kg. Four to twelve hours of water restriction is usually sufficient in this setting with a weight loss of 1.0 to 2.5 kg. A longer period is frequently necessary in patients with primary polydipsia, however, who may be water overloaded at the start of the test. These patients must be observed carefully to avoid unusual sources of surreptitious water intake, for example, from a flower pot.

The accuracy of this indirect test (in which the urine osmolality is used as an index of ADH secretion or effect) has been compared to the "gold standard," or direct measurement of plasma ADH levels [10]. The water restriction test established the correct diagnosis in 80 percent of patients, with the major error occurring in the distinction between partial central DI and primary polydipsia. Some patients with the former condition appear to have increased sensitivity to ADH (by an unknown mechanism). As a result, they are polyuric at a normal plasma osmolality of 280 to 290 mosmol/kg when ADH secretion is low but excrete a maximally concentrated urine at a plasma osmolality of 295 mosmol/kg when their ADH secretion is higher but still subnormal. Thus, a diagnosis of primary polydipsia will be made since exogenous ADH will be without effect. Establishing the correct diagnosis is particularly important in this setting because *treatment for central DI in a patient who actually has primary polydipsia* can lead to marked water retention and possibly life-threatening hyponatremia. Plasma ADH levels can be obtained to distinguish between these disorders; this test, however, is expensive and an accurate radioimmunoassay is not widely available. A simpler alternative is to institute a trial of dDAVP (see below) in patients in whom primary polydipsia seems less likely from the history. Rapid relief of polyuria and polydipsia will occur if central DI is present; however, careful monitoring to prevent hyponatremia is essential.

Etiology and Treatment of Diabetes Insipidus
The most common causes of central DI are probaby idiopathic (which may, in some cases, be induced by autoantibodies against the ADH secreting cells), head trauma, and hypoxic encephalopathy [11,12]. Less often, this disorder begins after surgical hypophysectomy or is due to infiltrative or neoplastic diseases in the area of the hypothalamus.

A typical triphasic response may be seen following surgery or trauma [12]. An initial period of polyuria lasts 4 to 5 days and probably represents inhibition of ADH release due to hypothalamic dysfunction. From days 6 to 11, an antidiuretic phase represents slow release of stored hormone from the degenerating posterior pituitary. During this time, excess water intake can lead to hyponatremia in a manner similar to the syndrome of inappropriate ADH secretion. This phase is typically followed by permanent central DI once neurohypophyseal stores are depleted.

As described previously, polyuria due to nephrogenic DI in adults is most often due to lithium toxicity, hypercalcemia, and hypokalemia* [12-15]. Each of these causes is due at least in part to reduced ADH effect on the collecting tubular cells [12,16]. Lithium, for example, can ultimately produce polyuria in 20 to 30 percent of patients [14]. This toxic effect appears to result from lithium entry into the collecting tubular cells through a sodium channel in the luminal membrane [13;16]. This observation has important clinical implications since blocking this channel with the potassium-sparing diuretic amiloride can minimize and possibly prevent the development of polyuria, presumably due to diminished cellular accumulation of lithium [13]. Discontinuation of lithium or correction of hypercalcemia or hypokalemia usually leads to resolution of the polyuria [12]. The recovery, however, may be incomplete, particularly with prolonged lithium therapy [14].

Determinants of Polyuria
In addition to the severity of the concentrating defect, the degree of polyuria in both central and nephrogenic DI is also dependent on the patient's volume status and solute intake. In particular, hypovolemia can substantially lower the urine volume. This effect is presumably mediated by increased proximal reabsorption, which diminishes distal flow. This slowing of flow allows relatively more fluid to equilibrate across the collecting tubules even in the absence of ADH effect [17]. Thus, patients with DI who are volume depleted (or poorly perfused due to coexistent anterior pituitary disease and cortisol deficiency) may not complain of polyuria until the DI is unmasked by fluid or cortisol repletion [12,17]. Conversely, the induction of mild hypovolemia with a thiazide diuretic can substantially lower the urine volume in both central and nephrogenic DI [18,19]. This modality constitutes an important form of therapy in these disorders.

When the urine osmolality is relatively fixed in DI, *the rate of solute excretion becomes the primary determinant of the urine output.* If, for example, the urine osmolality is 150

---

*Less common causes include congenital nephrogenic DI (in infants), sickle cell disease, Sjögren's syndrome, and amyloidosis [12]. Although concentrating ability is also uniformly reduced in renal insufficiency, this does not lead to polyuria since the urine osmolality typically remains above 300 mosmol/kg.

Table 3-2. Major forms of therapy in central diabetes insipidus

---

ADH preparations
  Aqueous vasopressin (short-acting, used primarily for diagnosis)
  dDAVP nasal spray
Drugs that increase ADH release
  Clofibrate
  Carbamazepine
Drugs that enhance the action of ADH
  Chlorpropamide
  Carbamazepine
Drugs not requiring ADH*
  Diuretics
  Nonsteroidal anti-inflammatory drugs

---

*Only these agents are effective in nephrogenic diabetes insipidus.

mosmol/kg, the daily urine output will be 6 liters if 900 mosmol of solute is excreted (900 mosmol/150 mosmol/kg equals 6 liters) but only 3 liters if 450 mosmol is excreted. Consequently, a low-sodium, low-protein diet can limit the degree of polyuria by diminishing solute excretion.

Treatment of Central Diabetes Insipidus
The most physiologic therapy of central DI consists of hormone replacement with dDAVP, a synthetic two–amino acid substitute of ADH that is long-acting (requiring once- or twice-daily administration), has antidiuretic but no pressor activity, and is given by nasal insufflation [20]. The usual starting dose is 5 μg twice daily.

Aside from the occasional patient with an incomplete response to dDAVP, the major problem with this medication is its cost, which can exceed $100 per month. As a result, it may be desirable to try the other drugs listed in Table 3-2 that have been found to be effective in the treatment of central DI: chlorpropamide (used in diabetes mellitus); carbamazepine (used to treat seizures or tic douloureux); clofibrate (used in hyperlipidemic states); and a thiazide diuretic [21]. The first three drugs require some ADH to be present and are therefore *effective in partial, but not complete, central DI.*

Chlorpropamide (in a dose of 125–250 mg, once or twice daily) has been the most widely studied, often lowering the urine output by 50 percent or more in responsive patients [12,18]. It seems to act by increasing the responsiveness to ADH, an effect that may be mediated by enhanced membrane receptor affinity for ADH or by direct stimulation of sodium chloride reabsorption in the thick ascending limb of the loop of Henle, thereby raising medullary interstitial osmolality [22,23].

The major side effects with chlorpropamide are hypoglycemia and incomplete control of the polyuria. If, for example, the urine output is lowered from 12 to 6 liters/day, the patient, although much improved, will still be symptomatic. In this setting, chlorpropamide can be given with a thiazide diuretic (such as 25–50 mg once a day of hydrochlorothiazide). This combination is synergistic in terms of both efficacy (since the associated volume depletion limits the polyuria) and toxicity (since the thiazide tends to raise the plasma glucose concentration) [18]. Furthermore, the cost of this combination should be less than $15 per month and many patients can be controlled with once-daily drug administration. If necessary, any of the agents in Table 3-2 can also be used in combination with dDAVP.

Treatment of Nephrogenic Diabetes Insipidus
Treatment of nephrogenic DI is more limited since only modalities that act independent of ADH will be effective. The induction of mild volume depletion with a thiazide diuretic has been the mainstay of therapy, lowering the urine output by as much as 60 percent [19]. As discussed before, diminishing net solute excretion with a low-sodium, low-pro-

tein diet and using amiloride in patients taking lithium also may diminish the polyuria [13].

One additional possibility that has been effective in children with congenital nephrogenic DI is the inhibition of renal prostaglandin synthesis with a nonsteroidal anti-inflammatory drug (such as indomethacin or tolmetin), either alone or with a diuretic [24]. Renal prostaglandins have a variety of effects that impair concentrating ability including (1) a reduction in ADH-induced stimulation of adenyl cyclase and (2) a decrease in medullary interstitial osmolality by diminishing the accumulation of sodium and urea [25]. The latter effect appears to be due to inhibition of both sodium chloride reabsorption in the thick ascending limb of the loop of Henle and urea reabsorption in the inner medullary collecting tubule. The administration of a prostaglandin synthesis inhibitor reverses these effects and probably explains the efficacy of these drugs in nephrogenic DI where they can lower the urine output by more than 50 percent in some cases [24].

References

1. Arieff, AI, Carroll, HJ. Nonketotic hyperosmolar coma with hyperglycemia; Clinical features, pathophysiology, renal function, acid-base balance, plasma cerebrospinal fluid equilibria and the effects of therapy in 37 patients. *Medicine* 51:73, 1972.
2. Gault, MH, Dixon, ME, Doyle, M, Cohen, WM. Hypernatremia, azotemia, and dehydration due to high-protein tube feeding. *Ann Intern Med* 68:778, 1968.
3. Coleman, AJ, Arias, M, Carter, NW, Rector, FC, Jr., Seldin, DW. The mechanism of salt-wasting in chronic renal disease. *J Clin Invest* 45:1116, 1966.
4. Danovitch, GM, Bourgoignie, JJ, Bricker, NS. Reversibility of the "salt-losing" tendency of chronic renal failure. *N Engl J Med* 296:14, 1977.
5. Uribarri, J, Oh, MS, Carroll, HJ. Salt-losing nephropathy. Clinical presentation and mechanisms. *Am J Nephrol* 3:193, 1983.
6. Howard, SS. Post-obstructive diuresis: A misunderstood phenomenon. *J Urol* 110:537, 1973.
7. Bishop, MC. Diuresis and renal functional recovery in chronic retention. *Br J Urol* 57:1, 1985
8. Barlow, ED, de Wardener, HE. Compulsive water drinking. *Q J Med* 28:235, 1959.
9. Miller, M, Kalkos, T, Moses, AM, Fellerman, H, Streeten, D. Recognition of partial defects in antidiuretic hormone secretion. *Ann Intern Med* 73:721, 1970.
10. Zerbe, RL, Robertson, GL. A comparison of plasma vasopressin measurements with a standard indirect test in the differential diagnosis of polyuria. *N Engl J Med* 305:1539, 1981.
11. Leaf, A. Neurogenic diabetes insipidus. *Kidney Int* 15:572, 1979.
12. Rose, BD. *Clinical Physiology of Acid-Base and Electrolyte Disorders* (2nd ed.). New York: McGraw-Hill, 1987. Pp. 518-524.
13. Battle, DC, von Riotte, AB, Gaviria, M, Grupp, M. Amelioration of polyuria by amiloride in patients receiving long-term lithium therapy. *N Engl J Med* 312:408, 1985.
14. Boton, R, Gaviria, M, Battle, DC. Prevalence, pathogenesis, and treatment of renal dysfunction associated with chronic lithium therapy. *Am J Kid Dis* 10:329, 1987.
15. Schwartz, WB, Relman, AS. Effects of electrolyte disorders on renal structure and function. *N Engl J Med* 276:383,452, 1967.
16. Cogan, E, Abramow, M. Inhibition by lithium of the hydroosmotic action of vasopressin in the isolated perfused cortical collecting tubule of the rabbit. *J Clin Invest* 77:1507, 1986.
17. Valtin, H, Edwards, BR. GFR and the concentration of urine in the absence of vasopressin. Berliner-Davidson re-explored. *Kidney Int* 31:634, 1987.
18. Webster, B, Bain, J. Antidiuretic effect and complications of chlorpropamide therapy in diabetes insipidus. *J Clin Endocrinol Metab* 30:215, 1970.
19. Earley, LE, Orloff, J. The mechanism of antidiuresis associated with the administration of hydrochlorothiazide to patients with vasopressin-resistant diabetes insipidus. *J Clin Invest* 41:1988, 1962.
20. Richardson, DW, Robinson, AG. Desmopressin. *Ann Intern Med* 103:228, 1985.
21. Rose, BD. *Clinical Physiology of Acid-Base and Electrolyte Disorders* (2nd ed). New York: McGraw-Hill, 1987. Pp. 538-541.

22. Moses, AM, Fenner, R, Schroeder, ET, Coulson, R. Further studies on the mechanisms by which chlorpropamide alters the action of vasopressin. *Endocrinology* 111:2025, 1982.
23. Kusano, E, Braun-Werness, JL, Vick, DJ, Keller, MJ, Dousa, TP. Chlorpropamide action on renal concentrating mechanism in rats with hypothalamic diabetes insipidus. *J Clin Invest* 72:1299, 1983.
24. Libber, S, Harrison, H, Spector, D. Treatment of nephrogenic diabetes insipidus with prostaglandin synthesis inhibitors. *J Pediatr* 108:305, 1986.
25. Stokes, JB. Integrated actions of renal medullary prostaglandins in the control of water excretion. *Am J Physiol* 240:F471, 1981.

4. DIURETICS: USES AND COMPLICATIONS

Diuretics are widely used in the treatment of edematous states, hypertension, and other disorders. Despite their proven efficacy, many questions remain unanswered concerning their mechanism of action, the metabolic complications that can occur, and the appropriate use of these agents in edematous states. This chapter will attempt to review these issues; the role of diuretics in the possible prevention of postischemic acute tubular necrosis and in patients with hypertension, calcium nephrolithiasis, diabetes insipidus, and the syndrome of inappropriate secretion of antidiuretic hormone is discussed in the appropriate sections elsewhere in the book.

Mechanism of Action
All diuretics act by inhibiting the tubular reabsorption of sodium, primarily by *diminishing the movement of sodium from the tubular lumen into the cell.* The different diuretics are usually classified by their primary site of action within the nephron: loop diuretics in the thick ascending limb of the loop of Henle; thiazide-type diuretics in the distal tubule; and potassium-sparing diuretics at the aldosterone-sensitive site in the cortical collecting tubule [1,2]. The site of action is important clinically since it determines both the diuretic potency and the concomitant effects on potassium and hydrogen excretion (Table 4-1)[2]. For example, the proximal tubule is responsible for the reabsorption of about 65 percent of the filtered sodium. Nevertheless, proximally acting diuretics (such as acetazolamide, the carbonic anhydrase inhibitor) are weak agents because most of the increase in sodium delivery out of the proximal tubule can be reabsorbed more distally, particularly in the loop of Henle, which has a high total reabsorptive capacity. In comparison, the capacity of the distal and collecting tubules is more limited. As a result, these segments can diminish but usually not seriously impair the diuretic response to a loop diuretic [2].

The general mechanism of sodium reabsorption is similar in each of the nephron segments. The sodium potassium–activated adenosine triphosphatase (Na-K-ATPase) pump in the basolateral (or peritubular) membrane transports sodium out of the cell into the peritubular capillary. This process maintains the cell sodium concentration at low levels, thereby allowing filtered sodium in the lumen to passively enter the cell via a carrier or channel in the luminal membrane. The different classes of diuretics act at specific sites within the nephron because *each nephron segment has a different sodium entry mechanism* [1].

Loop Diuretics
The loop diuretics, furosemide, bumetanide, and ethacrynic acid, are the most potent diuretics currently available, leading to the excretion of up to 25 percent of the filtered sodium when given in maximum dosage. They act in the medullary and cortical aspects of the thick ascending limb. At both sites, sodium entry is mediated by an electrically neutral *Na-K-2Cl carrier* in the luminal membrane that is most efficient when all four

Table 4-1. Characteristics of commonly used diuretics

Site of action	Carrier or channel inhibited	Filtered Na excreted (%)	Effect on K and H loss
Loop of Henle Furosemide Bumetanide Ethacrynic acid	Na-K-2Cl carrier	Up to 25	Increased
Distal tubule Thiazides Chlorthalidone Metolazone	Na-Cl carrier	Up to 3–5	Increased
Cortical collecting tubule Spironolactone Amiloride Triamterene	Na channel	1–2	Decreased

sites are occupied [3]. Furosemide, bumetanide, and possibly ethacrynic acid appear to inhibit net sodium transport by competing for the chloride site on this carrier* [3].

The loop diuretics also diminish calcium reabsorption, which is passively linked to sodium chloride reabsorption in the ascending limb [5]. This effect is clinically important since increasing urinary calcium excretion with saline and a loop diuretic is the mainstay of therapy for hypercalcemia [5].

Thiazide-Type Diuretics
The primary site of action of the thiazide-type diuretics is the early distal tubule [2,6,7]. This segment has a smaller quantitative effect than the loop of Henle; as a result, the thiazide diuretics in maximum dosage inhibit the reabsorption of only 3 to 5 percent of the filtered sodium. This decrease in potency limits the use of these drugs in edematous states but is not a problem in the treatment of uncomplicated hypertension since a large diuresis is neither necessary nor desirable in this setting.

The sodium entry mechanism in the distal tubule is a simple *Na-Cl carrier* that is inhibited by the thiazides [6]. In addition, the thiazides (by an unknown mechanism) also appear to directly stimulate calcium reabsorption in this segment [7]. The ensuing fall in calcium excretion (of up to 150 mg/day) presumably accounts for the apparent effectiveness of the thiazides in diminishing new calcium stone formation in patients with hypercalciuria (see Chap. 54).

Potassium-Sparing Diuretics
In comparison to the more proximal segments, sodium reabsorption in the cortical collecting tubule occurs through a selective *sodium channel,* rather than being carrier-mediated [8]. The reabsorption of cationic sodium creates an electrical gradient that then favors the secretion of potassium (through a selective potassium channel) and hydrogen. These processes are stimulated by aldosterone, in part by increasing the number of open sodium and potassium channels in the luminal membrane [9]. Thus, both aldosterone and the distal delivery of sodium and water are the primary physiologic regulators of distal potassium secretion, the major mechanism by which potassium is excreted in the urine [10].

---

*A second entry mechanism, which is also inhibited by at least furosemide and bumetanide, may account for as much as one-half of sodium entry in the *cortical* ascending limb: parallel Na/H and Cl/HCO$_3$ exchangers [4]. In this setting, cellular carbon dioxide and water combine to form carbonic acid and then H and HCO$_3$: the former then exchanges with Na and the latter with Cl. The net effect is NaCl reabsorption; the H and HCO$_3$ that enter the tubular lumen reform carbon dioxide and water.

Table 4-2. Major metabolic complications of diuretic therapy

Volume depletion
Azotemia
Hyponatremia, primarily with the thiazides
Hypokalemia, often with metabolic alkalosis
Hyperkalemia, with potassium-sparing diuretics
Hyperuricemia
Hypomagnesemia
Hyperlipidemia
Hyperglycemia

The effect of diuretics on potassium and hydrogen secretion is dependent on their site of action. The loop diuretics and the thiazides inhibit sodium and water reabsorption proximal to the secretory site. The ensuing rise in distal delivery plus the hypovolemia-induced hyperaldosteronism promote both potassium and hydrogen loss [2], often leading to hypokalemia and metabolic alkalosis.

In comparison, the potassium-sparing diuretics act in the cortical collecting tubule; the associated decline in sodium reabsorption limits the secretion of both potassium and hydrogen, frequently leading to a rise in the plasma potassium concentration and mild metabolic acidosis [1,2]. The three diuretics that act at this site have somewhat different modes of action. Amiloride and perhaps triamterene specifically block the sodium channel in the luminal membrane [11]. In contrast, spironolactone is a direct antagonist of aldosterone, competitively binding to the cytosolic aldosterone receptor [12]. The ensuing reduction in aldosterone effect decreases the number of open sodium and potassium channels in the luminal membrane [9]. Spironolactone is unique among the diuretics in that it enters the cell by moving from the plasma across the basolateral membrane; it does not require access to the luminal fluid [12].

The potassium-sparing diuretics have relatively weak natriuretic activity, leading to the maximum excretion of only 1 to 2 percent of the filtered sodium. As a result, they are most often used in conjunction with a thiazide or loop diuretic, both to potentiate the diuresis and to minimize urinary potassium loss [2,13].

An interesting example of how knowledge of the mechanism of action of a diuretic can have unsuspected clinical utility occurs in lithium-induced nephrogenic diabetes insipidus. This complication appears to result from lithium accumulation in the collecting tubular cells by movement *through the sodium channel* in the luminal membrane. Blocking this channel with amiloride has been shown to partially reverse and may even prevent the concentrating defect, presumably by limiting lithium entry into the cells [14].

Time Course of Diuretic Complications
Diuretic therapy may be associated with a variety of fluid, electrolyte, and metabolic disturbances (Table 4-2) [15]. These problems, including the possibility that diuretics may actually *increase coronary mortality* when used to lower the blood pressure in some patients with mild hypertension, are discussed in the appropriate sections elsewhere in the book (see Chap. 13). It is useful, however, to review at this point the *time course* of the diuretic effects on both the daily sodium excretion and the development of fluid and electrolyte complications.

The administration of a short-acting diuretic such as furosemide has a dramatic effect on the pattern of daily sodium excretion. Sodium excretion increases markedly during the 6-hour period of diuretic action. However, the associated volume depletion activates sodium-retaining mechanisms, resulting in an antinatriuresis and sodium retention during the remainder of the day (Fig. 4-1) [16]. The end result may be *no net sodium loss* in patients on a high-sodium diet. In this setting, the desired negative sodium balance can be achieved in one of three ways: (1) by restricting sodium intake to minimize

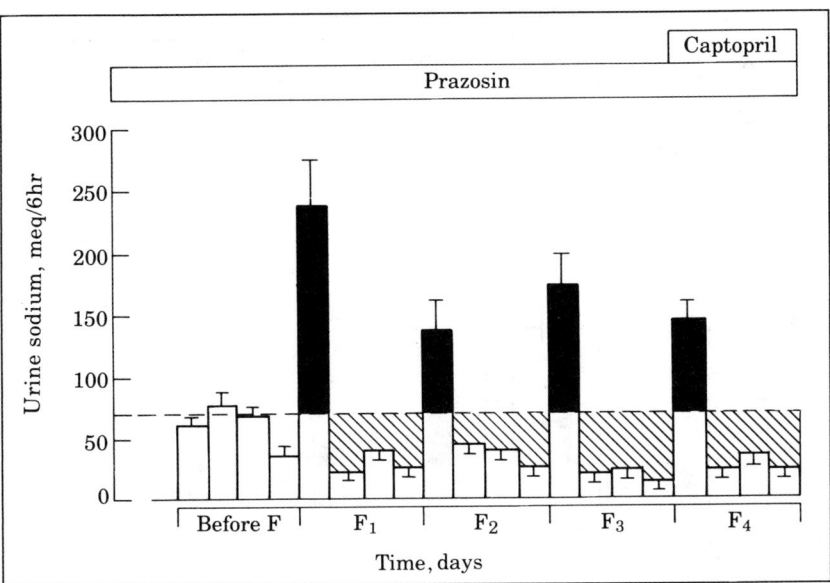

Fig. 4-1. Values for 6-hourly rates of sodium excretion in normal subjects ingesting 270 meq of sodium per day after being given furosemide. The dashed horizontal line represents the average rate of sodium excretion during the control period and is roughly equal to intake. Sodium excretion exceeded intake after the diuretic but fell below control levels (shaded areas) when the diuretic effect dissipated. The end result was no net diuresis. Blocking the renin-angiotensin-aldosterone system with captopril and the effect of norepinephrine with the α_1-adrenergic blocker prazosin did not alter this response. (From Wilcox, CS, Guzman, NJ, Mitch, WE, Kelly, RA, Maroni, BJ, Souney, PF, Rayment, CM, Braun, L, Colucci, R, Loon, NR. *Kidney Int* 31:135, 1987. Reprinted by permission from Kidney International.)

sodium retention once the diuretic has worn off (the most preferable way); (2) by increasing the dose of the diuretic, although the larger initial diuresis may lead to symptomatic hypovolemia; or (3) by giving the diuretic twice a day.

Studies in normal subjects have helped to elucidate the mechanisms responsible for the compensatory sodium retention. Although activation of the renin-angiotensin-aldosterone and sympathetic nervous systems is an obvious candidate to contribute to this response, the administration of both captopril (which blocks the formation of angiotensin II and aldosterone) and the alpha$_1$-adrenergic blocker prazosin did not prevent the antinatriuresis (Fig. 4-1). However, the mean blood pressure fell by about 12 mm Hg in the absence of the vasoconstrictive effects of angiotensin II and norepinephrine [16], a hemodynamic change that directly promotes sodium retention [17]. In comparison, the blood pressure is maintained after furosemide in the intact patient; in this setting, the tubular effects of angiotensin II, aldosterone, and possibly norepinephrine (rather than hypotension) are probably responsible for the diminution in sodium excretion.

Even if a net diuresis occurs initially, these neurohumoral sodium-retaining mechanisms lead to a response that is short-lived (assuming that the *diuretic dose and sodium intake are relatively constant,* as occurs, for example, in most patients with essential hypertension and in many patients with stable heart failure or hepatic cirrhosis). This limitation should be recognized as *appropriate,* since marked hypovolemia and shock would eventually ensue if the rate of sodium excretion remained above intake. What is

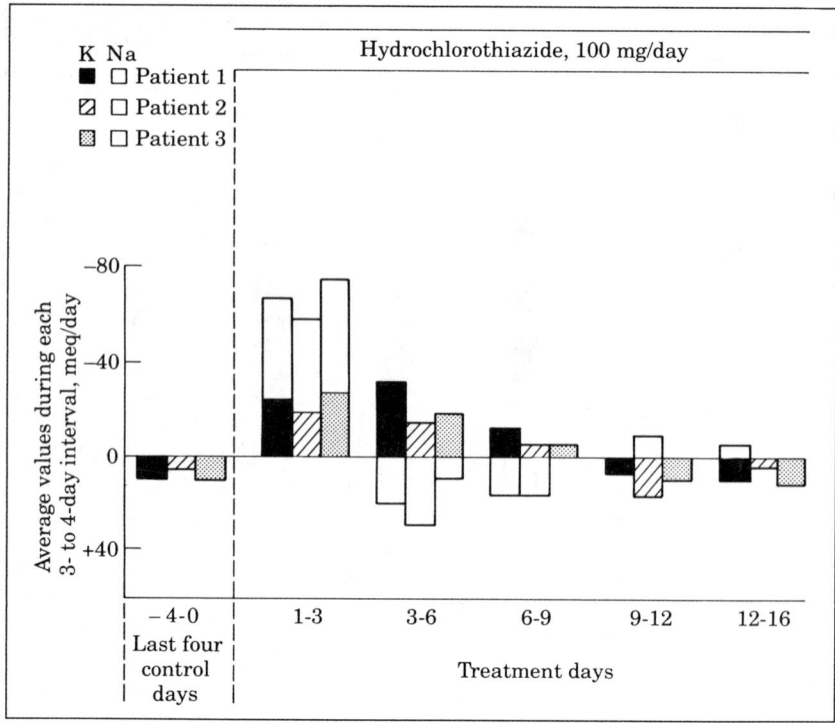

Fig. 4-2. Sodium and potassium balance in three nonedematous patients started on 100 mg of hydrochlorothiazide per day. Data are presented for each patient as the average balance during each 3- or 4-day period. Net loss of sodium occurred for 3 days and of potassium for 6 to 9 days before a new steady state was established. (Adapted from Maronde, RF, Milgrom, M, Vlachakis, ND, Chan, L. *J Am Med Assoc* 249:237, 1983. Copyright 1983, American Medical Association.)

generally underappreciated is how quickly this new steady state, in which intake and output are equal, is achieved. Figure 4-2 illustrates the response of three normal subjects to the administration of 100 mg of hydrochlorothiazide, a high initial dose. Sodium loss occurs for only 3 days and potassium loss occurs for 6 to 9 days even though the diuretic is continued. In this setting, the decrease in sodium reabsorption in the distal tubule is counteracted by increased reabsorption at hormone-sensitive sites in the proximal tubule (via angiotensin II and norpinephrine) and the cortical collecting tubule (via aldosterone) [17,18].

These findings are very important clinically. As long as the diuretic dose and dietary intake are relatively constant, *all of the diuretic-induced fluid and electrolyte abnormalities are most likely to occur within the first few weeks of drug administration* [13,15,19]. Suppose for example, that a patient with essential hypertension is begun on 50 mg of hydrochlorothiazide per day. At 3 weeks, blood pressure, volume status, plasma creatinine, sodium, and potassium concentrations are normal. In this setting, late volume depletion, hyponatremia, or hypokalemia is unlikely unless some new problem is superimposed, such as vomiting or an increase in drug dosage.

Diuretic Use in Edematous States: Cirrhotic Ascites
The most common generalized edematous states are congestive heart failure, hepatic cirrhosis, the nephrotic syndrome, and renal failure. In these disorders, diuretic therapy

is generally begun with a loop diuretic, and negative fluid balance is continued until at least much of the excess fluid is removed. However, hepatic cirrhosis is associated with some unique problems that illustrate the difficulties that may occur.

How Rapidly Should Edema Fluid Be Removed?

The fluid that is lost when diuretics are administered initially comes from the plasma volume. This results in a reduction in venous pressure and therefore in intracapillary pressure, a change that promotes *repletion of the plasma volume* by the movement of edema fluid from the interstitium into the vascular space.

In most patients with generalized edema, the edema fluid can be mobilized rapidly and 2 liters or more can be removed in 24 hours without much reduction in the plasma volume. An important exception occurs in the patient with cirrhosis and ascites but *no peripheral edema*. In this setting, the edema fluid can only be mobilized by the peritoneal capillaries, a process that is rate limited with an average maximum of 300 to 500 ml/day if hypovolemia is to be avoided [20]. More rapid fluid removal can lead to plasma volume depletion, a decline in renal function (as evidenced by a rise in the blood urea nitrogen [BUN]), and, in some patients, the hepatorenal syndrome [20]. In patients with tense ascites, a safe and perhaps more rapid alternative is daily paracentesis followed by dietary sodium restriction and diuretic therapy to minimize the reaccumulation of ascites [21].

In heart failure, a different mechanism may be responsible for diuretic-induced azotemia. Fluid removal results in a reduction in intravascular and intracardiac pressures. These changes lead to relief of peripheral and pulmonary edema and usually to an improvement in the patient's sense of well-being. However, the fall in left heart pressure via the Frank-Starling relationship can reduce cardiac contractility and the cardiac output (see Chap. 22). If tissue perfusion becomes significantly diminished in this setting, as evidenced by a rise in BUN, further diuresis should be withheld and treatment aimed at improving cardiac function with vasodilators or inotropic agents. On the other hand, it can be assumed that there is no important decline in cardiac output if the BUN remains stable as fluid is removed.

Which Diuretic is Likely to be Most Effective?

Although loop diuretics are generally the most potent, as many as one-half of cirrhotic patients may be furosemide resistant. In comparison, almost all patients are responsive to spironolactone [22]. One possible explanation for this seemingly paradoxical finding is that marked hyperaldosteronism can result in the cortical collecting tubule reclaiming most of the excess sodium delivered out of the loop of Henle. The observation that furosemide-resistant patients often have a markedly elevated plasma renin activity is consistent with this hypothesis [22]. However, many patients with heart failure also have secondary hyperaldosteronism yet resistance to a loop diuretic is unusual in the absence of advanced disease in which renal perfusion is markedly impaired.

A second, more likely possibility is that cirrhosis is associated with reduced furosemide entry into the urine [23]. Furosemides (and most other loop and thiazide diuretics) are highly protein bound in the plasma. As a result, they enter the urine primarily by secretion by the organic acid secretory pump in the proximal tubule, rather than by glomerular filtration. Furosemide excretion appears to be delayed in many patients with cirrhosis, an effect that could result from impaired secretion due, perhaps, to competition from other organic acids such as bile salts* [23]. Spironolactone might be uniquely

---

*Decreased furosemide excretion also may explain the diuretic resistance that occurs in some patients with marked hypoalbuminemia [23a]. Protein binding normally limits furosemide to the vascular space, thereby promoting its secretion into the urine. When binding is decreased due to a reduction in the plasma albumin concentration, furosemide has a relatively large extravascular volume of distribution, with less drug being presented to the kidney. In this setting, the diuretic resistance can be overcome by administering albumin-bound furosemide, which has been prepared by mixing the drug with albumin prior to infusion [23a].

effective in this setting since it is the only diuretic that does not have a luminal effect and therefore does not require access to the tubular fluid; in comparison to all other diuretics, spironolactone acts by entering the tubular cell from the plasma across the basolateral membrane [12]. It is therefore possible that another potassium-sparing diuretic such as amiloride would not be as effective in this setting.

Spironolactone may have an additional advantage in hepatic cirrhosis, being *safer* than the loop and thiazide diuretics. As described previously, the latter agents often lead to hypokalemia and metabolic alkalosis. This combination can produce hepatic coma in severe hepatic disease via two mechanisms [24]:

1. Hypokalemia increases renal ammonia production and subsequent release into the renal vein [24,25], an effect that is thought to be related to transcellular ionic exchange. As hypokalemia develops, potassium moves out of the cells to replete the extracellular stores; to maintain electroneutrality, extracellular hydrogen and sodium enter the cells. The ensuing intracellular acidosis in proximal tubular cells promotes ammonia production [25].

2. The effect of metabolic alkalosis can be appreciated from the Henderson-Hasselbalch equation for the ammonia-ammonium system:

$$pH = 9.2 + \log[NH_3]/[NH_4{}^+]$$

An increase in the arterial pH will increase the concentration of lipid-soluble ammonia (and possibly other toxic amines), which can then diffuse down a concentration gradient across the blood-brain barrier into the brain.

Avoidance of Nonsteroidal Anti-inflammatory Drugs

Patients treated with diuretics for hepatic cirrhosis, heart failure, or hypertension often have increased renin and norepinephrine release. In this setting of high circulating vasoconstrictors, renal perfusion is in part protected by increased production of vasodilator prostaglandins. Thus, reducing prostaglandin synthesis with a nonsteroidal anti-inflammatory drug can induce renal vasoconstriction, a moderate to marked reduction in glomerular filtration rate, and diminished diuretic responsiveness [26–28]. The last effect may be due both to the decline in renal perfusion and to reversal of the normal inhibitory action of renal prostaglandins on NaCl reabsorption in the loop of Henle and perhaps other segments (see Chap. 23) [27,28].

These findings suggest that nonsteroidal anti-inflammatory drugs should be avoided if possible in patients receiving a diuretic. There is, however, one possible exception. Sulindac appears to be somewhat unique in that it is less likely than other drugs to diminish renal prostaglandin synthesis and therefore is less likely to impair renal function or the response to diuretics (see Chap. 23) [26]. This is only a relative protection, however, and careful monitoring is still required.

Refractory Edema

Infrequently, an edematous patient is resistant to conventional diuretic therapy, including use of a loop diuretic at maximum dosage (such as 320 mg of furosemide given orally or slowly intravenously). Table 4-3 lists the possible causes of this problem and a sequential approach to inducing an effective diuresis [15]. In some patients, for example, the distal tubule reclaims most of the excess sodium delivered out of the loop of Henle, thereby minimizing the response to a loop diuretic alone. In this setting, the addition of a thiazide diuretic will block this distal compensation, often leading to a marked diuresis [29,30].

When combination diuretic therapy is used, the patient must be carefully monitored because an *excessive* response may be seen in which the urine volume can reach 5 liters/day and potassium losses can exceed 200 meq/day [30]. These potential problems can be minimized by concurrent use of a potassium-sparing diuretic and by beginning with a low dose of a thiazide (such as 25 mg of hydrochlorothiazide).

Table 4-3. Pathogenesis and treatment of refractory edema

Problem	Treatment
Excess sodium intake	Measure urine sodium excretion; attempt more rigorous dietary restriction if > 100 meq/day.
Decreased or delayed intestinal drug absorption	Bowel-wall edema can reversibly impair oral drug absorption; switch to intravenous loop diuretic if high-dose oral therapy is ineffective.
Increased distal reabsorption	Add thiazide-type diuretic or potassium-sparing diuretic, or both.
Decreased loop sodium delivery due to low GFR or enhanced proximal reabsorption, or both	Attempt to increase delivery out of proximal tubule with acetazolamide or rarely corticosteroids.
Decreased drug entry into tubule lumen	Trial of spironolactone in cirrhosis; albumin and loop diuretic if marked hypoalbuminemia; massive doses of loop diuretic or dialysis or hemofiltration in severe heart failure or renal failure.

References

1. Friedman, PA, Hebert, SC. Mechanism of action of diuretics. In BM Brenner and JH Stein (Eds.), *Contemporary Issues in Nephrology. Body Fluid Homeostasis* (Vol. 16). New York: Churchill Livingstone, 1987.
2. Hropot, M. Fowler, N, Karlmark, B, Giebisch, G. Tubular action of diuretics: Distal effects on electrolyte transport and acidification. *Kidney Int* 28:477, 1985.
3. Hebert, SC, Andreoli, TE. Control of NaCl transport in the thick ascending limb. *Am J Physiol* 246:F745, 1984.
4. Friedman, PA. Bumetanide inhibition of $[CO_2 + HCO_3]$-dependent and -independent equivalent electrical flux in renal cortical thick ascending limbs. *J Pharmacol Exp Therap* 238:407, 1986.
5. Sutton, RAL. Diuretics and calcium metabolism. *Am J Kid Dis* 5:4, 1985.
6. Velasquez, H, Wright, FS. Effect of diuretic drugs on Na, Cl, and K transport in the rat renal distal tubule. *Am J Physiol* 250:F1012, 1986.
7. Costanzo, LS. Localization of diuretic action in microperfused rat distal tubules: Ca and Na transport. *Am J Physiol* 248:F527, 1985.
8. Koeppen, BM, Biagi, BA, Giebisch, G. Intracellular microelectrode catheterization of the rabbit cortical collecting duct. *Am J Physiol* 244:F35, 1983.
9. Sansom, SC, O'Neil, RG. Mineralocorticoid regulation of apical cell membrane Na^+ and K^+ transport of the cortical collecting duct. *Am J Physiol* 248:F858, 1985.
10. Rose, BD. *Clinical Physiology of Acid-Base and Electrolyte Disorders* (2nd ed.). New York: McGraw-Hill, 1984. Pp 256-265.
11. Benos, DJ. Amiloride: A molecular probe of sodium transport in tissues and cells. *Am J Physiol* 242:C131, 1982.
12. Corvol, P, Claire, M, Oblin, ME, Geering, K. Rossier. B. Mechanism of the antimineralocorticoid effects of spironolactones. *Kidney Int* 20:1, 1981.
13. Ridgeway, NA, Ginn, DR, Alley, K. Outpatient conversion of treatment to potassium-sparing diuretics. *Am J Med* 80:785, 1986.
14. Battle, DC, von Riotte, AM, Gaviria, M, Grupp, M. Amelioration of polyuria by amiloride in patients receiving long-term lithium therapy. *N Engl J Med* 312:408, 1985.
15. Rose, BD. Clinical use of diuretics. In BM Brenner and JH Stein (Eds.), *Contemporary Issues in Nephrology. Body Fluid Homeostatis* (Vol. 16). New York: Churchill Livingstone, 1987.
16. Wilcox, CS, Guzman, NJ, Mitch, WE, Kelly, RA, Maroni, BJ, Souney, PF, Rayment,

CM, Braun, L, Colucci, R, Loon, NR. Na$^+$, K$^+$ and BP homeostasis in man during furosemide; Effects of prazosin and captopril. *Kidney Int* 31:135, 1987.

17. Rose, BD. *Clinical Physiology of Acid-Base and Electrolyte Disorders* (2nd ed.). New York: McGraw-Hill, 1987. Pp. 178-186.
18. Dirks, JH, Cirksena, WJ, Berliner, RW. Micropuncture study of the effects of various diuretics on sodium reabsorption in the proximal tubules of the dog. *J Clin Invest* 45:1875, 1966.
19. Morgan, DB, Davidson, C. Hypokalemia and diuretics: An analysis of publications. *Br Med J* 1:905, 1980.
20. Pockros, PJ, Reynolds, TB. Rapid diuresis in patients with ascites from chronic liver disease: The importance of peripheral edema. *Gastroenterology* 90:1827, 1986.
21. Quintero, E, Gines, P, Arroyo, V, Rimola, A, Bory, F, Planas, R, Viver, J, Cabrera, J, Rodes, J. Paracentesis versus diuretics in the treatment of cirrhotics with tense ascites. *Lancet* 2:611, 1985.
22. Perez-Ayuso, RM, Arroyo, V, Planas, R, Gaya, J, Bory, F, Rimola, A, Rivera, F, Rodes, J. Random comparative study of efficacy of furosemide vs. spironolactone in nonazotemic renin-aldosterone system. *Gastroenterology* 84:961, 1983.
23. Pintani, M, Daskalopoulos, G, Laffi, G, Gentilini, P, Zipser, RD. Altered furosemide pharmacokinetics in chronic alcoholic liver disease with ascites contributes to diuretic resistance. *Gastroenterology* 92:296, 1987.
23a. Inoue, M, Okajima, K, Itoh, K, Ando, Y, Watanabe, N, Yasaka, T, Nagase, S, Morino, Y. Mechanism of furosemide resistance in analbuminemic rats and hypoalbuminemic patients. *Kidney Int* 32:198, 1987.
24. Gabuzda, GJ, Hall, PW, III. Relation of potassium depletion to renal ammonium metabolism and coma. *Medicine* 45:481, 1966.
25. Jaeger, P, Karlmark, B, Giebisch, G. Ammonium transport in the rat cortical tubule: Relation to potassium metabolism. *Am J Physiol* 245:F593, 1983.
26. Patrono, C, Dunn, MJ. The clinical significance of inhibition of renal prostaglandin synthesis. *Kidney Int* 32:1, 1987.
27. Brater, DC. Analysis of the effect of indomethacin on the response to furosemide in man: Effect of dose of furosemide. *J Pharmacol Exp Therap* 210:386, 1979.
28. Kirchner, KA. Indomethacin antagonizes furosemide's intratubular effects during loop segment microperfusion. *J Pharmacol Exp Therap* 243:881, 1987.
29. Wollam, GL, Tarazi, RC, Bravo, EL, Dustan, HP. Diuretic potency of combined hydrochlorothiazide and furosemide therapy in patients with azotemia. *Am J Med* 72:929, 1982.
30. Oster, JR, Epstein, M, Smoller, S. Combination therapy with thiazide-type diuretic and loop diuretic agents for resistant sodium retention. *Ann Intern Med* 99:405, 1983.

5. METABOLIC ACIDOSIS

Metabolic acidosis refers to a reduction in arterial pH induced by a fall in the plasma bicarbonate concentration. This can be produced either by the addition of a metabolic (noncarbonic) acid, such as lactic acid, or by the loss of bicarbonate, as with diarrhea. The process causing the acidemia leads to a decrease in the blood pH below the normal value of 7.40 unless there is a coexisting disorder that tends to raise the pH.

The fall in pH that occurs in metabolic acidosis is minimized, but not prevented, by body buffers. When, for example, the excess H^+ ions combine with HCO_3^- or with cellular phosphates or proteins, there is only a small increment in the *free H^+ concentration,* as illustrated by the following reactions:

$$H^+ + HCO_3^- \rightarrow H_2CO_3 \rightarrow CO_2 + H_2O$$
$$H^+ + HPO_4^= \rightarrow H_2PO_4^-$$

In addition to buffering, the change in pH is also limited acutely by respiratory compensation. Acidemia stimulates ventilation which, by lowering the PCO_2, raises the pH toward normal. This process is defined by the Henderson-Hasselbalch equation:

$$pH = 6.1 + \log [HCO_3^-]/0.03(P_{CO_2})$$

These responses, however, do not restore normal acid-base balance. In most cases, correction of the acidosis requires *excretion of the excess acid in the urine,* either as titratable acidity or NH_4^+. This process generally requires 3 to 4 days to reach maximum levels.

Anion Gap

Many disorders can cause metabolic acidosis. From a diagnostic viewpoint, calculation of the anion gap (AG) is extremely helpful in narrowing the differential diagnosis to only a few conditions.

The AG (measured in meq/L) refers to the difference between the plasma concentrations of the major measured cation (sodium) and the major measured anions (bicarbonate and chloride):

$$\text{Anion gap} = [Na^+ - (HCO_3^- + Cl^-)]$$

The normal AG varies between 8 and 12 meq/L. It is composed primarily of the plasma proteins that are negatively charged at the normal arterial pH of about 7.40. The ionic charges of other cations (K^+, Mg^{2+}, Ca^{2+}) and anions ($HPO_4^=$, urate$^-$) tend to balance out.

Albumin normally comprises most of the AG. A decrease in the serum albumin concentration from 4.0 gm/dl to 2.0 gm/dl, therefore, may reduce the AG by as much as 6 meq/L, since each 1 gm/dl of albumin has a negative charge of about 2.0 to 2.8 meq/L [1,2][1]

Calculation of the AG is helpful in differentiating metabolic acidosis into two major types: (1) *acidosis with an increased gap,* in which the titration of H^+ by bicarbonate leads to accumulation of the associated "unmeasured" acid anion (such as lactate or β-hydroxybutyrate); and (2) *acidosis with a normal gap*[2] (also called a hyperchloremic acidosis), in which retention of hydrochloric acid or loss of sodium bicarbonate results in the replacement of HCO_3^- by Cl^- and therefore no change in either the sum of measured anions or the AG:

$$HA + NaHCO_3 \rightarrow NaA \text{ (high AG)}$$
$$HCl + NaHCO_3 \rightarrow NaCl \text{ (normal AG)}$$

It is important to note than an increased AG is not always due to metabolic acidosis. In metabolic alkalosis, for example, there is often volume depletion (due to vomiting or diuretic use), leading to hemoconcentration and a rise in the plasma protein concentration. Moreover, the elevation in blood pH in this setting increases the negative charge on most plasma proteins, as the following reaction is driven to the right by the fall in free H^+ concentration:

$$HPr \rightarrow H^+ + Pr^-$$

The combination of a higher protein concentration and a greater anionic charge per molecule can lead to an increase in the AG that is usually relatively small (up to 7–8 meq/L)[2]. Large increases in the AG, therefore, are almost always the result of a concomitant metabolic acidosis.

---

[1]A small decrease in AG can also be caused by a reduction in other unmeasured anions, as with hypophosphatemia. The same effect can be achieved by an increase in an unmeasured cation. In multiple myeloma, for example, the monoclonal paraprotein may be positively charged, leading to a fall in the AG.

[2]In this setting, calculation of the *urine* anion gap may be helpful in determining whether urinary acidification is normal (as with diarrhea) or impaired (as with renal tubular acidosis; see Chap. 8)

Table 5-1. Causes of metabolic acidosis with increased anion gap

Etiology	Major circulating anions	Characteristic features
Ketoacidosis	β-hydroxybutyrate, acetoacetate	See Chap. 7.
Lactic acidosis	Lactate > pyruvate	See Chap. 6.
Renal failure	Sulfate, phosphate, variety of organic acids	Bicarbonate usually > 12 meq/L; AG usually < 23 meq/L.
Rhabdomyolysis		PO_4, others (?): Increased creatinine phosphokinase, phosphate, urinary myoglobin; hypocalcemia.
TOXINS		
Methanol	Formate	Increased osmolal gap*; hyperemic optic disk with retinal sheen.
Ethylene glycol	Glycolate, lactate	Increased osmolal gap*; acute renal failure; urinary oxalate crystals; hypocalcemia. Coma and pulmonary edema can occur in severe cases.
Salicylates	Variety of organic acids, salicylate	Concomitant respiratory alkalosis; tinnitus.
Toluene	?Hippurate	Can also cause distal renal tubular acidosis.
Paraldehyde	?Acetate	Rare; previous cases may have been misdiagnosed patients with alcoholic ketoacidosis.

*The normal osmolal gap (obtained by subtracting the calculated from the measured plasma osmolality) is <10 and consists mainly of calcium, lipids, and proteins. The P_{osm} can be calculated from the following formula:

$$P_{osm} \text{ (calculated)} = 2[Na] + [glucose]/18 + BUN/2.8$$

An elevated osmolal gap in a patient with metabolic acidosis can be induced by methanol, ethylene glycol, or acute renal failure [3]. In these settings, the gap is due to the accumulation of small solutes such as methanol or formate.

Metabolic Acidosis with an Increased AG
The major causes of a high AG metabolic acidosis are listed in Table 5-1, with lactic acidosis, ketoacidosis, and renal failure being the most common [3]. It should be empha-sized, however, that mild elevations in the AG (AG ≤ 20 meq/L) are somewhat nonspe-cific in that the source of the excess unmeasured anion can be identified in only about 30 percent of cases [2,4]. The factors responsible for this change are not well understood; hyperproteinemia and hyperphosphatemia, for example, may contribute in some cases [5]. In contrast, a detectable organic anion is almost always present when the AG is greater than 25 to 30 meq/L.

Metabolic Acidosis with a Normal AG
The major causes of metabolic acidosis with a normal AG are listed in Table 5-2, with diarrhea and renal failure being the most common [3]. Diarrhea leads to the loss of $NaHCO_3$ in the stool; the ensuing volume depletion leads to compensatory NaCl reten-tion by the kidney. The net effect is replacement of HCO_3^- by Cl^- and no change in the

Table 5-2. Causes of metabolic acidosis with normal anion gap

Normal or elevated plasma K^+	Normal or low plasma K^+

Hydrochloric acid infusion
  Hyperalimentation
  NH_4Cl, HCl, Cholestyramine HCl
	Gastrointestinal disorders
	  Diarrhea; pancreatic, intestinal, or biliary
	  fistulae

Posthypocapnia	Ureteral diversions
	  Ureterosigmoidostomy
	  Ileal bladder (if obstructed)

Hypoaldosteronism (see Chap. 11)
  Selective hypoaldosteronism
  Adrenal insufficiency
  Aldosterone resistance or potassium-
  sparing diuretics
	Renal tubular acidosis (RTA)
	  Proximal RTA
	  Distal RTA
	  Recovery from ketoacidosis

Adapted from Arieff, AI, DeFronzo, RA (eds). *Fluid, Electrolyte, and Acid-Base Disorders,* New York: Churchill Livingstone, 1985.

AG. Severe diarrhea, however, can on occasion be associated with a rise in the AG when marked volume loss leads to both hyperproteinemia (due to hemoconcentration) and excess lactic acid production [5].

Renal failure presents an interesting example of the potential overlap between a normal and an elevated AG acidosis. The daily acid load, generated primarily by the metabolism of sulfur-containing amino acids into sulfuric acid, is about 50 to 100 meq/day on a typical American diet. This acid is immediately buffered by $NaHCO_3$:

$$H_2SO_4 + 2NaHCO_3 \rightarrow Na_2SO_4 + 2CO_2 + 2H_2O$$

The excess sulfate is excreted in the urine, with the rate being determined by the difference between glomerular filtration and tubular reabsorption; in comparison, the excess acid is excreted by the tubular secretion of H^+. If glomerular and tubular function decline in parallel, then both the H^+ and the $SO_4^=$ will be retained, producing metabolic acidosis with a high AG. If, however, there is more prominent tubular dysfunction, the excretion of acid will be diminished but that of sulfate may be maintained due to reduced reabsorption of filtered sulfate. The net effect is that sulfate is excreted as Na_2SO_4, and metabolic acidosis occurs without a rise in AG[6].

Clinical Manifestations

A frequent finding on physical examination in patients with metabolic acidosis is the presence of deep (Kussmaul) respirations, induced by stimulation of the respiratory center in the brain stem by the low blood pH. As acidemia becomes more severe, nausea and vomiting or mental status changes, including coma, may be seen.

Secondary hypotension also may be observed in severely acidemic patients [7]. The reduced blood pressure in this setting is the result of depressed myocardial contractility and arterial vasodilation, both induced by the low blood pH. Initially, the cardiovascular effects of acidemia are antagonized by elevated levels of circulating catecholamines; however, the effect of acidemia often predominates below a blood pH of 7.15.

A common accompanying electrolyte disturbance in metabolic acidosis is relative hyperkalemia. This results from a transcellular shift of potassium in exchange for H^+, which enters the cells to be buffered by cell phosphates and proteins. Infusions of mineral acid characteristically cause this finding, whereas this shift does not appear to occur with organic acidoses, such as lactic and ketoacidosis [8]. The reason for this apparent difference is not known; in experimental animals, stimulation of insulin release by organic substrates, such as lactate and β-hydroxybutyrate, appears to counteract the effect of acidemia, as insulin drives potassium into the cells (see Chap. 11) [9].[1] However, the applicability of these findings to humans remains to be proved.

Treatment

The treatment of metabolic acidosis is directed at the cause of the disturbance, such as restoring tissue perfusion in lactic acidosis, as well as at correction of the acidemia itself. Bicarbonate therapy should be considered in patients with moderate-to-severe metabolic acidosis.[2] The initial goal of alkali therapy is to raise the arterial blood pH to 7.20, a generally safe level at which the patient is not at risk of cardiovascular compromise [7]. One does not need to correct the pH back to normal, since the potential risks of bicarbonate therapy (hypernatremia, hypercapnia, cerebrospinal fluid (CSF), acidosis, and overshoot alkalosis) [3] are likely to outweigh the benefits, as long as renal function (and therefore acid-excretory ability) is relatively intact.

Calculation of the bicarbonate deficit is useful in estimating the quantity of bicarbonate required. For example, in a patient with an arterial pH of 7.10, a plasma HCO_3^- concentration of 6 meq/L, and a P_{CO_2} of 20 mm Hg, the quantity of bicarbonate required to increase the blood pH to 7.20 can be calculated using the Henderson equation (the non-logarithmic form of the Henderson-Hasselbalch equation) [3]:

$$[H^+] = 24 \times P_{CO_2}/[HCO_3^-]$$

The H^+ concentration at a pH of 7.20 is 63 nanomol/L. As bicarbonate is given, the P_{CO_2} is likely to increase by about 5 mm Hg (to 25 mm Hg) as the drive to hyperventilation diminishes due to correction of the acidemia. Thus:

$$63 = 24 \times 25/[HCO_3^-]$$
$$[HCO_3^-] = 10 \text{ meq/L}$$

As a result, only a 4 meq/L rise in the serum bicarbonate concentration from 6 to 10 meq/L is required to increase the blood pH to the relatively "safe" level of 7.20.

The amount of bicarbonate needed to produce this change in pH can be determined by estimating the effective volume of distribution of bicarbonate. The apparent bicarbonate space is about 40 to 50 percent of lean body weight (similar to total body water) in normal subjects and those with mild-to-moderate metabolic acidosis. In severe metabolic acidosis, however, *cellular and bone buffering become more prominent* due to the marked reduction in the quantity of available extracellular buffer (primarily bicarbonate). This preferential entry of H^+ into cells causes the HCO_3^- space to expand to about 70 percent of lean body weight [10].

Using these calculations, the quantity of bicarbonate required to raise the plasma bicarbonate concentration from 6 to 10 meq/L in a 70-kg subject can be estimated:

$$\text{Bicarbonate deficit} = \text{volume of distribution} \times \text{deficit/L}$$
$$= 0.7 \times 70 \times (10 - 6) = 196 \text{ meq}$$

Thus, 196 meq of $NaHCO_3$ should be given over the first few hours. If the blood pH remains at or above 7.20, more bicarbonate may not be necessary, since the kidney will eventually excrete the excess acid. It is important to emphasize, however, that these calculations are estimates that assume (not always correctly) that there is no further acid production and that the bicarbonate space is 70 percent of body weight. Consequently, this formula is not a substitute for serial measurements of the blood pH and bicarbonate concentration to ascertain the efficacy of therapy.

---

[1]Hyperkalemia is often seen in lactic and ketoacidosis, but factors other than acidemia may be involved. In ketoacidosis, for example, insulin deficiency impairs potassium uptake by the cells; furthermore, hyperosmolality enhances potassium exit from cells (perhaps by solvent drag, as water moves out of the cells down an osmotic gradient).

[2]Recent studies have questioned the use of alkali in the treatment of lactic and ketoacidosis, since exogenous alkali may not raise the plasma bicarbonate concentration in these settings due to a concurrent increase in lactic acid or ketoacid production (see p. 43). Furthermore, correction of the underlying abnormality usually leads to spontaneous restoration of acid-base balance as metabolism of the excess organic anions results in the generation of bicarbonate.

Ingestions
In addition to the administration of $NaHCO_3$, treatment also must be aimed at removal of circulating toxins in patients with a severe aspirin, methanol, or ethylene glycol overdose [3]. This can be most efficiently achieved with hemodialysis.

Another important aspect of therapy in methanol or ethylene glycol intoxication is minimizing the formation of the toxic metabolites (formate and glycolate, respectively) that are primarily responsible for many of the associated complications. This can usually be achieved by the oral or intravenous administration of ethanol, which has a much greater affinity for alcohol dehydrogenase, the enzyme that also catalyzes the metabolism of the parent compound [3]. Some patients accidently self-treat themselves by ingesting both methanol (or ethylene glycol) and ethanol; the net effect is severe methanol poisoning but no blindness, metabolic acidosis, or elevation in the AG[11].

Mixed Acid-Base Disorders
Patients with metabolic acidosis may also have a second acid-base disturbance (respiratory acidosis or alkalosis, or metabolic alkalosis). An understanding of the normal respiratory compensation in patients with metabolic acidosis as well as careful examination of the AG can reveal these mixed acid-base disorders.

Mixed Metabolic Acidosis and Respiratory Acidosis or Alkalosis
A simple metabolic acidosis is associated with a reduced blood pH, which stimulates the brain stem respiratory center. The net effect is a reduction in the P_{CO_2} that, in uncomplicated metabolic acidosis, can be estimated from the following equation [12]:

$$\text{Expected } P_{CO_2} \text{ (mm Hg)} = [(1.5 \times [HCO_3^-]) + 8] \pm 2$$

A PCO_2 that is substantially different from the predicted value indicates a superimposed respiratory acidosis or alkalosis.* The usefulness of this calculation can be seen in the following example:

CASE HISTORY: A 24-year-old man is admitted to the hospital with tinnitus and diaphoresis. Laboratory studies identify the presence of a high–AG metabolic acidosis.

$$\text{Arterial pH} = 7.28$$
$$P_{CO_2} = 20 \text{ mm Hg (normal } = 40 \text{ mm Hg)}$$
$$HCO_3^- = 14 \text{ meq/L (normal } = 25 \text{ meq/L)}$$
$$AG = 23 \text{ meq/L}$$

Comment. The expected arterial P_{CO_2} at this plasma HCO_3^- concentration is about 29 mm Hg $[(1.5 \times 14) + 8 = 29]$. Thus, the measured value of 20 mm Hg indicates the presence of a secondary primary acid-base disorder, a respiratory alkalosis. Based on the history and acid-base evaluation, an aspirin overdose was suspected. A toxic salicylate level was subsequently found and appropriate therapy was begun.

It is important to emphasize that although the P_{CO_2} begins to fall at the inception of metabolic acidosis, full respiratory compensation may not occur for 12 to 36 hours [13]. Consequently, an erroneous diagonsis of a superimposed respiratory acid-base disturbance may be made if the above calculation is applied before the fall in P_{CO_2} has stabilized.

Increment in AG/Decrement in Bicarbonate Concentration
Examination of the ratio of the *increment in AG* above baseline to the *decrement in the plasma bicarbonate concentration* below normal (referred to as the Δ/Δ) may be useful in detecting the presence of a second acid-base disorder, such as a concurrent metabolic alkalosis [14].

---

*Other formulas have been developed that are equally effective in predicting the respiratory response in metabolic acidosis. For example, each 1 meq/L decrease in the plasma HCO_3^- concentration is normally associated with a compensatory 1.2 mm Hg fall in the PCO_2 [12].

Suppose, for example, that 10 meq of lactic acid was added to each liter of extracellular fluid. In this setting, one might expect that the AG would increase by 10 meq/L (from 12 up to 22 meq/L) due to the accumulation of lactate anions, and that the plasma HCO_3^- concentration would decrease by 10 meq/L (from 25 down to 15) due to buffering of the excess H^+ ions. However, the Δ/Δ in lactic acidosis is normally higher (about 1.6 : 1.0) [15]. It is thought that this finding results at least in part from hydrogen ion buffering *within cells,* a process that will not lower the plasma HCO_3^- concentration. Since lactate largely remains in the extracellular space, the rise in AG will exceed the fall in the plasma HCO_3^- concentration. By comparison, patients with ketoacidosis often have a Δ/Δ that is close to 1 : 1. In this disorder, the effect of intracellular acid buffering is counteracted by the loss of ketoacid anions in the urine [15].

The net effect is that the Δ/Δ in an uncomplicated high–AG metabolic acidosis is usually between 1 and 2. Lower values suggest an accompanying normal–AG acidosis (as with diarrhea), whereas higher values suggest a concurrent metabolic alkalosis. These principles can be appreciated in the following example:

CASE HISTORY: A 43-year old woman is admitted with a 3-day history of nausea, vomiting, and flank pain. Her blood pressure is 90/60 (120/75 being the previous level) and her temperature is 39°C. The urinalysis reveals marked pyuria and bacteriuria. A clinical diagnosis of acute pyelonephritis with probable bacteremia is made. Admission blood tests reveal:

$$Na^+ = 140 \text{ meq/L}$$
$$K^+ = 34 \text{ meq/L}$$
$$Cl^- = 77 \text{ meq/L}$$
$$HCO_3^- = 9 \text{ meq/L}$$
$$\text{Arterial pH} = 7.23$$
$$P_{CO2} = 22 \text{ mm Hg}$$
$$AG = 54 \text{ meq/L}$$
$$\text{Creatinine} = 1.3 \text{ mg/dL}$$
$$\text{Serum ketones — negative}$$

Comment. This patient has a high–AG metabolic acidosis. The cause is most likely lactic acidosis, since the patient is hypotensive and there is no renal failure, ketonemia, or a history of an ingestion. However, the AG of 54 meq/L is markedly increased (42 meq/L above baseline), whereas there is a much smaller decrement (16 meq/L) in the plasma HCO_3^- concentration ($\Delta/\Delta = 42 : 16 = 2.6 : 1.0$). This disparity can be explained by a concomitant metabolic alkalosis due to vomiting. This disorder would raise the plasma HCO_3^- concentration without affecting the AG. The underlying metabolic alkalosis in this case was confirmed by observing the response to fluid repletion. The ensuing metabolism of the excess lactate anions resulted in the generation of HCO_3^- and a rise in the plasma HCO_3^- concentration to 38 meq/L.

References

1. Emmett, M, Narins, RG. Clinical use of the anion gap. *Medicine* 56:38, 1977.
2. Gabow, PA: Disorders associated with an altered anion gap. *Kidney Int* 27:472, 1985.
3. Rose, BD: *Clinical Physiology of Acid-Base and Electrolyte Disorders* (2nd ed). New York: McGraw-Hill, 1984, Chap. 19.
4. Gabow, PA, Kaehny, WD, Fennessey, PV, Goodman, SI, Gross, PA, Schrier, RW. Diagnostic importance of an increased serum anion gap. *N Engl J Med* 303:854, 1980.
5. Wang, F, Butler, T, Rabbani, GH, Jones, PK. The acidosis of cholera. Contributions of hyperproteinemia, lactic acidemia, and hyperphosphatemia to an increased anion gap. *N Engl J Med* 315:1591, 1986.
6. Wallia, R, Greenberg, A, Piraino, B, Mitro, R, Puschett, JB. Serum electrolyte patterns in end-stage renal disease. *Am J Kid Dis* 8:98, 1986.
7. Mitchell, JH, Wildenthal, K, Johnson, RL, Jr. The effect of acid-base disturbances on cardiovascular and pulmonary function. *Kidney Int* 1:375, 1973.

8. Adrogue, HJ, Madias, NE. Changes in plasma potassium concentration during acute acid-base disturbances. *Am J Med* 71:456, 1981.
9. Adrogue, HJ, Chap, Z, Ishida, T, Field, JB. Role of endocrine pancreas in the kalemic response to acute metabolic acidosis in conscious dogs. *J Clin Invest* 75:798, 1985.
10. Adrogue, HJ, Brensilver, J, Cohen, JJ, Madias, NE. Influence of steady-state alterations in acid-base equilibrium on the fate of administered bicarbonate in the dog. *J Clin Invest* 71:867, 1983.
11. Palmisano, J, Gruver, C, Adams, ND. Absence of anion gap metabolic acidosis in severe methanol poisoning: A case report and review of the literature. *Am J Kid Dis* 9:441, 1987.
12. Bushinsky, DA, Coe, FL, Katzenberg, C, Szidon, JP, Parks, JH. Arterial PCO_2 in chronic metabolic acidosis. *Kidney Int* 22:311, 1982.
13. Pierce, NF, Fedson, DS, Brigham, KL. The ventilatory response to acute base deficit in humans. Time course during development and correction of metabolic acidosis. *Ann Intern Med* 72:633, 1970.
14. Rose, BD. *Clinical Physiology of Acid-Base and Electrolyte Disorders* (2nd ed), New York: McGraw-Hill, 1984, Pp. 401-402.
15. Oh, MS, Carroll, HJ, Goldstein, DA, Fein, IA. Hyperchloremic acidosis during the recovery phase of diabetic ketosis. *Ann Intern Med* 89:925, 1978.

6. Lactic Acidosis

Lactic acidosis is the most common cause of metabolic acidosis in hospitalized patients. It is associated with an elevated anion gap (AG) and a plasma lactate concentration above 4 meq/L. Impaired tissue oxygenation, leading to anaerobic metabolism, appears to be responsible for the rise in lactate production in most cases.

Pathophysiology
A review of the biochemistry of lactate generation and metabolism is important in understanding both the pathogenesis of lactic acidosis and the implications of the various therapies used in this disorder. Both *overproduction* and *underuse* of lactate appear to be operative in most patients with established lactic acidosis [1,2].

Lactate Production
In normal subjects, the primary sites of lactate synthesis are the brain, red blood cells, skeletal muscle, and skin [1]. Lactate is synthesized reversibly from pyruvate in a reaction catalyzed by lactate dehydrogenase (LDH) and involving the conversion of NADH into NAD^+:

$$Pyruvate^- + NADH + H^+ \underset{\longleftarrow}{LDH} Lactate^- + NAD^+$$

The normal rate of lactate production is 15 to 20 meq/kg/day, most of which occurs via the glycolytic pathway or the deamination of alanine (Fig. 6-1). Glycolysis, which converts glucose to pyruvate, occurs in the cytoplasm. A small amount of this pyruvate is then converted into lactate. However, the majority of the pyruvate that is generated is transferred into mitochondria, where, in the presence of oxygen, it is metabolized either into carbon dioxide and water (via an initial reaction catalyzed by pyruvate dehydrogenase [PDH]) or back to glucose (via an initial reaction catalyzed by pyruvate carboxylase [PC]) (Fig. 6-1).

These oxidative pathways of pyruvate metabolism become markedly impaired in states of mitochondrial dysfunction (such as those induced by tissue hypoperfusion). Furthermore, oxidative metabolism is also required to regenerate NAD^+ from the NADH that is produced during glycolysis. Both the fall in oxidative pyruvate metabolism and the accumulation of NADH promote the conversion of pyruvate into lactate.

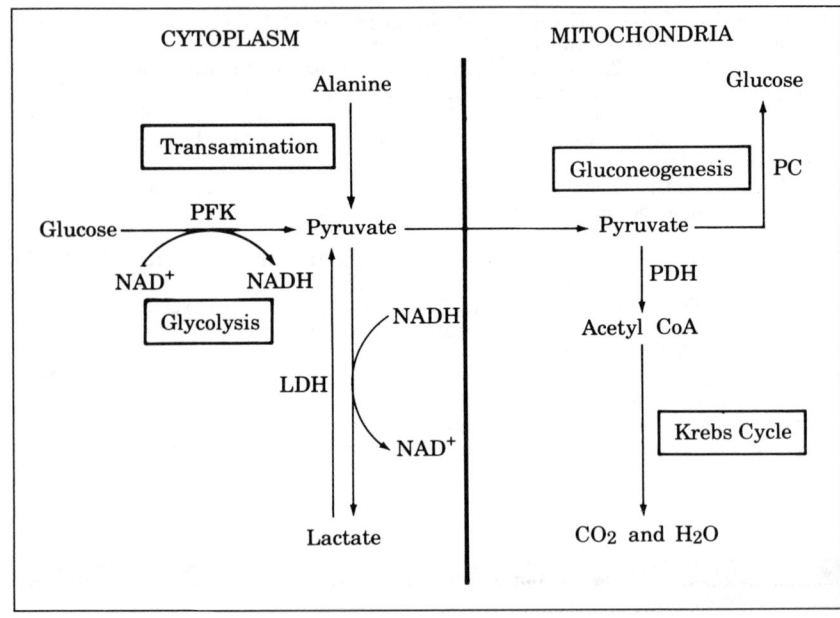

Fig. 6-1. Lactate generation and metabolism. PFK = phosphofructokinase; PDH = pyruvate dehydrogenase; PC = pyruvate carboxylase; and LDH = lactate dehydrogenase.

Lactate Metabolism
The liver and to a lesser degree the kidney are the major organs that remove lactate from the circulation. In both organs, lactate is converted back to pyruvate (in a reaction catalyzed by LDH) and then to carbon dioxide and water or to glucose (Fig. 6-1).

The normal maximal rate of lactate metabolism can reach 320 meq/hour, a rate that is usually greater than that of lactate production in lactic acidosis [1]. These findings suggest that, in most cases, there must be some component of impaired lactate use for lactic acid to accumulate [2]. For example, in shock this could result from the marked reduction in hepatic perfusion. Decreased lactate metabolism probably also explains the increased incidence of lactic acidosis in patients with advanced hepatic disease.

Etiology and Clinical Features
The causes of lactic acidosis can be divided into those associated with impaired tissue oxygenation (type A) and those in which a systemic impairment in oxygenation is not apparent (type B) (Table 6-1). Most patients with type A disease, for example, are in shock as manifested by a low systemic blood pressure; cool, clammy extremities; oligoanuria; and impaired mental status. These findings of systemic hypoperfusion are not apparent in type B lactic acidosis; in some cases, however, there is a toxin-induced impairment of cellular metabolism or probably regional areas of ischemia. With malignancy, for example, anaerobic metabolism by dense clusters of tumor cells in the liver may play a central role.

It might be expected that the marked reduction in pH that often occurs in lactic acidosis would lead to potassium movement out of the cells and hyperkalemia. In comparison to patients with mineral acid-induced acidemia (as with diarrhea or renal failure), the plasma potassium concentration does not predictably rise in the organic acidoses, such as lactic acidosis or ketoacidosis (see Chap. 11) [3,4]. When hyperkalemia does occur in lactic acidosis, it usually represents the cellular release of potassium due to ischemic cell breakdown. Cellular release also accounts for the commonly observed hy-

Table 6-1. Classification of lactic acidosis

Type A	Type B
Increased oxygen demand	Acquired
Generalized convulsions	Diabetes mellitus
Severe exercise	Certain malignancies
Hypothermic shivering	Hypoglycemia
Reduced oxygen delivery	D-Lactic acidosis
Shock	Toxins
Low cardiac output	Ethanol
Cardiac arrest	Methanol
Sepsis	Ethylene glycol
Severe hypoxemia (P_{O_2} < 25–30 mm Hg)	Phenformin
Carbon monoxide poisoning	Pheochromocytoma
Cyanide intoxication	Liver disease
	Acute respiratory alkalosis, including salicylates
	Congenital, e.g., glycogen storage disease, type 1

perphosphatemia in lactic acidosis [4]. This finding could reflect diminished cell use of phosphate due to an ischemia-induced inability to regenerate adenosine triphosphate (ATP) from adenosine diphosphate (ADP).

Diagnosis
The diagnosis of lactic acidosis is made by the findings of a high–AG metabolic acidosis and an elevated plasma lactate concentration (over 4 meq/L). In most cases, however, the history, physical examination, and response to therapy are also helpful. For example, the combination of initial hypotension and correction of the acidemia with fluid replacement is strongly suggestive of lactic acidosis.

An unusual and different disorder, in which intestinal bacteria generate D-lactate rather than L-lactate, is seen in some patients with intestinal bacterial overgrowth. In this setting, the diagnosis is made with a different enzymatic assay (which must be specifically requested) using D-lactate dehydrogenase [5]. The normal human enzyme, L-lactate dehydrogenase, does not recognize D-lactate.

Treatment
Correction of the underlying disorder is the primary therapy for lactic acidosis. For example, reversal of circulatory failure, hypoxemia, or sepsis reduces the rate of lactate production and enhances its removal.

The use of *alkali therapy in the treatment of lactic acidosis is controversial*. The benefits of bicarbonate therapy in metabolic acidosis are reviewed in Chap. 5, and mainly involve maintenance of normal cardiovascular homeostasis. This potential benefit must be weighed against the possible deleterious effects, such as volume overload, hypernatremia (5% $NaHCO_3$ contains almost 900 meq of sodium/L) and overshoot alkalosis after the restoration of tissue perfusion. The last problem results from the regeneration of bicarbonate when the excess lactate is metabolized, either to carbon dioxide and water or to glucose. For example:

$$CH_3—CHOH—COO^- \text{ (lactate)} + 3O_2 \rightarrow 2CO_2 + 2H_2O + HCO_3^-$$

In addition to these usual risks, bicarbonate therapy may be relatively ineffective, producing only a transient elevation in the plasma bicarbonate concentration [6–8]. Experimental studies suggest that this lack of efficacy is due to an associated *increase in net lactate production* (which leads to a further rise in the AG). This change in lactate metabolism appears to result from the accumulation of the CO_2 generated as the excess hydrogen ions are buffered by bicarbonate. The local rise in P_{CO_2} can exacerbate the intracellular acidosis, since CO_2 rapidly enters cells [8]. This can lead to decreased lactate use in hepatic cells and a decline in contractility by cardiac cells. The latter effect can reduce the cardiac output, a change that will promote further lactate production [6,8].

This problem of CO_2 accumulation may be masked clinically by the reduction in pulmonary blood flow that often occurs during cardiopulmonary resuscitation [8,9]. In this setting, blood entering the pulmonary circulation may be normally cleared of CO_2, leading to a relatively normal *arterial* P_{CO_2}. However, the *mixed venous* P_{CO_2}, which represents blood that has not yet entered the pulmonary circulation, may be markedly elevated because of both the increased rate of CO_2 production and the low cardiac output that slows the return of CO_2-carrying venous blood from the tissues to the lungs. In one study, patients with a mean arterial pH of 7.42 and P_{CO_2} of 32 mm Hg had mixed venous values of 7.15 and 74 mm Hg, respectively [9]. This problem appeared to be more prominent when $NaHCO_3$ was given and therefore the rate of CO_2 production was enhanced. If the mixed venous results more closely reflect the pH at the cellular level, then the arterial values may lead to the mistaken assumption that the pH is being well controlled.

Despite these arguments against the administration of bicarbonate in lactic acidosis, many physicians continue to support its use [10,11]. They contend that there are no human models showing a consistent adverse effect of bicarbonate and that the studies in animals with lactic acidosis (induced by hypoxemia or phenformin) may not have relevance to humans. Moreover, the well-documented deleterious effects of acidemia on cardiac output and blood pressure may be observed in this setting.

As a result of these conflicting findings, no definite recommendations can be made at the present time. One possible approach is to administer $NaHCO_3$ when the pH is below 7.10 to 7.15, since more severe acidemia may result in sudden cardiovascular collapse. However, the quantity of bicarbonate given must be closely titrated to minimize side effects, with the aim being to maintain the arterial pH above 7.20 until normal circulatory hemodynamics can be restored. If no hemodynamic improvement or rise in blood pH is observed, or if adverse effects of bicarbonate therapy (such as hypernatremia) occur, then further bicarbonate administration should probably be avoided. This is particularly true in patients with chronic malignancy-induced lactic acidosis, in whom alkali therapy (by increasing protein breakdown to provide alanine for lactate production) can also cause loss of lean body mass [12].

There are two possible future alternatives to bicarbonate therapy. One is the administration of dichloroacetate (DCA). DCA stimulates PDH activity in many tissues, thereby limiting lactate production by increasing the oxidation of pyruvate to acetyl CoA (Fig. 6-1). This investigational drug has shown promise experimentally and in some patients with lactic acidosis [13,14]. The second is the use of Na_2CO_3 (sodium carbonate) as a source of alkali; buffering of excess hydrogen ions by this compound will lead to the generation of bicarbonate, not CO_2 which, as described above, can worsen the intracellular acidosis [8].

References

1. Kreisberg, RA. Lactate homeostasis and lactic acidosis. *Ann Intern Med* 92:227, 1980.
2. Arieff, AI, Park, R, Leach, WJ, Lazarowitz, VC. Pathophysiology of experimental lactic acidosis in dogs. *Am J Physiol* 239:F135, 1980.
3. Adrogue, HJ, Madias, NE. Changes in plasma potassium concentration during acute acid-base disturbances. *Am J Med* 71:456, 1981.
4. Orringer, CE, Eustace, JC, Wunsch, CD, Gardner, LB. Natural history of lactic acidosis after grand mal seizures: a model for the study of an anion gap acidosis not associated with hyperkalemia. *N Engl J Med* 297:796, 1977.
5. Stolberg, L, Rolfe, R, Gitlin, N, Merritt, J, Mann, L, Linder, J, Finegold, S. D-Lactic acidosis due to abnormal gut flora. *N Engl J Med* 306:1344, 1982
6. Graf, H, Leach, W, Arieff, AI. Evidence for a detrimental effect of bicarbonate therapy in hypoxic lactic acidosis. *Science* 227:754, 1985.

7. Stacpoole, PW. Lactic acidosis: The case against bicarbonate therapy. *Ann Intern Med* 105:276, 1986.
8. Bersin, RM, Arieff, AI. Improved hemodynamic function during hypoxia with carbicarb, a new agent for the management of acidosis. *Circulation* 77:227, 1988.
9. Weil, MH, Rackow, EC, Trevino, R, Grundler, W, Falk, JL, Griffel, MI. Differences in acid-base state between venous and arterial blood during cardiopulmonary resuscitation *N Engl J Med* 315:153, 1986.
10. Madias, NE. Lactic acidosis. *Kidney Int* 29:752, 1986.
11. Narins, RG, Cohen, JJ. Bicarbonate therapy for organic acidosis: The case for its continued use. *Ann Intern Med* 106:615,1987.
12. Fields, ALA, Wolman, SL, Halperin, ML. Chronic lactic acidosis in a patient with cancer: Therapy and metabolic consequences. *Cancer* 47:2026, 1981.
13. Graf, H, Leach, W, Arieff, AI. Effects of dichloroacetate in the treatment of hypoxic lactic acidosis in dogs. *J Clin Invest* 76:919, 1985.
14. Stacpoole, PW, Harman, EM, Curry, HS, Baumgartner, TG, Misbin, RI. Treatment of lactic acidosis with dichloroacetate. *N Engl J Med* 309:390, 1983.

7. KETOACIDOSIS

Ketoacidosis develops when glucose use is impaired either by fasting or by insulin deficiency or resistance. In these settings, the production of ketone bodies (acetoacetic acid, β-hydroxybutyric acid, and acetone) serves as an alternative source of energy for many cells. Ultimately, the accumulation of acetoacetic acid and β-hydroxybutyric acid causes metabolic acidosis, usually with an increased anion gap (AG).

Pathogenesis

The development of ketoacidosis depends on two factors: (1) the release of free fatty acids (FFA) from fat cells, and (2) their subsequent metabolism into ketone bodies in the liver. Both *insulin deficiency* and *glucagon excess* play important roles in this process. Insulin normally inhibits lipolysis [1]; thus, insulin deficiency or resistance leads to increased release of FFA into the circulation where they are then transported to the liver.

Glucagon, which is secreted in response to insulin deficiency, appears to be the most important hormone regulating hepatic ketone production [2]. The rate-limiting step in this process is mediated by the enzyme carnitine acyltransferase (CAT); this enzyme catalyzes the conversion of fatty acyl CoA into fatty acyl carnitine, which can then be transported into the mitochondria, the site of ketone synthesis (Fig. 7-1) [1]. CAT activity in turn is normally inhibited by malonyl CoA, which is synthesized from acetyl CoA by acetyl CoA carboxylase [3]. High glucagon levels have two major effects on this process: glycolysis is inhibited, thereby reducing the amount of acetyl CoA produced; and the activity of acetyl CoA carboxylase is directly impaired. Both of these changes reduce malonyl CoA production, thereby increasing CAT activity and promoting FFA conversion into ketones.

In comparison, malonyl CoA is relatively abundant in the fed state where there are high insulin and low glucagon levels. As a result, CAT activity is low, and FFA remain in the cytoplasm where they are esterified into triglycerides.

Ketoacidosis most often occurs in poorly controlled diabetes mellitus, but also may be observed in patients who are fasting or ingesting large amounts of alcohol. Plasma glucose and insulin levels are low with fasting, leading to hyperglucagonemia and, ultimately, to ketone production. In addition to decreased carbohydrate intake, other factors also contribute to alcoholic ketoacidosis. Ethanol is initially metabolized to acetaldehyde in a reaction that generates NADH from NAD^+:

$$\text{Ethanol} + NAD^+ \rightarrow \text{acetaldehyde} + NADH + H^+ \rightarrow \text{acetyl CoA}$$

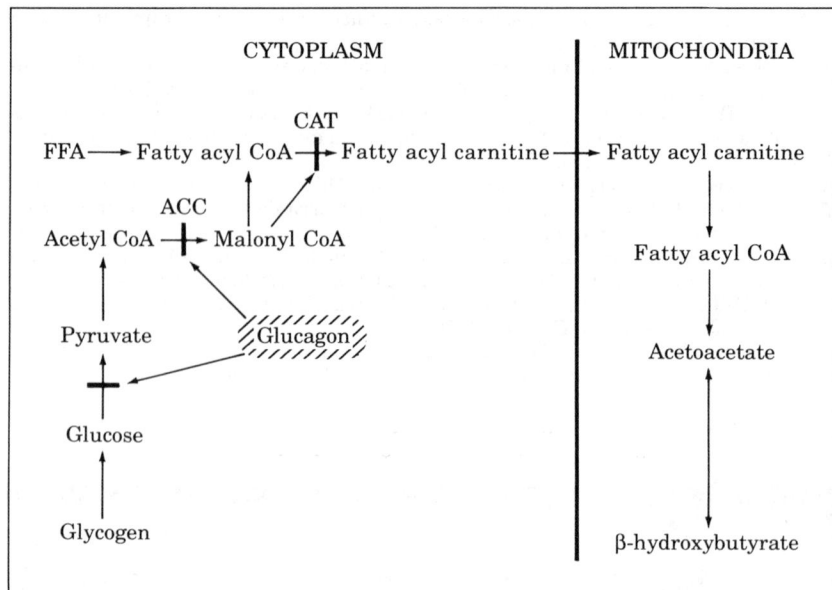

Fig. 7-1. Schematic representation of the roles of malonyl CoA and glucagon in hepatic ketogenesis. When malonyl CoA levels are high in the fed state, carnitine acyltransferase activity (CAT) is low; as a result, FFA remain in the cytoplasm and are esterified into triglycerides. Ketogenesis occurs only if the FFA enter the mitochondria, a process that is facilitated by glucagon-mediated changes in malonyl CoA and CAT activity. Glucagon lowers malonyl CoA levels, in part by inhibiting the enzyme acetyl CoA carboxylase (ACC); this removes the negative feedback of malonyl CoA on CAT activity, thereby promoting ketone production.

Thus, alcohol ingestion can lead to depletion of NAD$^+$ stores. If glucose ingestion is also impaired, then glucose production initially occurs by glycogenolysis, rather than by gluconeogenesis, which is dependent on availability of NAD$^+$. Relative hypoglycemia may then ensue when glycogen stores become depleted. The resulting low insulin and high glucagon state leads to ketone formation; alcohol may also contribute to this process directly by promoting the release of FFA from adipose tissue.

Clinical Features
The physical examination may disclose signs or symptoms suggestive of ketoacidosis. These include a sweet odor to the breath, principally due to the presence of acetone in expired air; and findings directly attributable to acidemia, such as hyperventilation (see Chap. 5). Patients with marked hyperglycemia due to uncontrolled diabetes mellitus may also have problems induced by (1) the associated osmotic diuresis, such as polyuria, polydipsia, volume depletion, and weight loss, and (2) the elevation in plasma osmolality, such as lethargy or coma.

The AG characteristically increases in ketoacidosis [4]. β-hydroxybutyrate and acetoacetate are the major unmeasured anions that accumulate in this setting, although a concomitant lactic acidosis may occasionally be observed. The AG may be markedly elevated (> 30 meq/L) in diabetic ketoacidosis; in comparison, the acidemia is generally mild and the AG is rarely greater than 18 meq/L in starvation ketosis. These findings appear to be due to ketone-induced release of insulin, which limits the degree of lipolysis and ketogenesis [5]. The ratio of the elevation in AG to the decline in plasma bicarbonate concentration is usually about 1 : 1 in ketoacidosis (see p. 40)[4].

In addition to the acid-base abnormalities, changes in the plasma sodium, creatinine, potassium, and phosphate concentrations are also commonly detected, both at presentation and after the initiation of therapy. The rise in plasma osmolality induced by hyperglycemia should lower the plasma sodium concentration as water moves out of the cells down an osmotic gradient. The expected change is a *1.6 meq/L decline in the plasma sodium concentration for each 100 mg/dl elevation in the plasma glucose concentration* [6]. Additional factors, however, are often present that can alter this expected relationship. The glucosuria-induced osmotic diuresis, for example, causes water loss in excess of sodium, tending to raise the plasma sodium concentration. Continued water intake, on the other hand, can counteract this effect. Thus, the plasma sodium concentration can range from hyponatremic levels to those that are actually greater than normal. These hypernatremic patients are extremely hyperosmolar and often have impaired mental status.

The plasma creatinine concentration is typically increased above baseline levels in ketoacidosis. Volume depletion, resulting in prerenal azotemia, usually plays a major role. To some degree, however, the elevation may be an *artifact* of the method used to make the measurement. With the most common alkaline picrate method, acetoacetate is sensed as creatinine, raising the measured plasma creatinine concentration in some patients by 1 to 2 mg/dl or more [7]. This change is rapidly reversed with correction of the ketosis by insulin administration.

Potassium stores are usually depleted in diabetic ketoacidosis, due in part to the osmotic diuresis. Despite these losses, the plasma potassium concentration is generally normal or, in about one-third of cases, elevated. This apparently paradoxical finding results from the shift of potassium out of the cells into the extracellular fluid. Insulin deficiency (which limits potassium entry into cells) and hyperosmolality (which pulls water and by solvent drags potassium out of cells) are primarily responsible for this change [8]. In comparison, ketoacidosis does not seem to have a major effect on potassium distribution (see Chap. 5) [9].

The plasma phosphate concentration is also often elevated at presentation due to cell catabolism. Once again, however, total body stores are typically depleted due to the osmotic diuresis and to acidemia (which directly impairs tubular phosphate reabsorption). It is important to emphasize that both the hyperkalemia and hyperphosphatemia are rapidly reversed with insulin therapy, unmasking the total body deficits. In some patients, for example, the plasma phosphate concentration can fall to 1.5 mg/dl or less [10].

Diagnosis
The diagnosis of ketoacidosis is usually made using the nitroprusside reaction. This test will identify acetone and acetoacetate but not β-hydroxybutyrate. The ratio of β-hydroxybutyrate to acetoacetate is usually about 3 : 1. However, higher levels of β-hydroxybutyrate (and, therefore, a possible *negative serum or urine nitroprusside reaction*) may be found in patients with concurrent lactic acidosis or alcoholic ketoacidosis, since a high ratio of NADH/NAD$^+$ is found in these settings (see above and Chap. 6). As a result, the following reaction will be driven to the right:

$$\text{Acetoacetate}^- + \text{NADH} + \text{H}^+ \rightarrow \beta\text{-hydroxybutyrate}^- + \text{NAD}^+$$

An indirect way to get around this problem is to add a few drops of hydrogen peroxide to a urinary specimen; this will shift the reaction to the left, resulting in the generation of the detectable acetoacetate.

Therapy
Insulin administration (usually by continuous low-dose intravenous infusion) and volume replacement are the initial therapeutic modalities in patients with diabetic ketoacidosis. Insulin will diminish FFA release and will reduce glucagon levels, leading to a resumption of normal carbohydrate metabolism with less ketoacid production. Furthermore, ketone use is promoted by insulin, thereby reducing acidemia, since metabolism of the ketoacid anions results in the regeneration of bicarbonate. *Insulin should not be given* in alcoholic or starvation ketoacidosis, since the plasma glucose concentration is usually normal or reduced in these disorders; glucose alone is usually sufficient since it will stimulate endogenous insulin secretion without the risk of hypoglycemia.

The fluid deficit in diabetic ketoacidosis is usually 3 to 6 liters. In general, one liter of isotonic saline should be rapidly administered *before insulin therapy,* since the latter will produce further extracellular volume depletion by driving glucose and secondarily water into the cells. Thereafter, half-isotonic saline is usually preferred, since this will tend to correct the hyperosmolality as well. However, isotonic saline should be continued in patients with severe hypovolemia until adequate perfusion is restored.

The administration of intravenous fluids and insulin in diabetic ketoacidosis is rarely associated with the development of cerebral edema during the first 24 hours of therapy [11]. In experimental animals, the use of insulin to rapidly lower the plasma glucose concentration can lead to the generation of new (idiogenic) osmoles within the brain cells; this rise in brain osmolality then promotes water movement into the brain. It may be possible to reduce the risk of this unusual complication by discontinuing regular insulin and beginning dextrose administration when the plasma glucose concentration falls below 300 mg/dl.

As described above, insulin therapy also drives potassium and phosphate into cells, possibly unmasking relatively large deficits of these ions. As a result, careful monitoring is essential and potassium supplementation should begin (20–40 meq/L) once the plasma potassium concentration falls below 4.5 to 5.0 meq/L. In comparison, studies have not shown a beneficial effect of routine phosphate replacement in this disorder, even when marked (but asymptomatic) hypophosphatemia has developed during therapy [10].

Bicarbonate administration is not indicated in most patients with ketoacidosis, since metabolism of the ketoacid anions results in the regeneration of bicarbonate and spontaneous correction of the acidosis [12,13]. However, small amounts of sodium bicarbonate may be beneficial when there is either *severe acidemia* (pH < 7.0–7.1) or a *relatively small rise in the AG* ($\leq$ 5 meq/L) due to the loss of ketoacid anions in the urine [13,14]. The latter situation is most likely to be seen in patients who remain well hydrated with relatively normal renal function [14]. In this setting, the marked urinary loss of β-hydroxybutyrate means that the bicarbonate deficit can be repaired only by the regeneration of new bicarbonate by renal acid excretion, a relatively slow process that takes several days to reach maximal levels.

References

1. Cahill, GF, Jr. Ketosis. *Kidney Int* 20:416, 1983.
2. Miles, JM, Haymond, MW, Nissen, SL, Gerich, JE. Effects of free fatty acid availability, glucagon excess, and insulin deficiency on ketone body production in postabsorptive man. *J Clin Invest* 71: 1554, 1983.
3. McGarry, JD, Mannaerts, GP, Foster, DW. A possible role for malonyl-CoA in the regulation of hepatic fatty acid oxidation and ketogenesis. *J Clin Invest* 60:265, 1977.
4. Paulson, WD. Anion gap-bicarbonate relation in diabetic ketoacidosis. *Am J Med* 81:995, 1986.
5. Owen, OE, Reichard, GA, Jr. Human forearm metabolism during progressive starvation. *J Clin Invest* 50:1536, 1971.
6. Katz, M. Hyperglycemia-induced hyponatremia: calculation of expected serum sodium depression. *N Engl J Med* 289:843, 1973.
7. Molitch, ME, Roidman, E, Hirsch, CA, Dubinsky, E. Spurious serum creatinine elevations in ketoacidosis. *Ann Intern Med* 93:280, 1980.
8. Viberti, GC. Glucose-induced hyperkalemia: A hazard for diabetics. *Lancet* 1:690, 1978.
9. Adrogue, HJ, Madias, NE. Changes in plasma potassium concentration during acute acid-base disturbances. *Am J Med* 71:456, 1981.
10. Wilson, HK, Kever, SP, Lea, AS, Boyd, AE, Eknoyan, G. Phosphate therapy in diabetic ketoacidosis. *Arch Intern Med* 142:517, 1982.
11. Rose, BD. *Clinical Physiology of Acid-Base and Electrolyte Disorders* (2nd ed). New York: McGraw-Hill, 1984. P. 560.

12. Morris, LR, Murphy, MB, Kitabachi, AE. Bicarbonate therapy in severe diabetic ketoacidosis. *Ann Intern Med* 105:836, 1986.
13. Foster, DW, McGarry, JD. The metabolic derangements and treatment of diabetic ketoacidosis. *N Engl J Med* 309:159, 1983.
14. Adroqué, HJ, Wilson, H, Boyd, AE, et al. Plasma acid-base patterns in diabetic ketoacidosis. *N Engl J Med* 307:1603, 1982.

8. RENAL TUBULAR ACIDOSIS

Renal tubular acidosis (RTA) refers to those forms of metabolic acidosis that are caused either by diminished acid excretion per nephron or by the renal loss of bicarbonate. This disorder can be separated mechanistically into three principal categories: type 1 (distal) RTA; type 2 (proximal) RTA, and type 4 (hypoaldosteronism) RTA* (Table 8-1). Many patients with chronic renal failure also have an associated metabolic acidosis. However, the defect in the latter setting is a reduction in the number of functioning nephrons; the acid excretion rate per functioning nephron is actually elevated in an appropriate attempt to correct the acidemia. Thus, renal failure is not generally classified as a form of RTA.

Type 1 RTA

Type 1 RTA is characterized by a defect in the ability to maximally acidify the urine [1-3]. Normally, the urine pH can be lowered to 4.5 to 5.0 in the collecting tubules in the presence of an acid load; this represents a hydrogen ion concentration that is almost *1000* times greater than that in the plasma where the pH is about 7.40. In comparison, patients with type 1 RTA cannot lower the urine pH below 5.3, even with severe acidemia. In most cases, this defect results in an inability to excrete the dietary acid load, which is primarily derived from the metabolism of sulfur-containing amino acids to sulfuric acid. The net effect is a progressive metabolic acidosis, with a plasma bicarbonate concentration that may fall below 10 meq/L if untreated.

An *incomplete* form of distal RTA has also been described in which the urine cannot be acidified, but the plasma bicarbonate concentration and pH remain normal. In this setting, ammonia production is markedly increased, so that acid excretion is adequate even though the efficiency of ammonium trapping in the tubules is impaired by the relatively high urine pH. It is unclear why patients with the complete form are unable to make a similar adaptation; it may be that they have later or more advanced disease with a greater impairment in tubular function.

Pathogenesis and Etiology

Acidification in the collecting tubules primarily occurs by hydrogen secretion via a H^+-ATPase pump in the luminal membrane of the *intercalated* cells in the cortical and medullary collecting tubules [4]. These cells do not participate in sodium transport, which occurs in the *principal* cells in the cortical collecting tubule and in the cells in the inner medullary collecting tubule, in part under the influence of aldosterone [4]. Sodium reabsorption in the principal cells indirectly influences net hydrogen secretion by making the lumen electronegative, thereby favoring the movement of hydrogen ions from the adjacent intercalated cells into the tubular lumen [3,4].

There are three mechanisms by which this distal acidification process can be impaired: (1) a defect in the hydrogen pump, which appears to account for most cases; (2) increased permeability of the collecting tubules, so that the large pH gradient cannot be maintained because of back diffusion; and (3) reduced sodium reabsorption, so that the

---

*Type 3 RTA refers to what is now considered to be an infantile variant to type 1 RTA.

Table 8-1. Characteristics of types 1, 2, and 4 RTA

	Type 1 (distal)	Type 2 (proximal)	Type 4
Basic defect	Decreased distal acidification	Decreased proximal HCO_3^- reabsorption	Aldosterone deficiency or resistance
Urine pH	> 5.3	Variable: > 5.3 if above reabsorptive threshold; ≤ 5.3 if below	Usually ≤ 5.3
Plasma $[HCO_3^-]$ (untreated)	May be below 10 meq/L	Above 12 meq/L	Above 15 meq/L
Fractional excretion of bicarbonate when plasma $[HCO_3^-]$ > 20 meq/L*	< 3%	> 15–20%	< 3%
Diagnosis	Response to $NaHCO_3$ or ammonium chloride	Response to $NaHCO_3$	Measure plasma aldosterone concentration
Plasma $[K^+]$	Usually reduced or normal; rarely elevated	Normal or reduced	Elevated
Therapeutic amount of $NaHCO_3$ required to normalize plasma $[HCO_3^-]$	1–3 meq/kg/day	10–15 meq/kg/day	1–3 meq/kg/day, may require no alkali if correct hyperkalemia
Nonelectrolyte complications	Nephrocalcinosis and renal stones; osteomalacia uncommon	Rickets in children, osteomalacia or osteopenia in adults; calculi rare unless taking carbonic anhydrase inhibitor	None

*Fractional excretion HCO_3^- (%) = $\dfrac{\text{urine } [HCO_3^-] \times \text{plasma [creatinine]} \times 100}{\text{plasma } [HCO_3^-] \times \text{urine [creatinine]}}$

This formula, which can be calculated from a random urine specimen collected under oil (to minimize the evaporative loss of CO_2), is similar to that for the fractional excretion of sodium used in the differential diagnosis of acute renal failure (see Chap. 19).

electrical gradient favoring hydrogen secretion is diminished [1-3]. The last defect is often accompanied by hyperkalemia, since the electrical gradient created by sodium transport is also an important determinant of potassium secretion and subsequent excretion (see Chap. 10) [3,5].

The disorders that have been described to cause type 1 RTA are listed in Table 8-2. Autoimmune diseases such as Sjögren's syndrome are probably the major causes of this rare condition in adults, whereas hereditary RTA is most common in children.

Clinical Features and Diagnosis

The classic feature of type 1 RTA is the presence of a normal–anion gap metabolic acidosis with a urine pH that is persistently above 5.3. In addition to this defect in acid-base balance, potassium homeostasis is also frequently abnormal in this disorder. In most cases *hypokalemia* is observed. This problem is largely related to sodium reabsorption. Filtered sodium is either reabsorbed with chloride or, to maintain electroneutrality, reabsorbed in exchange for hydrogen or potassium. Since net distal hydrogen secretion is impaired in type 1 RTA, more sodium must be reabsorbed in the cortical collecting tubule in exchange for potassium [6]. This defect is largely corrected by the administration of $NaHCO_3$; by increasing the filtered bicarbonate load and therefore the pH in the tubular fluid, more hydrogen ions can now be secreted without reaching the limiting urine pH, thereby allowing potassium secretion to fall [6].

In comparison, patients in whom the primary abnormality is a limitation in sodium reabsorption tend to become hyperkalemic [3,5]. *Urinary tract obstruction* and *sickle cell nephropathy* are the major causes of this complication.

In addition to these electrolyte disturbances, type 1 RTA is frequently associated with *renal calculi* and *nephrocalcinosis* [7]. Several factors appear to contribute to this problem, including: (1) increased urinary excretion of calcium and phosphorus (due both to the release of these ions from bone during buffering of the excess acid and to a direct inhibition of tubular calcium and phosphorus reabsorption by acidemia) [7,8]; (2) the elevated urine pH (which promotes calcium phosphate precipitation); and (3) hypocitraturia (urinary citrate is a potent inhibitor of crystallization because it combines with calcium to form a soluble calcium citrate complex). Citrate is normally filtered and then reabsorbed in the proximal tubule by a sodium-citrate cotransporter. Metabolic acidosis of any cause tends to increase citrate metabolism within the renal tubular cells, thereby lowering the cell citrate concentration. This creates a more favorable gradient for luminal citrate to enter the cells, leading to a fall in citrate excretion [9].

The diagnosis of type 1 RTA should be suspected in any patient with *metabolic acidosis and a urine pH above 5.3*. Urinary tract infection caused by a urea-splitting organism must first be excluded, however; this type of infection can raise the urine pH in the renal pelvis or bladder because the generation of ammonia from urea lowers the hydrogen concentration (without affecting net acid excretion) by driving the following reaction to the right:

$$NH_3 + H^+ \rightarrow NH_4^+$$

In addition, patients with other forms of metabolic acidosis (such as diarrhea) who are severely volume depleted also may have a reversible defect in urinary acidification [10]. In this setting, enhanced proximal reabsorption limits the amount of sodium available for reabsorption and subsequent stimulation of hydrogen secretion in the distal nephron. The result is an inability to lower the urine pH below 5.3, an abnormality that can be corrected with volume replacement. Thus, the diagnosis of type 1 RTA should not be made if the urine sodium concentration is below 10 to 15 meq/L unless the defect persists after euvolemia has been restored.

In the absence of infection or volume depletion, the differential diagnosis of a normal–anion gap metabolic acidosis with a high urine pH consists of type 1 and type 2 RTA. These disorders can easily be distinguished by infusing $NaHCO_3$ to raise the plasma bicarbonate concentration to just below the normal range (20–22 meq/L) and then measuring the urine pH and the fraction of the filtered bicarbonate that is excreted (Table 8-1). The urine pH will be unchanged in type 1 RTA and the fractional excretion of

Table 8-2. Causes of type 1 RTA

Primary
  Idiopathic or sporadic
Genetic
  Familial
  Marfan's syndrome
  Wilson's disease
  Ehler-Danlos syndrome
Disorders of calcium metabolism with nephrocalcinosis
  Idiopathic hypercalciuria
  Hypervitaminosis D
  Chronic hyperparathyroidism
Hypergammaglobulinemic states
  Amyloidosis*
  Multiple myeloma*
  Cryoglobulinemia
Drugs and toxins
  Amphotericin B
  Lithium carbonate
  Toluene
Autoimmune diseases
  Sjögren's syndrome*
  Thyroiditis
  Chronic active hepatitis
  Primary biliary cirrhosis
Miscellaneous
  Cirrhosis
  Medullary sponge kidney
Associated with hyperkalemia
  Urinary tract obstruction
  Sickle cell anemia
  Systemic lupus erythematosus
  Renal transplant rejection*

*May also cause type 2 RTA

bicarbonate will remain below 3 percent, since bicarbonate reabsorption, which is largely a proximal function, is not impaired in this condition. In comparison, raising the plasma bicarbonate concentration above the reabsorptive threshold in type 2 RTA will induce a marked bicarbonate diuresis with the urine pH rising above 7 and the fractional excretion of bicarbonate exceeding 10 percent (see below).

A different approach is required to make the diagnosis of incomplete type 1 RTA [11]. This disorder is associated with no or little decline in the plasma bicarbonate concentration or pH; as a result, it is most commonly manifested clinically by the combination of calcium stone formation and a persistently elevated urine pH [12]. The diagnosis can be established by giving an acid load as ammonium chloride in a dose of 0.1 gm/kg [11]. Maintenance of the urine pH above 5.3 is indicative of an underlying acidification defect.

URINE ANION GAP. Measurement of the urine pH can generally distinguish between the 2 most common forms of a normal–anion gap metabolic acidosis with relatively normal renal function: gastrointestinal losses, such as diarrhea, in which urine acid excretion as *ammonium* is normal; and RTA in which ammonium excretion is impaired.

In some patients with diarrhea, however, the urine pH may be above 5.3, similar to that in RTA. This is most often due to hypokalemia; in this setting, potassium moves out of the cells to replace extracellular losses and, to maintain electroneutrality, extracellular hydrogen and sodium move into the cells. The ensuing intracellular acidosis in renal tubular cells increases *ammonia* production; as some of the excess ammonia diffuses into the tubular lumen, it raises the urine pH (or lowers the hydrogen concentration) by driving the following reaction to the right:

$$NH_3 + H^+ \rightarrow NH_4^+$$

Despite the high urine pH, ammonium excretion is appropriately elevated, since hydrogen secretion is intact.

One way to estimate the amount of urinary ammonium (which is an unmeasured cation) is to calculate the *urine anion gap* [12a]:

$$\text{Urine anion gap} = ([Na^+] + [K^+]) - [Cl^-]$$

When acidification is normal, as in most cases of diarrhea, there is a relatively large quantity of ammonium, which is excreted with chloride. As a result, the urine anion gap has a *negative* value, since the chloride concentration exceeds that of sodium plus potassium. In comparison, a positive value indicates impaired ammonium excretion and is suggestive of one of the forms of RTA. The uses and limitations of this simple measurement are reviewed in reference 12a.

Treatment

The acidemia in type 1 RTA can be corrected by the administration of bicarbonate or a bicarbonate precursor such as citrate. The usual dose is 1 to 3 meq/kg/day, which should be sufficient to buffer that fraction of the daily acid load (which averages 50–100 meq/day) that is not being excreted. Correction of the acidemia also tends to raise the plasma potassium concentration in patients who are hypokalemic [6], to allow normal growth in children [13] and, when present, to diminish the tendency for stone formation [7,12]. Several factors contribute to the latter effect since raising the systemic pH decreases the release of calcium and phosphorus from bone, enhances the tubular reabsorption of these ions (both of which will lower their rate of excretion), and increases urinary citrate by reducing its rate of reabsorption in the proximal tubule [7–9,12]. The administration of alkali is also effective in stone formers with incomplete type 1 RTA [12].

In some patients, however, increased urinary calcium excretion appears to be the primary abnormality, with secondary tubular damage then limiting distal acidification [14]. In this setting, therapy of stone disease must also be directed toward lowering calcium excretion with a thiazide-type diuretic (see Chap. 54).

When treating stone disease, it is important that alkali be given as the *potassium,* rather than the sodium, salt (assuming that hyperkalemia is not a problem). Tubular calcium reabsorption tends to passively follow that of sodium and water in the proximal tubule and loop of Henle. Thus, decreasing sodium reabsorption in these segments by the administration of sodium bicarbonate or citrate can result in a parallel decline in calcium transport [15]; this calciuric effect may prevent the expected reduction in stone formation with alkali therapy. In comparison, potassium salts do not influence calcium handling.

Although bicarbonate is the usual form of alkali therapy administered, large doses can cause gastrointestinal symptoms due to gas formation, as gastric acid is titrated to form carbonic acid and then CO_2 and water. This problem can be minimized by the use of citrate (which is ultimately metabolized in the body to bicarbonate). Solutions are available that contain 1 to 2 meq/ml of sodium, potassium, or sodium and potassium citrate. Sodium alone should be used in hyperkalemic patients (since increasing distal sodium delivery can enhance potassium secretion*), potassium alone when there is stone disease, and potassium alone or with sodium in patients who are potassium depleted.

---

*If alkali therapy alone is ineffective, a low–potassium diet and a loop or thiazide diuretic can also be used to lower the plasma potassium concentration [1,2]. Mineralocorticoids are not indicated since plasma aldosterone levels are normal or elevated in this disorder [6].

Type 2 RTA

Type 2 renal tubular acidosis is another uncommon problem. Although also associated with abnormal acid handling, this disorder has substantially different clinical characteristics from type 1 RTA.

Pathophysiology

Type 2 RTA is caused by a defect in the proximal tubular reabsorption of bicarbonate. The renal threshold for bicarbonate is normally set so that, in euvolemic patients, bicarbonate does not appear in the urine until the plasma concentration is above 25 meq/L. This is appropriate, since it prevents bicarbonate loss unless the plasma concentration is above normal. In contrast, patients with type 2 RTA have a reduced proximal tubular reabsorptive capacity for bicarbonate. If, for example, only 18 meq/L of filtered bicarbonate can be reabsorbed, the plasma level will decrease until it reaches 18 meq/L. At this point, the patient will again be in a steady state since all of the filtered bicarbonate can be reabsorbed. This explains why the *urine pH is variable* in type 2 RTA. It will be greater than 5.3 (as in type 1 RTA) if the plasma bicarbonate concentration is above the reabsorptive threshold, since bicarbonate wasting will be present. However, the urine can be normally acidified (with the urine pH falling below 5.3) once the plasma bicarbonate concentration is at or below threshold.

This observation explains why, in the absence of a complicating disorder such as diarrhea, the acidemia in type 2 RTA is limited. The plasma bicarbonate concentration *should not fall below bicarbonate reabsorptive capacity* in this disorder; once the filtered load reaches a level at which all of the filtered bicarbonate can be reabsorbed, excretion of the daily acid load as ammonium and titratable acidity can proceed normally. Therefore, the severe, progressive acidemia that can be seen in type 1 RTA does not occur as the plasma bicarbonate concentration usually stabilizes between 13 and 20 meq/L. This limited fall in the plasma bicarbonate concentration presumably reflects the maximum reabsorptive capacity of the distal nephron, so that even complete loss of proximal bicarbonate transport produces no more than a 50 percent reduction in the plasma bicarbonate concentration [16].

Etiology, Clinical Features, and Diagnosis

The disorders causing type 2 RTA are listed in Table 8-3, with vitamin D deficiency-induced chronic hypocalcemia (both the fall in the plasma calcium concentration and the ensuing secondary hyperparathyroidism impair proximal bicarbonate reabsorption) and light chain toxicity in multiple myeloma being most common in adults. The proximal tubular defect is usually not limited to bicarbonate transport; other findings that are often seen include glucosuria, aminoaciduria, phosphaturia, uricosuria, and increased excretion of organic anions such as citrate.

Hypokalemia is common in type 2 RTA. Urinary potassium losses are initiated by decreased bicarbonate reabsorption in the proximal tubule, which causes more sodium bicarbonate to be presented to the cortical collecting tubule [17]. In this segment, the excess bicarbonate acts as a poorly reabsorbable anion; therefore, some of the sodium must be reabsorbed in exchange for potassium. As a result, alkali therapy aggravates the tendency toward hypokalemia by raising the plasma bicarbonate concentration, thereby allowing more bicarbonate to reach the distal potassium secretory site. In comparison, untreated patients at or below the reabsorptive threshold no longer waste bicarbonate, and potassium losses are markedly diminished [6,17].

Type 2 RTA is not usually associated with renal calculi or nephrocalcinosis [7]. This difference from type 1 RTA is probably related to two major factors: the urine pH is often acid (which increases the solubility of calcium phosphate); and urinary citrate levels may be normal as the proximal reabsorptive defect offsets the expected reduction induced by the acidemia [7].

Patients with type 1 RTA are, however, at risk of developing bone disease. This is manifested in up to 20 percent of cases as rickets in children and osteomalacia or osteopenia in adults [7]. Proximal phosphate wasting and possibly diminished proximal formation of 1,25-dihydroxyvitamin D_3 are thought to contribute to this complication. In addition, even a mild degree of acidemia can impair growth in children [13].

Table 8-3. Causes of type 2 RTA

Hereditary disorders	Acquired disorders
Cystinosis	Multiple myeloma*
Tyrosinemia	Vitamin D deficiency
Wilson's disease	Nephrotic syndrome
Glycogen storage disease, type 1	Amyloidosis*
Pyruvate carboxylase deficiency	Renal transplant rejection*
Galactosemia	Sjögren's syndrome*
	Toxins and drugs
	Lead
	Cadmium
	Mercury
	Uranium
	Copper (Wilson's disease)
	Acetazolamide
	Outdated tetracycline
	Streptozotocin

*May also cause type 1 RTA.

The diagnosis of type 2 RTA should be considered in any patient with an otherwise unexplained normal–anion gap metabolic acidosis, particularly if the urine pH is above 5.3. As described above, the diagnosis can be confirmed by the marked increase in urine pH (to above 7) and in fractional excretion of bicarbonate that follows the administration of sodium bicarbonate (Table 8-1).

Treatment
The initial step in the management of type 2 RTA is to determine if a treatable underlying disorder is present, such as vitamin D deficiency, multiple myeloma, or the use of a carbonic anhydrase inhibitor, such as acetazolamide (Table 8-3). Even if no specific therapy is available, correction of the acidemia may not be required in adults if the patient is asymptomatic and there is only a small reduction in the plasma bicarbonate concentration. In comparison, treatment is always indicated in children since restoring acid-base balance can permit normal growth to resume [13].

Treatment is somewhat more difficult than in type 1 RTA because much larger doses of alkali are required. As soon as the plasma bicarbonate concentration begins to rise, it will exceed the reduced reabsorptive threshold and the excess bicarbonate will be rapidly excreted in the urine. Thus, doses of alkali (usually given as the better-tolerated citrate salt) as high as *10 to 15 meq/kg/day* are often required to keep ahead of urinary excretion. Thiazide diuretics are sometimes useful as adjunctive therapy. These agents diminish sodium chloride reabsorption in the distal tubule; the ensuing mild volume depletion results in a compensatory increase in proximal sodium transport (in part mediated by angiotensin II), thereby minimizing the degree of proximal bicarbonate wasting [18].

Alkali therapy tends to aggravate the tendency toward hypokalemia by allowing more sodium to reach the potassium secretory sites in the distal nephron. Consequently, a combination of potassium and sodium citrate (such as Polycitra) is often required.

Type 4 RTA
Type 4 RTA is observed when aldosterone deficiency or resistance leads to defective secretion of both hydrogen and potassium. Patients with hypoaldosteronism usually acidify the urine normally (urine pH < 5.3) and have a relatively mild degree of acidemia,

in comparison to the hyperkalemic form of type 1 RTA. This difference may occur because hypoaldosteronism primarily impairs transport in the cortical collecting tubule; medullary function may be relatively well maintained, allowing a normal transtubular pH gradient to be established [2,3]. In comparison, conditions associated with hyperkalemic type 1 RTA, such as urinary tract obstruction or sickle cell nephropathy, are likely to affect tubular function in both the cortex and medulla [3,5].

Since hyperkalemia is the most prominent manifestation of hypoaldosteronism, this disorder is discussed in detail in Chapter 11. As will be seen, the acidemia in this setting is primarily due to decreased tubular production of ammonia, thereby limiting the excretion of acid as ammonium.

References

1. Kurtzman, NA. Renal tubular acidosis: A constellation of syndromes. *Hosp Prac* 22 (11):131, 1987.
2. Batlle, DC, Sehy, JT, Roseman, MK, et al. Clinical and physiologic spectrum of acquired distal renal tubular acidosis. *Kidney Int* 20:389, 1981.
3. Batlle, DC. Segmental characterization of defects in collecting tubule acidification. *Kidney Int* 30:546, 1986.
4. Levine, DZ, Jacobson, HR. The regulation of renal acid excretion: New observations from studies of distal nephron segments. *Kidney Int* 29:1099, 1986.
5. Batlle, DC, Arruda, JAL, Kurtzman, NA. Hyperkalemic distal renal tubular acidosis associated with obstructive uropathy. *N Engl J Med* 304:373, 1981.
6. Sebastian, A, McSherry, E, Morris, RC Jr. Renal potassium wasting in renal tubular acidosis (RTA); Its occurrence in types 1 and 2 RTA despite sustained correction of systemic acidosis. *J Clin Invest* 50:667, 1971.
7. Brenner, RJ, Spring, DB, Sebastian, A, et al. Incidence of radiographically evident bone disease, nephrocalcinosis, and nephrolithiasis in various types of renal tubular acidosis. *N Engl J Med* 307:217, 1982.
8. Sutton, RAL, Wong, NLM, Dirks, JH. Effects of metabolic acidosis and alkalosis on sodium and calcium transport in the dog. *Kidney Int* 15:520, 1979.
9. Simpson, DP. Citrate excretion: A window on renal metabolism. *Am J Physiol* 244:F223, 1983.
10. Batlle, DC, von Riotte, A, Schlueter, W. Urinary sodium in the evaluation of hyperchloremic metabolic acidosis. *N Engl J Med* 316:140, 1987.
11. Kurtzman, NA. Acquired distal renal tubular acidosis. *Kidney Int* 24:807, 1983.
12. Preminger, GM, Sakhaee, K. Skurla, C, Pak, CYC. Prevention of renal calcium stone formation with potassium citrate therapy in patients with distal renal tubular acidosis. *J Urol* 134:20, 1985.
12a. Batlle, DC, Hizon, M, Cohen, E, et al. The use of the urinary anion gap in the diagnosis of hyperchloremic metabolic acidosis *N Engl J Med* 318:594, 1988.
13. McSherry, E, Morris, RC, Jr. Attainment and maintenance of normal stature with alkali therapy in infants and children with classic renal tubular acidosis. *J Clin Invest* 61:509, 1978.
14. Buckalew, VM, Jr. Purvis, M, Shulman, M, Herndon, CN, Rudman, D. Hereditary renal tubular acidosis. *Medicine* 53:229, 1974.
15. Sakhaee, K. Nicar, M, Hill, K, Pak, CYC. Contrasting effects of potassium citrate and sodium citrate therapies on urinary chemistries and crystallization of stone-forming salts. *Kidney Int* 24:348, 1983.
16. Manz, F, Waldherr, R, Fritz, HP, et al. Idiopathic de Toni-Debre-Fanconi syndrome with absence of proximal tubular brush border. *Clin Nephrol* 22:149, 1984.
17. Sebastian, A, McSherry, E, and Morris, RC, Jr. On the mechanism of renal potassium wasting in renal tubular acidosis associated with the Fanconi syndrome (type 2 RTA). *J Clin Invest* 50:231, 1971.
18. Donckerwolcke, RA, van Stekelenberg, GJ, Tiddens, HA. Therapy of bicarbonate-losing renal tubular acidosis. *Arch Dis Child* 45:774, 1970.

9. METABOLIC ALKALOSIS

Primary metabolic alkalosis is characterized by an increase in the plasma bicarbonate concentration and an arterial pH above 7.40. Hyperbicarbonatemia alone, however, is not diagnostic of this disorder since it can also represent the appropriate renal compensation to chronic respiratory acidosis. These conditions can easily be distinguished by measurement of the arterial pH, which is reduced in respiratory acidosis.

Pathophysiology and Etiology

The evaluation and treatment of metabolic alkalosis is made easier by first reviewing the pathophysiology of this disorder. Two steps are involved in the development of metabolic alkalosis; the alkalosis must first be *generated* and then it must be *maintained* [1,2]. With regard to generation, a primary elevation in the plasma bicarbonate concentration can be induced by one or more of three mechanisms: (1) the loss of acid from the gastrointestinal tract or in the urine; (2) the administration of bicarbonate (or another organic anion, such as citrate, that is metabolized into bicarbonate); or (3) the loss of fluids with a high chloride / low bicarbonate concentration. In the last setting, which has been called a *contraction* alkalosis, the extracellular volume contracts around a relatively constant quantity of extracellular bicarbonate, thereby raising the plasma bicarbonate concentration [3]. In comparison, loss of fluid with an electrolyte composition similar to plasma, as occurs with gastrointestinal bleeding, produces volume depletion but no direct change in the plasma bicarbonate concentration.

Under normal circumstances, the excess bicarbonate generated by one of the above mechanisms would be rapidly excreted in the urine. Thus, there must also be an *impairment in renal bicarbonate excretion* to allow the alkalosis to persist. This is most often due to volume and chloride depletion and is usually correctable with the administration of chloride (as NaCl, KCl, or NCl). In comparison, giving chloride is ineffective when hyperaldosteronism, marked hypokalemia, or renal failure is responsible for the defect in bicarbonate excretion.

Chloride-Responsive Metabolic Alkalosis

The two most common causes of metabolic alkalosis are the loss of gastric secretions (due to vomiting or nasogastric suction) and diuretic therapy (Table 9-1) [1,2]. The process of gastric acid secretion results in the retention of 1 meq of HCO_3^- for each meq of H^+ that is secreted, since both of these ions are derived from the intracellular dissociation of carbonic acid:

$$H_2CO_3 \rightarrow HCO_3^- + H^+$$

This does not lead to metabolic alkalosis in normal subjects, since the 80 to 200 meq of HCl secreted by the stomach each day enters the duodenum where it stimulates an equivalent amount of bicarbonate secretion from the pancreas. When vomiting or nasogastric suctioning is present, however, the H^+ secreted by the stomach cannot stimulate pancreatic bicarbonate secretion, thereby leading to net retention of HCO_3^-.

Thiazide-type and loop diuretics also can generate a metabolic alkalosis, whether given to treat hypertension or an edematous state. The primary mechanism is enhanced urinary H^+ loss, which is induced by the increase in sodium delivery to the collecting tubules and subsequent stimulation (in part by secondary hyperaldosteronism) of distal Na^+-H^+ (as well as Na^+-K^+) exchange [3]. To the degree that the urinary anion losses are primarily chloride, a component of contraction alkalosis can contribute as well. Contraction can also play a role in the metabolic alkalosis observed with vomiting (even in patients with achlorhydria in whom NaCl replaces HCl in the gastric secretions) and with some forms of diarrhea, in which chloride is the predominant anion that is lost [4].

Acute reversal of chronic respiratory acidosis is another cause of metabolic alkalosis. Compensatory mechanisms normally activated during chronic hypercapnia induce HCl loss in the urine; the ensuing rise in the plasma bicarbonate concentration is appropriate in that it returns the arterial pH toward normal [5]. If, however, the hypercapnia is

Table 9-1. Major causes of metabolic alkalosis

Hydrogen loss
  Gastrointestinal loss
    Removal of gastric secretions (vomiting or nasogastric suction)*
    Chloride-losing diarrheal states
  Renal loss
    Loop or thiazide-type diuretics*
    Mineralocorticoid excess*
    Postchronic hypercapnia
    Hypercalcemia and hyperparathyroidism (including the milk-alkali syndrome)
    High-dose intravenous carbenicillin or other penicillin derivative
    Bartter's syndrome
  Hydrogen movement into cells
    Hypokalemia
Bicarbonate retention
  Massive blood transfusion (citrate is metabolized to bicarbonate)
  Administration of NaHCO$_3$ (as during cardiopulmonary resuscitation)
  Milk-alkali syndrome
Contraction alkalosis
  Diuretics*
  Loss of high chloride / low-bicarbonate gastrointestinal secretions (vomiting and
    some diarrheal states)

---

*Most common causes.

rapidly corrected (most often by artificial ventilation), the excess bicarbonate that has been generated persists and the pH rises from acidemic to alkalemic levels.

MAINTENANCE OF METABOLIC ALKALOSIS. The normal kidney can excrete over 1000 meq of bicarbonate per day without a substantial rise in the plasma bicarbonate concentration [6]. In patients with chloride-responsive metabolic alkalosis, both a reduction in glomerular filtration rate and, more importantly, an increase in tubular sodium bicarbonate reabsorption limit bicarbonate excretion and allow the rise in the plasma bicarbonate concentration to persist [2,7,8]. Chloride is normally the major anion reabsorbed with sodium. In the setting of chloride depletion, however, the sodium that is retained in an attempt to restore euvolemia must, because of electroneutrality, be reabsorbed in part with bicarbonate. Thus, the need to preserve volume prevents correction of the alkalosis [7,8].

Hypokalemia, which is often present due to concurrent renal or gastrointestinal losses, also can enhance bicarbonate reabsorption and contribute to maintenance of the alkalosis [9]. When potassium is lost from the extracellular fluid due, for example, to diuretics or vomiting, potassium moves out of the cells to partially replete the extracellular stores. This is accompanied by sodium and hydrogen movement into the cells to maintain electroneutrality [10]. The ensuing *intracellular acidosis* can, in renal tubular cells, stimulate H$^+$ secretion and therefore bicarbonate reabsorption. Furthermore, the transcellular shift of H$^+$ out of the extracellular fluid can directly raise the plasma bicarbonate concentration and exacerbate the alkalosis [10].

Chloride-Resistant Metabolic Alkalosis
Metabolic alkalosis that is unresponsive to chloride administration can be observed in patients with primary mineralocorticoid excess, severe potassium depletion, or Bartter's syndrome. In these disorders, hyperaldosteronism and hypokalemia are usually responsible for maintenance of the alkalosis by their ability to enhance renal H$^+$ excretion and therefore bicarbonate reabsorption. Volume depletion is generally absent, thereby explaining the lack of dependence on chloride.

MINERALOCORTICOID EXCESS. Mineralocorticoids act in the collecting tubules to increase the reabsorption of sodium and the secretion of both potassium and hydrogen

[11,12]. Thus, the overproduction of endogenous mineralocorticoids (such as hyperaldosteronism due to an adrenal adenoma) or the administration of substances with mineralocorticoid activity (such as glycyrrhizic acid in licorice) can produce both metabolic alkalosis and hypokalemia [2]. Hypertension is common in these disorders but edema does not occur. Although there is initial sodium retention and volume expansion, a spontaneous natriuresis (or "escape") occurs within a few days, returning the extracellular volume toward normal. It is possible that atrial natriuretic peptide, released in response to volume expansion, contributes to this phenomenon [13].

In addition to the direct effect of aldosterone on H^+ secretion, concurrent *hypokalemia* also is essential if a substantial rise in the plasma bicarbonate concentration is to occur [14]; as described above, this is largely due to the intracellular acidosis induced by transcellular potassium-hydrogen exchange, a change that enhances H^+ secretion and HCO_3 reabsorption [9].

SEVERE HYPOKALEMIA.   In addition to lowering the renal tubular cell pH, severe hypokalemia (plasma potassium concentration usually < 2 meq/L) can also impair (via an unknown mechanism) distal chloride reabsorption [14]. Thus, some of the Na^+ that is reabsorbed occurs in exchange for H^+ rather than with Cl^-. In this setting, the urine chloride concentration is typically above 15 meq/L even in the presence of volume depletion, a change that is reversible only after partial repletion of the potassium deficit [15].

BARTTER'S SYNDROME.   Bartter's syndrome is a rare disorder that is most often seen in patients under the age of 25. Most studies suggest that the primary defect is *impaired chloride reabsorption* in the loop of Henle or distal tubule, leading to an initial tendency toward volume depletion with subsequent increases in renin and aldosterone secretion [16]. This results in enhanced distal H^+ and K^+ losses, similar to that seen with loop or thiazide diuretics.

For reasons that are not completely understood, renal prostaglandin production is markedly stimulated in this disorder; the prostaglandins then stimulate further release of renin and secondarily aldosterone, producing further H^+ and K^+ loss. Thus, blocking prostaglandin synthesis with a nonsteroidal anti-inflammatory drug in this condition diminishes the activity of the renin-angiotensin-aldosterone system, leading to amelioration but not correction of the metabolic alkalosis and hypokalemia [16].

Respiratory Compensation
The increased arterial pH in metabolic alkalosis leads to a compensatory rise in the P_{CO_2}, due to direct suppression of the medullary respiratory center by alkalemia [17]. This response is appropriate in that it tends to lower the pH toward normal. In general, the P_{CO_2} rises about 0.7 mm Hg for each 1 meq/L increase in the plasma bicarbonate concentration, up to a P_{CO_2} of about 60 mm Hg; values above this level are unusual because further hypoventilation is limited by the development of hypoxemia. The finding of a P_{CO_2} substantially different from the predicted value suggests a concurrent respiratory acidosis or alkalosis.

Clinical Manifestations
Patients with metabolic alkalosis are often asymptomatic and complaints, when present, are usually due to volume depletion (weakness, muscle cramps, postural dizziness) or hypokalemia (muscle weakness, polyuria, polydipsia). Alkalemia can increase neuromuscular excitability, leading to paresthesias, carpopedal spasm, or lightheadedness. These findings, however, are much more frequently seen with acute respiratory alkalosis, since lipid-soluble CO_2 crosses the blood-brain barrier more rapidly than the charged bicarbonate ion [18].

Diagnosis
The etiology of the metabolic alkalosis is usually apparent from the history. Patients in whom there is no obvious cause will almost always have *surreptitious vomiting, surreptitious diuretic ingestion,* or one of the forms of *primary mineralocorticoid excess* [2].

Measurement of the urinary chloride concentration is useful in differentiating between these disorders (Table 9-2) [1,2]. The urinary chloride concentration is typically less than 15 meq/L with hypovolemia due to vomiting* or diuretic therapy (if the effect of the diuretic has worn off). In comparison, higher values are seen if the diuretic is still active, in Bartter's syndrome or severe hypokalemia (due to the associated defects in chloride reabsorption) [15,16], and in primary mineralocorticoid excess, which is associated with mild volume expansion and, in most cases, low plasma renin levels. Screening the urine for diuretics is indicated if surreptitious ingestion is suspected.

The urine chloride is used in metabolic alkalosis because there may be a *tendency to sodium wasting*, particularly in the first few days. As the plasma bicarbonate concentration and therefore the filtered bicarbonate load increases during the generation of metabolic alkalosis, the renal threshold for bicarbonate reabsorption is, at least initially, exceeded. The resulting loss of bicarbonate in the urine must be accompanied by a cation (predominantly sodium) to maintain electroneutrality. In this setting, the urinary sodium concentration may be greater than 20 meq/L, despite the presence of volume depletion. In contrast, renal chloride conservation is unimpaired, and the urinary chloride concentration is low due both to chloride and volume loss.

When present, bicarbonate wasting can be detected by measurement of the urine pH, which will be above 7.0 to 7.5. This loss of bicarbonate is usually transient; within 3 to 5 days, hypovolemia enhances the capacity for tubular sodium bicarbonate reabsorption, primarily in the proximal tubule. At this time, the desire to conserve sodium results in a urine that is virtually free of sodium and bicarbonate, leading to the characteristic "paradoxical aciduria" with the urine pH often being below 5.5 [20].

These sequential changes in $NaHCO_3$ excretion result in parallel changes in potassium excretion [20]. In the early stages, some of the sodium that leaves the proximal tubule with bicarbonate is then reabsorbed distally in exchange for potassium. These *urinary losses are primarily responsible for the hypokalemia seen with vomiting*; gastric losses are usually less important, since they have a potassium concentration below 10 meq/L. The later phase of increased proximal reabsorption results in a fall in distal sodium delivery and an abrupt decline in further urinary potassium losses [20].

Treatment

Correction of metabolic alkalosis is not usually a medical emergency due to the general lack of adverse effects directly related to the rise in pH. As a result, there is usually time to identify the cause of the disorder and then to gradually reduce the plasma bicarbonate concentration toward normal. Exogenous sources of alkali (such as bicarbonate, acetate, lactate, and citrate) can exacerbate the alkalemia and should be avoided.

Chloride-Responsive Metabolic Alkalosis

The primary treatment of a chloride-responsive metabolic alkalosis is the *administration of chloride, either as NaCl or KCl*. These modalities act in several ways to allow the renal excretion of the excess bicarbonate: (1) more sodium can now be reabsorbed with chloride, rather than in exchange for hydrogen; (2) volume repletion removes the stimulus to sodium retention, permitting $NaHCO_3$ excretion in the urine; and (3) potassium repletion results in potassium entry into and hydrogen movement out of cells, thereby raising the cell pH and decreasing renal H^+ excretion. The efficacy of therapy in this setting can often be determined simply by *monitoring the urine pH*. Most patients will begin with an acid urine (pH < 6) because of the need to conserve sodium. However, the urine pH will rise to above 7.0 to 7.5 as bicarbonate begins to be lost in considerable amounts.

The transcellular exchange of hydrogen for potassium seen with potassium repletion also directly corrects the alkalosis, independent of any changes in renal excretion; the new extracellular H^+ is buffered by HCO_3^-, thereby lowering the plasma bicarbonate concentration [10].

---

*In addition to the low urine chloride concentration, the presence of self-induced vomiting also may be suggested by findings on physical examination such as dental erosions (due to repeated exposure to gastric acid) and calluses and scarring on the dorsum of the hand [19].

Table 9-2. Urine chloride concentration in major causes of metabolic alkalosis

< 15 meq/L	> 20 meq/L
Vomiting	Mineralocorticoid excess
Nasogastric suction	During diuretic therapy
Postdiuretic therapy	Alkali loading*
Posthypercapnia	Severe hypokalemia
Alkali loading*	

*Metabolic alkalosis induced by the administration of alkali will be associated with a urinary chloride concentration below 15 meq/L if there is underlying hypovolemia. If, however, the reduced renal bicarbonate clearance is due to a primary reduction in glomerular filtration rate (as in acute tubular necrosis), volume expansion will ensue and the urinary chloride concentration will be higher.

Patients with vomiting or nasogastric suction may also benefit from H$_2$ blockers, such as cimetidine or ranitidine. These medications reduce gastric acid secretion, thereby minimizing further hydrogen loss. They are, however, not a substitute for chloride repletion, which still is necessary to correct the already present chloride deficit.

The treatment of metabolic alkalosis is more complex in the edematous patient with congestive heart failure, hepatic cirrhosis, or the nephrotic syndrome. Renal perfusion is often reduced in these disorders (see Chap. 26), and the urine chloride concentration is typically below 15 meq/L. However, saline administration will exacerbate the edema and will not sufficiently expand the effective circulating volume to permit excretion of the excess bicarbonate. In this setting, the carbonic anhydrase inhibitor acetazolamide may be extremely effective. This agent primarily impairs NaHCO$_3$ reabsorption in the proximal tubule; the net effect is the loss of NaHCO$_3$, which will tend to correct both the metabolic alkalosis and, to a lesser degree, the edema. Acetazolamide does, however, increase urinary potassium excretion due to increased sodium delivery to the exchange site in the cortical collecting tubule. Thus, careful monitoring of the plasma potassium concentration is required and potassium-sparing diuretics (such as amiloride) should be added, if necessary.

If these combined modalities are ineffective, HCl can be given intravenously to lower the plasma bicarbonate concentration. The standard 0.1N hydrochloric acid solution contains 100 meq of H$^+$ per liter. The amount of HCl needed to reduce the serum bicarbonate concentration can be estimated from the product of the volume of distribution of bicarbonate (about 40% of lean body weight) and the bicarbonate deficit per liter. Thus, to lower the plasma bicarbonate concentration from 45 to 35 meq/L in a 70-kg man:

$$\text{Bicarbonate excess} = 0.4 \times 70 \times (45 - 35) = 280 \text{ meq}$$

This would require about 2.8 liters of the 0.1 N HCl solution. The very low pH of this solution is corrosive to veins; thus, administration should occur over 12 to 24 hours into a large bore (central) vein.

Dialytic therapy (either as hemodialysis with ultrafiltration [21] or continuous arteriovenous hemofiltration [22]; see Chap. 59) may be useful in the occasional patient with metabolic alkalosis, volume overload, and renal failure. The fluid that is removed is replaced, if necessary, with a solution containing chloride, but no alkali.

Chloride-Resistant Metabolic Alkalosis

Patients who have a urine chloride concentration greater than 15 meq/L are unlikely to respond to sodium chloride with correction of the metabolic alkalosis. The administered chloride in this setting is excreted in the urine since chloride deficiency is not a limiting factor in bicarbonate excretion. Furthermore, the high sodium intake will enhance urinary potassium losses (by increasing Na$^+$K$^+$ exchange in the cortical collecting tubule) and exacerbate the hypokalemia in patients with primary mineralocorticoid excess.

The ideal treatment of one of the latter conditions (such as primary hyperaldosteronism) is discussed in detail in Chap. 10. Summarized briefly, removal of the source of mineralocorticoid and use of potassium-sparing diuretics can restore normal electrolyte balance in most patients.

The primary defect in Bartter's syndrome, impaired tubular chloride reabsorption, cannot be corrected with therapy [16]. Thus, treatment is aimed at decreasing the activity of the renin-angiotensin-aldosterone system as a means of decreasing urinary potassium and hydrogen losses. Nonsteriodal anti-inflammatory drugs (since prostaglandins promote renin secretion in this disorder), converting enzyme inhibitors, and potassium-sparing diuretics singly or in combination are usually effective in returning the plasma potassium and bicarbonate concentrations to or near normal [16,23].

Last, partial correction of severe hypokalemia can reverse the associated chloride reabsorptive defect and make the alkalosis responsive to NaCl. Continued KCl administration is also required to repair the potassium deficit.

References

1. Black, RM. Metabolic acid-base disturbances. In JM Rippe, RS Irwin, JS Alpert, JE Dalen (Eds.), *Intensive Care Medicine.* Boston: Little, Brown, 1985.
2. Rose, BD. *Clinical Physiology of Acid-Base and Electrolyte Disorders* (2nd ed.). New York: McGraw-Hill, 1984. Pp. 374-393.
3. Garella, S, Chang, BS, Kahn, SI. Dilution acidosis and contraction alkalosis: Reviews of a concept. *Kidney Int* 8:279, 1975.
4. Perez, GO, Oster, JR, Rogers, A. Acid-base disturbances in gastrointestinal disease. *Dig Dis Sci* 32: 1033, 1987.
5. Polak, A, Haynie, GD, Hays, GM, Schwartz, WB. Effects of chronic hypercapnia on electrolyte and acid-base equilibrium: I. Adaptation. *J Clin Invest* 40:1223, 1961.
6. Van Goidsenhoven, G, Gray, OV, Price, AV, Sanderson, PH. The effect of prolonged administration of large doeses of sodium bicarbonate in man. *Clin Sci* 13:383, 1954.
7. Jacobson, HR, Seldin, DW. On the generation, maintenance, and correction of metabolic alkalosis. *Am J Physiol* 245:F425, 1983.
8. Berger, BE, Cogan, MG, Sebastian, A. Reduced glomerular filtration and enhanced bicarbonate reabsorption maintain metabolic alkalosis in humans. *Kidney Int* 26:105, 1984.
9. Hernandez, RE, Schambelan, M, Cogan, MG, et al. Dietary NaCl determines the severity of potassium depletion-induced metabolic alkalosis. *Kidney Int* 31:1356, 1987.
10. Cooke, RE, Segar, W, Cheek, DB, Corville, F, Darrow, D. The extrarenal correction fo alkalosis associated with potassium deficiency. *J Clin Invest* 31:798, 1952.
11. Sansom, S, Muto, S, Giebisch, G. Na-dependent effects of DOCA on cellular transport properties of CCDs from ADX rabbits. *Am J Physiol* 253:F753, 1987.
12. Stone, DK, Seldin, DW, Kokko, JP, Jacobson, HR. Mineralocorticoid modulation of rabbit medullary collecting duct acidification: a sodium-independent effect. *J Clin Invest* 72:77, 1983.
13. Capuccio, FP, Markandu, ND, Buckley, MG, et al. Changes in the plasma levels of atrial natriuretic peptides during mineralocorticoid escape in man. *Clin Sci* 72:531, 1987.
14. Hulter, HN, Sigala, JF, Sebastian, A. K^+ deprivation potentiates the renal alkalosis-producing effect of mineralocorticoid. *Am J Physiol* 235:F298, 1978.
15. Garella, S, Chazan, JA, Cohen, JJ. Saline-resistant metabolic alkalosis or "chloride-wasting nephropathy." *Ann Intern Med* 73:31, 1970.
16. Stein, JH. The pathogenetic spectrum of Bartter's syndrome. *Kidney Int* 28:85, 1985.
17. Javaheri, S, Shore, NS, Rose, BD, Kazemi, H. Compensatory hypoventilation in metabolic alkalosis. *Chest* 81:296, 1982.
18. Narins, RG, Jones, ER, Townsend, R, Goodkin, DA, Shay, RJ. Metabolic acid-base disorders: Pathophysiology, classification, and treatment. In AI Arieff, RA DeFronzo (Eds.), *Fluid, Electrolyte, and Acid-Base Disorders.* New York: Churchill Livingstone, 1985.

19. Mitchell, JE, Seim, HC, Colon, E, Pomeroy, C. Medical complications and medical management of bulimia. *Ann Intern Med* 107:71, 1987.
20. Kassirer, JP, Schwartz, WB. The response of normal man to selective depletion of hydrochloric acid. *Am J Med* 40:10, 1966.
21. Swartz, RD, Jabobs, JF. Modified dialysis for metabolic alkalosis. *Ann Intern Med* 88:432, 1978.
22. Kaplan, AA, Longnecker, RE, Folkert, VW. Continuous arteriovenous hemofiltration. *Ann Intern Med* 100:358, 1984.
23. Hene, RJ, Koosmans, HA, Dorhout Mees, EJ, et al. Correction of hypokalemia in Bartter's syndrome by enalapril. *Am J Kid Dis* 9:200, 1987.

10. HYPOKALEMIA

Potassium is the major intracellular cation, with an average cellular concentration of 125 to 140 meq/L. In comparison, only about 2 percent of the body potassium is located in the extracellular fluid, where the concentration is much lower at 3.5 to 5.0 meq/L. This concentration difference, which is a major determinant of membrane excitability, is preserved by the Na^+-K^+-ATPase pump in the cell membrane that actively transports sodium out of and potassium into almost all cells.

This and the following chapter will discuss the major clinical disorders causing either hypokalemia or hyperkalemia. It is useful, however, to first review the extrarenal and renal mechanisms involved in the maintenance of normal potassium balance.

Potassium Homeostasis
Potassium intake in the United States generally varies between 50 and 100 meq/day. Under normal circumstances, about 90 percent of dietary potassium is excreted in the urine, while the remainder is eliminated in the stool. However, gastrointestinal excretion of potassium can increase to up to 35 percent of dietary intake, when urinary excretion is limited because of severe, chronic renal failure (glomerular filtration rate < 5 ml/min). This process is influenced in part by aldosterone, which promotes potassium secretion from the colonic mucosal cell into the intestinal lumen [1].

Although the kidney is the major site of potassium excretion, only about 50 percent of an oral or intravenous potassium load appears in the urine during the first 4 hours [1]. As a result, a marked and potentially life-threatening rise in the plasma potassium concentration could occur if the retained potassium were confined to the extracellular fluid. To prevent this problem, most of the potassium load is initially translocated into cells.

There are several factors that promote this intracellular movement of potassium, the most important being *insulin* and β_2-*adrenergic receptor stimulation* [1,2], both of which appear to enhance the activity of the Na^+-K^+-ATPase pump [3]. The effect of insulin is independent of its action on glucose transport. If, for example, basal insulin secretion is inhibited by somatostatin, there will be a greater than normal increment in the plasma potassium concentration after a potassium load [4]. This impairment in potassium tolerance is unrelated to changes in urinary excretion and can be reversed by insulin replacement.

A similar defect in acute potassium handling can be induced by interfering with the β_2-adrenergic receptors with a nonselective β-blocker such as propranolol [5,6]. In contrast, the α-adrenergic receptors have an opposite, although lesser, effect on potassium distribution, slightly impairing cellular potassium uptake [6].

Renal Regulation of Potassium Excretion
Potassium is freely filtered at the glomerulus and is then largely reabsorbed in the proximal tubule and loop of Henle; the net effect is that only 10 percent remains in the tubular lumen by the early distal tubule. Therefore, renal excretion of dietary potassium occurs almost exclusively by *secretion* in the distal nephron [7].

The *principal cells* in the cortical collecting tubule are the primary site of potassium secretion, a model of which is depicted in Fig. 10-1. The movement of potassium from the tubular cell into the lumen is primarily passive and is predominantly controlled by the following factors:

1. Dietary potassium intake, which presumably acts by producing parallel changes in the plasma and renal tubular cell potassium concentrations.
2. The rate of sodium reabsorption, which creates a lumen-negative electrical gradient that promotes potassium secretion.
3. The rate of distal flow, which, by supplying more potassium-free fluid from the loop of Henle, maintains a low tubular fluid potassium concentration and therefore a favorable gradient for continued secretion.
4. Aldosterone, the release of which is directly increased by a rise in the plasma potassium concentration.

Aldosterone acts primarily by opening sodium channels on the luminal side of the principal cell, thus promoting the entry of luminal sodium into the tubular cell (Fig. 10-1) [8,9]. The resulting increase in the cell sodium concentration then stimulates the Na^+-K^+-ATPase pump on the basolateral (or peritubular) membrane, transferring sodium into the peritubular fluid in exchange for potassium. The ensuing rise in the cell potassium concentration favors the secretion of potassium into the lumen down the electrochemical gradient that has been created. Aldosterone may also have a later effect to increase the number of open potassium channels in the luminal membrane [9].

This sequence is reversed in states of potassium depletion. Not only is potassium secretion markedly reduced in this setting, but there is net *potassium reabsorption* in the collecting tubules. This process occurs in the *intercalated cells* in the cortical and outer medullary collecting tubule and appears to be mediated by an active K^+-ATPase pump in the luminal membrane [10]. The signal that activates this pump is not well understood. It is possible, for example, that a decrease in the cell potassium concentration plays an important role.

Hypokalemic Disorders

Hypokalemia (plasma potassium concentration < 3.5 meq/L) can be caused by transcellular shifts of potassium from the plasma into cells, by ingestion of a low-potassium diet, or, most commonly, by potassium losses from the gastrointestinal tract, skin, or kidneys.

Altered Potassium Distribution
Translocation of potassium into the cells can reduce the plasma potassium level without any change in total body stores. The major causes of this problem are listed in Table 10-1.

Metabolic, and to a much lesser degree, acute respiratory *alkalosis* may be associated with hypokalemia [11]. The principal mechanism operating in this setting is the transfer of H^+ out of cells as part of a buffering response to minimize the rise in the extracellular pH; electroneutrality is then maintained in part by potassium entry into the cells. The relationship between the degree of hypokalemia and the increase in blood pH is highly variable, averaging 0.1 to 0.4 meq/L for every 0.1 pH unit rise [11]. Increased gastrointestinal or renal potassium losses due to vomiting or diuretic therapy also contribute to the potassium depletion that is commonly seen with metabolic alkalosis.

A *catecholamine* surge (as occurs with stresses such as an acute myocardial infarction) can cause an acute intracellular shift of potassium due to stimulation of the β_2-adrenergic receptors [12,13]. This phenomenon, in which epinephrine can convert mild into severe hypokalemia [12], may contribute to the apparent increase in coronary mortality observed in diuretic-treated patients with mild hypertension and left ventricular hypertrophy (see Chap. 13). Release of epinephrine also may explain the transient hypokalemia that is often associated with delirium tremens [14].

The plasma potassium concentration typically falls during *insulin administration* in diabetic ketoacidosis, despite a normal or increased level on presentation. This finding results in part from insulin-stimulated transfer of potassium into cells. A similar problem can occur when intravenous dextrose is given; in hypokalemic patients, for example, the administration of 20 meq of potassium in 1 liter of dextrose and water can produce

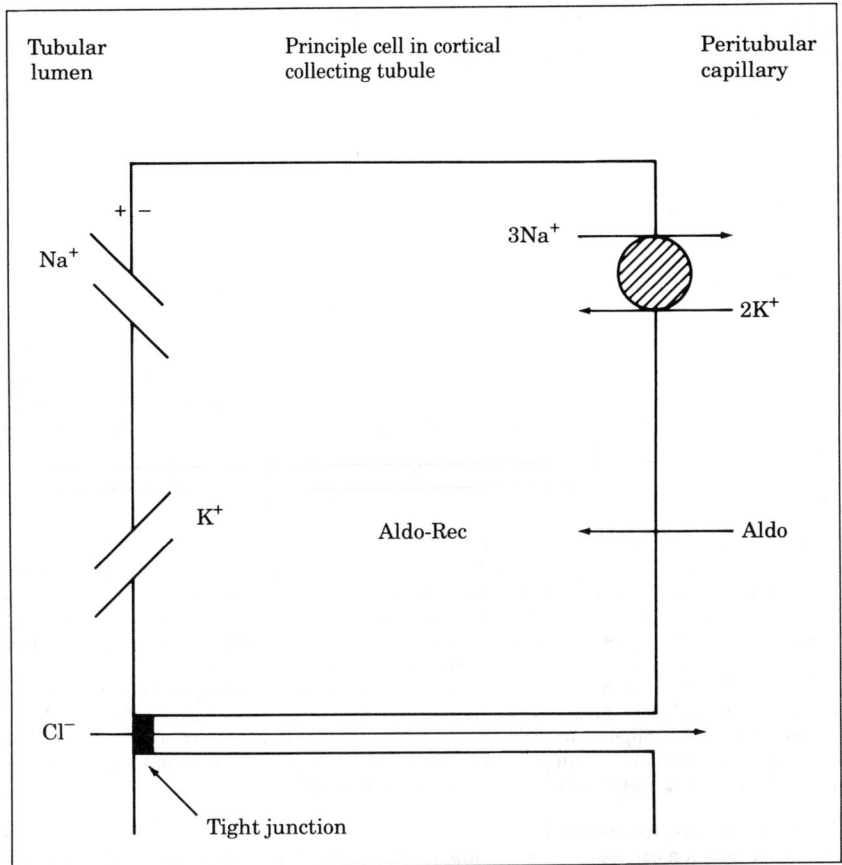

Fig. 10-1. Schematic analysis of the major pathways of sodium and potassium transport in the principal cell of the cortical collecting tubule. As in other nephron segments, the Na^+-K^+-ATPase pump in the basolateral (or peritubular) membrane plays a central role by (1) returning reabsorbed sodium to the systemic circulation, (2) pumping extracellular potassium into the cell, and (3) maintaining a low cell sodium concentration. The last effect allows filtered sodium to passively enter the cell through a sodium channel in the luminal membrane (channels or carriers are required since ions cannot pass directly through the lipid bilayer in the cell membrane). The lumen-negative electrical gradient created by the transport of cationic sodium then promotes potassium secretion into the lumen through a separate potassium channel. Aldosterone, which enters the cell and combines with a cytosolic receptor (Aldo-Rec), stimulates these processes by increasing the number of open sodium (and later potassium) channels. In comparison, chloride reabsorption appears to occur across the tight junction and then between the cells, driven again by the electrical gradient induced by the reabsorption of sodium.

Table 10-1. Hypokalemia due to cellular translocation

Metabolic, and to a lesser degree, acute respiratory alkalosis
β_2-adrenergic stimulation as with a myocardial infarction or delirium tremens
Insulin administration, particularly in ketoacidosis
Increased cell proliferation during the treatment of megaloblastic anemia
Hypokalemic periodic paralysis
Barium poisoning

a transient *worsening* of the hypokalemia with the possible development of cardiac arrhythmias [15].

Rare causes of redistribution-induced hypokalemia include folic acid or vitamin B_{12} treatment of megaloblastic anemias (in which rapid production of new red cells results in the uptake of potassium from the extracellular fluid), hypokalemic periodic paralysis, and poisoning with barium salts (which block potassium channels in cell membranes that normally allow potassium to leave the cells) [16–18]. Patients undergoing radiographic procedures are not at risk for the last problem, since barium sulfate used in gastrointestinal studies is not absorbed into the systemic circulation.

Low Potassium Intake
Potassium depletion due to inadequate intake is rare because potassium, the major intracellular cation, is abundant in most foods. Furthermore, urine and intestinal losses can be reduced to below 15 meq/day if intake is diminished. This probably explains why hypokalemia is infrequent in patients with eating disorders such as anorexia nervosa or bulimia, as long as severe vomiting is not present [19].

In some rural areas in the southeastern United States, however, two dietary factors can combine to produce potassium depletion. First, potassium intake may be only about 25 meq/day in this population, due in part to the relatively high cost of potassium-containing foods. Second, chronic clay ingestion, which is a not uncommon practice, binds potassium in the gut, thereby limiting its absorption [20].

Potassium Losses from the Body
The most common causes of hypokalemia are due to potassium losses from the gastrointestinal tract, skin, or kidneys (Table 10-2).

EXTRARENAL LOSSES.   The gastrointestinal tract may be an important site of potassium wasting, particularly with vomiting or diarrhea. However, the potassium concentration in gastric secretions (5–10 meq/L) is much lower than that seen in intestinal secretions, where it can reach 75 meq/L. As a result, enormous gastric losses would be required to produce substantial potassium depletion. The fall in the plasma potassium concentration that is seen with vomiting is primarily due to increased *urinary,* rather than gastric, losses (see below) [21].

There are two settings where *cutaneous* potassium losses can cause hypokalemia: exercise in a hot, humid climate; and severe burns. Patients who undergo intense physical exercise may lose over 10 liters of sweat per day [22]. This can lead to significant potassium depletion even though the potassium concentration in sweat is only about 5 meq/L [23]. By comparison, the potassium concentration of fluid lost through the skin after burns may greatly exceed the plasma level because of local tissue breakdown, which leads to the release of potassium from cells.

RENAL LOSSES.   The most common causes of renal potassium wasting are *diuretic therapy* and *vomiting*. In both settings, extracellular volume contraction stimulates the release of aldosterone, which directly promotes distal potassium secretion. Hyperaldosteronism is not sufficient, however, because distal flow must also be maintained. This is achieved by decreased sodium and water reabsorption in more proximal segments due to the direct effect of the diuretic or, with vomiting, to an increase in the filtered bicar-

Table 10-2. Causes of hypokalemia due to potassium losses

Extrarenal losses
    Gastrointestinal
        Vomiting and nasogastric suction*
        Diarrhea, including villous adenoma
    Skin
        Profuse sweating
        Extensive burns
Renal losses
    Normotensive
        Loop or thiazide diuretics
        Vomiting
        Hypomagnesemia
        Nonreabsorbable anions (bicarbonate, high-dose penicillins)
        Tubular disorders
            Renal tubular acidosis
            Bartter's syndrome
            Drugs (cisplatin, aminoglycosides)
            Lysozymuria in leukemia
    Hypertensive, with mineralocorticoid excess
        Low plasma renin activity
            Primary hyperaldosteronism due to adrenal adenoma or hyperplasia
        High or normal plasma renin activity
            Renal artery stenosis
            Malignant hypertension
            Cushing's syndrome

*Concomitant renal potassium losses also contribute to hypokalemia (see text).

bonate load that initially exceeds reabsorptive capacity [21]. In the latter setting, bicarbonate also behaves as a *nonreabsorbable anion*; as sodium is reabsorbed in the principal cells in the collecting tubule, bicarbonate cannot follow, thereby necessitating an increase in potassium secretion to maintain electroneutrality. This mechanism also explains the renal potassium wasting observed after therapy with high doses of intravenous sodium carbenicillin (or, less often, with other penicillin derivatives).

Hypomagnesemia is a relatively common finding in hypokalemia, being observed in up to 40 percent of patients [24]. In some cases, the abnormality causing potassium depletion (such as hyperaldosteronism or cisplatin therapy) also impairs renal magnesium reabsorption. In addition, experimental and human observations have shown that magnesium depletion alone can produce renal potassium wasting and that the ensuing potassium depletion cannot be corrected without restoring magnesium balance [25–27]. Hypomagnesemia-induced hyperaldosteronism may contribute to this response [27].

Primary hyperaldosteronism is a rare condition that should be considered in patients with hypertension, otherwise unexplained hypokalemia, and urinary potassium wasting. The most common causes of this disorder are an adrenal adenoma and adrenal hyperplasia [28,29].

A variety of diseases in which tubular function is impaired can also cause urinary potassium losses. These include renal tubular acidosis (see Chap. 8), Bartter's syndrome (see Chap. 9), drugs such as cisplatin and aminoglycosides (which also cause magnesium wasting) [30], and lysozymuria associated with acute and less often chronic leukemia [31]. Decreased sodium reabsorption, which increases both distal flow and aldosterone secretion, plays an important role in many of these disorders.

Clinical Manifestations
Most hypokalemic patients have a relatively small decline in the plasma potassium concentration and no symptoms attributable to potassium depletion. The major clinical manifestations that may be seen with more marked potassium losses are the result of

changes in cardiovascular, neuromuscular, and renal function. Cardiac toxicity is typically manifested by the development of potentially serious arrhythmias [32]. The fall in the plasma potassium concentration hyperpolarizes the cell membrane (i.e., the resting potential becomes more electronegative), a change that prolongs the duration of the refractory period and increases the susceptibility to reentrant arrhythmias. Hypokalemia also predisposes to arrhythmias by increasing automaticity, particularly in patients being treated with digitalis [32].

Hyperpolarization of the cell membrane also slows nerve conduction and muscle contraction. This can contribute to such symptoms as muscle weakness, cramps, and paresthesias, which usually do not become apparent until the plasma potassium concentration is below 2.5 meq/L. Severe hypokalemia also can lead to rhabdomyolysis, due to impairments in muscle metabolism and perfusion [33]. Exercising cells normally release potassium, which then acts as a local vasodilator and contributes to the appropriate increase in tissue perfusion. This response is diminished in hypokalemia, potentially leading to ischemic damage to the muscle cells [33].

Polyuria, due to a reduced ability to concentrate the urine, and polydipsia are the primary renal manifestations of marked hypokalemia. The renal defect in water reabsorption is due to resistance to antidiuretic hormone and therefore is a form of nephrogenic diabetes insipidus. The associated polydipsia may reflect both direct stimulation of the hypothalamic thirst center by hypokalemia and an appropriate secondary response to the rise in urine output [34].

Diagnosis

In most patients, the cause of hypokalemia is apparent from the history and physical examination. Measurement of urinary electrolytes and looking for concurrent acid-base disorders are often useful in patients in whom the differential diagnosis is uncertain. Urinary potassium excretion of more than 25 meq/day, for example, is indicative of at least a contributory role for potassium wasting. A lower level, on the other hand, suggests either extrarenal losses or diuretic-induced hypokalemia at a time when the diuretic effect has worn off.

Many patients with unexplained hypokalemia will also have metabolic alkalosis. The differential diagnosis in this setting in normotensive patients includes self-induced vomiting, surreptitious diuretic therapy, and rarely Bartter's syndrome. Measurement of the urine chloride concentration is often helpful in distinguishing between the first two disorders (see p. 60). This value is appropriately low (< 15 meq/L) in vomiting but is usually elevated despite volume depletion in the patient taking diuretics. A positive screen of the urine for diuretics can be used to confirm the diagnosis.

The evaluation of the hypertensive patient with unexplained hypokalemia is beyond the scope of this discussion, but is outlined in Fig. 10-2. As can be seen, measurement of the plasma renin activity is very helpful once urinary potassium wasting has been demonstrated. This value is elevated in renovascular disease or diuretic therapy but is appropriately reduced by mild volume expansion in primary hyperaldosteronism [28,29]. Distinguishing between an adrenal adenoma and adrenal hyperplasia as the cause of hypersecretion of aldosterone is extremely important because the former can usually be cured by surgery, whereas the latter should be treated medically with a potassium-sparing diuretic such as amiloride or spironolactone [28,29]. This distinction can be achieved by CT scanning of the adrenal glands (looking for a unilateral mass) or by measurement of adrenal vein aldosterone levels, which will lateralize in the presence of an adenoma.

Treatment

Potassium replacement is indicated in most hypokalemic patients, unless the cause has been corrected (as with diarrhea), allowing restoration of potassium balance to be achieved by normal dietary intake. In the past, there has been controversy about the necessity to treat mild diuretic-induced hypokalemia (plasma potassium concentration 3.0–3.4 meq/L) in patients with essential hypertension. However, as reviewed in Chap. 13, there is suggestive evidence that potassium depletion can lead to complex ventricular arrhythmias, particularly in patients with underlying left ventricular hypertrophy.

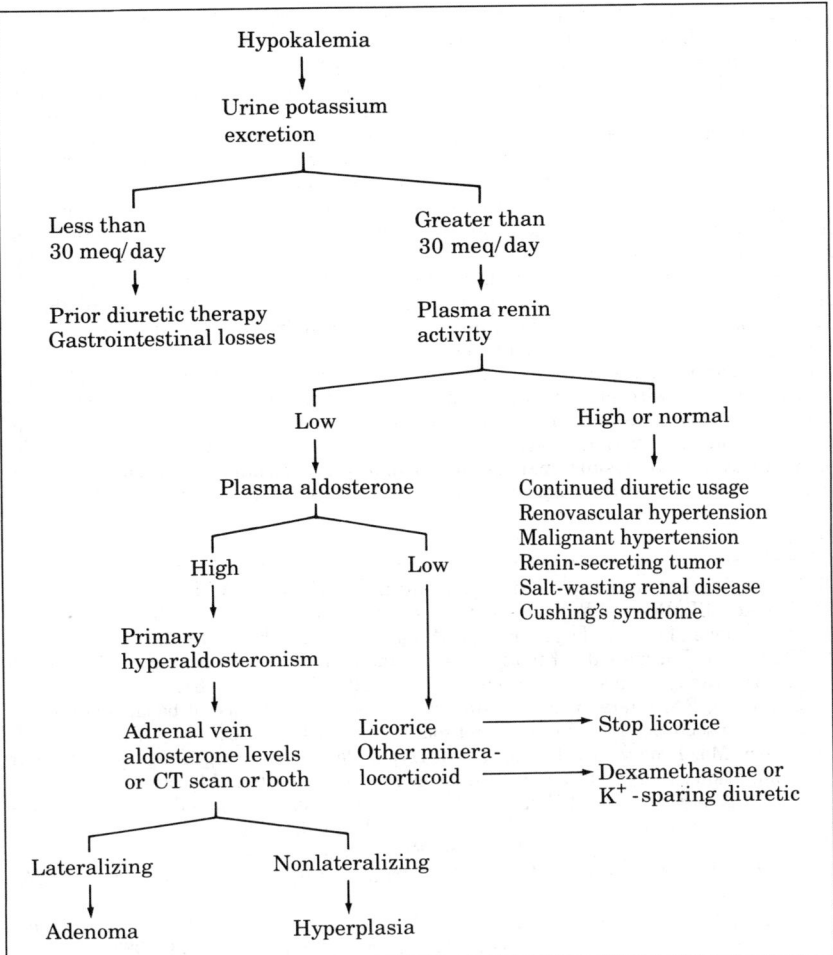

Fig. 10-2. Stepwise approach to the hypertensive patient with unexplained hypokalemia. (From Rose, BD. *Clinical Physiology of Acid-Base and Electrolyte Disorders* 2nd ed. New York: McGraw-Hill, 1984. P. 589).

The quantity of potassium needed to normalize the plasma level is often uncertain, since the plasma potassium concentration does not always correlate with the total deficit. In the absence of factors that cause transcellular shifts of potassium, however, a relatively predictable relationship exists between the degree of hypokalemia and the extent of total body potassium depletion [35]. For each 1 meq/L decrement in the serum potassium concentration, potassium stores decrease by about 200 to 400 meq until the plasma level falls below 2.0 meq/L. At this point, the total deficit may exceed 1000 meq.

Once a decision to begin potassium replacement is made, the route of replacement (oral or parenteral) must be chosen. With either route, potassium must enter the plasma before it can be transferred into cells (the site of greatest K⁺ depletion). As a result, potassium supplementation carries the risk of hyperkalemia if the dose is too large or is administered too rapidly (particularly by the intravenous route). When possible, therefore, potassium supplements should be given orally.

Oral potassium replacement can be administered as potassium-rich foods (such as bananas, which contain about 8 meq each) or as one of a variety of potassium salts (chloride, phosphate, bicarbonate, or a bicarbonate precursor such as citrate). In metabolic acidosis, potassium bicarbonate or potassium citrate is often the agent of choice, since both the plasma potassium concentration and the pH can be returned toward normal. In contrast, metabolic alkalosis, which is much more common, will respond only to KCl (see p. 60).* Any other anion will be nonreabsorbable in the collecting tubules, thereby promoting continued potassium loss as sodium is reabsorbed.

Potassium also can be administered intravenously into peripheral veins in concentrations as high as 40 meq/L; higher concentrations can cause phlebitis and should be infused only into a large vein (femoral or subclavian). The rate of administration, except in unusual settings such as severe hypokalemia with intractable arrhythmias, should probably never exceed 20 to 40 meq/hour. Glucose-containing solutions should also be avoided since the associated rise in insulin release can drive potassium into cells and transiently exacerbate the hypokalemia [15].

Finally, chronic potassium wasting is seen in patients treated with a loop or thiazide diuretic or those with primary hyperaldosteronism not receiving surgical therapy. In these settings, a potassium-sparing diuretic, such as amiloride or spironolactone, represents an alternative that is often better tolerated than oral potassium salts [37]. The *combination* of a potassium-sparing diuretic and dietary potassium supplementation should generally be *avoided* because of an increased risk of developing hyperkalemia.

References

1. Brown, RS. Extrarenal potassium homeostasis. *Kidney Int.* 30:116, 1986.
2. Minaker, EL, Rowe, JW. Potassium homeostasis during hyperinsulinemia: Effect of insulin level, beta-blockage, and age. *Am J Physiol* 242:E373, 1982.
3. Clausen, T, Flatman, JA. Effect of insulin and epinephrine on Na^+-K^+-ATPase and glucose transport in soleus muscle. *Am J Physiol* 252:E492, 1987.
4. DeFronzo, RA, Sherwin, RS, Dillingham, M, et al. Influence of basal insulin and glucagon secretion on potassium and sodium metabolism. *J Clin Invest* 61:472, 1978.
5. Brown, MJ, Brown, DC, Murphy, MB. Hypokalemia resulting from beta$_2$-receptor stimulation by circulating epinephrine. *N Engl J Med* 309:1414, 1983.
6. Williams, ME, Gervino, EV, Rosa, RM, et al. Catecholamine modulation of rapid potasium shifts during exercise. *N Engl J Med* 312:823, 1985.
7. Wright, FS. Renal potassium handling. *Sem Nephrol* 7:174, 1987.
8. Stanton, BA. Regulation of Na^+ and K^+ transport by mineralocorticoids. *Sem Nephrol* 7:82, 1987.
9. Sansom, S, Muto, S, Giebisch, G. Na-dependent effects of DOCA on cellular transport properties of CCDs from ADX rabbits. *Am J Physiol* 253:F753, 1987.
10. Doucet, A, Marsy, S. Characterization of K-ATPase activity in distal nephron: Stimulation by potassium depletion. *Am J Physiol* 253:F418, 1987.
11. Adrogue, HJ, Madias, NE. Changes in plasma potassium concentration during acute acid-base disturbances. *Am J Med* 71:456, 1981.
12. Struthers, AD, Whitesmith, R, Reid, JL. Prior thiazide diuretic treatment increases adrenaline-induced hypokalemia. *Lancet* 1:358, 1983.
13. Morgan, DB, Young, RM. Acute transient hypokalemia: New interpretation of a common event. *Lancet* 2:751, 1982.
14. Wadstein, J, Skude, G. Does hypokalemia precede delirium tremens? *Lancet* 2:549, 1978.
15. Kunin, AS, Surawicz, B, Sims, EAH. Decrease in serum potassium concentration and appearance of cardiac arrhythmias during infusion of potassium with glucose in potassium-depleted patients. *N Engl J Med* 266:228, 1962.
16. Lawson, DH, Murray, RM, Parker, JLW. Early mortality in the megaloblastic anemias. *Q J Med* 41:1, 1972.

---

*Foods rich in potassium (such as bananas and oranges) often have relatively little chloride, as citrate and phosphate are the major anions [36]. Thus, patients with diuretic-induced hypokalemia generally cannot be corrected solely by dietary means.

17. Layzer, RB. Periodic paralysis and the sodium-potassium pump. *Ann Neurol* 11:547, 1982.
18. Berning, J. Hypokalemia of barium poisoning. *Lancet* 1:110, 1975.
19. Mitchell, JE, Seim, HC, Colon, E, Pomeroy, C. Medical complications and medical management of bulimia. *Ann Intern Med* 107:71, 1987.
20. Gonzalez, JJ, Owens, W, Ungaro, PC, et al. Clay ingestion: A rare cause of hypokalemia. *Ann Intern Med* 97:65, 1982.
21. Kassirer, JP, Schwartz, WB. The response of normal man to selective depletion of hydrochloric acid: Factors in the genesis of persistent gastric alkalosis. *Am J Med* 40:10, 1966.
22. Knochel, JP, Dotin, LN, Hamburger, RJ. Pathophysiology of intense physical conditioning in hot climate: I. Mechanism of potassium depletion. *J Clin Invest* 51:242, 1972.
23. Quinton, PM. Physiology of sweat secretion. *Kidney Int* 32 (suppl 21):S-102, 1987.
24. Whang, R, Oei, TO, Aidawa, JK, et al. Magnesium and potassium interrelationships. Experimental and clinical. *Acta Med Scand* 647 (suppl):139, 1981.
25. Smith, JD, Bia, MJ, DeFronzo, RA. Clinical disorders of potassium metabolism. In Arieff, AI, DeFronzo, RA (Eds.), *Fluid, Electrolyte, and Acid-Base Disorders.* New York: Churchill Livingstone, 1985. Pp. 471-472.
26. Whang, R, Flink, EB, Dyckner, T, Wester, PO, Aikawa, JK, Ryan, MP. Magnesium depletion as a cause of refractory potassium depletion. *Arch Intern Med* 145:1686, 1985.
27. Dirks, JH. The kidney and magnesium regulation. *Kidney Int* 23:771, 1983.
28. Melby, JC. Primary aldosteronism. *Kidney Int* 26:769, 1984.
29. Bravo, EL, Tarazi, RC, Dustan, HP, et al. The changing clinical spectrum of primary aldosteronism. *Am J Med* 74:641, 1983.
30. Schilsky, RL, Anderson, T. Hypomagnesemia and renal magnesium wasting in patients receiving cisplatin. *Ann Intern Med* 90:929, 1979.
31. Evans, JJ, Bozdech, MJ. Hypokalemia in nonblastic chronic myelogenous leukemia. *Arch Intern Med* 141:786, 1981.
32. Helfant, RH. Hypokalemia and arrhythmias. *Am J Med* 80 (suppl 4A):13, 1986.
33. Knochel, JP. Neuromuscular manifestations of electrolyte disorders. *Am J Med* 72:521, 1982.
34. Berl, T, Linas, SL, Aisenbrey, GA, et al. On the mechanism of polyuria in potassium depletion. The role of polydipsia. *J Clin Invest* 60:620, 1977.
35. Stern, RH, Cox, M, Fieg, PU, et al. Internal potassium balance and the control of the plasma potassium concentration. *Medicine* 60:339, 1981.
36. Kopyt, N, Dalal, F, Narins, RG. Renal retention of potassium in fruit (letter). *N Engl J Med* 313:582, 1985.
37. Griffing, GT, Cole, AG, Aurecchia, SA, et al. Amiloride in primary hyperaldosteronism. *Clin Pharmacol Therap* 31:57, 1982.

11. HYPERKALEMIA

Hyperkalemia is a common electrolyte disorder. It is often iatrogenic and therefore preventable, since a variety of commonly used medications can interfere with normal potassium homeostasis [1]. This chapter will discuss the approach to the patient with hyperkalemia; it is important, however, for the reader to first review the renal and extrarenal factors involved in potassium balance presented in the preceding chapter.

Etiology
Potassium enters the body by oral intake or intravenous infusion, is stored in the cells (where it is the major cation), and is then excreted primarily in the urine. An abnormality of any of these processes can lead to an elevation in the plasma potassium concentration (Table 11-1). Although uncommon, the presence of an incorrect potassium

Table 11-1. Causes of hyperkalemia

Pseudohyperkalemia
    Traumatic hemolysis during blood drawing
    Thrombocytosis
    Marked leukocytosis
Increased intake (oral or intravenous)
    May contribute when impaired renal potassium excretion
    Acute load can cause hyperkalemia even with normal renal function
Altered internal distribution
    Insulin deficiency
    Hyperosmolality (most often due to hyperglycemia)
    β-adrenergic blockade
    Acute metabolic acidosis
    Cell breakdown
        Rhabdomyolysis
        Trauma
        Cell lysis syndrome after chemotherapy
    Marked exercise (transient, rapidly resolves with rest)
    Massive digitalis intoxication
    Succinylcholine
    Arginine
    Hyperkalemic periodic paralysis
Impaired renal potassium excretion
    Oligoanuric renal failure*
    Marked volume depletion
    Hypoaldosteronism (type 4 RTA)*
    Hyperkalemic type 1 (distal) RTA

*Most common causes of chronic hyperkalemia.

measurement (pseudohyperkalemia) should be excluded before the patient is considered to be hyperkalemic.

Pseudohyperkalemia
Pseudohyperkalemia refers to those disorders in which a high plasma potassium concentration is due to release of K^+ from cells *occurring after the blood specimen has been obtained*. Hemolysis due to traumatic blood drawing is the most frequent cause of this problem and is identified by the presence of a red tint in the plasma due to the release of hemoglobin. Clotting can also lead to the release of potassium from white cells or platelets. The elevation in the measured serum potassium concentration is normally less than 0.5 meq/L; however, the potassium concentration can reach 9 meq/L in some patients with marked thrombocytosis (platelet count $> 10^6/\mu l$) or leukocytosis (WBC $>$ 100,000/μl) [2,3].
    The diagnosis of pseudohyperkalemia in these settings can be made by demonstrating that the potassium concentration is normal in a nonhemolyzed *plasma* sample, in which clotting is prevented by drawing the blood into a heparinized tube [4]. No diagnostic evaluation or therapy is indicated for this problem, since potassium balance is normal.

Increased Intake
The elevation in the plasma potassium concentration that occurs after an acute K^+ load (either oral or intravenous) is dependent on four factors: the quantity of potassium taken in; the ability of some of the excess potassium to enter the cells; urinary potassium excretion; and the preceding level of potassium intake. The rise in the plasma potassium concentration is *minimized if potassium intake has been slowly increased*. This adaptation is due to increased efficiency of both renal excretion and perhaps cellular entry [5,6]. Enhanced release of aldosterone and increased Na^+-K^+-ATPase activity in the cortical collecting tubule play important roles in this process: the latter by promoting

potassium uptake by the tubular cells, and the former by increasing the luminal membrane permeability to sodium and potassium, thereby facilitating potassium secretion into the tubular lumen, both directly and by the lumen-negative potential generated by the reabsorption of sodium (see Chap. 10).

Even in the absence of adaptation, the excess potassium is ultimately, although more slowly, excreted by the kidney. Thus, hyperkalemia due to an acute load is *transient, unless renal potassium excretion is concomitantly reduced.*

Redistribution between Cells and Extracellular Fluid

As discussed in Chap. 10, approximately one-half of dietary potassium is translocated into the cells before being excreted in the urine [7]. Both *insulin* and *catecholamines* (via the β_2-adrenergic receptors) promote this cellular transfer of potassium. As a result, either insulin deficiency or the administration of a nonselective β-adrenergic blocker (such as propranolol) can lead to an elevation in the plasma potassium concentration, particularly if there is an increased potassium load or some other abnormality in potassium handling. In hemodialysis patients, for example, propranolol (but not the β_1-selective agent, atenolol) can raise the plasma potassium concentration by about 1 meq/L [8]. On the other hand, insulin deficiency, along with the rise in plasma osmolality (which pulls water and therefore potassium out of the cells) plays an important role in the hyperkalemia often found in diabetic ketoacidosis [9,10].

Acute *acidemia* also can raise the plasma potassium concentration via a transcellular shift. As some of the excess acid enters the cells to be buffered, cellular potassium moves into the extracellular fluid in order to maintain electroneutrality. This problem is important only in metabolic acidosis, particularly with a nonorganic acidosis (such as renal failure) [11]. In comparison, organic acidoses such as lactic acidosis or ketoacidosis do not appear to be associated with prominent potassium shifts [11,12]. The reason for this difference is incompletely understood; it is possible, for example, that different hormonal responses may play a role or that the organic anions are able to follow hydrogen into the cell, thereby minimizing the need for potassium exit [11,13].

Massive *cell breakdown* can lead to acute and potentially life-threatening hyperkalemia, due to release of potassium from the damaged cells. This is most often seen with rhabdomyolysis, trauma, or cell lysis following chemotherapy (particularly with leukemia or lymphoma).

Less commonly, clinically significant redistribution-induced hyperkalemia may be observed with exercise to exhaustion (the released potassium acts as a local vasodilator, thereby enhancing perfusion to the exercising muscle) [14], massive digitalis intoxication (due to partial inhibition of the Na^+-K^+-ATPase pump) [15], succinylcholine administration (which depolarizes the cell membrane, allowing K^+ to leak out of cells) [16], arginine HCl infusion (due to entry of cationic arginine into the cells, partially in exchange for potassium) [17], and the rare hyperkalemic form of periodic paralysis [18].

Impaired Urinary Excretion

The kidney is the major site of potassium excretion, with a marked ability to increase the rate of excretion as the plasma potassium concentration rises [5]. Thus, *sustained hyperkalemia is virtually always associated with some impairment in renal potassium excretion.* Distal hydrogen secretion is usually diminished as well, often leading to a normal–anion gap metabolic acidosis (see the following).

OLIGOANURIC RENAL FAILURE.   Although renal failure predisposes to potassium retention, excretion of dietary potassium is usually maintained in chronic renal disease until the glomerular filtration rate falls below 5 to 10 ml/min. This adaptation, which is less efficient in acute renal failure, can occur because most of urinary potassium is derived from tubular secretion, not glomerular filtration [19]. Thus, both aldosterone and a rise in Na^+-K^+-ATPase activity in the cortical collecting tubule allows increased distal secretion per functioning nephron [5,6]. Aldosterone-induced *colonic* potassium secretion can also play an important role in the maintenance of potassium balance in this setting [20].

The maintenance of adequate *distal delivery* of sodium and water is essential for this response to occur. For example, sodium reabsorption in the cortical collecting tubule generates a lumen-negative potential difference that promotes potassium secretion [19]. On the other hand, potassium excretion is limited and hyperkalemia usually ensues when distal delivery is reduced in oligoanuric patients.

EFFECTIVE VOLUME DEPLETION.   Distal delivery and therefore potassium excretion may also be impaired with effective circulating volume depletion (as with marked fluid loss or severe heart failure). Both a fall in glomerular filtration and a rise in proximal reabsorption (mediated in part by angiotensin II) can contribute in this setting.

HYPOALDOSTERONISM (TYPE 4 RENAL TUBULAR ACIDOSIS).   Some patients are noted to have persistent hyperkalemia in the absence of any apparent cause, such as advanced renal failure, an offending drug, or a potassium load. In this setting, aldosterone deficiency (or resistance) is responsible in over 75 to 85 percent of cases [21–23].

Hypoaldosteronism is also associated with diminished hydrogen excretion. Both the aldosterone deficiency (since aldosterone can directly promote distal hydrogen secretion) and hyperkalemia contribute to this problem [24]. The latter effect is related to a change in intracellular pH. As some of the excess potassium enters the cells, hydrogen and sodium leave the cells to maintain electroneutrality. The ensuing *intracellular alkalosis* reduces ammonia production and hydrogen secretion by the renal tubular cells (in contrast to the fall in cell pH and increase in ammonia production seen with metabolic acidosis). The net effect is an impairment in net acid excretion and a modest fall in the plasma bicarbonate concentration, which generally remains above 15 meq/L. The urine pH, however, can still be appropriately lowered to below 5.3 (Table 11-2), perhaps because lack of aldosterone impairs cortical but not medullary collecting tubular function.

The major causes of hypoaldosteronism are listed in Table 11-3, with the hyporeninemic form being the most common [21–23]. This syndrome is characterized by a low plasma renin activity and most often occurs in patients with mild-to-moderate renal insufficiency. The underlying renal disease is usually diabetic nephropathy or chronic interstitial nephritis. In addition to the associated renal damage, medications can also contribute, particularly nonsteroidal anti-inflammatory drugs and converting enzyme inhibitors [25].

The pathophysiology of hypoaldosteronism in this disorder is incompletely understood [26]. Decreased renin secretion is clearly important, since angiotensin II and potassium are the major physiologic stimuli to aldosterone release. There is, however, suggestive evidence that there may also be a concurrent *adrenal defect* in at least some cases. Anephric patients, for example, have no renal renin; nevertheless, aldosterone secretion still increases appropriately with hyperkalemia, suggesting that low angiotensin II levels alone may not be sufficient to cause hypoaldosteronism [26].

The factors responsible for the renal and possibly adrenal defects are at present not known. One possibility is prostacyclin deficiency, which has been demonstrated in some patients [27]. Prostacyclin normally increases renin release and may also play a role in aldosterone secretion. Alternatively, increased release of atrial natriuretic peptide (ANP) can also explain all of the features of this disorder, since this hormone is a potent inhibitor of both renin and aldosterone release [26]. Patients with mild-to-moderate renal insufficiency may, for example, be volume expanded, leading to the secondary release of ANP. This hypothesis, however, is as yet unproved.

In other cases of hypoaldosteronism, there is a direct impairment in adrenal function. Heparin (or perhaps its preservative, chlorbutol) is a potent inhibitor of aldosterone production, even when given subcutaneously in low doses [28,29]. The reason that heparin is not widely associated with hyperkalemia is that moderate aldosterone deficiency is not sufficient to cause significant potassium retention in the great majority of patients who still have normal renal function. Hyperkalemia can occur, however, if there is underlying renal disease, similar to that seen in the hyporeninemic form.

HYPERKALEMIC TYPE I (DISTAL) RENAL TUBULAR ACIDOSIS.   Although most patients with type 1 renal tubular acidosis have a normal or reduced plasma potassium concentration, a subset develops hyperkalemia (see Chap. 8). This disorder, which is most often seen with urinary tract obstruction or sickle cell nephropathy, can be distinguished from hy-

Table 11-2. Urinary pH, sodium excretion, and aldosterone levels
in hyperkalemic patients with impaired potassium excretion

Disorder	Urine pH	Urine Na, meq/L	Plasma aldosterone
Renal failure	< 5.3	> 20	Variable
Marked volume depletion	Variable	< 20	Increased
Hypoaldosteronism	< 5.3	> 20	Low
Hyperkalemic type 1 RTA	> 5.3	> 20	Normal or elevated

Table 11-3. Causes of hypoaldosteronism or aldosterone resistance

Low aldosterone levels
  Reduced activity of the renin-angiotensin system
    Hyporeninemic hypoaldosteronism (diabetes mellitus most common)
    Nonsteroidal anti-inflammatory drugs (with possible exception of sulindac)
    Converting enzyme inhibitors
    Cyclosporine
    Acquired immunodeficiency syndrome
  Reduced adrenal synthesis
    Low cortisol
      Primary adrenal insufficiency
      Enzyme deficiencies (primarily congenital adrenal hyperplasia)
    Normal cortisol
      Heparin
      Post-removal of adrenal adenoma for primary aldosteronism
      Enzyme deficiencies
Normal or increased aldosterone levels
  Aldosterone resistance
    Potassium-sparing diuretics
    Pseudohypoaldosteronism (hereditary or acquired resistance to aldosterone)

poaldosteronism by the persistently alkaline urine pH (above 5.3) and a normal or increased plasma aldosterone level (Table 11-2).

In rare cases, a selective potassium secretory defect can be seen in the absence of any abnormality in urinary acidification or aldosterone release. This has been described with lupus nephritis and transplant rejection and presumably reflects a direct effect on the potassium secretory process [30].

Clinical Manifestations

Hyperkalemic patients are usually asymptomatic until the plasma potassium concentration is above 6.5 to 7.0 meq/L. The principal findings that may occur are due to alterations in the electrical excitability of the cell membrane. The resting transmembrane potential difference is normally about -85 mV and is determined primarily by the ratio of the potassium concentrations in the intracellular and extracellular fluids. When the plasma potassium concentration rises, the resting membrane potential becomes less negative, moving closer to the threshold for excitation (Fig. 11-1). This change is also associated with delayed depolarization due to a decrease in membrane sodium permeability.

The most important clinical effects of hyperkalemia involve the heart and neuro-muscular system. A variety of changes may be seen on the electrocardiogram (ECG), beginning with peaked T waves and progressing to prolongation of the PR interval and widening of the QRS complexes (which reflect a slower rate of depolarization). Ultimately, ventricular fibrillation or asystole may appear if the patient is untreated.

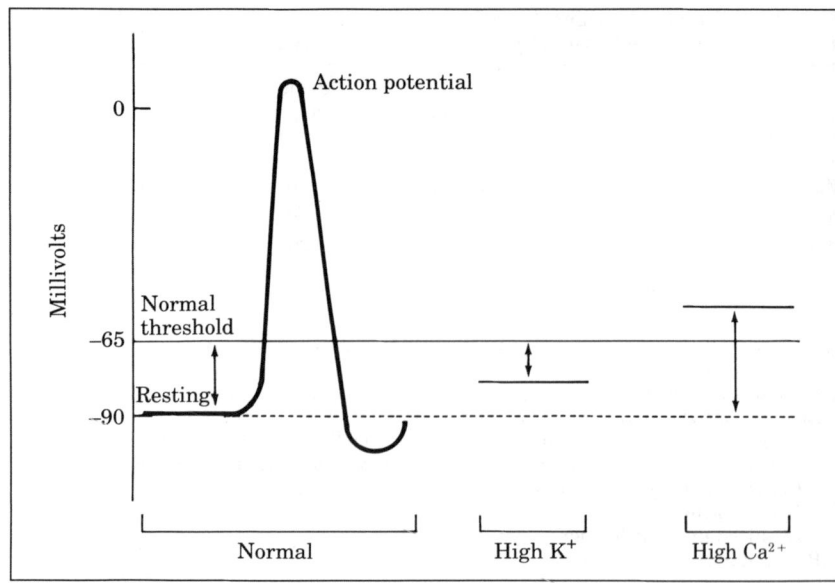

Fig. 11-1. Effects of hyperkalemia on the resting membrane potential of excitable tissues. The increased plasma potassium concentration brings the resting potential closer to threshold. Calcium administration, on the other hand, raises the threshold potential, minimizing the toxicity of hyperkalemia by returning the difference between the resting and threshold potentials toward normal. (Adapted from Leaf, A, Cotran, RS. *Renal Pathophysiology* (2nd ed.). New York: Oxford University Press, 1980.)

The first ECG abnormalities are not usually seen until the plasma potassium concentration is above 6.0 meq/L and are most likely to occur when hyperkalemia has developed rapidly [31]. There is, however, no absolute predictive relationship between the severity of the electrolyte disturbance and the ECG; in rare cases, the ECG can remain unchanged even with a plasma potassium concentration of 9 meq/L [32].

The neuromuscular manifestations of hyperkalemia are nonspecific and are similar to those observed with potassium deficiency. The earliest symptoms are paresthesias and weakness, which can progress to an ascending paralysis that can eventually affect the respiratory muscles [33]. Cranial nerve function is usually spared.

Diagnosis
Once the diagnosis of pseudohyperkalemia has been excluded, the cause of hyperkalemia (increased intake, release from cells, or reduced urinary excretion) can almost always be elicited from the clinical history (looking for dietary sources and possible offending medications) and laboratory studies. One of the disorders that reduces renal potassium excretion (Table 11-1) should be suspected in any patient with chronic hyperkalemia, since normal renal excretory function should prevent a persistent rise in the plasma potassium concentration. The causes of impaired potassium excretion can be differentiated on the basis of renal function, urine pH, urinary sodium concentration, and the plasma aldosterone level (Table 11-2). The plasma cortisol concentration should also be obtained if the plasma aldosterone concentration is low to exclude the presence of primary adrenal insufficiency.

Treatment
Patients with mild hyperkalemia can be treated conservatively by reducing potassium intake (below 2gm/day) and, if indicated, by the use of a loop or thiazide diuretic. This

Table 11-4. Treatment of hyperkalemia

Antagonism of membrane effects of hyperkalemia
  Calcium
Potassium movement into the cells
  Glucose (with or without insulin)
  Sodium bicarbonate
Removal of potassium from the body
  Loop or thiazide diuretics
  Cation exchange resin (Kayexalate)
  Peritoneal dialysis or hemodialysis

regimen is usually effective in patients with renal insufficiency or hypoaldosteronism. Although mineralocorticoid replacement (up to 0.2 mg/day of fludrocortisone) can also lower the plasma potassium concentration in the latter setting, this therapy is often undesirable because of concomitant hypertension. Other general recommendations include discontinuation of medications that can impair potassium homeostasis, such as a nonselective β-blocker, converting enzyme inhibitor, or nonsteroidal anti-inflammatory drug, and treatment of any underlying disorder such as diabetic ketoacidosis.

Drug therapy should be initiated if the plasma potassium concentration has risen *acutely* to 6.0 meq/L or above, particularly if ECG changes of hyperkalemia are present. Drug intervention may act via three different mechanisms: antagonism of the effects of potassium at the cell membrane; transfer of potassium into the cells; and removal of potassium from the body (Table 11-4) [34]. In most circumstances, several modalities should be started simultaneously.

An infusion of *calcium* is the most rapid treatment available, working within minutes by opposing the effects of hyperkalemia at the cell membrane without changing the plasma potassium concentration. As illustrated in Fig. 11-1, calcium makes the threshold potential less electronegative; in the presence of hyperkalemia, this change returns membrane excitability (the difference between the resting and threshold potentials) toward normal. Calcium should be administered* only if ominous ECG manifestations of hyperkalemia are present (such as widening of the QRS complex), since these may herald the onset of ventricular fibrillation. Ten ml of a 10% calcium gluconate solution should be infused over 2 to 5 minutes and may be repeated in 5 minutes if a positive response (assessed by improvement in the ECG) has not been elicited [34]. A beneficial response to calcium may only persist for 1 hour or less; consequently, measures that will lower the plasma potassium concentration are also necessary.

Sodium bicarbonate and *insulin* reduce the degree of hyperkalemia by causing movement of potassium from the plasma into cells. The effect of bicarbonate, which may be mediated by a transcellular hydrogen-potassium exchange, is only partially dependent on its ability to raise the blood pH [35]. A decrease in the plasma potassium concentration is observed within 15 minutes and lasts for 1 to 2 hours. Excess alkalinization should be avoided, since the rise in blood pH can decrease the ionized calcium level, possibly exacerbating the adverse membrane effects of hyperkalemia (Fig. 11-1).

Insulin promotes potassium movement into cells by stimulating the Na^+-K^+-ATPase pump [36]. This effect can be achieved in nondiabetics by simply giving 25 gm of glucose intravenously, which rapidly stimulates endogenous insulin release. Alternatively, insulin can be given with glucose (6–8 units of insulin with 25gm of glucose), a regimen that has the disadvantage of producing hypoglycemia in some patients [37]. Insulin and glucose are necessary, however, in diabetics to be certain both that insulin availability is enhanced and that the plasma glucose concentration does not rise, since the latter change can pull potassium out of the cells and worsen the hyperkalemia [9]. A reduction in the plasma potassium concentration with insulin is typically observed within 30 to 60 minutes and may last several hours.

*Calcium can exacerbate or precipitate cardiac glycoside-induced arrhythmias. As a result, it should be used only when necessary and with great care in patients taking digitalis.

As with the use of calcium, sodium bicarbonate and insulin are also temporizing measures, since the excess potassium has not been removed from the body. Thus, further therapy is required to prevent return of the plasma potassium concentration to pretreatment levels. Diuretics can be tried, but renal insufficiency usually limits the effectiveness of these agents. On the other hand, the *sodium-potassium cation exchange resin*, Kayexalate, can be administered orally or as a retention enema (30–50 gm in sorbitol every 3–4 hours), and is almost always effective. This modality can be used as *sole therapy* with asymptomatic hyperkalemia; it requires 2 to 4 hours to work, however, and therefore, calcium, sodium bicarbonate, and insulin are given when symptoms or ECG changes are present, to provide protection until the excess potassium can be removed. Finally, dialysis should also be used in severe cases; hemodialysis is preferred acutely because it removes potassium much more quickly than peritoneal dialysis.

References

1. Rimmer, JM, Horn, JF, Gennari, FJ. Hyperkalemia as a complication of drug therapy. *Arch Intern Med* 147:867, 1987.
2. Hartmann, RC, Auditore, JV, Jackson, DP. Studies on thrombocytosis: I. Hyperkalemia due to release of potassium from platelets during coagulation. *J Clin Invest* 37:699, 1958.
3. Chumbley, LC. Pseudohyperkalemia in acute myelocytic leukemia. *J Am Med Assoc* 211:1007, 1970.
4. Hyman, D, Kaplan, NM. The difference between serum and plasma potassium (letter). *N Engl J Med* 313,:642, 1985.
5. Hayslett, JP, Binder, HJ. Mechanism of potassium adaptation. *Am J Physiol* 243:F103, 1982.
6. Stanton, B, Pan, L, Deetjen, et al. Independent effects of aldosterone and potassium on induction of potassium adaptation in rat kidney. *J Clin Invest* 79:198, 1987.
7. Brown, RS. Extrarenal potassium homeostasis. *Kidney Int* 30:116, 1986.
8. Sterns, RH, Spital, A. Disorders of internal potassium balance. *Sem Nephrol* 7:206, 1987.
9. Viberti, GC. Glucose-induced hyperkalemia: A hazard for diabetics. *Lancet* 1:690, 1978.
10. Adrogue, HJ, Leaderer, ED, Suki, WN, Eknoyan, G. Determinants of plasma potassium levels in diabetic ketoacidosis. *Medicine* 65:163, 1986.
11. Adrogue, HJ, Madias, NE. Changes in plasma potassium concentration during acute acid-base disturbances. *Am J Med* 71:456, 1981.
12. Oster, JR. Perez, GO, Castro, A, et al. Plasma potassium response to metabolic acidosis induced by mineral and nonmineral acids. *Min Elect Metab* 4:28, 1980.
13. Adrogue, HJ, Chap, Z, Ishida, T. Field, JB. Role of endocrine pancreas in the kalemic response to acute metabolic acidosis in conscious dogs. *J Clin Invest* 75:798, 1985.
14. Williams, ME, Gervino, EV, Rosa, RM, et al. Catecholamine modulation of rapid potassium shifts during exercise. *N Engl J Med* 312:823, 1985.
15. Reza, MJ, Kovick, RB, Shine, KI, Pearce, ML. Massive intravenous digoxin overdosage. *N Engl J Med* 291:777, 1974.
16. Cooperman, LH. Succinylcholine-induced hyperkalemia in neuro-muscular disease. *J Am Med Assoc* 213:1867, 1970.
17. Bushinsky, DA, Gennari, FJ. Life-threatening hyperkalemia induced by arginine. *Ann Intern Med* 89:632, 1978.
18. Clausen, T, Wang, P, Orskov, H, Kristen, O. Hyperkalemic periodic paralysis: Relationship between changes in plasma water, electrolytes, insulin, and catecholamines during attacks. *Scand J Clin Lab Invest* 40:211, 1980.
19. Wright, FS. Renal potassium handling. *Sem Nephrol* 7:174, 1987.
20. Raju, SF, Kiley, JE, Johnson, BB, et al. Hyperkalemia in a hemodialysis patient without a colon. *Dial Transpl* 9:1086, 1980.
21. Kurtzman, NA. Renal tubular acidosis: A constellation of syndromes. *Hosp Prac* 22 (11):131, 1987.

22. Tan, SY, Burtson, M. Hyporeninemic hypoaldosteronism: An overlooked cuase of hyperkalemia. *Arch Intern Med* 141:30, 1981.
23. Kokko, JP. Primary acquired hypoaldosteronism. *Kidney Int* 27:690, 1985.
24. Harrington, JT, Hulter, HN, Cohen, JJ, Madias, NE. Mineralocorticoid-stimulated renal acidification: The critical role of dietary sodium. *Kidney Int* 30:43, 1986.
25. Zimran, A, Dramer, M, Plaskin, M, Hershko, C. Incidence of hyperkalaemia induced by indomethacin in a hospital population. *Br Med J* 291:107, 1985.
26. Williams, GH. Hyporeninemic hypoaldosteronism. *N Engl J Med* 314:1041, 1986.
27. Nadler, JL, Lee, FO, Hsueh, W, Horton, R. Evidence of prostacyclin deficiency in the syndrome of hyporeninemic hypoaldosteronism. *N Engl J Med* 314:1015, 1986.
28. Sherman, RA, Ruddy, MC. Suppression of aldosterone production by low-dose heparin. *Am J Nephrol* 6:165, 1986.
29. Sequeira, SJ, McKenna, TJ. Chlorbutol, a new inhibitor of aldosterone biosynthesis identified during examination of heparin effect on aldosterone production. *J Clin Endocrinol Metab* 63:780, 1986.
30. DeFronzo, RA, Cooke, CR, Goldberg, M, et al. Impaired renal tubular potassium secretion in systemic lupus erythematosus. *Ann Intern Med* 86:268, 1977.
31. Surawicz, B, Chlebus, H, Mussoleni, A. Hemodynamic and electrocardiographic effects of hyperpotassemia. Differences in response to slow and rapid increases in concentration of plasma K. *Am Heart J* 73:647, 1967.
32. Szerlip, HM, Weiss, J, Singer, I. Profound hyperkalemia without electrocardiographic manifestations. *Am J Kid Dis* 7:461, 1986.
33. Epstein, FH. Signs and symptoms of electrolyte disorders. In MH Maxwell, CR Kleeman (Eds.), *Clinical Disorders of Fluid and Electrolyte Metabolism* (3rd ed.). New York: McGraw-Hill, 1980.
34. Black, RM. Disorders of serum sodium and serum potassium. In JM Rippe, RS, Irwin, JS Alpert, JE Dalen (Eds.), *Intensive Care Medicine*. Boston: Little, Brown, 1985.
35. Fraley, DS, Adler, S. Correction of hyperkalemia by bicarbonate despite constant blood pH. *Kidney Int* 12:354, 1977.
36. Clausen, T, Flatman, JA. Effect of insulin and epinephrine on Na^+-K^+-ATPase and glucose transport in soleus muscle. *Am J Physiol* 252:E492, 1987.
37. Fisher, KF, Lees, JA, Newman, JH. Hypoglycemia in hospitalized patients. Causes and outcomes. *N Engl J Med* 315:1245, 1986.

II. HYPERTENSION

12. ESSENTIAL HYPERTENSION: WHO SHOULD BE TREATED?

Although lowering the systemic blood pressure (BP) is clearly beneficial to many patients, several questions remain unanswered including: (1) Which BP measurement is the most accurate indicator of cardiovascular risk—office versus ambulatory?; (2) At what level of diastolic BP should therapy be instituted?; (3) When should antihypertensive therapy be administered to elderly patients?; and (4) Should isolated systolic hypertension be treated? This chapter will attempt to address these issues even though definitive answers cannot as yet be given.

Measurement of the Blood Pressure
Although measurement of the BP is a simple procedure, several potential sources of error must be avoided if an accurate reading is to be obtained. These include [1]:

1. The patient should sit quietly for 5 minutes before the BP is measured. The cuff should be inflated to a level above systolic pressure and then deflated slowly at a rate of 2 to 3 mm Hg per heartbeat. The systolic pressure is equal to the pressure at which the pulse is first heard (phase I), and the diastolic pressure is equal to the disappearance (phase V) not the muffling of sound (phase IV). The point of muffling should be used only in the occasional "hyperdynamic" patient (with anemia or aortic regurgitation, for example) in whom there is greater than a 10 mm Hg difference between muffling and disappearance.
2. The BP cuff should be the proper size: the length of the bladder should be 75 to 80 percent of the circumference of the upper arm and the width of the bladder should be more than 50 to 60 percent of the length. Use of a cuff that is too small, as in an obese patient, can overestimate the true BP by as much as 10 to 50 mm Hg.
3. The BP in the sitting or standing position should be taken with the arm held at the level of the heart. If the arm is allowed to hang down, the brachial artery will be approximately 15 cm below the heart. This will raise the measured BP by 10 mm Hg due to the added hydrostatic pressure imposed by gravity.
4. The BP should be determined in both arms since a falsely low BP can be obtained in one arm if there is an atherosclerotic lesion in the ipsilateral axillary or subclavian artery.

The Effect of the Physician
Many patients are apprehensive when seeing the physician, resulting in an increase in sympathetic tone that can substantially elevate the BP. As an example, this effect was studied in hospitalized patients undergoing continuous BP monitoring with an intraarterial catheter. A visit by a new physician led to an acute rise in BP that averaged 22/14 mm Hg [2]. This hypertensive response, which also occurred during three subsequent visits by the same physician, was largely dissipated within 10 minutes and was much less prominent following a nurse's visit.

A similar process of acclimatization occurs in the outpatient setting. In one study, patients with mild hypertension had a mean fall in BP of 14/7 mm Hg between the first and third visits to a new physician, with no further change on subsequent visits [3]. Thus, the *decision to label a given patient as having mild or moderate hypertension should be delayed for at least three visits* to allow a more accurate assessment of the true BP (unless there is evidence of end-organ damage).

Even after multiple visits, however, many patients will have a BP in the physician's office that is as much as 10 to 15 mm Hg higher than that obtained with 24-hour ambulatory monitoring [4] or with a casual ambulatory value determined at work or at home [5]. Furthermore, several studies utilizing 24-hour ambulatory monitoring suggest that the cardiovascular morbidity from hypertension *correlates better with the ambulatory BP than with that measured by the physician* [4,6]. This may seem somewhat surprising since all of the large studies that have demonstrated a benefit from antihypertensive therapy have been based on office BP measurements. As will be discussed below, however, the clearly positive trials were performed in patients with at least moderate diastolic hypertension (diastolic BP $\geq$ 105 mm Hg) whose ambulatory values would also be likely to be elevated. In comparison, it is probable that at least some patients with mild office hypertension (diastolic BP 90–104 mm Hg) are actually normotensive for much of the day. This could explain why it has been more difficult to demonstrate a positive effect of therapy in this setting.

Devices for 24-hour monitoring are not widely available at the present time. A possible alternative is to base clinical decisions on casual (rather than continuous) values obtained by the patient at work or at home; this measurement appears to correlate more closely with the 24-hour mean level than the BP taken in the physician's office [5]. Thus, it may be elected to withhold further antihypertensive therapy from a patient whose BP is 150/100 in the office but only 130/85 on multiple casual determinations. If this course is chosen, it is important for the physician to ascertain that the person taking the BP is properly trained and that the machine used is accurate. It is also essential to carefully monitor the patient for signs of end-organ damage. For example, an elevation in the QRS voltage on the electrocardiogram suggests an increase in left ventricular mass, indicating that the patient's BP is not under adequate control.

What Level of Diastolic Pressure Should Be Treated?
Over the past 25 years, a series of studies have demonstrated that the treatment of malignant, severe diastolic (115–129 mm Hg) and moderate diastolic (105–114 mm Hg) hypertension with oral antihypertensive agents leads to a marked reduction in cardiovascular morbidity and mortality [7–9]. In patients with moderate hypertension, for example, the proportion of patients developing some cardiovascular complication at 5 years was 55 percent in the placebo group but only 15 percent in the treated group [9]. Thus, *40 percent of treated patients had a demonstrable benefit within only 5 years.*

The issue that remains unsettled is the necessity for therapy in patients with mildly elevated diastolic pressures of 90 to 104 mm Hg. A number of studies, including the Hypertension Detection and Follow-up Program (HDFP) suggested that therapy was also effective in this setting [10,11]. However, two more recent large studies, the Medical Research Council (MRC) trial and the Multiple Risk Factor Intervention Trial (MRFIT), have revealed less clear-cut evidence of benefit [12,13]. The following findings deserve emphasis (Table 12-1):

1. The incidence of total morbid events in the control group was only 4.1 percent (and only 7–8% in the HDFP) at 5 years [12]. This is in contrast to the 55 percent incidence found in moderate hypertension [9]. Thus, mild hypertension is a substantially less severe disease and therefore the *absolute benefit* must be much less. Part of the reason for this difference may be that many patients initially labelled as having mild hypertension are actually normotensive. In the MRC trial, for example, about 20 percent of placebo-treated patients became normotensive with a diastolic BP that was persistently under 90 mm Hg [12]; this proportion may approach 50 percent if normotension is defined as a diastolic BP less than 95 mm Hg [14].

2. The 46 percent reduction in cerebrovascular events (which comprised almost all the total benefit in Table 12-1) represents an absolute decline of only 0.6 percent (from 1.3–0.7%). Thus, only about 1 in every 200 patients did not have a stroke because of antihypertensive therapy. This is in marked contrast to the 40 percent absolute benefit in moderate hypertension.

3. The decreased incidence of stroke is consistent with all other studies [8–11], a reflection of the observation that *hypertension is the single major risk factor for cerebrovascular disease* [15]. In comparison, mild hypertension alone produces only a minor increase in the risk of coronary disease unless accompanied by one or both of the other major predisposing conditions: hypercholesterolemia and smoking [16], factors that seem to be less important in stroke [15]. This pathogenetic difference may explain why it has been difficult in most studies of mild hypertension to demonstrate a beneficial effect of antihypertensive therapy on coronary morbidity (Table 12-1). An additional contributing problem may be the adverse effects on plasma lipids that can be seen with the commonly used thiazides and β-adrenergic blockers: the former raise low-density lipoprotein (LDL) cholesterol by 5 to 15 percent whereas the latter lower the "cardioprotective" high-density lipoprotein (HDL) cholesterol by about 10 percent [17].

Table 12-1. Complications in control and treated groups
in the MRC and MRFIT trials of mild hypertension

Complication	Control (%)	Treated (%)	Improvement (%)
All cardiovascular events*	4.1	3.3	20
Cerebrovascular events*	1.3	0.7	46
Total mortality	1.9	1.8	—
Coronary mortality	1.4	1.5	—

Note: Data from refs. 12 and 13 involving over 25,000 patients followed for 5 to 7 years. The control patients received either no (MRC) or less (MRFIT) antihypertensive therapy.
*The incidence of nonfatal events is derived only from the MRC trial; MRFIT presented data only on fatal events.

The inability of the MRC and MRFIT trials to demonstrate a more pronounced benefit of therapy may also be related in part to different responses among subgroups of patients. This can be illustrated by the following observations from the MRC trial, in which patients were randomized to therapy with placebo, propranolol, or a thiazide diuretic [12]. Propranolol produced a 50 percent reduction in stroke and a 33 percent reduction in coronary events in *nonsmokers,* when compared to placebo. By a mechanism that is not understood, propranolol lowered the BP but had *no effect on cardiovascular morbidity in smokers.* This finding raises questions concerning the continued use of propanolol and perhaps other β-blockers in smokers with hypertension.

In comparison, the efficacy of thiazide therapy was not influenced by smoking; however, the pattern of the response was different from that to propranolol. Thiazides lowered the frequency of stroke but had *no benefit on coronary morbidity* as was seen with propranolol in nonsmokers. This observation suggests that the thiazide diuretics may have an adverse effect on coronary risk that counteracts the benefit of BP reduction [13]. As will be reviewed in the next chapter, diuretics may actually *increase coronary mortality* in some patients with underlying heart disease, as evidenced by an abnormal electrocardiogram [13].

In summary, it is difficult to make definitive recommendations in terms of when antihypertensive therapy should be begun, particularly when the cost, inconvenience, and side effects associated with antihypertensive therapy are taken into account [18]. Thus, there is a need for flexibility in deciding which patients require treatment. The guidelines presented in Table 12-2 seem to represent a reasonable compromise with respect to diastolic hypertension [1,19]. Most physicians treat a diastolic BP that is persistently 95 mm Hg or above. In comparison, the value of drug therapy remains controversial in an otherwise low-risk patient with a diastolic BP in the 90 to 94 mm Hg range; it is probably worthwhile, however, to try nonpharmacologic measures in this setting, since they can safely lower the BP into the normal range in many patients (see Chap. 13). Drug therapy can also be attempted, particularly if control can be achieved with one medication and no side effects.

The general aim of therapy is to lower the diastolic BP to about 85 mm Hg [19,20]; a lesser reduction to 90 to 95 mm Hg seems to offer less complete protection against hypertensive complications [20]. However, patients with active coronary or cerebrovascular disease may represent an exception to these recommendations, since an excessive reduction in pressure can lead to diminished tissue perfusion. In these settings, the goal diastolic pressure should probably be 85 to 90 mm Hg; going below this level, for example, may impair coronary filling during diastole in some patients, leading to a possible *increase* in coronary mortality [21,21a]. Similarly, lowering the systolic pressure below 130 mm Hg in elderly patients with symptomatic cerebrovascular disease can lead to a deterioration in mental function [22].

The decision as to whether a diastolic BP of 90 or 95 mm Hg represents the level at which therapy should be initiated is not trivial, since approximately 11 percent of the

Table 12-2. Recommendations for antihypertensive therapy
in patients with mild hypertension

1. The decision should be based on measurement of the BP on at least three separate
   visits.
2. Nonpharmacologic therapy can be used initially (see Chap. 13).
3. Medical therapy should be begun if:
   a. Diastolic BP persistently 95 mm Hg or above
   b. Diastolic BP between 90 and 94 mm Hg if:
      1. Evidence of end-organ damage
      2. Family history of complications
      3. Other risk factors for coronary disease
   c. Systolic BP above 160 mm Hg, independent of diastolic BP
4. The same considerations apply to the elderly.
5. Therapeutic decisions may be based on ambulatory BP measurements, which may
   be lower than those obtained in the physician's office. In this setting, careful
   monitoring for end-organ damage is essential.

adult population in the United States has a diastolic BP in the 90 to 94 mm Hg range
[23]. Even if treatment is initially withheld, careful follow-up is essential since many
patients will have a rise in diastolic BP with time [12].

Treatment of the Elderly

The BP often rises with age. If, for example, hypertension is defined as a BP greater
than or equal to 160/95, then the incidence of hypertension in patients over the age of
65 reaches 45 percent overall and 60 percent in blacks [24]. These observations have led
some physicians to assume that hypertension may be part of aging and therefore may
represent a lesser risk in older than in younger patients. The incidence of drug-induced
side effects also increases with age due to reductions in renal and hepatic drug clearance
and to impairment of baroreceptor sensitivity, increasing the susceptibility to orthostatic hypotension. As a result, older hypertensive patients are often treated less aggressively.

However, results from the European Working Party on High Blood Pressure in the
Elderly (EWPHE) have demonstrated that mild-to-moderate hypertension is not a benign condition in these patients [25,26]. This study included 850 patients over the age
of 60 with a mean BP of 183/101. When compared to placebo, treatment produced a 19/
5 mm Hg reduction in BP. This was associated with a marked decrease in stroke and
total cardiovascular morbidity that, in absolute terms, was much greater than that seen
in younger patients in the MRC trial (patient age 35–64) [1,25]. In the latter study, for
example, the incidence of stroke in the placebo group was 0.26 percent per year (or 1.3%
at 5 years as in Table 12-1); a 46 percent reduction with therapy, therefore, benefited
only 0.12 percent of patients per year [12]. The comparable value in a placebo-treated
older patient (who is much more likely to have a stroke) was 3.7 percent per year; a 43
percent reduction with therapy now benefited 1.6 percent of patients, a *13-fold greater
absolute improvement* [25]. Similarly, the yearly decline in all cardiovascular complications with therapy was 4.3 percent in the elderly, versus only 0.15 percent in the MRC
trial.

Thus, the data in favor of therapy for mild-to-moderate hypertension are actually
more compelling in older (versus younger) patients [26]. However, antihypertensive
therapy should be initiated with lower-than-usual doses (such as 25 mg of hydrochlorothiazide or 250 mg of methyldopa) and the BP reduced slowly, since elderly patients are
more susceptible to volume depletion and other drug-induced side effects [27].

Treatment of Isolated Systolic Hypertension

All of the above studies stratified patients according to the level of the diastolic BP.
However, the systolic BP appears to be a separate risk factor for the development of
hypertensive complications, causing a two- to four-fold increase in myocardial infarction, stroke, and cardiovascular mortality, even at a normal diastolic pressure [28,29].

In the past, this relationship has been ascribed to systolic hypertension (BP $\geq$160/<90 mm Hg) representing decreased vascular compliance and therefore simply being a marker for underlying vascular disease. However, the Framingham study, using loss of the dicrotic notch in the carotid tracing as a sign of decreased vascular compliance, found that the systolic BP influences the risk of cardiovascular disease, independent of vascular stiffness [29]. The importance of the systolic BP (at least in the elderly) was also confirmed in the EWPHE study in which the risk of cardiovascular complications increased approximately four-fold as the systolic BP rose from 160 to 240 mm Hg but appeared to be *unaffected by the diastolic BP* over a range of 90 to 119 mm Hg [26].

Isolated systolic hypertension is primarily a finding in older patients, increasing in frequency from less than 4 percent under the age of 55 to 20 to 40 percent over the age of 75 [28,29]. There is as yet no proof that treating isolated systolic hypertension is beneficial, although studies are currently in progress. Nevertheless, the observations presented above suggest that it is reasonable to attempt to lower the systolic BP to 140 to 150 mm Hg as long as the diastolic BP does not fall below 75 to 80 mm Hg, a level at which coronary perfusion might become diminished [28,30].

References

1. Rose, BD. *Pathophysiology of Renal Disease* (2nd ed.). New York: McGraw-Hill, 1987. Pp. 509-522.
2. Mancia, G, Parati, G. Pomidossi, G, Grassi, G, Casadei, R, Zanchetti, A. Alerting reaction and rise in blood pressure during measurement by physician and nurse. *Hypertension* 9:209, 1987.
3. Hartley, RM, Velez, R, Morris, RW, DeSouza, MF, Heller, RF. Confirming the diagnosis of mild hypertension. *Br Med J* 286:287, 1983.
4. Perloff, D, Sokolow, M, Cowan, R. The prognostic value of ambulatory blood pressures. *J Am Med Assoc* 249:2792, 1983.
5. Kleinert, HD, Harshfield, GA, Pickering, TG, Devereux, RB, Sullivan, PA, Marion, RM, Mallory, WK, Laragh, JH. What is the value of home blood pressure measurements in patients with hypertension? *Hypertension* 6:574, 1984.
6. Brunner, HR, Waeber, B, Nussberger, J. Blood pressure recording in the ambulatory patient and evaluation of cardiovascular risk. *Clin Sci* 68:485, 1985.
7. Harrington, M, Kincaid-Smith, P, McMichael, J. Results in treatment of malignant hypertension: A seven-year experience in 94 cases. *Br Med J* 2:969, 1959.
8. Veterans Administration Cooperative Study Group on Antihypertensive Agents. Effects of treatment on morbidity in hypertension: Results in patients with diastolic blood pressure averaging 115 through 129 mmHg. *J Am Med Assoc* 202:1028, 1967.
9. Veterans Administration Cooperative Study Group on Antihypertensive Agents. Effects of treatment on morbidity in hypertension. II: Results in patients with diastolic blood pressure averaging 90 through 114 mmHg. *J Am Med Assoc* 213:1143, 1970.
10. Hypertension Detection and Follow-up Program Cooperative Group. The effect of treatment on mortality in "mild" hypertension. *N Engl J Med* 307:976, 1982.
11. Narins, RG. Mild hypertension: A therapeutic dilemma. *Kidney Int* 26:881, 1984.
12. Medical Research Council Working Party. MRC trial of treatment of mild hypertension: Principal results. *Br Med J* 291:97, 1985.
13. Multiple Risk Factor Intervention Trial Research Group. Baseline resting electrocardiographic abnormalities, antihypertensive treatment, and mortality in Multiple Risk Factor Intervention Trial. *Am J Cardiol* 55:1, 1985.
14. Management Committee: The Australian therapeutic trial in mild hypertension: Untreated mild hypertension. *Lancet* 1:185, 1982.
15. Dauber, TR. *The Framingham Study. The Epidemiology of Artherosclerotic Disease.* Cambridge: Harvard, 1980. Chaps. 7 and 8.
16. Madhavan, S, Alderman, MH. The potential effect of blood pressure reduction on cardiovascular disease. A cautionary note. *Arch Intern Med* 141:1583, 1981.
17. Weinberger, MH. Antihypertensive therapy and lipids: Paradoxical influences on cardiovascular disease risk. *Am J Med* 80 (suppl 2A):64, 1986.
18. Hyman, D, Kaplan, NM. Treatment of patients with mild hypertension. *Hypertension* 7:165, 1985.

19. Memorandum from the WHO/ISH. 1986 guidelines for the treatment of mild hypertension. *Hypertension* 8:957, 1986.
20. Taguchi, J, Freis, ED. Partial reduction of blood pressure and prevention of complications in hypertension. *N Engl J Med* 291:329, 1974.
21. Editorial. How far to lower blood pressure. *Lancet* 2:251, 1987.
21a. Samuellson, O, Wilhelmsen, L, Andersson, OK, Pennert, K. Berglund, G. Cardiovascular morbidity in relation to changes in blood pressure and serum cholesterol levels in treated hypertension. Results from the Primary Prevention Trial in Göteberg, Sweden. *J Am Med Assoc* 258:1768, 1987.
22. Meyer, JS, Judd, BW, Tawaklna, T, Rogers, RL, Mortel, KF. Improved cognition after control of risk factors for multi-infarct dementia. *J Am Med Assoc* 256:2203, 1986.
23. Hypertension Detection and Follow-up Program Cooperative Group. Mild hypertensives in the Hypertension Detection and Follow-up Program. *Ann NY Acad Sci* 304:254, 1979.
24. The Working Group on Hypertension in the Elderly. Statement on hypertension in the elderly. *J Am Med Assoc* 256:70, 1986.
25. Amery, A, Birkenhager, W, Brixko, R, Bulpitt, C, Clement, D, Deruyttere, M, De Schaepdryver, A, Dollery, C, Fagard, R, Forette, F. Mortality and morbidity results from the European Working Party on High Blood Pressure in the Elderly trial. *Lancet* 1:349, 1985.
26. Amery, A, Birkenhager, W, Brixko, R, et al. Efficacy of antihypertensive drug treatment according to age, sex, blood pressure, and previous cardiovascular disease in patients over the age of 60. *Lancet* 2:589, 1986.
27. Shannon, RP, Wei, JY, Rosa, RM, Epstein, FH, Rowe, JW. The effect of age and sodium depletion on cardiovascular response to orthostasis. *Hypertension* 8:438, 1986.
28. Gifford, RW, Jr. Isolated systolic hypertension in the elderly. Some controversial issues. *J Am Med Assoc* 247:781, 1982.
29. Kannel, WB, Wolf, PA, McGee, DL, Dawber, TR, McNamara, P, Castelli, WP. Systolic blood pressure, arterial rigidity, and risk of stroke. The Framingham study. *J Am Med Assoc* 245:1225, 1981.
30. Rowe, JW. Systolic hypertension in the elderly. *N Engl J Med* 309:1246, 1983.

13. ESSENTIAL HYPERTENSION: INITIAL THERAPY

Once it has been decided that treatment to lower the blood pressure (BP) is indicated (see Chap. 12) both nonpharmacologic and drug therapies can be used. Nonpharmacologic therapies are often used initially and may be particularly helpful in patients with mild hypertension, frequently lowering the BP into the normal range.

Nonpharmacologic Therapy

A variety of non-drug regimens have been reported to be effective in patients with hypertension (Table 13-1) [1,2]. These therapies, many of which are also beneficial from a general health viewpoint, have the advantages of low cost, safety, and lack of side effects. They do, however, often require *difficult to sustain* changes in diet and life-style. Furthermore, only sodium restriction, weight reduction in the obese, and restriction of alcohol intake have been definitely proved to have an important antihypertensive effect [1].

The potential impact of intensive nutritional modification in the treatment of hypertension is illustrated in Fig. 13-1. Antihypertensive therapy was discontinued in two groups of patients whose BP had previously been well controlled for at least 1 year with medical therapy: sodium restriction (to about 2 gm/day), weight reduction (averaging 3 kg), and avoidance of excessive alcohol ingestion were instituted in group 1 whereas no dietary modification was made in group 2. At 4 years, almost no patients in group 2 versus *39 percent* in group 1 remained normotensive (defined as a diastolic BP under 90 mm Hg).

Table 13-1. Nonpharmacologic therapy of hypertension

Dietary changes
    Moderate sodium restriction
    Weight reduction, if obese
    Restrict alcohol intake, if excessive
    Increased potassium intake (?)
    Calcium supplementation (?)
    High-fiber, low-saturated fat, or vegetarian diet(?)
Aerobic exercise
Relaxation techniques

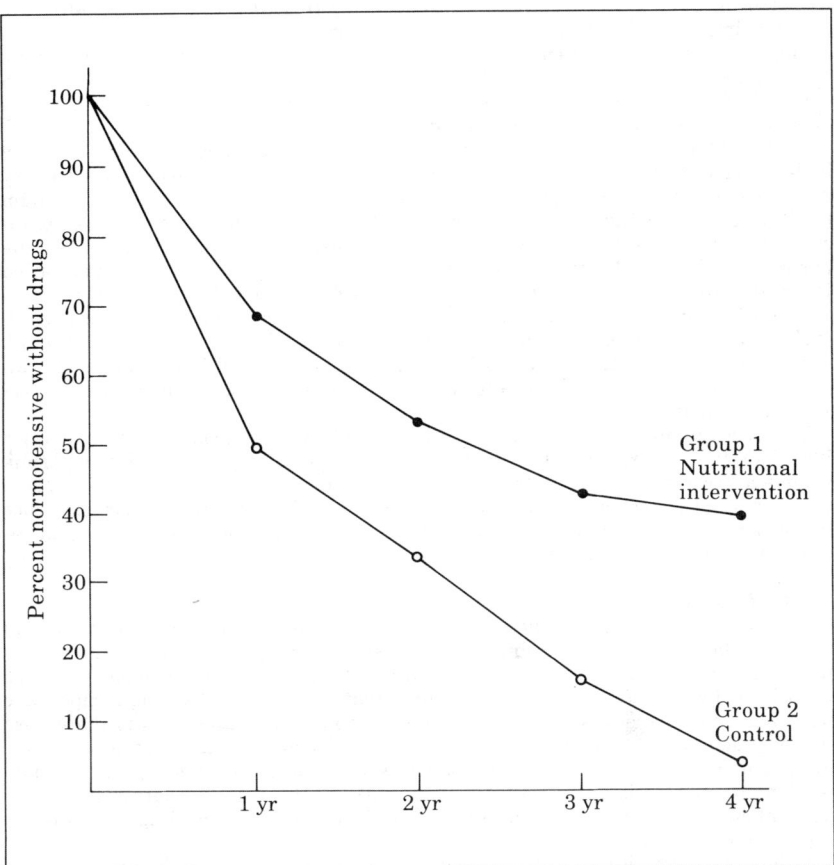

Fig. 13-1. Percentage of patients remaining normotensive after withdrawal of antihypertensive therapy from 93 patients treated with (Group 1; n = 50) or without (Group 2; n = 43) dietary modification. (From Stamler, R, Stamler, J, Grimm, R, Gosch, FC, Elmer, P, Dyer, A, Berman, R, Fishman, J, Van Heel, N, Civinelli, J, McDonald, A. *J Am Med Assoc* 257:1484, 1987. Copyright 1987, American Medical Association.)

Sodium Restriction

Forty to sixty percent of patients with essential hypertension are sodium sensitive, as evidenced by a rise in BP with sodium loading and a reduction in BP (often exceeding 10 mm Hg) with sodium restriction [3]. Furthermore, limiting sodium intake may be beneficial even in those patients who do not have a fall in BP. To the degree that a hypotensive response in this setting is limited by activation of the renin-angiotensin system, the patient will be more sensitive to the subsequent use of a converting enzyme inhibitor [4].

The direct relationship between sodium intake and the systemic BP appears to be steepest between 70 and 120 meq/day. Thus, a daily sodium intake of 70 to 80 meq is probably optimal. More marked sodium restriction is relatively unpalatable and frequently produces little further change in BP, presumably because continued volume depletion leads to increased formation of angiotension II [4].

Patient adherence to dietary recommendations is often an important limiting factor with sodium restriction (as well as with other antihypertensive therapies). Compliance can be tested by measuring sodium excretion with a 24-hour or overnight urine collection. This method is effective even in patients being treated with a diuretic. Although diuretics initially increase sodium excretion above intake, this response is self-limited. Within *3 to 7 days,* most patients are back in balance as neurohumoral sodium-retaining forces counteract the effect of the diuretic (see Chap. 4). Thus, plasma volume depletion generally occurs only during the first 1 to 2 weeks of therapy, as long as diuretic dose and dietary sodium intake are relatively constant.

The mechanism by which sodium intake affects the systemic BP is incompletely understood. Both experimental and human studies suggest that there may be a primary defect in renal function in hypertension, leading to a relative inability to excrete sodium [5,6]. As a result, a high-sodium diet can initially lead to sodium retention and extracellular volume expansion. However, this does not explain how the BP rises, since the major hemodynamic abnormality in established essential hypertension is an elevation in vascular resistance, not in plasma volume or cardiac output [5].

One possibility is that hypervolemia promotes the release of an *endogenous digital-islike natriuretic hormone* (which is different from the atrial natriuretic peptides) [7,7a]. This hormone, by inhibiting Na-K-ATPase, can raise the intracellular sodium and calcium concentrations; the latter change in vascular smooth muscle cells can produce vasoconstriction and a rise in BP.

This as yet unproved model can be reversed by sodium restriction or diuretic therapy. With diuretics, for example, the fall in BP is initially mediated by a decline in plasma volume and cardiac output. Within 1 to 2 months, however, cardiac output increases toward normal as the hypotensive response is maintained by a fall in vascular resistance [8]. This vasodilation could result from a reduction in secretion of the putative natriuretic hormone by the early volume depletion.

Weight Reduction

Obesity is associated with an increased incidence of hypertension. At least two factors may contribute to this relationship: increased sympathetic activity; and insulin resistance, leading to enhanced secretion of insulin [9-11a]. Insulin, for example, can raise the BP by directly promoting renal sodium retention and by enhancing sympathetic tone. The latter change may be in part adaptive in that a sympathetically mediated rise in thermogenesis increases energy output and limits further weight gain; the price, however, is an elevation in BP [11a]. Conversely, weight reduction can lower the BP independent of any associated decline in sodium intake [9,10]. This is generally a dose-dependent effect as the BP can fall by an average of 1 mm Hg for every 1 kg of weight lost [10].

Weight reduction, if achievable and sustainable, is also beneficial because of its favorable effect on plasma lipids, lowering the plasma cholesterol concentration by as much as 5 to 10 percent [12]. In comparison, commonly used antihypertensive agents often have a deleterious effect: the thiazides tend to raise low-density lipoprotein (LDL) cholesterol by 5 to 15 percent; and the β-adrenergic blockers tend to lower high-density lipoprotein (HDL) cholesterol by about 10 percent [12,13]. Although these changes appear small, they may be clinically important since every 1 percent elevation in the plasma cholesterol level can increase coronary risk by approximately 2 percent [14].

Limiting Alcohol Intake
Excess alcohol intake is another important dietary factor predisposing to the development of hypertension. The risk increases when daily intake exceeds two drinks per day and is most prominent above five drinks per day [15]. Conversely, decreasing or eliminating the intake of alcohol often leads to a long-lasting reduction in BP. The mechanism by which these changes occur is uncertain but a direct effect of alcohol to increase the sensitivity of vascular smooth muscle to vasoconstrictors such as angiotensin II and norepinephrine may be involved [15].

Potassium and Calcium Supplementation
Low dietary potassium and calcium intakes may be additional factors promoting the development of essential hypertension [16,17]. On the other hand, increasing dietary potassium can lower the BP by an average of about 5 percent, perhaps by increasing sodium excretion or by decreasing the vascular responsiveness to norepinephrine [5,18]. Although this effect is relatively modest, maintaining potassium intake above 60 meq/day may have an additional advantage, apparently decreasing the incidence of stroke by up to 40 percent; this poorly understood effect appears to be independent of the systemic BP or other cardiovascular risk factors [19].

Calcium also appears to play an important role in essential hypertension. As described before, the cell calcium concentration is elevated in hypertensive patients (perhaps due in part to a digitalislike natriuretic hormone [7]), roughly paralleling the rise in BP [20]. Furthermore, lowering the BP with a diuretic, β-adrenergic blocker, or calcium channel blocker is associated with a proportionate fall in cell calcium [20]. In addition, a variety of other abnormalities in calcium balance have been described including decreased calcium intake, a reduced plasma concentration of ionized calcium, secondary hyperparathyroidism, elevated plasma calcitriol levels, and the presence of a circulating factor that directly promotes calcium entry into cells [17,21,22]. Although the mechanisms responsible for these findings are not well understood, calcium supplementation may lower the BP in some patients [17,21]. However, the efficacy and safety of this regimen remains unproved [23]; as an example, increasing calcium intake can, in some patients, produce a substantial *rise* in the systemic BP [21].

Drug Therapy
Antihypertensive medications are required if the above modalities are ineffective. In the stepped-care approach that has been widely used, medical therapy begins with a thiazide diuretic or a β-adrenergic blocker. A variety of recent findings, however, have questioned these recommendations in terms of both safety and effects on the "quality of life" [24]. As a result, alternative agents are being increasingly used for initial therapy, particularly converting enzyme inhibitors and calcium channel blockers.

Diuretics
Thiazide diuretics have been one of the mainstays of antihypertensive therapy. However, recent studies in patients with mild hypertension (diastolic BP 90–104 mm Hg) have raised some serious questions about the safety of these agents. In the Multiple Risk Factor Intervention Trial (MRFIT), for example, antihypertensive therapy led to a 25 percent reduction in coronary mortality in patients who began with a normal electrocardiogram (ECG). In those patients with an abnormal ECG, however, therapy was associated with a *68 percent increase in coronary mortality* [25]. This trend toward increased risk has been confirmed in other studies, including the Hypertension Detection and Follow-up Program [26].

Further analysis of the MRFIT results indicated that the elevation in coronary risk (due entirely to sudden death) was *limited to those patients who received diuretic therapy* [25,27]. Findings in the Medical Research Council trial also suggested an adverse effect of diuretic therapy: in nonsmokers, the incidence of coronary events was reduced by one-third in patients treated with propranolol (when compared to placebo); this beneficial response was not seen in those receiving a thiazide even though there was a comparable reduction in BP [28].

The mechanism by which diuretics may be harmful* to some patients with mild hypertension is uncertain: hypokalemia, hypomagnesemia, hyperlipidemia, and hyperglycemia all could contribute [13,24]. The role of any of these factors is, of course, difficult to prove. For example, hypokalemia (defined as a plasma potassium concentration $\leqslant$ 3.5 meq/L) occurs in up to 50 percent of patients treated with the equivalent of 50 to 100 mg of hydrochlorothiazide per day. Mild hypokalemia, however, can become severe hypokalemia during a stress response; this effect appears to be mediated by epinephrine, which drives potassium into the cells via activation of the β-adrenergic receptors [30]. As illustrated in Fig. 13-2, infusion of epinephrine to achieve a plasma concentration similar to that occurring during an acute myocardial infarction lowered the plasma potassium concentration in normal subjects from 3.8 to 3.2 meq/L. If, however, these patients were pretreated with a thiazide diuretic to induce mild hypokalemia, epinephrine now lowered the plasma potassium concentration to below 2.5 meq/L in some subjects [31].

It is possible that the combination of diuretic- and epinephrine-induced hypokalemia could predispose to serious ventricular arrhythmias, particularly during an episode of coronary ischemia. There is some evidence in support of this hypothesis as patients with an acute myocardial infarction who are hypokalemic on admission seem to have an increased incidence of ventricular fibrillation [32]. Furthermore, hypertensive left ventricular hypertrophy alone (the most common cause of an abnormal ECG in the MRFIT) may be an important risk factor for sensitivity to potassium depletion, since this disorder is associated with a substantial increase in the incidence of simple and complex ventricular arrhythmias [32a].

In addition to possibly increasing coronary risk, diuretics also produce symptoms that may interfere with the quality of life [33]. It is not generally appreciated, for example, that thiazides are more likely than β-blockers to cause impotence in men [28].

At present, it is uncertain what conclusions should be drawn concerning diuretic therapy in uncomplicated hypertension. At the least, these agents should be used if *cost* is an issue and in those settings in which they are particularly likely to be effective: in *blacks* (who respond much better to monotherapy with a diuretic than with a β-blocker or a converting enzyme inhibitor) [34,35]; and in patients already treated with a *converting enzyme inhibitor* [36], since it is the hypovolemia-induced rise in angiotensin II that normally limits the hypotensive efficacy of diuretic therapy [37].

If a diuretic is administered, it should be used in the lowest effective dose such as 25 to 50 mg of hydrochlorothiazide per day [34]. Furthermore, hypokalemia should probably be treated to minimize the risk of arrhythmias and to possibly lower the BP and reduce the incidence of stroke [18,19]. The use of a potassium-sparing diuretic (such as amiloride or triamterene) may be the preferred way to raise the plasma potassium concentration, since these agents also diminish diuretic-induced magnesium loss [37a]. This may be beneficial because magnesium deficiency can contribute to the increased incidence of arrhythmias seen with diuretic use, an effect that may be in part mediated by the induction of cellular potassium depletion that is correctable only with the restoration of magnesium balance [37a]. How magnesium affects potassium homeostasis is not well understood.

β-Adrenergic Blockers

Problems with the use of β-blockers and other sympatholytic agents (such as methyldopa, clonidine, and prazosin) are more related to symptoms than to safety. By *interfer-*

---

*The inability to demonstrate these findings in earlier studies may have been related to the severity of the hypertension. With moderate hypertension (diastolic BP of 105–114 mm Hg), for example, as many as 40 percent of patients may be protected from a cardiovascular complication within 5 years by antihypertensive therapy [29]. In this setting in which treatment is of great benefit, any adverse drug effect would be masked. In comparison, the risk and therefore the total benefit are much less in mild hypertension (see p. 84).

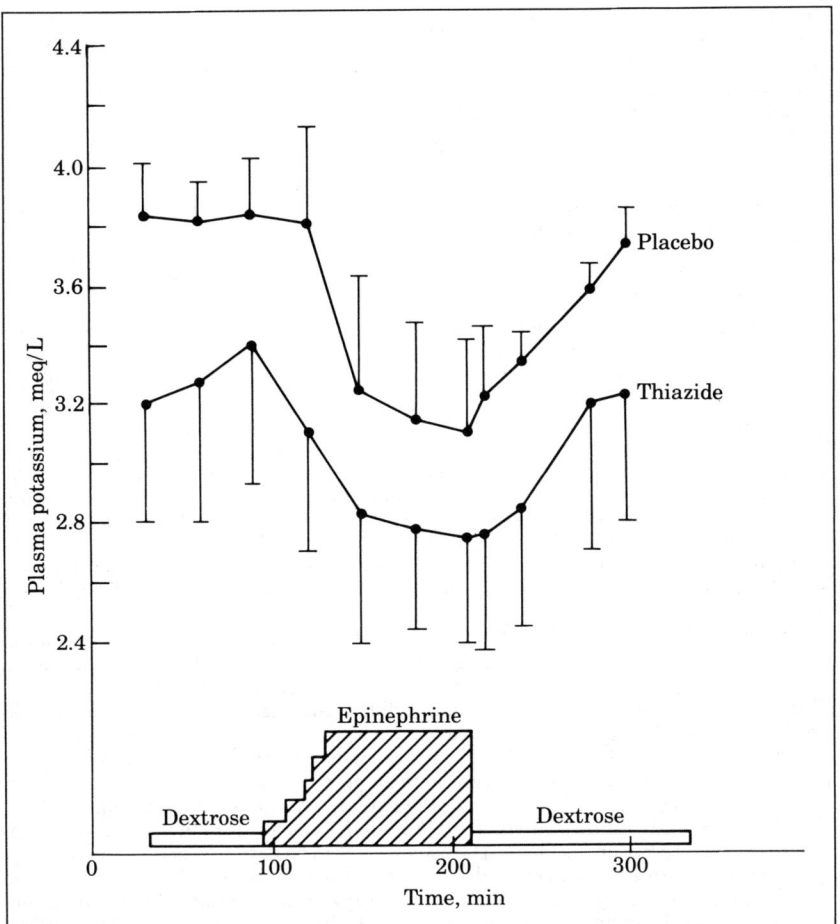

Fig. 13-2. Plasma potassium concentration during an infusion of epinephrine in six patients pretreated with a placebo or a thiazide for 7 days. (From Struther, A, Whitesmith, R, Reid, JL. *Lancet* 1:1358, 1983.)

ing with normal sympathetic functioning, these drugs are more likely to produce symptoms such as lethargy, fatigue, depression, and decreased work performance [33,38]. In the MRC trial, for example, 20 to 25 percent of patients discontinued propranolol within 5 years because of suspected adverse affects (versus < 5% withdrawal from placebo therapy) [28]. Furthermore, questioning patients' spouses suggests that the actual incidence of side effects may be much higher than reported by the patient [39].

Thus, the efficacy of the β-blockers must be weighed against their deleterious effects on patient well-being. Although they can lower the BP and, at least in nonsmokers*, can reduce cerebrovascular and perhaps cardiovascular complications [28], these agents produce too many side effects that are a *predictable result of their mechanism of action* to

---

*An unexpected finding in the MRC trial was that propranolol lowered the BP but did not reduce coronary or cerebrovascular morbidity in smokers [28]. The mechanism by which this occurs is not known.

be considered optimal first-line agents. Nevertheless, there are patients who may particularly *benefit from treatment with* β-*blockers,* including those with angina pectoris, a recent myocardial infarction, heart failure due to diastolic dysfunction (in which systolic function as assessed by the ejection fraction is normal) [40], or evidence of increased sympathetic tone such as resting tachycardia or isolated systolic hypertension in a young patient [41].

Converting Enzyme Inhibitors
The converting enzyme inhibitors offer two major advantages as first-line therapy for mild-to-moderate hypertension:

1. They are effective as monotherapy in mild hypertension [24,33,36], lowering the BP to normal in up to 65 to 70 percent of patients (except for blacks) [35].
2. They lack the metabolic side effects of the diuretics and do not interfere with sympathetic function. As a result, these agents are often associated with an improved sense of well-being and tend to be better tolerated than other antihypertensive drugs [33].

Side effects do occur with the converting enzyme inhibitors and can be divided into two general groups: those that represent a toxic or idiosyncratic reaction; and those that are directly due to the decrease in angiotensin II formation [24]. The former include neutropenia, rash, abnormal taste, and proteinuria. These problems were most prominent when captopril was initially used in high doses, up to 450 to 600 mg/day. It is now clear, however, that the maximum effective dose of captopril is 100 to 150 mg/day [36]; at these levels, the incidence of side effects is *markedly reduced* [42]. Furthermore, enalapril and lisinopril, which lack the sulfhydryl group present in captopril, seem even less likely to produce these problems.

Inhibition of angiotensin II production can lead to side effects that also can be minimized by appropriate use of the drug. *Hypotension,* particularly following the first dose, is a potentially serious problem as acute reductions exceeding 50 mm Hg may occur. This is most likely to occur in hypovolemic, diuretic-treated patients. As a result, diuretics should optimally be discontinued for 3 to 5 days prior to institution of a converting enzyme inhibitor. *Hyperkalemia* (due to diminished angiotensin II–induced aldosterone secretion) and *acute renal failure with bilateral renal artery stenosis* (see next chap.) also may occur but are unusual in the patient with mild hypertension.

Two final recently recognized problems are *cough* (which occurs in about 2–5% of patients) [43] and rarely angioedema. The cough tends to be dry and hacking in nature, is not associated with any pulmonary disease, and is readily reversible with a reduction in dosage or, if necessary, discontinuation of therapy. It may be related to the high concentration of angiotensin converting enzyme in the lung and may be mediated secondarily by an increase in local prostaglandin production. This possibility is suggested by preliminary observations that prostaglandin synthesis inhibitors lead to cessation of cough despite continuation of converting enzyme inhibitor therapy [43a]. It is also possible that captopril, perhaps because of its shorter duration of action and therefore more intermittent inhibition of converting enzyme activity, is less likely to produce this problem than enalapril [43].

In summary, converting enzyme inhibitors are both effective and generally well tolerated. Those patients who do not respond to monotherapy with a converting enzyme inhibitor often become normotensive with the addition of a low dose of a thiazide diuretic (such as 12.5–50 mg of hydrochlorothiazide) [36]. This combination is often synergistic because the converting enzyme inhibitor prevents the rise in angiotensin II that normally limits the response to the diuretic* [37]. Furthermore, the converting enzyme inhibitor has the additional advantages of minimizing both diuretic-induced hypokalemia (by its inhibitory effect on aldosterone release) and hypercholesterolemia (via an unknown mechanism) [45].

---

*This sequence should be reversed in blacks, who respond best to initial therapy with a diuretic [35]. If additional therapy is required, a converting enzyme inhibitor often leads to a substantial reduction in BP [44].

Calcium Channel Blockers
Calcium channel blockers, like the converting enzyme inhibitors, offer the advantages of lack of metabolic changes and lack of interference with the sympathetic nervous system [46–48]. They also may be correcting one of the major abnormalities in essential hypertension, a rise in the cell calcium concentration that promotes increased arteriolar tone [20].

Verapamil, diltiazem, and nifedipine are the calcium channel blockers that are currently available. These drugs are most effective in older patients [47,48]; they lower the BP primarily by reducing vascular resistance (particularly nifedipine), although verapamil and diltiazem also may reduce the cardiac output because of their negative inotropic effects.

Verapamil, which is now available in once-daily tablets, and diltiazem are generally well tolerated by most patients. In comparison, nifedipine is short-acting, producing acute, marked vasodilation that often leads to headache, flushing, a feeling of hot limbs, and reflex tachycardia [47]. Edema may also occur with this drug. This problem appears to be primarily related to the redistribution of fluid between the vascular space and the interstitium, rather than to renal sodium retention [49]. Vasodilation at the precapillary arteriole could be responsible by raising the intracapillary pressure, thereby favoring the movement of fluid into the interstitium.

Summary
There is at this time no clear consensus regarding the optimal means by which antihypertensive therapy should be begun. The optimal drug should be effective, taken once or at most twice daily, have few toxic or metabolic side effects, and not interfere with the patient's quality of life. For the reasons outlined previously, converting enzyme inhibitors seem to come closest to meeting these criteria among the currently available antihypertensive agents. A thiazide diuretic or long-acting calcium channel blocker can then be added if goal BP (diastolic BP of about 85 mm Hg in most but not all patients; see p. 85)[50] is not attained with the converting enzyme inhibitor.

These recommendations apply primarily to patients with uncomplicated hypertension. In selected cases, however, other agents may be preferable. Examples include thiazide diuretics in blacks or patients in whom cost is an issue, and β-blockers in patients with angina, a recent myocardial infarction, heart failure with diastolic dysfunction, or evidence of increased sympathetic tone [40,41].

References

1. Final Report of the Subcommittee on Nonpharmacological Therapy of 1984 Joint National Committee on Detection, Evaluation, and Treatment of High Blood Pressure. Nonpharmacological approaches to the control of high blood pressure. *Hypertension* 8:444, 1986.
2. Kaplan, NM. Non-drug treatment of hypertension. *Ann Intern Med* 102:359, 1985.
3. MacGregor, GA. Sodium is more important than calcium in essential hypertension. *Hypertension* 7:628, 1985.
4. Navis, G, de Jong, PA, Donker, AbJM, van der Hem, GK, de Zeeuw, D. Moderate sodium restriction in hypertensive subjects: Renal effects of ACE-inhibition. *Kidney Int* 31:815, 1987.
5. Rose, BD. *Pathophysiology of Renal Disease* (2nd ed.). New York: McGraw-Hill, 1987. Pp. 469-488.
6. Curtis, JJ, Luke, RG, Dustan, HP, Kashgarian, M, Whelchel, JD, Jones, P, Dietheim, AG. Remission of essential hypertension after renal transplantation. *N Engl J Med* 309:1009, 1983.
7. Haddy, FJ. Endogenous digitalis-like factor or factors. *N Engl J Med* 316:621, 1987.
7a. Haber, E, Haupert, GT, Jr. The search for a hypothalamic Na$^+$, K$^+$-ATPase inhibitor. *Hypertension* 9:315, 1987.

8. van Brummelen, P, Man in't Veld, AJ, Schalekamp, MADH. Hemodynamic changes during long-term thiazide treatment of essential hypertension in responders and nonresponders. *Clin Pharmacol Therap* 27:328, 1980.
9. Reisin, E, Frohlich, ED, Messerli, FH, Dreslinksi, GR, Dunn, FG, Jones, MM, Batson, HM, Jr. Cardiovascular changes after weight reduction in obesity hypertension. *Ann Intern Med* 98:315, 1983.
10. Tuck, ML, Sowers, J, Dornfeld, L. Kledzik, G, Maxwell, M. The effect of weight reduction on blood pressure, plasma renin activity, and plasma aldosterone levels in obese patients. *N Engl J Med* 304:930, 1981.
11. Modan, M, Halkin, H, Almog, S. Lusky, A, Eshkol, A, Shefi, M, Shitrit, A, Fuchs, Z. Hyperinsulinemia. A link between hypertension obesity and glucose intolerance. *J Clin Invest* 75:809, 1985.
11a. Landsberg, L. Diet, obesity and hypertension: An hypothesis involving insulin, the sympathetic nervous system, and adaptive thermogenesis. *Q J Med* 61:1081, 1986.
12. MacMahon, SW, MacDonald, GJ, Bernstein, L, Andrews, G, Blacket, RB. Comparison of weight reduction with metoprolol in treatment of hypertension in young overweight patients. *Lancet* 1:1233, 1985.
13. Weinberger, MH. Antihypertensive therapy and lipids: Paradoxical influences on cardiovascular disease risk. *Am J Med* 80 (suppl 2A):64, 1986.
14. Lipid Research Clinics Program. The Lipid Research Clinics Coronary Primary Prevention Trial results. I. Reduction in incidence of coronary heart disease; II. The relation of reduction in incidence of coronary heart disease to cholesterol lowering. *J Am Med Assoc* 251:351,365, 1984.
15. MacMahon, SW, Norton, RN. Alcohol and hypertension: Implications for prevention and treatment. *Ann Intern Med* 105:124, 1986.
16. Langford, HG. Dietary potassium and hypertension: Epidemiologic data. *Ann Intern Med* 98:770, 1983.
17. McCarron, DA. Is calcium more important than sodium in the pathogenesis of essential hypertension? *Hypertension* 7:607, 1985.
18. Bianchetti, MG, Weidmann, P, Beretta-Piccoli, C, Ferrier, C. Potassium and norepinephrine- or angiotensin-mediated pressor control in hypertension. *Kidney Int* 31:956, 1987.
19. Khaw, K-T, Barrett-Connor, E. Dietary potassium and stroke-associated mortality: A 12-year prospective population study. *N Engl J Med* 316:235, 1987.
20. Erne, P, Bolli, P, Burgisser, E, Buhler, FR. Correlation of platelet calcium with blood pressure. Effect of antihypertensive therapy. *N Engl J Med* 310:1084, 1984.
21. Resnick, LM, Muller, FB, Laragh, JL. Calcium-regulating hormones in essential hypertension. Relation to plasma renin activity and sodium metabolism *Ann Intern Med* 105:649, 1986.
22. Lindner, A, Kenny, M, Meacham, AJ. Effects of a circulating factor in patients with essential hypertension on intracellular free calcium in normal platelets. *N Engl J Med* 316:509, 1987.
23. Kaplan, NM, Meese, RB. The calcium deficiency hypothesis of hypertension: A critique *Ann Intern Med* 105:947, 1986.
24. Rose, BD. *Pathophysiology of Renal Disease* (2nd ed.). New York: McGraw-Hill, 1987. Pp. 526-538.
25. Multiple Risk Factor Intervention Trial Research Group. Baseline resting electrocardiographic abnormalities, antihypertensive treatment, and mortality in Multiple Risk Factor Intervention Trial. *Am J Cardiol* 55:1, 1985.
26. Hypertension Detection and Follow-up Program Cooperative Research Group. The effect of antihypertensive drug treatment on mortality in the presence of resting electrocardiographic abnormalities: The HDFP experience. *Circulation* 70:996, 1984.
27. Grimm, RH, Jr. The drug treatment of mild hypertension in the Multiple Risk Factor Intervention Trial. A review. *Drugs,* 31 (suppl 1):13, 1986.
28. Medical Research Council Working Party. MRC trial of treatment of mild hypertension: Principal results. *Br Med J* 291:97, 1985.
29. Veterans Administration Cooperative Study Group on Antihypertensive Agents. Effects of treatment on morbidity in hypertension, II: Results in patients with diastolic

blood pressure averaging 90 through 114 mm Hg. *J Am Med Assoc* 213:1143, 1970.
30. Brown, MJ, Brown, DC, Murphy, MB. Hypokalemia from beta₂-receptor stimulation by circulating epinephrine. *N Engl J Med* 309:1414, 1983.
31. Struthers, A. Whitesmith, R, Reid, JL. Prior thiazide diuretic treatment increases adrenaline-induced hypokalaemia. *Lancet* 1:1358, 1983.
32. Nordrehaug, JE, von der Lippe, G. Hypokalemia and ventricular fibrillation in acute myocardial infarction. *Br Heart J* 50:525, 1983.
32a. McLenachan, JM, Henderson, E, Morris, KI, Dargie, HJ. Ventricular arrhythmias in patients with hypertensive left ventricular hypertrophy. *N Engl J Med* 317:787, 1987.
33. Croog, SH, Levine, S, Testa, MA, Brown, B, Bulpitt, CJ, Jenkins, CD, Klerman, GL, Williams, GH. The effects of antihypertensive therapy on the quality of life. *N Engl J Med* 314:1657, 1986.
34. Veterans Administration Cooperative Study Group on Antihypertensive Agents. Comparison of propranolol and hydrochlorothiazide for the initial treatment of hypertension. II. Results of long-term therapy. *J Am Med Assoc* 248:2004, 1982.
35. Moser, M, Lunn, J. Responses to captopril and hydrochlorothiazide in black patients with hypertension. *Clin Pharmacol Therap* 32:307, 1982.
36. Veterans Administration Cooperative Study Group on Antihypertensive Agents. Captopril: Evaluation of low doses, twice-daily doses, and the addition of diuretic for the treatment of mild to moderate hypertension. *Clin Sci* 63 (suppl 8):443s, 1982.
37. Vaughan, ED, Jr, Carey, RM, Peach, MJ, Ackerly, JA, Ayers, CR. The renin response to diuretic therapy: A limitation of antihypertensive potential. *Circ Res* 42:376, 1978.
37a. Dyckner, T, Wester, PO. Potassium/magnesium depletion in patients with cardiovascular disease. *Am J Med* 82 (suppl 3A):11, 1987.
38. Avorn, J, Everitt, DE, Weiss, S. Increased antidepressant use in patients prescribed β-blockers. *J Am Med Assoc* 255:357, 1986.
39. Jachuck, SJ, Brierley, H, Jachuck, S, Wilcox, PM. The effect of hypotensive drugs on the quality of life. *J R Coll Gen Pract* 32:103, 1982.
40. Topol, EJ, Traill, TA, Fortuin, NJ. Hypertensive hypertrophic cardiomyopathy of the elderly. *N Engl J Med* 312:277, 1985.
41. Simon, AC, Safar, MA, Levenson, JA, Kheder, AM, Levi, BI. Systolic hypertension: Hemodynamic mechanism and choice of antihypertensive treatment. *Am J Cardiol* 44:505, 1979.
42. Dombey, S. Optimal dose of captopril in hypertension (letter). *Lancet* 1:529, 1983.
43. Coulter, DM, Edwards, IR. Cough associated with captopril and enalapril. *Br Med J* 294:1521, 1987.
43a. Nicholls, MG, Gilchrist, NL. Sulindac and cough induced by converting enzyme inhibitors (letter). *Lancet* 1:872, 1987.
44. Frier, PA, Wollam, GL, Hall, WD, Unger, DJ, Douglas, MD, Bain, RP. Blood pressure, plasma volume, and catecholamine levels during enalapril therapy in blacks with hypertension. *Clin Pharmacol Therap* 36:731, 1984.
45. Weinberger, MH. Influence of an angiotensin converting-enzyme inhibitor on diuretic-induced metabolic effects in hypertension. *Hypertension* 5 (suppl III):III-132, 1983.
46. Halperin, AK, Cubeddu, LX. The role of calcium channel blockers in the treatment of hypertension. *Am Heart J* 111:363, 1986.
47. Massie, BM, Hirsch, AT, Inouye, IK, Tubau, JF. Calcium channel blockers as antihypertensive agents. *Am J Med* 77 (suppl 4A):135, 1984.
48. Massie, B, MacCarthy, P, Ramanathan, KB, et al. Diltiazem and propranolol in mild to moderate essential hypertension as monotherapy or with hydrochlorothiazide. *Ann Intern Med* 107:150, 1987.
49. Marone, C, Luisoli, S, Bomio, F, Beretta-Piccoli, C, Bianchetti, MG, Weidmann, P. Blood sodium-blood volume state, aldosterone, and cardiovascular responsiveness after calcium entry blockade with nifedipine. *Kidney Int* 28:658, 1985.
50. Editorial. How far to lower blood pressure. *Lancet* 2:251, 1987.

14. HYPERTENSION: RENAL ARTERY STENOSIS

Renal artery stenosis and renal disease are probably the two most common causes of secondary (or nonessential) hypertension (Table 14-1). Establishing the diagnosis of one of these conditions is particularly important since the underlying disorder can often be corrected, leading to a reduction in the systemic blood pressure (BP) and possible cure of the hypertension.

This chapter will review the diagnosis and treatment of renovascular hypertension. The renal arterial lesions are usually due to *atherosclerosis* or *fibromuscular dysplasia,* conditions with different clinical characteristics (Table 14-2) [1]. Atherosclerosis primarily affects men over the age of 45, usually is at the aortic orifice or the proximal one-third of the renal artery, and frequently leads to progressive stenosis. In comparison, fibromuscular dysplasia most often affects females under the age of 40, primarily involves the distal two-thirds of the main renal artery and the proximal intrarenal branches, and progression is uncommon. Both disorders can also affect extrarenal vessels.

Diagnosis
Secondary hypertension is probably less common than previously suspected. This is particularly true in patients with mild hypertension in whom the incidence may be under 1 percent [2]. As a result, it is not feasible to evaluate every patient for one of the disorders in Table 14-1. There are, however, certain characteristics that are uncommon in essential hypertension, which is generally a slowly progressive disorder that begins between the ages of 20 and 50 and is usually associated with a positive family history of hypertension (Table 14-3). As an example, the incidence of renal artery stenosis rises to 10 to 40 percent in patients with an *acute elevation in BP* over a previously stable baseline or with *severe or refractory hypertension* [3,4]. Furthermore, the combination of marked hypertension and otherwise unexplained renal insufficiency (plasma creatinine concentration above 1.5 mg/dl) may be associated with bilateral atherosclerotic renovascular disease in almost one-half of cases [4]. For reasons that are not well understood, however, renal artery stenosis is uncommon in blacks, even in the presence of a severe elevation in BP [3].

Patients with a history suggestive of secondary hypertension should also be evaluated for symptoms or signs of the less common disorders listed in Table 14-1:

1. An elevated blood urea nitrogen (BUN) and plasma creatinine concentration with an abnormal urinalysis are suggestive of *primary renal disease.*

2. *Pheochromocytoma* should be suspected in a patient with paroxysmal hypertension, particularly if associated with the triad of headache (usually pounding), palpitations, and sweating [5].

3. Hypertension, hypokalemia, and urinary potassium wasting (potassium excretion > 30 meq/day) can be seen with renovascular disease, malignant hypertension, concurrent diuretic use, or one of the causes of *primary mineralocorticoid excess* (an aldosterone-producing adrenal adenoma being most common). Only the last disorder is also associated with a low plasma renin activity [6].

4. *Cushing's syndrome* (including that due to corticosteroid administration) should be suspected in those patients with the classic physical findings of cortisol excess: cushingoid facies, central obesity, ecchymoses, and muscle weakness [7].

Evaluation for Renal Artery Stenosis
Renal arteriography is the "gold standard" for the diagnosis of renal artery stenosis. However, the invasive nature of this test has led to the search for a simpler screening procedure. A rapid-sequence intravenous pyelogram (IVP), for example, may reveal a unilateral decrease in renal size or a delayed calyceal appearance time, or both. Unfortunately, this test is normal in 20 to 25 percent of patients with unilateral disease and probably is normal in a higher percentage of patients with bilateral disease in whom there may be a smaller difference in function between the two kidneys [8]. Thus, *a non-*

Table 14-1. Major causes of secondary hypertension in adults

Renal artery stenosis—unilateral or bilateral
Renal disease
Oral contraceptives
Pheochromocytoma
Primary mineralocorticoid excess
Cushing's syndrome
Pregnancy
Hypercalcemia

Table 14-2. Distinction between atherosclerotic renal artery stenosis
and fibromuscular dysplasia

Characteristic	Atherosclerosis	Fibromuscular dysplasia
Typical age at onset	> 45	< 40
Gender	Primarily men	80% female
Distribution of lesions	Aortic orifice and proximal main renal artery	Distal main renal artery and intrarenal branches
Progression of lesions	Common, may lead to complete occlusion	May occur, but total occlusion is rare

Table 14-3. Findings suggestive of secondary hypertension

An acute rise in BP over a previously stable baseline
Severe or refractory hypertension, including retinal hemorrhages or papilledema
Proven age of onset < 20 (especially if before puberty) or > 50
Unexplained hypokalemia
Negative family history of hypertension
Systolic-diastolic abdominal bruit, particularly in a young patient

lateralizing IVP cannot reliably exclude the presence of renovascular hypertension. A false-negative rate of 10 to 15 percent has also limited the utility of sequential radionuclide scanning and *intravenous* digital subtraction angiography [8].

It is possible, however, that the accuracy of renal scanning can be substantially improved by the prior administration of a converting enzyme inhibitor. Diminishing the formation of angiotensin II can increase the likelihood of a lateralizing scan by enhancing the difference in filtration rate between the two kidneys [9]: the glomerular filtration rate (GFR) tends to rise in the nonstenotic kidney because flow is enhanced, whereas it frequently falls in the stenotic kidney because maintenance of the intraglomerular pressure distal to the stenosis requires the vasoconstrictor effect of angiotensin II on the efferent arteriole [10]. The role of the converting enzyme inhibitor–*GFR scan* remains to be defined. If the patient is not already taking a converting enzyme inhibitor, diuretic therapy should first be discontinued for 3 to 5 days to minimize the risk of first-dose hypotension.

Measurement of the plasma renin activity under controlled conditions has been proposed as an alternative to the aforementioned radiologic screening procedures. As an example, the change in the plasma renin activity can be determined 1 hour after the administration of 25 mg of captopril [11]. Patients with renal artery stenosis have a marked rise in the plasma renin activity versus a relatively small elevation in patients with essential hypertension. This difference may be related to enhanced sensitivity of the stenotic kidney to a reduction in the systemic BP. However, the accuracy of this test is limited by a low-sodium diet and diuretic therapy, both of which must be discontinued for at least 1 to 2 weeks. Furthermore, some risk may be involved as some patients have an acute reduction in BP that can exceed 50 mm Hg.

In summary, there is at this time no safe and sufficiently accurate noninvasive radiologic or serologic screening test that, if negative, can reliably exclude the diagnosis of renal artery stenosis. Thus, the *clinical index of suspicion* remains the primary determinant of the extent of the work-up. A renal arteriogram or *intraarterial* digital subtraction angiogram (both of which can be performed in the outpatient setting) should be the initial test when the history is strongly suggestive of secondary hypertension (as with an acute rise in BP over a previously stable value or severe or refractory hypertension). A GFR scan (with prior converting enzyme inhibitor therapy) or intravenous digital subtraction angiogram can be used if the history is only moderately suggestive, with further evaluation being performed if a positive result is obtained.

RENAL VEIN RENIN LEVELS. Documenting the presence of a renal arterial lesion does not prove that the stenosis is responsible for the elevation in BP. The *physiologic importance* of the stenosis has been most often assessed by simultaneous measurement of the plasma renin activity in blood from each of the renal veins. Renin secretion should be increased in the stenotic kidney but suppressed by the hypertension in the contralateral kidney. The criteria for a positive test are the following [12]:

1. The renal venous renin activity in the stenotic kidney is more than 1.5 times that in the contralateral kidney.
2. Suppression of renin secretion in the nonstenotic kidney can be demonstrated by a venous-arterial difference in plasma renin activity that is close to zero. Arterial renin activity can be estimated from a sample obtained from the infrarenal inferior vena cava, since the extrarenal circulations do not secrete or metabolize renin. Contralateral suppression is considered to be present if the ratio of the renal vein to inferior vena cava renin activity is ⩽ 1.2.

The frequency of normalization or a marked reduction in BP following correction of unilateral renal artery stenosis is over 90 percent if there are lateralizing renal vein renins [12]. In many studies, however, a positive response to percutaneous angioplasty or surgery also occurs in 50 to 75 percent of patients with a nonlateralizing renal venous study [12]. A variety of methodologic and technical problems (such as the effect of concurrent antihypertensive therapy on renin release and assay or collection errors) may explain these findings. In addition, the high success rate in patients with nonlateralizing findings probably represents in part selection bias, since only those patients with a strong clinical history were likely to have undergone correction of the stenosis. Nevertheless, it is hard to escape the conclusion that renal vein renin determinations are not sufficiently sensitive; thus, *a negative test should not preclude correction of the stenosis* if the history is highly suggestive of secondary hypertension.

Renal vein renin measurements may be more helpful in patients with *bilateral* renal artery stenosis. The kidney with the higher renal vein renin activity probably is more ischemic and should be corrected first.

Treatment

There are three forms of therapy that can be used in renovascular hypertension: antihypertensive medications and correction of the stenosis by either percutaneous transluminal angioplasty or surgery [13–17]. The choice among these modalities is dependent on a variety of factors, including the cause of the stenosis (atherosclerosis versus fibromuscular dysplasia), the presence of unilateral or bilateral involvement, the ability of

Table 14-4. Factors determining response to correction of renal artery
stenosis by angioplasty or surgery

Factor	Favorable	Less favorable
Cause	Fibromuscular dysplasia	Atherosclerosis
Duration of hypertension	< 5 years	> 5 years
Degree of involvement	Unilateral	Bilateral
Degree of stenosis	Partial	Complete
Renal vein renins	Lateralizing	Nonlateralizing

medical therapy to control the BP with minimal side effects, and the patient's overall
health (Table 14-4).

Medical Therapy
Antihypertensive medications are frequently able to control the BP in patients with
renovascular hypertension. Converting enzyme inhibitors, either alone or with concomitant diuretic therapy, are particularly effective, a finding that is consistent with the
primary role of angiotensin II in this setting [14]. There are, however, two potential
problems with medical treatment: *progression of the stenosis* and *renal failure*.

Serial observations in patients with atherosclerotic lesions suggest that progressive
stenosis occurs in 45 to 60 percent (within 4–7 years), despite adequate control of the
BP [18]. Furthermore, total occlusion develops in 10 to 15 percent of all arteries and in
up to 40 percent of those with greater than a 75 percent narrowing of the vascular lumen. In some patients with bilateral disease, the decline in renal perfusion is so marked
that maintenance dialysis is required unless the stenoses can be corrected [19]. In comparison, the course appears to be much more benign in fibromuscular dysplasia: progression occurs in approximately one-third of patients but total occlusion is unusual
[18].

Despite the efficacy of converting enzyme inhibitors, their use is occasionally limited
by the development of acute renal failure in patients with bilateral disease or unilateral
stenosis in a solitary functioning kidney. [13,14]. When the systemic BP is lowered toward normal, the pressure distal to the stenosis that is perfusing the glomeruli tends to
fall below normal. In this setting, maintenance of the GFR is dependent on angiotensin
II, which raises the intraglomerular pressure by constricting the efferent arteriole.
Blocking this response with a converting enzyme inhibitor can, therefore, lead to a decline in renal function in 30 to 60 percent of patients. This is most likely to occur with
concurrent diuretic therapy since the associated volume depletion makes the glomerular
filtration rate more angiotensin II–dependent [20].

These observations do not mean that converting enzyme inhibitors are contraindicated in patients with bilateral renovascular disease. Most patients will have an excellent antihypertensive response without an important decrease in renal function [14].
Furthermore, the renal failure is readily reversible by discontinuing the diuretic [20] or,
if necessary, the converting enzyme inhibitor.

It is also important to appreciate that the autoregulatory response can protect the
GFR only over a limited pressure range, even in the presence of angiotensin II. As a
result, *any antihypertensive drug* can impair renal function if the bilateral stenoses are
sufficiently severe or if there is an excessive drop in the systemic BP [21].

Therapy with a converting enzyme inhibitor can also have a deleterious effect in unilateral renal artery stenosis. This problem is often masked because the presence of the
contralateral kidney usually prevents any decline in renal function [14]. If, however, a
GFR scan is performed before and after therapy with a converting enzyme inhibitor, up
to 50 percent of patients with unilateral disease will have a nearly complete cessation
of filtration in the stenotic kidney [22]. The long-term importance of this finding is un-

clear; in animals, prolonged hypofiltration eventually leads to irreversible tubular atrophy and interstitial fibrosis [23].

Percutaneous Angioplasty
Percutaneous transluminal angioplasty has the potential advantage of allowing nonsurgical correction of the stenosis [15]. This procedure is most effective in fibromuscular dysplasia, curing the hypertension in 50 to 80 percent and lowering the BP in most of the remaining patients [15,24]. Its efficacy is substantially lower in atherosclerotic disease, however. The cure rate with unilateral renal artery stenosis is only about 30 percent, with up to 50 percent having no fall in BP. Furthermore, recurrent stenosis and hypertension may occur in 5 to 50 percent of successful studies.

The antihypertensive response is largely determined by whether or not the vessel can be dilated [15]. The optimal lesion is partially occluding, noncalcified, and in the main renal artery. Ostial and totally occluded lesions are generally *resistant to dilation,* and angioplasty should probably not be attempted in this setting.

Percutaneous angioplasty should also be avoided in most patients with bilateral atherosclerotic renovascular disease. The success rate is only about 10 percent [15], and there is a significant risk of inducing an irreversible decline in renal function due to atheroembolic disease.

Complications occur in 5 to 15 percent of patients following percutaneous angioplasty. These are usually not serious but can include radiocontrast media-induced acute renal failure, atheroemboli, renal artery dissection or thrombosis, and rarely, rupture of the balloon or vessel [15].

Surgery
The stenotic lesion can usually be successfully bypassed by surgery. Cure or improvement in the hypertension occurs in 65 to 90 percent of patients [13,16,17]. The response varies within subgroups, however, as depicted in Table 14-4. The unfavorable effect of prolonged hypertension, for example, is probably related to the development of nephrosclerosis in the contralateral kidney that is chronically perfused at a high pressure [25].

Surgery may also be performed for a second reason in *bilateral* renal artery stenosis: *preservation of renal function.* In patients with progressive renal insufficiency, the GFR can be stabilized and often improved by correction of the stenoses. Even patients who initially require dialysis frequently recover enough function to allow dialysis to be discontinued [19]. In general, only the more severely stenotic kidney (as identified from the arteriogram or renal vein renin levels) is corrected at the initial operation to minimize the operative risk. An exception may occur in patients in whom one of the kidneys is markedly atrophic with a totally occluded artery. In this setting, unilateral nephrectomy plus bypass on the other side can be performed at the same time.

The risk of surgery is dependent on the patient's age and the presence or absence of other cardiovascular disease. Healthy young patients with fibromuscular dysplasia have very little operative morbidity. In comparison, older patients with diffuse atherosclerosis are at higher risk, with a mortality rate between 2 and 9 percent [13,16,17].

Recommendations
The optimal therapy for renovascular hypertension is uncertain because each of the therapeutic modalities has disadvantages in selected patients. The recommendations in Table 14-5 attempt to define the procedure that is likely to be both effective and safe with the different forms of renovascular disease. Percutaneous angioplasty, for example, is the preferred therapy in unilateral or bilateral fibromuscular dysplasia: it is highly effective in this condition, has little morbidity, and lifelong medical therapy is less desirable in these typically young patients [15,24].

Probably the greatest controversy concerns the preferred therapy for unilateral atherosclerotic renal artery stenosis. There are, at present, no definitive studies comparing the outcomes with medical therapy, percutaneous angioplasty, or surgery. Recent preliminary data confirm older observations that, despite control of the BP with antihypertensive medications, progressive stenosis (as evidenced by a decrease in renal size or a rise in the plasma creatinine concentration) occurs in up to 40 percent of cases [26]. These findings suggest that surgery or, depending on the anatomy of the lesion, angio-

Table 14-5. Preferred therapy in renovascular hypertension

Setting	Therapy
Fibromuscular dysplasia	Percutaneous angioplasty.
Atherosclerosis	
Bilateral with declining renal function	Surgery, if operative candidate. Angioplasty less likely to be successful and increased risk of atheroemboli.
Bilateral with stable renal function	Medical therapy can be tried, with careful monitoring due to risk of progressive stenosis. Surgery if antihypertensive therapy is unsuccessful or leads to renal insufficiency.
Unilateral	Medical therapy can be tried, preferably with a converting enyzme inhibitor; posttreatment GFR scan should be obtained to assess function of stenotic kidney.
	Angioplasty (with partial, nonostial lesion) or surgery if patient preference, failure of medical therapy, or evidence of progressive disease such as a decrease in renal size or a rise in the plasma creatinine concentration.

plasty is preferable in relatively low-risk younger patients (below the age of 50); in contrast, medical therapy, beginning with a converting enzyme inhibitor and (if necessary) a diuretic, can be tried in patients who are older or who refuse an invasive procedure. Lack of BP control, loss of filtration in the stenotic kidney [22], or evidence of progressive stenosis [18,26] indicate the need for a corrective procedure.

References

1. Simon, N, Franklin, SS, Bleifer, KH, Maxwell, MH. Clinical characteristics of renovascular hypertension. *J Am Med Assoc* 220:1209, 1972.
2. Levin, A, Blaufox, MD, Castle, H, Entwisle, G, Langford, H. Apparent prevalence of curable hypertension in Hypertension Detection and Follow-up Program. *Arch Intern Med* 145:424, 1985.
3. Davis, BA, Crook, JE, Vestal, RE, Oakes, JA. Prevalence of renovascular hypertension in patients with grade III or IV hypertensive retinopathy. *N Engl J Med* 301:1273, 1979.
4. Ying, CY, Tifft, CP, Gavras, H, Chobanian, AV. Renal revascularization in the azotemic hypertensive patient resistant to therapy. *N Engl J Med* 311:1070, 1984.
5. Bravo, EL, Gifford, RW, Jr. Pheochromocytoma: Diagnosis, localization, and management. *N Engl J Med* 311:1298, 1984.
6. Melby, JC. Primary aldosteronism. *Kidney Int* 26:769, 1984.
7. Gold, EM. The Cushing's syndromes: Changing views of diagnosis and treatment. *Ann Intern Med* 90:829, 1979.
8. Havey, RJ, Krumlovsky, F, del Greco, F, Martin, HG. Screening for renovascular hypertension. Is renal digital-subtraction angiography the preferred noninvasive test? *J Am Med Assoc* 254:388, 1985.
9. Fommei, E, Ghione, S, Palla, L, Mosca, F, Ferrari, M, Palombo, C, Giaconi, S, Gazetti, P, Donato, L. Renal scintigraphic captopril test in the diagnosis of renovascular hypertension. *Hypertension* 10:212, 1987.
10. Huang, WC, Navar, LG. Effects of unclipping and converting enzyme inhibition on bilateral renal function in Goldblatt hypertensive rats. *Kidney Int* 23:816, 1983.

11. Muller, FB, Sealey, JE, Case, AB, Atlas, SA, Pickering, TG, Pecker, MS, Preibisz, JJ, Laragh, JH. The captopril test for identifying renovascular disease in hypertensive patients. *Am J Med* 80:633, 1986.
12. Rudnick, MR, Maxwell, MH. Diagnosis of renovascular hypertension: Limitations of renin assays. In RG Narins (Ed), *Controversies in Nephrology*. New York: Churchill Livingstone, 1984.
13. Rose, BD. *Pathophysiology of Renal Disease* (2nd ed). New York: McGraw-Hill, 1987. Pp 563-569.
14. Franklin, SS, Smith, RD. Comparison of effects of enalapril plus hydrochlorothiazide versus standard triple therapy on renal function in renovascular hypertension. *Am J Med* 79(suppl 3C):14, 1985.
15. Sos, TA, Pickering, TG, Sniderman, K, Sadekni, S, Case, DB, Silane, MF, Vaughan, ED, Jr, Laragh, JH. Percutaneous transluminal angioplasty in renovascular hypertension due to atheroma or fibromuscular dysplasia. *N Engl J Med* 309:274, 1983.
16. Novick, AC, Straffon, RA. The current status of surgery for renovascular disease. *Am J Kid Dis* 1:188, 1981.
17. Stanley, JC, Fry, WJ. Surgical treatment of renovascular hypertension. *Arch Surg* 112:1291, 1977.
18. Pohl, MA, Novick, AC. Natural history of atherosclerotic and fibrous renal artery disease: Clinical implications. *Am J Kid Dis* 5:A120, 1985.
19. Novick, AC, Textor, SC, Bodie, B, Khauli, RB. Revascularization to preserve renal function in patients with atherosclerotic renovascular disease. *Urol Clin N Am* 11:477, 1984.
20. Hricik, DE. Captopril induced renal insufficiency and the role of sodium balance. *Ann Intern Med* 103:222, 1985.
21. Textor, SC, Novick, AC, Tarazi, RC, Klimas, V, Vidt, DG, Pohl, M. Critical perfusion pressure for renal function in patients with bilateral atherosclerotic renal vascular disease. *Ann Intern Med* 102:308, 1985.
22. Wenting, GJ, Tan-Tjiong, HL, Derkx, FHM, de Bruyn, JHB, Man in't Veld, AJ. Split renal function after captopril in unilateral renal artery stenosis. *Br Med J* 288:886, 1984.
23. Michel, J-B, Dussaule, J-C, Choudat, L, Auzan, C, Nochy, D, Corvol, P, Menard, J. Effect of antihypertensive treatment in one-clip, two kidney hypertension in rats. *Kidney Int* 29:1011, 1986.
24. Council on Scientific Affairs. Percutaneous transluminal angioplasty. *J Am Med Assoc* 251:764, 1984.
25. Hughes, JS, Dove, HG, Gifford, RW, Jr, Feinstein, AF. Duration of blood pressure elevation in accurately predicting surgical cure of renovascular hypertension. *Am Heart J* 101:408, 1981.
26. Dean, RH. Comparison of medical and surgical treatment of renovascular hypertension. *Nephron* 44 (suppl 1):101, 1986.

15. HYPERTENSIVE URGENCIES AND EMERGENCIES

The majority of patients with hypertension have a relatively mild elevation in systemic blood pressure (BP). However, severe hypertension (usually defined as a diastolic BP above 115 mm Hg) is observed in about 10 percent of cases [1]. Many such patients will be asymptomatic, but a *hypertensive emergency* is considered to be present if there is new or progressive vascular damage that requires a prompt reduction in BP (within minutes or hours) to prevent irreversible injury or death. In comparison, severe hypertension that is associated with minimal or no obvious acute vascular injury, but that may put the patient at risk if the BP is not controlled within hours to days, constitutes a *hypertensive urgency* (Table 15-1).

Table 15-1. Hypertensive emergencies and urgencies

Emergencies
    Malignant hypertension
    Hypertensive encephalopathy
    Intracranial hemorrhage
    Acute aortic dissection
    Acute pulmonary edema with hypertension
    Pheochromocytoma crisis
    Severe preeclampsia or eclampsia (see Chap. 44)
Urgencies
    Uncontrolled hypertension in patients requiring emergency surgery
    Severe postoperative hypertension
    Withdrawal of antihypertensive medications
    Acute head injury
    Severe hypertension without acute end-organ damage

Hypertensive Emergencies

Any condition capable of causing hypertension may be associated with a hypertensive emergency. It is usually the *level* of BP that is the most important determinant of organ damage. Thus, most patients with malignant hypertension have a diastolic BP above 125 to 130 mm Hg. However, the *rate of rise* in BP may also be important, particularly in patients who were previously normotensive as, for example, occurs in preeclampsia.

Malignant Hypertension and Hypertensive Encephalopathy

Malignant hypertension is generally characterized by the presence of extreme hypertension complicated by fibrinoid necrosis that primarily involves the arterioles and capillaries. These changes are most often manifested in the retina by hemorrhages, exudates, and, in some cases, papilledema, and in the kidney by acute renal insufficiency and an active urine sediment containing red cells and granular and cellular casts [2-4].

The primary event in the development of these lesions is damage to the vascular wall by a marked and often rapid rise in BP [4]. Disruption of the vascular endothelium then allows plasma constituents (including fibrinoid material) to enter the vascular wall, leading to narrowing or obliteration of the vascular lumen. Renal vascular damage can also contribute to worsening of the hypertension, because of activation of the renin-angiotensin system by renal ischemia.

The likelihood of developing fibrinoid necrosis is related to the degree to which the systemic pressure is transmitted to the capillary. As the BP begins to rise, the capillary is initially protected by constriction of the precapillary sphincter, a process called *autoregulation*. With marked elevations in BP, however, autoregulation eventually fails, leading to intracapillary hypertension and vascular damage [5,6]. In addition to the absolute BP level, the degree of elevation above the previous baseline is also important. Thus, even moderate hypertension can produce fibrinoid necrosis in a previously normotensive patient; this may explain why malignant hypertension can occur in preeclampsia or acute glomerulonephritis with diastolic pressures as low as 100 mm Hg [5]. Failure of autoregulation also appears to be involved in the development of *hypertensive encephalopathy* [6], which is associated with fibrinoid necrosis in the cerebral vessels.

The physical examination in malignant hypertension typically reveals severe hypertension, retinal lesions and, if hypertensive encephalopathy is present, nonlocalizing signs and symptoms, such as restlessness, headache, nausea, vomiting, or confusion. Focal neurologic findings may also be present in some cases [7]. These neurologic abnormalities are usually *reversible within 24 to 48 hours* with effective antihypertensive therapy, although the retinal hemorrhages and exudates may not completely resolve for weeks or months.

TREATMENT. Malignant hypertension should be treated in the hospital where the BP can be rapidly reduced and where damage to target organs can be closely monitored. The goal of therapy is to reduce the diastolic BP to a safe level (between 100 and 105 mm Hg) rather than to return the pressure to normal, since perfusion to vital organs may be compromised by the luminal narrowing produced by the acute vascular disease [7,8].

Parenteral therapy is usually initiated with either nitroprusside or diazoxide, with conventional oral therapy being added once the BP is controlled (Table 15-2). Oral therapy alone may be successful but its use should be limited to those patients with malignant hypertension who are less acutely ill and who may, therefore, be treated as a hypertensive urgency (Table 15-3).

In comparison, hypertensive encephalopathy is an acute, life-threatening illness that requires immediate BP reduction. Nitroprusside is the drug of choice in this setting, since its very short duration of action allows minute-to-minute control of the BP. If, for example, the neurologic findings deteriorate as the BP falls, the dose of nitroprusside can be lowered, thereby allowing the BP to rise to a level that maintains cerebral function. Further neurologic evaluation (such as CT scanning) should also be instituted, since a thrombotic stroke or an intracerebral hemorrhage should be excluded.

Establishing the cause of the neurologic dysfunction is important because the indications for therapy are somewhat different for a thrombotic stroke [4]. The BP commonly rises shortly *after* a stroke, presumably reflecting an appropriate attempt to maintain blood flow to borderline ischemic areas [9]. Thus, reducing the BP in this setting can cause further ischemia and an increase in the size of the stroke. Since the level of hypertension at the time of the ischemic event poses little acute risk to the patient, antihypertensive therapy should be withheld unless the patient has heart failure, a diastolic BP above 120 to 130 mm Hg, or there is evidence of hypertensive encephalopathy [10].

Hypertension and Intracerebral Bleeding
In contrast to the hypertensive patient with an ischemic stroke, an intracerebral hemorrhage requires a *rapid, but controlled reduction in BP* to avoid further bleeding [10]. There is, however, still a risk of exacerbating the ischemia in surrounding brain tissue and increasing the neurologic deficit. Thus, nitroprusside is again the agent of choice, pending the preferred treatment of surgical decompression.

Acute Aortic Dissection
Dissection of the aorta is initiated by a tear in the aortic intima through which blood flows into the aortic media, ultimately resulting in separation of the intima from the adventitia. The principal cause of mortality in this disorder is not the intimal tear itself; rather, it is caused by aortic rupture usually into the pericardial space or left pleural cavity or by occlusion of a vessel supplying a major organ [11].

A dissecting aneurysm is most commonly observed in the elderly male patient with chronic hypertension, who typically presents with severe, persistent chest or back pain [11]. Asymmetric distal pulses, focal neurologic deficits, and oliguric renal failure also may be present, depending on the level of dissection and possible occlusion of a major artery.

The radiologic diagnosis of acute aortic dissection is suggested by a double aortic contour or widening of the mediastinum on chest x ray. Although aortography is the definitive test to define the extent of aortic disease, echocardiography (accuracy of 70–90%) and contrast-enhanced CT scanning or magnetic resonance imaging (both of which have a diagnostic accuracy of 90%) allow rapid, noninvasive diagnosis of this disorder in most patients [11].

TREATMENT. The initial short-term management of a suspected acute aortic dissection consists of prompt reduction of BP to the lowest level that will still maintain adequate cerebral, coronary, and renal perfusion. However, direct vasodilators such as nitroprusside or diazoxide *should not be used alone*, since these drugs reflexly stimulate ventricular contractility, thereby increasing the aortic shearing forces and possibly aggravating the dissection. The most commonly used regimen consists of nitroprusside plus a β-adrenergic blocker [11]. Intravenous labetolol or trimethaphan, in comparison, can be used as monotherapy since they directly diminish β-receptor activity (Table 15-2).

Table 15-2. Parenteral therapy of hypertensive urgencies and emergencies

Drug	Onset	Duration	Comments
VASODILATORS			
Nitroprusside	Seconds	3–5 min	Thiocyanate toxicity if prolonged use (> 48h), especially if renal failure. Should not be used without a β-blocker in acute aortic dissection and should not be used in pregnancy (toxic to fetus). Requires careful BP monitoring.
Diazoxide	1–5 min	4–24 h	Extravasation can be caustic since pH = 11. Risk of acute hypotension can be reduced by using lower (30–75mg) doses initially. Should not be given if angina, acute myocardial infarction, dissecting aneurysm, or acute CVA. Since peak action occurs in about 15–30 minutes, minute-to-minute BP monitoring not usually necessary. A loop diuretic should also be given to prevent volume retention that can limit drug effectiveness.
Nitroglycerine	1–5 min	3–5 min	May be especially useful in hypertension complicating acute myocardial infarction or after cardiac surgery.
ADRENERGIC INHIBITORS			
Trimethaphan	1–5 min	10 min	Can be used *alone* for acute aortic dissection. Tachyphylaxis common.
Labetolol	10–30 min	2–4 h	β-blocking activity dominates with increasing plasma concentration.
Phentolamine	5–30 min	1–2 h	Specifically indicated for pheochromocytoma or tyramine-induced catecholamine crises.

Table 15-3. Acute nonparenteral therapy for hypertensive urgencies

Drug	Dose	Onset	Comments
ADRENERGIC INHIBITORS			
Clonidine	0.1–0.2 mg PO initially; then 0.05–0.1 mg/1–2h, up to 0.7 mg total	30–120 min	Sedation prominent; hypotension can occur.
CALCIUM BLOCKERS			
Nifedipine	2.5–10.0 mg sublingual or orally	5–15 min	Can precipitate angina or myocardial infarction if hypotensive response is excessive.
Diltiazem	30–60 mg orally	15–60 min	Less acute drop in BP than with nifedipine.
CONVERTING ENZYME INHIBITORS			
Captopril	6.25–12.5 mg sublingual or orally	15 min	Renin-dependent states (such as malignant hypertension) generally most responsive; hypotension can occur, particularly if volume depleted.
VASODILATORS			
Isosorbide dinitrate	10 mg sublingual	15–30 min	Hypotension uncommon. No reflex tachycardia.

Once the BP has been stabilized, subsequent definitive treatment can be planned. Surgery should be considered when there is an acute proximal aortic lesion or when there is major vascular occlusion; more distal dissections can be treated either medically or surgically [11].

Hypertension and Acute Left Ventricular Failure
When severe hypertension develops in or causes congestive heart failure, the increased afterload raises myocardial oxygen requirements. Immediate BP control in this setting reduces the risk of myocardial ischemia while it simultaneously improves both cardiac output and the symptoms of pulmonary congestion.

TREATMENT. Prompt BP reduction can be achieved in this setting with antihypertensive agents given intravenously (nitroprusside or nitroglycerine), orally (calcium channel blockers or converting enzyme inhibitors), or sublingually (isosorbide dinitrate) [1,8,12]. In comparison, diazoxide or hydralazine should not be used since they increase cardiac work by reflexly stimulating both the heart rate and myocardial contractility [13]. It is also important to remember that an excessive reduction in BP can *exacerbate coronary ischemia or cause myocardial infarction,* a problem that has been observed, for example, with nifedipine [14].

In contrast to therapy in left ventricular failure, there is controversy about the importance of acute BP reduction in the patient with *myocardial ischemia or infarction, but without heart failure.* It has been suggested that moderate to severe hypertension in the setting of acute myocardial infarction is transient and does not exert any adverse effect on the cardiac course [15]. However, other studies have observed a significantly higher mortality rate and a higher incidence of cardiac failure when severe systolic hypertension complicates an acute infarction [16]. It seems reasonable, therefore, to reduce the BP gradually in this setting with intravenous nitroprusside or nitroglycerine, being careful to avoid a decrease in diastolic BP below 90 to 100 mm Hg, since a further reduction might compromise coronary perfusion.

Pheochromocytoma Crisis
Pheochromocytoma is a rare cause of secondary hypertension that may be associated with acute, severe hypertension, occasionally with minimal or no elevation in BP between episodes.

TREATMENT. The intravenous α-adrenergic blocker, phentolamine, has been the antihypertensive agent of choice in patients with catecholamine-induced hypertension. Oral prazosin is also useful but may not produce adequate acute control [17]. Effective alternatives to pure α-blocking agents include intravenous labetolol and nitroprusside.

It must be emphasized that the use of β-blockers alone in patients with catecholamine-induced hypertension can result in *unopposed α-adrenergic stimulation* of vascular smooth muscle, possibly causing further vasoconstriction and more severe hypertension. As a result, β-blockers (except labetolol, which has concomitant α- and β-blocking activity) should be avoided in this setting unless tachyarrhythmias are present, in which case an α-blocking agent should be administered first.

Hypertensive Urgencies
Hypertensive urgencies are conditions in which a markedly increased BP has not yet caused immediate harm to the patient, but where BP control over a period of hours or days is desired to prevent the development of end-organ damage (Table 15-1). BP reduction in this setting often does not require intravenous therapy, but the potential adverse effects of hypertension are too serious for the BP to be managed routinely.

Preoperative Hypertension
Uncontrolled hypertension in the patient requiring emergency surgery is a fairly common occurrence. In the absence of significant coronary or myocardial dysfunction, the BP elevation does not appear to contribute to the cardiovascular risk of *noncardiac* surgery [18]. As a result, it is important to avoid an excessive preoperative reduction of BP in patients in whom the duration of hypertension is unknown. If, for example, the BP is

acutely reduced to normotensive levels in the patient with chronic, poorly controlled hypertension, decreased perfusion to vital organs may ensue.

When intraoperative BP control is required, the use of an agent that can give minute-to-minute control, such as nitroprusside, is often desirable, since general anesthesia can cause wide swings in the BP. This drug has the additional advantage of rapid clearance in the event of a sudden drop in BP during surgery.

The severely hypertensive patient who is scheduled for immediate *arteriography* presents a relatively unique problem. Acute BP control is helpful in this setting to minimize the risk of uncontrolled bleeding. A reasonable approach is to begin by placing the patient in a quiet, darkened room for 30 to 60 minutes before the procedure, since the BP may fall spontaneously. In a study of 84 patients, for example, 23 who had initial diastolic BPs of 135 mm Hg experienced a mean reduction in arterial pressure of about 30 mm Hg[19]. Oral agents can then be administered if the BP remains at a level that precludes safe arterial puncture. A calcium blocker is usually effective in reducing the BP but nifedipine may result in a hypotensive response in some patients [14]; diltiazem, which is more slowly absorbed, may be less likely to cause this problem. Alternatively, sublingual isosorbide dinitrate is an effective acute antihypertensive agent, and hypotension appears to be infrequent [12]. Angiotensin converting enzyme inhibitors also may be used, but they can produce marked hypotension in some patients, particularly those who are volume depleted with a high plasma renin activity [20]. Finally, nitroprusside can be used if other modalities fail to achieve adequate BP control.

Postoperative Hypertension
Postoperative hypertension, which may be severe, is observed in about one-third of patients who have undergone open-heart surgery. This problem usually begins within the first 2 hours and lasts 4 to 6 hours [21]. The elevation in BP appears to reflect an increase in sympathetic activity [22], which may act both directly and by stimulation of the renin-angiotensin system [23]. Severe hypertension in this setting has been successfully treated with nitroglycerine, nitroprusside, calcium channel blockers, and β-blockers.

Hypertension may also develop after any surgical procedure if chronic antihypertensive therapy is discontinued preoperatively. When the hypertension is severe, the BP should be treated promptly to reduce the risk of acute organ damage [24]. Nitroprusside is usually administered in this setting because of its ability to be regulated closely and because patients in the early postoperative period often cannot take medications orally.

Rebound Hypertension After Withdrawal of Antihypertensive Drugs
In most patients, withdrawal of antihypertensive therapy causes a return of the BP to pretreatment levels; this can occur within a few days or take 1 year or more [25,26]. However, acute overshoot of the BP to above the baseline level, often with symptoms and signs of sympathetic overactivity, may be seen in patients who had been taking sympatholytic agents. This "discontinuation syndrome" is most commonly observed with clonidine [26,27] and may reflect upregulation of α-adrenergic receptors during the period of sympathetic blockade. The short duration of action of clonidine probably also contributes, since the drug effect rapidly dissipates. Longer-acting drugs, such as methyldopa, seem to be much less likely to produce this problem.

The consequences are somewhat different with abrupt discontinuation of β-blocker therapy. In this setting, increased β-adrenergic receptor activity can lead to accelerated angina, myocardial infarction, or sudden death, changes that are again thought to result from receptor upregulation [28].

TREATMENT.   A mild increase in BP does not generally require acute therapy. More severe elevations, especially if associated with evidence of a catecholamine surge, should be treated promptly to prevent end-organ damage.

The ideal therapy is prevention by gradually tapering antihypertensive medications, although this does not offer absolute protection [29]. Once the withdrawal syndrome appears, reinstitution of the previously administered drug usually results in rapid resolution of symptoms. If this is unsuccessful or cannot be done, therapy with another sympatholytic agent or a vasodilator should be instituted (Tables 15-2 and 15-3). β-blockers should not be used alone, since unopposed α-adrenergic stimulation can lead to an exacerbation of the hypertension.

Acute Head Injury

Severe head injuries are commonly associated with acute, severe hypertension. This response may be mediated by the medullary vasomotor centers, which, in the presence of ischemia, cause reflex activation of the sympathetic nervous system [7,30].

The dilemma in these patients is whether to lower the BP acutely, since treatment could aggravate an existing reduction in cerebral perfusion. On the other hand, sustained hypertension could increase the tendency toward cerebral edema. As a result, rigid recommendations cannot be made, and the goal of therapy, if instituted, should be to *gradually* reduce the diastolic BP to, but not below, 100 mm Hg.

Severe Hypertension without Acute End-Organ Damage

Some patients have severe hypertension (diastolic BP above 130–140 mm Hg) but no evidence of malignant hypertension or other life-threatening complications requiring parenteral therapy. In this setting, a controlled fall in BP that begins within a period of hours is a reasonable initial goal [1,31]. A variety of different medications have been used with some success, including 10 mg of sublingual or chewed nifedipine, 0.1 to 0.2 mg of oral clonidine (followed by 0.05–0.1 mg every 1–2 hours to a maximum of 0.7 mg), and 6.25 to 12.5 mg of oral captopril [1,4,31,32].

It is important to note, however, that these regimens can on occasion lead to an excessive antihypertensive response, occasionally producing coronary or cerebral ischemia or infarction [14,31]. As a result, it is probably safest to begin by having the patient lie in a quiet, dark room for 1 hour, a procedure that will lead to a significant fall in BP out of the dangerous range in many patients [19]. Ten mg of sublingual isosorbide dinitrate or 30 mg of oral diltiazem can also be given at this time, since hypotension is unusual with these agents [12]. Nifedipine, clonidine, or intravenous labetolol, which lowers the BP slowly, can be added if severe hypertension persists. Nifedipine, which has the most rapid onset of action, should be begun in low doses (2.5–5.0 mg; ¼–½ of the contents of the liquid in a 10-mg capsule) to minimize the risk of acute hypotension [14]. The dose can then be increased in 5-mg increments, if necessary, to a maximum of 10 to 20 mg. Conventional oral therapy should be initiated once the BP is controlled.

References

1. Houston, M. Hypertensive emergencies and urgencies: Pathophysiology and clinical aspects. *Am Heart J* 111:205, 1986.
2. Ramos, O. Malignant hypertension: The Brazilian experience, *Kidney Int* 26:209, 1984.
3. Kincaid-Smith, P, McMichael, J, Murphy, EA. The clinical course and pathology of hypertension with papilloedema. *Q J Med* 27:117, 1958.
4. Rose, BD. *Pathophysiology of Renal Disease*, 2d ed, New York: McGraw Hill, 1987, chap. 11.
5. Koch-Weser, J. Hypertensive emergencies, *N Engl J Med* 290:211, 1974.
6. Johansson, B, Strandgaard, S, Lassen, NA. On the pathogenesis of hypertensive encephalopathy: The hypertensive "breakthrough" of autoregulation of cerebral blood flow with forced vasodilatation, flow increase, and blood-brain-barrier damage, *Circ Res* 334:167, 1974.
7. Ram, CV, Hyman, D. Hypertensive crises. *J Intensive Care Med* 2:151, 1987.
8. Vidt, DG. Current concepts in treatment of hypertensive emergencies. *Am Heart J* 111:220, 1986.

9. Wallace, JD, Levy, LL. Blood pressure after stroke *J Am Med Assoc* 246:2177, 1981.

10. Lavin, P. Management of hypertension in patients with acute stroke. *Arch Intern Med* 146:66, 1986.

11. DeSanctis, RW, Doroghazi, RM, Austen, WG, Buckley, MJ. Aortic dissection. *N Engl J Med* 317:1060, 1987.

12. Fontanet, H, Garcia, JC, del Rio, J, Martinez-Maldonado, M. The use of isosorbide dinitrate in the treatment of severe, uncontrolled hypertension. *Arch Intern Med* 147:426, 1987.

13. Kumar, GK, Dastoor, FC, Robayo, JR, Razzaque, MA. Side effects of diazoxide. *J Am Med Assoc* 235:275, 1976.

14. O'Mailia, J, Sander, GE, Giles, TD. Nifedipine-associated myocardial ischemia or infarction in the treatment of hypertensive urgencies. *Ann Intern Med* 107:185, 1987.

15. Gibson, TAC. Blood pressure levels in acute myocardial infarction. *Am Heart J* 96:475, 1978.

16. Fox, KM, Tomlinson, JW, Portal, RW, Aber, CP. Prognostic significance of acute systolic hypertension after acute myocardial infarction. *Br Med J* 3:128, 1975.

17. Nicholson, JP, Vaughn, ED, Pickering, TG, Resnick, LM, Artusio, J, Kleinert, HD, Lopez-Overjero, JA, Laragh, JH. Pheochromocytoma and prazosin. *Ann Intern Med* 99:477, 1983.

18. Goldman, L. Cardiac risks and complications of noncardiac surgery. *Ann Intern Med* 98:504, 1983.

19. Nielsen, PE, Krogsgaard, A, McNair, A, Hilden, T. Emergency treatment of severe hypertension emulated in a randomized study: Effect of rest and furosemide and a randomized evaluation of chlorpromazine, dihydralazine and diazoxide. *Acta Med Scand* 208:473, 1980.

20. Hodsman, GP, Isles, CG, Murray, GD, Usherwood, TP, Webb, DJ, Robertson, JIS. Factors related to first dose hypotensive effect of captopril: Prediction and treatment. *Br Med J* 286:832, 1983.

21. Estafanous, FG, Tarazi, RC. Systemic arterial hypertension associated with cardiac surgery. *Am J Cardiol* 46:685, 1980.

22. Wallach, R, Karp, RB, Reves, JG, Oparil, S Smith, LR, James, TN. Pathogenesis of paroxysmal hypertension developing during and after coronary bypass surgery: A study of hemodynamic and humoral factors. *Am J Cardiol* 46:559, 1980.

23. Kaplan, NM. *Clinical Hypertension.* 4th ed, Baltimore: Williams and Wilkins, 1986. p. 442.

24. Katz, JD, Croneau, LH, Barash, PG. Postoperative hypertension: A hazard of abrupt cessation of antihypertensive medication in the preoperative period. *Am Heart J* 92:79, 1976.

25. Medical Research Council Working Party on Mild Hypertension. Course of blood pressure in mild hypertensives after withdrawal of long-term antihypertensive treatment. *Br Med J* 293:988, 1986.

26. Houston, MC. Abrupt cessation of treatment in hypertension: Consideration of clinical features, mechanisms, prevention, and management of the discontinuation syndrome. *Am Heart J* 102:415, 1981.

27. Metz, S, Klein, C, Morton, N. Rebound hypertension after discontinuation of transdermal clonidine therapy. *Am J Med* 82:17, 1987.

28. Lefkowitz, RJ, Caron, MG, Stiles, GL. Mechanisms of membrane-receptor regulation. Biochemical, physiological, and clinical insights derived from studies of the adrenergic receptors. *N Engl J Med* 310:1570, 1984.

29. Vanholder, R. Carpentier, J, Schurgers, M, Clement, DL. Rebound phenomenon during gradual withdrawal of clonidine. *Br Med J* 2:1138, 1977.

30. Clifton, GI, Robertson, CS, Kyper, K, Taylor, AA, Dhekne, RD, Grossman, RG. Cardiovascular response to severe head injury. *J Neurosurg* 59:447, 1983.

31. Anderson, RJ. Current concepts in treatment of hypertensive urgencies. *Am Heart J* 111:211, 1986.

32. Houston, MC. The comparative effects of clonidine hydrochloride and nifedipine in the treatment of hypertensive crisis. *Am Heart J* 115:152, 1988.

III. EVALUATION OF THE PATIENT WITH RENAL DISEASE

Patients with renal disease may present to the physician in a variety of ways. Some have symptoms that are directly referable to the kidney (flank pain, gross hematuria) or to associated extrarenal abnormalities (edema, hypertension, signs of uremia). Other patients are asymptomatic and are incidentally found to have an abnormal urinalysis or an elevated plasma creatinine concentration (P_{cr}).

Once renal disease is discovered, the primary goals are to establish the correct diagnosis and to assess and monitor the severity of the renal dysfunction. In addition to the history and physical examination, careful examination of the urine, particularly the urinalysis, is the major noninvasive tool available to the clinician. The urinalysis also may give some information about severity; in glomerular disease, for example, marked hematuria, red cell casts, and heavy proteinuria are likely to represent more severe disease than just mild hematuria (5–10 red blood cells/high power field) or mild proteinuria (1–2 + on the dipstick) alone. However, this relationship between the urinary findings and severity is not always present; the transition from acute glomerulonephritis to chronic disease with scarring is typically associated with decreased activity of the urine sediment that parallels the decline in glomerular inflammation.

This chapter will emphasize the diagnostic importance of the urinalysis, even in patients in whom there are no abnormal findings. The following chapter will then review the uses and limitations of the P_{cr} to estimate the glomerular filtration rate (GFR), the most commonly used method to assess severity and to monitor the course of the disease.

Etiology and Duration of Disease

The most common causes of renal disease (most of which are discussed separately in other sections of the book) are listed in Table 16-1, according to the commonly used "functional" classification: prerenal (decreased renal perfusion), postrenal (urinary tract obstruction), and renal (glomerular, vascular, tubular, interstitial).

As can be seen, the differential diagnosis can often be narrowed by knowing whether the disorder is acute or chronic. This can be done most accurately if past information is available. Chronic disease is most likely if, for example, the P_{cr} were 1.1 mg/dl 2 years ago, 1.6 mg/dl 1 year ago, and 2.3 mg/dl now. In comparison, a P_{cr} that begins to rise in the hospital is probably related to some event that had happened in the hospital. In patients in whom serial measurements have been obtained, the *day on which the P_{cr} began to rise can often be identified*. In this setting, either some acute insult happened on that day (such as the administration of radiocontrast media) or the cumulative effect of a nephrotoxin first became apparent (as with the chronic use of an aminoglycoside).

The initial distinction between acute and chronic is more difficult if previous data are not available. The history may, however, provide helpful information. A complaint of gross hematuria following an upper respiratory infection suggests an acute postinfectious glomerulonephritis. The presence of a low urine output (< 500 ml/day) also points toward an acute component since persistent oliguria rapidly leads to advanced renal failure.

Examination of the Urine

A complete examination of the urine consists of the urinalysis, estimation of the urine volume, and, in selected cases, measurement of the urine sodium concentration and osmolality. The urinalysis should always be performed on a fresh urine specimen that is examined within 30 to 60 minutes of voiding. A midstream specimen is adequate in men; in women, however, the external genitalia should first be cleaned to avoid contamination with vaginal secretions. The urine should be centrifuged at 3000 r/min for 3 to 5 minutes. The supernatant should then be carefully poured into a separate tube and the sediment completely resuspended by gently flicking the side of the tube. (When a large amount of sediment is present, 0.5 ml of urine can be added.) A small amount of sediment should be poured or transferred with a pipette onto a slide and covered with a

Table 16-1. Most common causes of renal disease

Prerenal
  True volume depletion
  Heart failure
  Hepatic cirrhosis (including the hepatorenal syndrome)
  Nonsteroidal anti-inflammatory drugs
  Bilateral renal artery stenosis (particularly after use of a converting enzyme
    inhibitor)
Postrenal (obstructive uropathy)
  Prostatic disease
  Pelvic or retroperitoneal malignancy
  Calculi
  Congenital abnormalities
Glomerular disease
  Glomerulonephritis
  Nephrotic syndrome
Vascular disease
  Acute
    Vasculitis
    Malignant hypertension
    Scleroderma
    Thromboembolic disease
  Chronic
    Nephrosclerosis
Tubular disease
  Acute
    Acute tubular necrosis
    Multiple myeloma
    Hypercalcemia
    Acute uric acid nephropathy
  Chronic
    Polycystic kidney disease
    Medullary sponge kidney
    Medullary cystic kidney disease
Interstitial disease
  Acute
    Interstitial nephritis (usually drug-induced)
    Pyelonephritis
  Chronic
    Pyelonephritis (due primarily to vesicoureteral reflux)
    Analgesic abuse

cover slip. Both the supernatant (which can be tested for protein, glucose, heme pigments, and concentration) and sediment are then ready for analysis.

Urinalysis
As depicted in Table 16-2, the value of the urinalysis lies in the association between different patterns of urinary findings and different renal diseases. In some, the changes are so characteristic that one or just a few diagnoses are suggested. As an example, the presence of red cell casts, heavy proteinuria, or lipiduria, or a combination of these is virtually diagnostic of glomerular disease or vasculitis. (The use of the urinalysis to help distinguish between the different forms of glomerular disease is reviewed in Chap. 25).

Even a normal or near-normal urinalysis is of diagnostic importance. If seen in a patient with chronic renal disease, for example, the most likely possibilities are prerenal disease, obstruction, tubular or interstitial diseases, and nephrosclerosis. At this point,

Table 16-2. Urinary findings and causes of renal disease

Urinary Findings	Etiology
Hematuria with red cell casts Heavy proteinuria (> 3.5 gm/ day or 50 mg/kg/day) Lipiduria	Any of these findings, singly or in combination, is virtually diagnostic of glomerular disease or vasculitis. The absence of these changes, however, does not exclude these diagnoses.
Renal tubular epithelial cells with granular and epithelial cell casts	In acute renal failure, strongly suggestive of acute tubular necrosis, although marked hyperbilirubinemia alone can produce similar findings.
Pyuria with white cell and granular or waxy casts and no or mild proteinuria	Suggestive of tubular or interstitial disease or obstruction.
Hematuria and pyuria with no or variable casts (excluding red cell casts)	May be seen in glomerular disease, vasculitis, obstruction, renal infarction, or acute interstitial nephritis. The last disorder may be associated with eosinophils in the urine.
Hematuria alone	Suggestive of vasculitis or obstruction in acute renal failure. May also be found with mild glomerular disease, polycystic kidney disease, or with extrarenal problems such as prostatic disease, calculi, or tumor (see Chap. 18).
Normal or near-normal (few cells with little or no casts or proteinuria; hyaline casts are not an abnormal finding)	Acute: may be found in prerenal disease, obstruction, hypercalcemia, myeloma,* some cases of acute tubular necrosis, or vascular diseases with glomerular ischemia but not infarction (scleroderma, atheroemboli, rare cases of polyarteritis nodosa). Chronic: may be seen in prerenal disease, obstruction, tubular or interstitial disorders, and nephrosclerosis.
Pyuria alone	Usually indicative of urinary tract infection (including tuberculosis); may occur with tubulointerstitial diseases.

*The dipstick is likely to be negative in multiple myeloma since it detects albumin but not immunoglobulin light chains.

knowledge of the characteristics of each of these disorders can further narrow the differential diagnosis. Prerenal disease is typically associated with a urine sodium concentration below 20 meq/L, a fractional excretion of sodium below 1 percent, a urine osmolality that may exceed 500 mosmol/kg, and one of the causes of decreased renal perfusion (see Chap. 19); urinary tract obstruction is characterized by hydronephrosis that is usually detectable by ultrasonography or, if necessary, CT scanning; and nephrosclerosis primarily occurs in patients with long-standing hypertension. If none of these findings is present, then a chronic tubulointerstitial disease such as analgesic abuse nephropathy becomes most likely.

Urine Volume
In contrast to the urinalysis, the urine volume is generally of little diagnostic value and may not be related to the severity of the underlying condition. Even patients with advanced disease may maintain an adequate urine output because the latter is determined not by the GFR alone but by the *difference* between the GFR and tubular reabsorption. Thus, a patient whose GFR has fallen from the normal of 180 liters/day (or 125 ml/min) down to near end-stage renal failure at 10 liters/day (or 7 ml/min) will still have a daily

urine output of 2 liters if only 8 liters of the filtrate is reabsorbed. The factors responsible for the relatively low rate of tubular reabsorption in this setting include volume expansion, the urea osmotic diuresis per nephron (if dietary intake is unchanged, the same quantity of urea now has to be excreted by fewer functioning nephrons), and direct tubular damage. The importance of hypervolemia and urea has been demonstrated by the use of dialysis in patients with advanced renal disease; removal of the excess fluid and urea frequently results in a marked reduction in, or even cessation of, the urine output [1].

As a result, patients with most forms of renal disease may be oliguric (urine volume < 500 ml/day) or have an output that is the same as or even greater than normal. One general exception occurs in prerenal disease, in which the appropriate retention of sodium and water usually keeps the urine output below 1 liter/day. Even this is not absolute, however, as patients with impaired concentrating ability can maintain a urine volume above 1 liter/day despite the presence of decreased renal perfusion and a low rate of sodium excretion [2].

The major setting in which the urine volume may be of diagnostic importance is in the patient with anuria (output < 50 ml/day). Common causes of acute renal failure such as prerenal disease and acute tubular necrosis are often accompanied by oliguria, but only rarely anuria. The two primary disorders associated with essentially no urine output are *shock* (typically accompanied by intense renal vasoconstriction and usually marked hypotension) and *complete and bilateral urinary tract obstruction.* Less often, severe glomerulonephritis or vasculitis, the hemolytic-uremic syndrome, renal cortical necrosis, or bilateral vascular occlusion (as with a dissecting aneurysm) is responsible.

Urine Sodium Excretion and Osmolality
Measurement of the urine osmolality and sodium excretion is most useful in the distinction between prerenal disease and acute tubular necrosis as the cause of acute renal failure. This topic is discussed in detail in Chap. 19. Reviewed briefly, the kidney appropriately attempts to retain sodium and water when renal perfusion is reduced; as a result, the urine sodium concentration and fractional excretion of sodium are usually low and, due to the hypovolemic stimulus to the release of antidiuretic hormone, the urine osmolality may exceed 500 mosmol/kg. These responses are impaired by tubular damage in acute tubular necrosis. Thus, urinary sodium excretion is relatively high and the urine osmolality tends to be isosmotic to that of the plasma (< 350 mosmol/kg).

Radiologic Studies
Radiologic studies can provide a great deal of useful information in selected patients with renal disease (Table 16-3). In general, a plain film of the abdomen and ultrasonography are the major tests used as part of the initial evaluation. The former can show renal size and shape and detect radiopaque calculi whereas the latter can reliably detect the presence of hydronephrosis due to urinary tract obstruction [3].

Urinary Tract Obstruction
Urinary tract obstruction, which is an important diagnosis to establish because it can often be *readily reversed,* displays a marked variability in presenting symptoms and signs. If the process is acute, as with prostatic disease or ureteral calculi, suprapubic or flank pain is often present. However, many patients with gradual obstruction, as with pelvic malignancies, have no symptoms referable to the urinary tract. Furthermore, the urinalysis is variable, ranging from normal to hematuria with calculi, pyuria with superimposed infection or chronic obstruction, or mild proteinuria (usually < 1 gm/day) due to secondary glomerular damage. The urine output, as described above, is also variable. Although anuria can be seen with complete obstruction, the secondary tubular injury resulting from chronic *partial* obstruction can impair reabsorptive capacity, thereby permitting maintenance of an adequate urine volume. The net effect of these protean manifestations is that, in the absence of other diagnostic findings such as red cell casts, *obstruction should be suspected and ultrasonography performed* in any patient who presents with unexplained renal insufficiency.

Table 16-3. Major uses of radiologic studies in renal disease

Test	Uses
Abdominal plain film	Kidney size and shape Diagnosis and monitoring of radiopaque stones
Intravenous pyelogram	Kidney size, shape, and calyceal anatomy Detection of site and cause of obstruction (ultrasound or CT scan preferable for screening) Diagnosis of disorders with anatomic changes such as chronic pyelonephritis, medullary sponge kidney, or papillary necrosis Screening for renovascular hypertension
Ultrasonography and CT scanning	Evaluation for possible urinary tract obstruction Evaluation for renal mass (cyst versus tumor) Early diagnosis of polycystic kidney disease Detection of radiolucent kidney stones
Radionuclide studies	Screening for renovascular hypertension Screening for renal thromboemboli Detection of vesicoureteral reflux
Renal arteriography	Direct visualization of renal arterial system for renovascular hypertension, polyarteritis nodosa, thromboemboli, or diagnosis of renal mass that seems noncystic on other studies
Voiding cystourethrogram	Detection of vesicoureteral reflux, the major cause of chronic pyelonephritis
Retrograde or antegrade pyelography	Determination of site of obstruction Relief of obstruction (catheters inserted)

Renal Biopsy

A renal biopsy is performed in patients with intrinsic renal disease when less invasive procedures are unable to establish the correct diagnosis or when the severity and activity of injury must be assessed directly to determine the appropriate mode of therapy that will be given. The latter is particularly important in patients with glomerular disease or vasculitis in whom the urinalysis, P_{cr}, and serologic studies frequently do not provide sufficient information.

Clinical Examples

The following case histories illustrate how the approach presented in this chapter can be used to arrive at a reasonable differential diagnosis and to design an appropriate plan for further evaluation. One such example has been presented above in which the combination of chronic renal insufficiency and a normal urinalysis led to a possible diagnosis of analgesic abuse nephropathy.

CASE HISTORY

A 47-year-old woman with a history of rheumatic heart disease presents with fever and a new heart murmur, and the diagnosis of bacterial endocarditis is confirmed. Therapy is begun (based on the blood culture results) with penicillin and an aminoglycoside, and the patient rapidly defervesces. The P_{cr} and the urinalysis are initially normal. On day 12, however, fever recurs, the P_{cr} is noted to be 2.9 mg/dl, and the urinalysis reveals trace protein on dipstick, 20 to 30 red and white cells per high-power field, and occasional white cell and granular but no red cell casts.

Comment: The urinary findings in this case of acute renal failure are compatible with glomerulonephritis, interstitial nephritis, or acute vascular disease. Thus, the urinalysis does not distinguish among the three major forms of renal disease found with bacterial endocarditis: an immune complex glomerulonephritis, drug-induced interstitial nephritis, and renal infarction due to embolic disease. The time course and history, however, are more helpful. The glomerulonephritis seen with endocarditis typically is most severe before antimicrobial therapy is instituted, with subsequent rapid improvement, in contrast to the late development in this patient. Renal emboli severe enough to produce renal failure is also unlikely; this problem can occur at any time but should lead to marked flank pain. Segmental perfusion defects on radionuclide scanning can confirm this diagnosis.

In comparison, drug-induced interstitial nephritis characteristically occurs after 1 to 3 weeks of treatment and may be associated with recurrent fever. This diagnosis is therefore the most likely cause of this patient's renal failure; consequently, another antimicrobial should be substituted for the penicillin. Although the time course in this patient is also compatible with aminoglycoside-induced acute tubular necrosis, granular and epithelial cell casts would be expected in the urine sediment, not hematuria and pyuria.

CASE HISTORY

A 71-year-old man is admitted for nonspecific complaints of weakness and fatigue. He has a past history of mild hypertension but is currently on no medications. Physical examination shows a blood pressure of 111/80 with slightly cool extremities but no signs of peripheral or pulmonary edema. Skin turgor is normal. During the first 36 hours, it is noted that the patient is oliguric and that the blood urea nitrogen (BUN) and P_{cr} have risen from 14/1.1 mg/dl to 49/1.7 mg/dl. The urinalysis is unremarkable (including a negative sulfosalicylic acid test), the urine sodium is < 10 meq/L, the fractional excretion of sodium is 0.4 percent, and the urine osmolality is 498 mosmol/kg. The hematocrit is unchanged at 39 percent.

Comment: This patient has acute renal failure with a normal urinalysis. The negative sulfosalicylic acid test is important in that it tends to exclude myeloma kidney in which the urine typically contains immunoglobulin light chains (which are not detected by the primarily albumin-sensitive dipstick; see Chap. 52). The high BUN/P_{cr} ratio, low urine sodium and fractional excretion of sodium, and high urine osmolality all favor the diagnosis of prerenal disease. It is not clear, however, *why* the patient is effectively volume depleted. There is no history of vomiting, diarrhea, or diuretic therapy, and there is neither history nor signs of hepatic cirrhosis, heart failure, or active bleeding. In this setting, an *occult cardiopulmonary event* must be excluded as the cause of the reduced renal perfusion. As a result, an electrocardiogram is obtained and demonstrates an acute anterior myocardial infarction. In retrospect, the apparently "normal" blood pressure of 110/80 is probably low for this patient with a past history of mild hypertension. In addition, the presence of cool extremities is another sign suggesting poor perfusion.

References

1. Yeh, BPY, Tomki, DJ, Stacy, WK, Bear, ES, Haden, HT, Falls, WF, Jr. Factors influencing sodium and water excretion in uremic man. *Kidney Int* 7:103, 1975.
2. Miller, PD, Krebs, RA, Neal, BJ, McIntyre, DO. Polyuric prerenal failure. *Arch Intern Med* 140:907, 1980.
3. Webb, JAW, Reznek, RH, White, FE, Cattell, WR, Kelsey Fry, I, Baker, LRI. Can ultrasound and computed tomography replace high-dose urography in patients with impaired renal function? *Q J Med* 53:411, 1984.

17. CREATININE AND GLOMERULAR FILTRATION RATE: USES AND LIMITATIONS

The preceding chapter described how the urinalysis can be used diagnostically in the patient with renal disease. In addition, two other important questions need to be answered in this setting:

1. How severe is the renal damage?
2. Is the disease progressing, stable, or improving?

Estimation of the glomerular filtration rate (GFR) is the major clinical modality used to address these questions. The GFR is important because it is equal to the sum of the filtration rates of all of the functioning nephrons. As a result, the loss of nephrons will ultimately lead to a fall in total GFR. This change in some patients will be the first detectable sign of renal disease. The urinalysis, for example, is normal in some conditions, and fluid and electrolyte handling may remain intact because of compensatory responses by the remaining functioning nephrons.

Measurement of the plasma creatinine concentration (P_{cr}) and calculation of the creatinine clearance have been the major methods used to estimate the GFR. This chapter will review the rationale underlying these tests, as well as the important limitations that are present. As will be seen, these parameters are often a *relatively inaccurate measure of the GFR*. Nevertheless, they may be very helpful in assessing the severity of the disease and in following its course.

Creatinine Clearance and GFR

Determination of the GFR in patients involves measurement of the rate of urinary excretion of certain compounds. Substances such as the polysaccharide inulin or isotopically labelled iothalamate or DTPA share the following properties: (1) they are freely filtered at the glomerulus; (2) they are able to achieve a relatively stable plasma concentration after intravenous infusion or subcutaneous injection; (3) they are not reabsorbed, secreted, or metabolized by the kidney. As a result, for inulin:

$$\text{Filtered inulin} = \text{excreted inulin} \tag{1}$$

The filtered inulin is equal to the GFR times the plasma inulin concentration (P_{in}), and the excreted inulin is equal to the product of the urine inulin concentration (U_{in}) and the urine flow rate (V, in ml/min or liters/day). Consequently,

$$\text{GFR} \times P_{in} = U_{in} \times V \tag{2}$$
$$\text{GFR} = U_{in} \times \frac{V}{P_{in}}$$

This formula ($U_{in} \times V$)/P_{in} is called the clearance of inulin* and is an accurate measure of the GFR. However, the clearance of inulin (as well as that of radioisotopes) is technically cumbersome and is not usually performed clinically.

The most widely used method to measure the GFR is the endogenous creatinine clearance. Creatinine is derived from the nonenzymatic metabolism of creatine (occurring primarily in skeletal muscle) and is released into the plasma at a relatively uniform rate. As a result, the P_{cr} tends to be stable, varying about 6 percent per day in serial observations in patients with stable renal function [1]. Like inulin, creatinine is freely filtered at the glomerulus and is neither reabsorbed nor metabolized by the kidney. However, a variable amount of creatinine enters the urine by tubular secretion in the proximal tubule. As a result, the *quantity of creatinine excreted exceeds the quantity filtered* by about 10 to 20 percent in patients with normal renal function [2]. Thus, the creatinine

---

*The inulin clearance, in ml/min, refers to that volume of plasma cleared of inulin by renal excretion. If, for example, 1 mg of inulin is excreted per minute ($U_{in} \times V$) and the P_{in} is 1.0 mg/dl (or to keep the units consistent, 0.01 mg/ml), then the clearance of inulin (or GFR) is 100 ml/min; in other words, 100 ml of plasma has been cleared of the 1 mg it contained.

clearance (C_{cr}), which is usually calculated using the results from a 24-hour urine collection,

$$C_{cr} = \frac{U_{cr} \times V}{P_{cr}} \tag{3}$$

will tend to exceed the true GFR by 10 to 20 percent [1]. Fortuitously, this is balanced by an error of almost equal magnitude in the measurement of the P_{cr}. The plasma, but not the urine, contains noncreatinine chromogens (acetone, proteins, ascorbic acid) that are measured as creatinine by the commonly used alkaline picrate colorimetric reaction. Since both the urine and plasma creatinine levels are elevated to roughly the same degree, the C_{cr} is a reasonably accurate estimate of the GFR *if the GFR is relatively normal* (95–120 ml/min in adults).

As the GFR begins to fall, however, the rise in P_{cr} enhances creatinine delivery to the secretory pump. This leads to a progressive increase in creatinine secretion since the pump is not yet saturated. As a result, the C_{cr} can substantially exceed the true GFR (see the following). To partially counteract this problem in patients with advanced renal disease (GFR below 30 ml/min), the GFR can more accurately be estimated from the average of the creatinine and urea clearances,

$$GFR = (C_{cr} + C_{urea}) / 2 \tag{4}$$

since the overestimation induced by creatinine secretion is counterbalanced by the underestimation of the urea clearance resulting from the reabsorption of 40 to 50 percent of the filtered urea [3].

The normal values for the C_{cr} in adults are approximately 125 ± 25 ml/min in men and 95 ± 20 ml/min in women. These values tend to decline with age, falling almost 1 ml/min/year over the age of 40.

Several errors, in addition to the problem of creatinine secretion, are involved in the determination of the creatinine clearance. Perhaps most important is an incomplete urine collection. Fortunately, the relative constancy of creatinine production and subsequent excretion can be used to assess the completeness of the collection. In adults, daily creatinine secretion (in mg/kg lean body weight) should be about ($28 - [0.2 \times$ age]) in men and 85 percent of this value or ($24 - [0.2 \times$ age]) in women [1,4]. Thus, creatinine excretion between the ages of 40 and 70 in a man should fall from approximately 20 down to 14 mg/kg/day, probably due to a reduction in skeletal muscle mass.[1] If total creatinine excretion is less than these normal values, then an incomplete collection is likely.

Even when great care is taken to collect all the urine, the coefficient of variation of the C_{cr} on serial measurements is still 15 to 25 percent [1,5]. Thus, a change in C_{cr} of as much as 20 ml/min in a patient with normal renal function may not represent any real change in GFR. Variations in measurement of the plasma and urine creatinine concentrations (the latter may be very high due to the removal of up to 99 % of the filtered water by tubular reabsorption) and in dietary meat intake are thought to be responsible for this problem.

Plasma Creatinine and GFR

Estimation of, and changes in, the GFR can also be ascertained from measurement of the P_{cr}, a simple test that does not require any urine collection. Use of the P_{cr} is related to the observation that creatinine excretion ($U_{cr} \times V$) tends to be relatively constant,[2] reflecting the stable rate of creatinine production in patients in the steady state (in

---

[1]A similar decrease in both muscle mass and creatinine excretion can occur with malnutrition from any cause.
[2]An important exception occurs once the P_{cr} exceeds 6 mg/dl [6]. Creatinine excretion falls progressively by 25 to 50 percent in this setting due to the combination of decreased glomerular filtration and increased extrarenal degradation of creatinine, possibly mediated by bacteria in the gut [7].

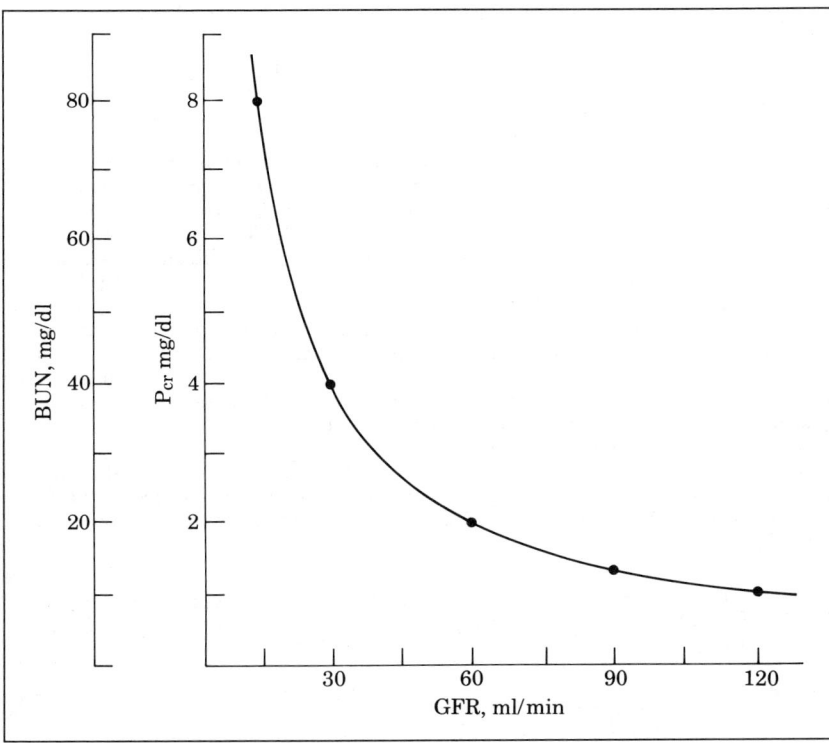

Fig. 17-1. Hypothetical steady-state relationship between the plasma creatinine concentration (P_{cr}), blood urea nitrogen (BUN), and glomerular filtration rate (GFR).

whom muscle mass and dietary meat intake do not change substantially). If we amend the formula for the C_{cr} in Eq 3 to reflect this relationship, then:

$$C_{cr} \sim \frac{\text{constant}}{P_{cr}} \tag{5}$$

Thus, the P_{cr} *varies inversely with the GFR.* If, for example, the GFR falls by 50 percent, there will be initial equivalent reductions in creatinine filtration and subsequent excretion to a level that is now below that of production. As a result, creatinine will accumulate in the plasma and the P_{cr} will rise until the filtered load again equals the rate of production. This will occur when the P_{cr} has doubled:

$$1/2 \text{ GFR} \times 2 \text{ P}_{cr} = \text{GFR} \times \text{P}_{cr} = \text{constant}$$

The normal P_{cr} in adults is 0.8 to 1.3 mg/dl in men and 0.6 to 1.0 mg/dl in women.

The reciprocal relationship between the GFR and the P_{cr} is depicted in Fig. 17-1. There are three points that deserve emphasis [8]:

1. The curve is valid only in the steady state. If a patient suddenly develops renal failure and the GFR falls from 100 to 10 ml/min, the P_{cr} will still be normal on day 1

since there has not been time for creatinine to accumulate in the plasma. After 7 to 10 days, however, the P_{cr} will stabilize at about 10 mg/dl, a level consistent with the reduced GFR. An understanding of this concept is particularly important when adjusting the dose of drugs that are excreted in the urine. If the above patient had been given the aminoglycoside gentamicin in full dosage initially because of the "normal" P_{cr}, potentially toxic plasma levels would have eventually ensued.

2. The shape of the curve relating the GFR to the P_{cr} is also important. In a woman with normal renal function, for example, *an apparently minor increase in the P_{cr} from 0.7 to 1.4 mg/dl can represent a marked 50 percent fall in GFR from 100 to 50 ml/min.* Thus, the initial elevation in P_{cr} represents a major loss in GFR. In comparison, the same woman with advanced renal disease has a high P_{cr} and a low GFR. In this setting, an apparently large increment in the P_{cr} from 5 to 10 mg/dl can reflect a relatively small reduction in GFR from 15 to 7.5 ml/min.

3. The relationship between the GFR and P_{cr} is also dependent on the rate of creatinine production. The latter is largely a function of muscle mass but can also be influenced in the short-term by marked changes in the intake of creatine (which is mostly present in meat products). Switching to a meat-free diet, for example, can lower the P_{cr} by as much as 15 percent whereas a transient rise in the P_{cr} of as much as 1.0 mg/dl can follow the ingestion of a large meat meal [9].

A normal GFR is associated with a P_{cr} of 1.0 mg/dl in Fig. 17-1. Although this may be true for a 70-kg man, a similar GFR in a small woman may be associated with a P_{cr} of only 0.6 mg/dl. In this setting, a P_{cr} of 1.0 mg/dl is not normal and represents a 40 percent fall in GFR.

The effects of body weight, age, and sex on muscle mass are taken into account by the following formula, which follows the C_{cr} (in ml/min) to be estimated from the P_{cr} in the steady state [4]:

$$C_{cr} = \frac{(140 - \text{age}) \times \text{lean body weight (in kg)}}{72 \times P_{cr}} \tag{6}$$

This formula is similar to that for direct measurement of the C_{cr} ($U_{cr}V/P_{cr}$) in that the term ([140 − age] × lean body weight / 72) represents an estimate of daily creatinine excretion (in units that allow the C_{cr} to be expressed in ml/min). The value obtained should be multiplied by 0.85 in women who have a lower fraction of body weight that is composed of muscle. Only estimated lean body mass should be used since adipose tissue contains essentially no creatinine.

The results obtained with this formula correlate fairly closely with a simultaneously measured creatinine clearance [4]. Its usefulness can be illustrated by the observation that a P_{cr} of 1.4 mg/dl represents a C_{cr} of 95 ml/min in an 80-kg, 20-year-old man,

$$C_{cr} = \frac{(140 - 20) \times 80}{72 \times 1.4}$$

but only a C_{cr} of 20 ml/min in a 40-kg, 80-year-old woman,

$$C_{cr} = \frac{(140 - 80) \times 40 \times 0.85}{72 \times 1.4}$$

This simple example calls attention to the risk of overdosing elderly patients in whom it is mistakenly assumed that a relatively normal P_{cr} represents a normal GFR. Although use of the above formula can minimize this problem, it should not replace appropriate monitoring of plasma drug levels when potentially toxic drugs are used.

A similar decrement in creatinine production can occur in malnourished patients with hepatic cirrhosis. In addition to the loss of muscle mass, decreased meat intake and possibly decreased hepatic production of creatine, the precursor of creatinine, may also play a contributory role. The net effect is that some cirrhotic patients with a "normal" P_{cr} of 1.0 to 1.3 mg/dl have a GFR (as measured by inulin clearance) as low as 10 to 20 ml/min [10]. The low protein intake and diminished hepatic production of urea also limit the rise in blood urea nitrogen (BUN) that should occur as the GFR falls.*

In summary, the P_{cr} tends to vary inversely with the GFR and is *best used to follow changes in renal function* in the patient with renal disease. A rise in the P_{cr} generally indicates disease progression whereas a fall in the P_{cr} suggests recovery of function (assuming that muscle mass and meat intake are relatively constant). It is also presumed that a stable P_{cr} means stable disease, although this may not be an accurate assumption.

Limitations in the Use of the Plasma Creatinine and Creatinine Clearance

A variety of studies have indicated that there may be *serious limitations* with use of the P_{cr} or the C_{cr} to estimate the GFR. In patients with a normal or near-normal GFR (above 60 ml/min), it is now clear that considerable *disease progression can occur with little or no change in the P_{cr}.* Three factors can contribute to this problem, two of which prevent or minimize any fall in true GFR and one of which (creatinine secretion) can prevent or minimize a rise in the P_{cr} when the GFR does fall:

1. Loss of nephrons leads to compensatory hyperfiltration in the remaining more-normal nephrons, thereby maintaining the total GFR despite continued disease activity (see Chap. 56).
2. Glomerular diseases damage the glomerular basement membrane, tending to lower the GFR by reducing net capillary permeability (a function of both the unit permeability of the basement membrane and the surface area available for filtration). This effect, however, is counteracted by a rise in glomerular capillary hydrostatic pressure that is produced by an unknown mechanism involving changes in glomerular arteriolar resistance [11]. As a result, progressive glomerular damage can occur without any initial reduction in GFR.
3. As the GFR begins to fall, the rise in the P_{cr} is lessened or prevented by an increase in tubular secretion by the proximal organic-base secretory pump [2,12,13]. As described above, approximately 15 percent of urinary creatinine is derived from secretion (rather than filtration) in patients with a normal GFR [2]. As the GFR falls to 40 to 80 ml/min, however, the *absolute amount of creatinine secreted can rise by more than 50 percent* with secretion now accounting for as much as 35 percent of urinary creatinine [2].

The net effect of these changes in 171 patients with glomerular disease is illustrated in Fig. 17-2. As shown by the idealized solid curve, a fall in inulin clearance from 120 to 60 ml/min should be associated with a rise in P_{cr} from 1.0 to 2.0 mg/dl (similar to Fig. 17-1). In many of the patients, however, there seems to be *little or no increase in P_{cr}* in this range of GFR because of enhanced creatinine secretion. Similar considerations apply to the C_{cr}, which may be normal (above 90 ml/min) in about one-half of patients with a true GFR of 61 to 70 ml/min and one-fourth of those with a GFR of 51 to 60 ml/min [13]. These findings also illustrate the marked individual variability that may be present; in some patients, *oversecretion of creatinine does not become prominent* and the P_{cr} and the C_{cr} remain relatively accurate estimates of the GFR. It is not possible, however, to predict the degree of secretion that occurs in a given patient.

With more advanced renal disease ($P_{cr} > 1.5$–2.0 mg/dl), the P_{cr} rises as expected in Fig. 17-2, since the creatinine secretory mechanism appears to become saturated. Creatinine secretion may, however, account for an increasing *fraction* of urinary creatine due to the fall in filtration. As a result, overestimation of the true GFR by the C_{cr} becomes progressively larger. Some patients with a GFR of 20 ml/min, for example, may have a C_{cr} as high as 40 to 60 ml/min [2,12]. The increments in creatinine secretion and therefore in the C_{cr} can be largely reversed by the acute intravenous administration of cimetidine, which competitively inhibits the secretory pump [2]. In this setting, the C_{cr} falls to a level near that of the true GFR.

---

*The BUN, like the P_{cr}, tends to vary inversely with the GFR (Fig. 17-1). However, the BUN is also affected by dietary protein intake and by tubular reabsorption. Approximately 40 to 50 percent of the filtered urea is normally reabsorbed by the tubules, a fraction that can increase with volume depletion. As a result, changes in the BUN do not necessarily reflect changes in GFR, making the BUN less accurate than the P_{cr}.

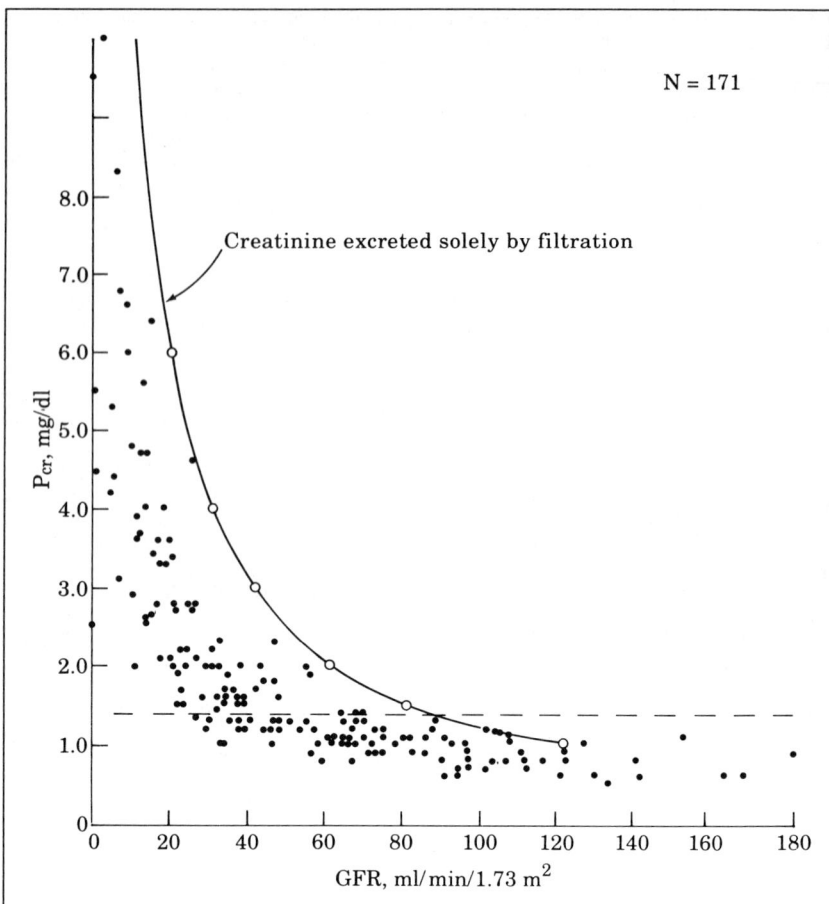

Fig. 17-2. Relationship between the plasma creatinine concentration (P_{cr}) and the true GFR (as measured by the inulin clearance, C_{in}) in 171 patients with glomerular disease. The open circles joined by a continuous line represent the hypothetical relationship shown in Fig. 17-1 in which creatinine is excreted solely by glomerular filtration; the dotted line represents the upper limit of "normal" for the P_{cr} of 1.4 mg/ dl. With the GFR varying between 120 and 60 ml/min in different patients, there is often little or no elevation in the P_{cr}, due primarily to enhanced tubular creatinine secretion. With more severe disease, the P_{cr} rises as expected from further reductions in GFR. (From Shemesh, O, Golbetz, H, Kriss, JP, Myers, BD. *Kidney Int* 28:830, 1985. Reprinted by permission from Kidney International.)

Table 17-1. Factors that can increase the P_{cr} without change in the GFR

Increased creatinine production
  High meat intake
  Massive rhabdomyolysis
Compounds that competitively decrease creatinine secretion
  Cimetidine
  Trimethoprim
Compounds measured as creatinine in certain assays
  Acetoacetate in ketoacidosis
  Cefoxitin
  Flucytosine

Errors in Interpretation of the Plasma Creatinine
Another problem, a rise in the measured P_{cr} without change in the GFR (or BUN) can also occur. This may be due to increased creatinine production, decreased creatinine secretion, or the presence of compounds in the plasma that are measured as creatinine (Table 17-1) [8]. Probably the most common problem is that the P_{cr} varies during the day, rising by as much as 0.5 to 1.0 mg/dl after a large meat meal and then returning slowly toward baseline [9]. Thus, it is most accurate to obtain blood samples either in the fasting state or after a nonmeat meal.

Acetoacetate is an example of a compound that is measured as a plasma noncreatinine chromogen by the alkaline picrate method. The presence of acetoacetate can raise the measured P_{cr} by 0.5 to 2.0 mg/dl or more in patients with ketoacidosis. This effect is rapidly reversed with correction of the ketonemia.

Cimetidine and trimethoprim, on the other hand, are organic bases that can competitively inhibit creatinine secretion [2,14]. The net effect is a mild elevation in the P_{cr} that is typically less than 0.5 mg/dl [14]. Ranitidine, a histamine (H_2)-receptor antagonist like cimetidine, is much less likely to interfere with creatinine secretion. Although it is also an organic base, ranitidine is generally given in much lower doses than cimetidine (300 versus 1200 mg/day) and therefore has a lesser renal effect.

Summary
Use of the C_{cr} or the P_{cr} to estimate the GFR or disease progression can often lead to erroneous conclusions. Even if the 24-hour urine collection is complete, for example, a "normal" C_{cr} can be associated with a GFR ranging from 50 ml/min to a truly normal value that can exceed 100 ml/min due to increased creatinine secretion [2,12,13]. The C_{cr} also becomes progressively less accurate in patients with renal insufficiency, being greater than the GFR by as much as two-fold or more [2,12]. Although the C_{cr} will be accurate in some patients, it is not possible to identify these patients without simultaneous measurement of an inulin or radioisotopic clearance.

Thus, the *major* accurate assumption that can be drawn from a single C_{cr} is that the value obtained represents an upper limit that the true GFR will not exceed. Serial measurements, however, may be more helpful in that changes in the C_{cr} should reflect the course of the disease. This may be particularly important in malnourished patients in whom the loss of muscle mass leads to a decline in creatinine production. As a result, the P_{cr} may remain stable or may even fall despite a reduction in GFR that can be detected by a decrease in C_{cr} [13].

Problems also exist in the interpretation of the P_{cr}, particularly when the GFR is above 60 ml/min. In this setting, compensatory hyperfiltration in less affected nephrons and enhanced creatinine secretion may combine to prevent any elevation in P_{cr} in some patients despite (1) continued disease activity or (2) as much as a 30 to 50 percent reduction in GFR (Fig. 17-2). It is also worth noting that, when the additive effect of compensatory hyperfiltration is considered, a 30 percent fall in GFR represents the loss of more than 30 percent (and perhaps as much as 50%) of functioning nephrons.

Thus, the maintenance of a normal or near-normal and stable P_{cr} in a patient with known renal disease (as with lupus nephritis, for example) *should not lead to the conclusion that the disease is necessarily stable or even mild.* In this setting in which serial monitoring of the true GFR can be accurately achieved only by cumbersome procedures such as inulin or radioisotopic iothalamate clearances, other parameters must also be carefully monitored to assess possible disease progression. For example, an increase in proteinuria, in the activity of the urine sediment, or in the systemic blood pressure all may be signs of continued activity of the underlying disease; this possibility can be confirmed by renal biopsy, if necessary.

These limitations, however, should not obscure those situations in which the P_{cr} is very helpful. In particular, *changes in the P_{cr}* generally reflect opposite changes in GFR, regardless of the severity of the disease. Furthermore, a stable P_{cr} does suggest stable disease once the P_{cr} is above 1.5 to 2.0 mg/dl. In this setting, creatinine secretion and compensatory hyperfiltration are already at near-maximal levels, and the P_{cr} should correlate closely with changes in the GFR (as depicted in Fig. 17-2).

Reciprocal of the P_{cr} versus Time
The inverse relationship between the GFR and P_{cr}

$$GFR \sim constant / P_{cr}$$

can be used to follow and to predict the course of chronic renal disease [1]. Many patients who progress do so at a relatively uniform rate, with the GFR declining in a linear fashion with time. As a result, plotting the GFR (which is cumbersome to measure accurately) or more simply the reciprocal of the P_{cr} ($1/P_{cr}$) versus time frequently reveals a linear relationship (Fig. 17-3). Determining the slope of this line allows the future course of the disease to be predicted and the efficacy of therapy to be evaluated; a decrease or plateau in the slope suggests that disease progression has been slowed.

The accuracy of using the reciprocal of the P_{cr} is greatest when the P_{cr} most closely reflects changes in the GFR. This generally occurs when the P_{cr} is between 1.5 and 6.0 to 7.0 mg/dl [1]. Below this range, enhanced tubular secretion of creatinine can, in some patients, prevent or minimize any change in P_{cr} despite a reduction in GFR (Fig. 17-2); above this range, increasing extrarenal metabolism of creatinine also can minimize the change in P_{cr} in the presence of progressive disease [6,7].

References

1. Mitch, WE. Measuring the rate of progression of renal insufficiency. In WE Mitch (Ed.), *Contemporary Issues in Nephrology. The Progressive Nature of Renal Disease.* (Vol. 14). New York: Churchill Livingstone, 1986.
2. Shemesh, O, Golbetz, H, Kriss, JP, Myers, BD. Limitations of creatinine as a filtration marker in glomerulopathic patients. *Kidney Int* 28:830, 1985.
3. Lubowitz, H, Slatopolsky, E, Shankel, S, Rieselbach, RE, Bricker, NS. Glomerular filtration rate: Determination in patients with chronic renal disease. *J Am Med Assoc* 199:252, 1967.
4. Cockroft, DW, Gault, MH. Prediction of creatinine clearance from serum creatinine. *Nephron* 16:13, 1976.
5. Rosano, TG, Brown, HH. Analytical and biological variability of serum creatinine and creatinine clearance: Implications for clinical interpretation. *Clin Chem* 28:2330, 1982.
6. Mitch, WE, Collier, VU, Walser, M. Creatinine metabolism in chronic renal failure. *Clin Sci* 58:327, 1980.
7. Mitch, WE, Walser, M. A proposed mechanism for reduced creatinine excretion in severe chronic renal failure. *Nephron* 21:248, 1978.
8. Rose, BD. *Pathophysiology of Renal Disease* (2nd ed.). New York: McGraw-Hill, 1987. Chapter 1.
9. Payne, RB. Creatinine clearance: A redundant clinical investigation. *Ann Clin Biochem* 23:243, 1986.

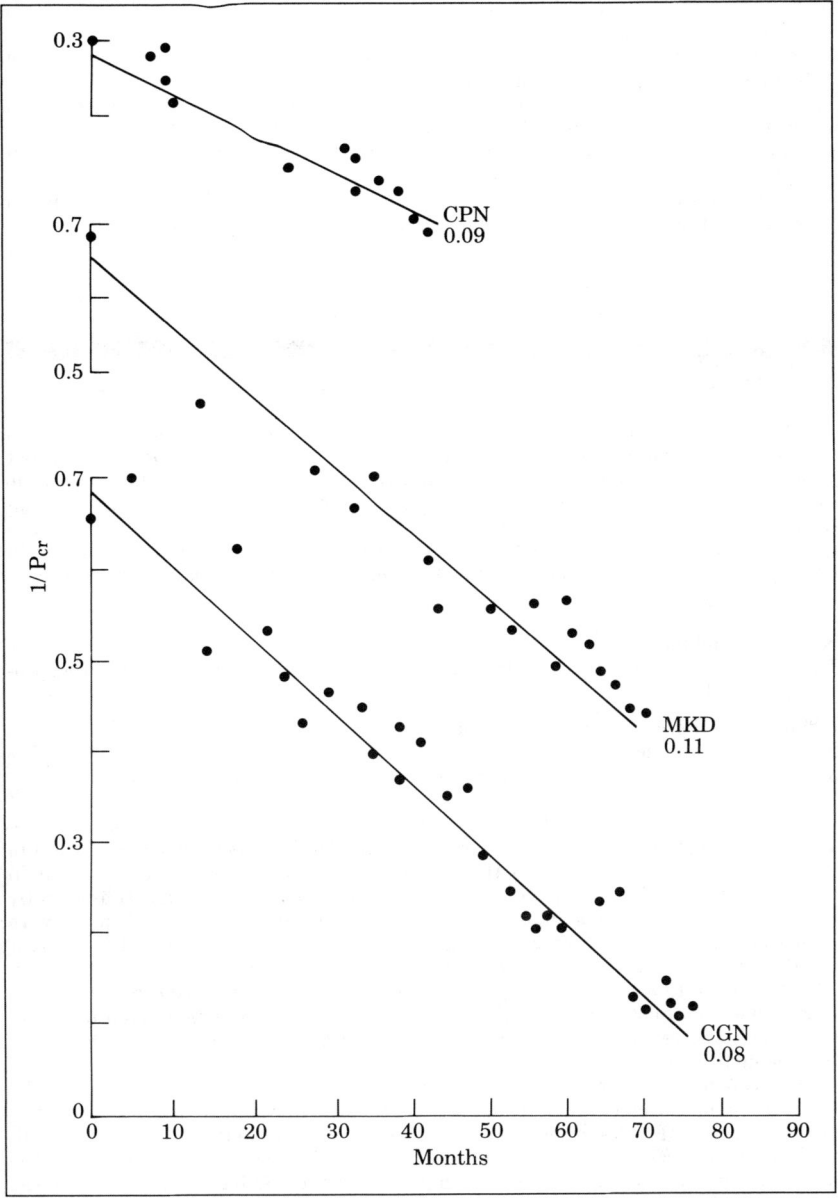

Fig. 17-3. Composite plot of the reciprocal of the P_{cr} versus months of observation in three patients with progressive renal disease due to chronic pyelonephritis (CPN), medullary cystic kidney disease (MKD), and chronic glomerulonephritis (CGN). (Adapted from Mitch, WE, Walser, M, Buffington, GA, Lemann, J, Jr. *Lancet* 2:1326, 1976.)

10. Papadakis, MA, Arieff, AI. Unpredictability of clinical evaluation of renal function in cirrhosis. Prospective study. *Am J Med* 82:945, 1987.
11. Kaizu, K, Marsh, D, Zipser, R, Glassock, RJ. Role of prostaglandins and angiotensin II in experimental glomerulonephritis. *Kidney Int* 28:629, 1985.
12. Bauer, JH, Brooks, CS, Burch, RN. Clinical appraisal of creatinine clearance as a measurement of glomerular filtration rate. *Am J Kid Dis* 2:337, 1982.
13. Kim, KE, Onesti, G, Ramirez, O, Brest, AN, Swartz, C. Creatinine clearance in renal disease. A reappraisal. *Br Med J* 4:11, 1969.
14. Dubb, JW, Stote, RM, Familiar, RG, Lee, K, Alexander, F. Effect of cimetidine on renal function in normal man. *Clin Pharmacol Therap* 24:76, 1978.

18. ISOLATED PROTEINURIA AND HEMATURIA

When a patient has an abnormal urinalysis in conjunction with an elevated plasma creatinine concentration, it is clear that some form of renal disease is present. It is not unusual, however, to find only mild proteinuria or microscopic hematuria on a routine examination. In children, for example, asymptomatic urinary abnormalities are relatively common but are almost always transient and not generally indicative of significant renal or extrarenal disease [1]. The prognosis may not be so benign, however, in adults as proteinuria or hematuria may be associated with potentially serious disease in the urinary tract [2].

Isolated Proteinuria

Three questions need to be answered when approaching the patient with isolated proteinuria (Table 18-1):

1. What type of protein is being excreted?
2. How much protein is excreted?
3. Under what conditions is protein excreted?

What Type of Protein is Being Excreted?
The glomerular capillary wall is both size-selective and charge-selective with respect to the filtration of macromolecules [3,4]. Thus, large and anionic proteins such as albumin are normally filtered to a very limited degree and most of this albumin is subsequently reabsorbed in the proximal tubule so that albumin excretion is under 15 mg/day. In comparison, smaller (or cationic) proteins, such as lysozyme and immunoglobulin light chains, are more easily filtered. These proteins are also largely reabsorbed in the proximal tubule, so that total protein excretion is normally less than 100 to 150 mg/day. Furthermore, 30 to 50 mg of this urinary protein represents Tamm-Horsfall mucoprotein, which is secreted by the cells in the thick ascending limb of the loop of Henle, rather than being filtered.

From this brief review, it can be seen that there are three general mechanisms by which proteinuria can occur: (1) *glomerular* proteinuria in which an increase in glomerular permeability results in the filtration and subsequent excretion of normally nonfiltered macromolecules, such as albumin and IgG; (2) *tubular* proteinuria in which proximal tubular reabsorptive function is impaired by tubulointerstitial disease or the Fanconi syndrome, resulting in the excretion of normally filtered proteins such as β_2-microglobulin and amino acids; and (3) *overflow* proteinuria in which overproduction of low-molecular-weight proteins, such as immunoglobulin light chains in multiple myeloma, overwhelms proximal reabsorptive capacity (Table 18-1) [2,5,6].

Distinguishing between these types of proteinuria is extremely important, since the prognosis and therapy of glomerular disease, for example, is very different from that of multiple myeloma. The excretion of low-molecular-weight proteins can usually be easily detected by testing the urine with both the dipstick, which primarily senses albumin, and sulfosalicylic acid, which senses all proteins. A negative or only trace-positive dip-

Table 18-1. Causes of isolated mild proteinuria

Glomerular proteinuria
    Transient or intermittent proteinuria
    Orthostatic proteinuria
    Benign persistent proteinuria
    Early or mild glomerular disease
Tubular proteinuria
    Tubulointerstitial diseases (aminoglycoside nephrotoxicity, chronic pyelonephritis)
    Fanconi's syndrome (often with amino aciduria and renal tubular acidosis)
Overflow proteinuria
    Multiple myeloma
    Acute leukemia (with lysozymuria)

stick with a 3 + or 4 + response with sulfosalicylic acid indicates the presence of non-albumin proteins. In patients in whom multiple myeloma is suspected, urinary immunoelectrophoresis can then be used to confirm the presence of monoclonal urinary light chains.

How Much Protein is Excreted?
In patients with glomerular proteinuria, the quantity of protein excreted often parallels the severity of the underlying disease. Measurement of the degree of protein excretion is best obtained with a 24-hour urine collection; in comparison, use of the dipstick or sulfosalicylic acid reflects only the protein concentration, which is also a function of the urine volume. Thus, oliguric patients may have a 3 + response on the dipstick without marked proteinuria being present.

A simpler alternative to a 24-hour urine collection is to measure the protein-creatinine ratio (mg/mg) in a random midday urine specimen [7]. This ratio correlates closely with total protein excretion; for example, a ratio of 3.2 represents daily protein excretion of approximately 3.2 gm/1.73 m² body surface area. Use of this ratio is particularly helpful in serial monitoring to determine, for example, if therapy is leading to a reduction in the degree of proteinuria.

Patients with the benign form of isolated proteinuria (which most often occurs in children) generally excrete less than 1 gm/day of protein, although as much as 2 gm/day may occasionally be seen [2,8]. Higher values generally indicate more serious renal disease. Even in patients with primary glomerular diseases (such as membranous nephropathy, focal glomerulosclerosis, and membranoproliferative glomerulonephritis), however, the degree of proteinuria is prognostically important: those patients with nonnephrotic-range proteinuria (<3.0 gm/day) have a much lesser rate of progressive renal insufficiency [9].

Considering the significance of the level of proteinuria, it is important to be aware that the quantity of protein excreted can be reduced by a decline in either glomerular filtration rate or the plasma albumin concentration. Patients excreting less than 2 gm/day generally do not become hypoalbuminemic since these losses can be replaced by increased hepatic synthesis. In some patients with the nephrotic syndrome, however, the associated reduction in the plasma albumin concentration can reduce protein excretion to less than nephrotic levels. Thus, the presence of otherwise unexplained hypoalbuminemia in a patient with moderate proteinuria (1.5–3.0 gm/day) is suggestive of one of the causes of the nephrotic syndrome (see Chap. 26). If necessary, this suspicion can be confirmed by an intravenous infusion of albumin that will raise the plasma albumin concentration and markedly enhance protein excretion [10,11].

Under What Conditions is Protein Excreted?
Mild, asymptomatic proteinuria can be divided into three categories: (1) *transient* or intermittent, (2) *orthostatic,* and (3) *persistent* [12]. Transient proteinuria is by far the most common, occurring in up to 4 percent of men and 7 percent of women on a single examination, but resolving on subsequent examinations in almost all patients [12].

Stresses such as fever and exercise are responsible in at least some cases, perhaps by neuro-humorally mediated changes in renal hemodynamics [2,13].

Orthostatic proteinuria occurs in 2 to 5 percent of adolescents but is rare over the age of 30 [12]. It is characterized by protein excretion that is increased in the upright position but is *normal during recumbency* (<50 mg/8 hours). Total protein excretion is generally below 1 gm/day but values in excess of 3 gm/day may occasionally be seen [14,15]. Increases in norepinephrine and angiotensin II with assumption of the upright position may be responsible for the mild increase in glomerular permeability.

Orthostatic proteinuria is a benign condition as renal function remains normal after as long as 40 to 50 years of follow-up [15]. The increase in protein excretion seems to disappear spontaneously in most patients, being present in only 49 percent at 10 years and 17 percent at 20 years [14].

Persistent proteinuria is a fixed disorder in which protein excretion is usually below 1 to 2 gm/day but is increased on all examinations and is present in both the upright and recumbent positions [2,8]. These patients are more likely to have some primary glomerular disease, such as mesangial proliferative glomerulonephritis [16]. In addition, hemodynamic disturbances, such as heart failure, also may be associated with persistent, mild proteinuria, again thought to be due to alterations in renal hemodynamics [17].

The prognosis of persistent proteinuria appears to vary with age. The course is typically benign under the age of 25 but may be associated with a variety of potentially serious renal diseases, such as diabetic nephropathy, membranous nephropathy, and nephrosclerosis, in older patients [2,18].

Diagnosis
The evaluation of the patient found to have mild proteinuria should begin by repeating the urinalysis on at least two other occasions, using both the dipstick and sulfosalicylic acid. No further evaluation is required if the proteinuria is found to be transient.

The urine sediment should also be carefully examined at these times. The finding of lipiduria, as manifested by free fat droplets, oval fat bodies, or fatty casts, is strongly suggestive of significant glomerular disease, since glomerular permeability must be enhanced to allow the filtration of large circulating lipoproteins.

The patient with persistent proteinuria should have a 24-hour urine collection to quantify the degree of protein excretion. In patients under the age of 25 to 30, the collection should be obtained as outlined in Table 18-2 to see if orthostatic proteinuria is present. It is important to emphasize that a postural rise in protein excretion is common in many glomerular diseases; the diagnosis of orthostatic proteinuria is made only if protein excretion is normal during the recumbent collection—less than 50 mg/8 hours (i.e., a rate < the upper limit of normal of 150 mg/day).

The diagnostic approach to patients with proteinuria throughout the day should begin with the exclusion of potentially responsible systemic disorders, such as diabetes mellitus, hypertension, or heart failure. A prior history of poststreptococcal glomerulonephritis may also be important; patients who apparently recover from the acute episode may have mild isolated proteinuria for many years, possibly a reflection of some irreversible glomerular damage [19].

If the history is not helpful, a renal ultrasound or intravenous pyelogram should be performed to exclude disorders that can produce mild proteinuria including polycystic kidney disease, chronic pyelonephritis, and urinary tract obstruction. Only periodic monitoring (consisting of a urinalysis and measurement of both the urine protein-creatinine ratio and the plasma creatinine concentration) is necessary if these procedures show no anatomic abnormality. A renal biopsy is generally not indicated in adults unless there is some sign of more serious renal disease, such as an elevation in the plasma creatinine concentration, persistent protein excretion in excess of 2 gm/day, or unexplained hypoalbuminemia.

Isolated Hematuria
Isolated hematuria is defined as the presence of more than two red cells per high-power field in the *absence of renal insufficiency or other urinary abnormalities* (such as red cell or other casts or proteinuria). It is a relatively common and frequently transient prob-

Table 18-2. Evaluation for orthostatic proteinuria

The first morning void is discarded.
A 16-hour collection is obtained between 7 A.M. and 11 P.M. with the patient
performing normal activities and finishing the collection by voiding just before
11 P.M.
The patient should be recumbent after 9 P.M. to prevent contamination of the
recumbent collection with urine formed in the upright position.
A separate 8-hour collection is obtained between 11 P.M. and 7 A.M.

Table 18-3. Major causes of isolated hematuria

Extrarenal bleeding
  Ureters: calculi
  Bladder: infection due to common bacteria or tuberculosis, carcinoma,
    catheterization, cyclophosphamide
  Prostate: hypertrophy, carcinoma, prostatitis
  Urethra: urethritis, trauma
Extraglomerular renal bleeding
  Pelvic calculi
  Crystalluria: hypercalciuria, rarely sulfonamides or mercaptopurine
  Carcinoma: renal cell, transitional cell (especially with analgesic abuse; see Chap.
    49)
  Sickle cell trait or disease
  Cystic diseases: polycystic kidney disease, medullary sponge kidney
  Coagulation disorders: anticoagulation therapy, hemophilia
  Trauma
  Vascular malformations: hemangiomas, varices, fistulas
  Vascular diseases: emboli, vasculitis
Glomerular bleeding
  Mild forms of glomerulonephritis: IgA nephropathy, hereditary nephritis, thin
    basement membrane disease (see Chap. 25)
  Long-distance running
  Malignant hypertension

lem. In one study of 1000 young men who had yearly urinalyses between the ages of 18
and 33, hematuria was seen in 39 percent on at least one occasion and 16 percent on
two or more examinations [20]. Hematuria has also been found in up to 13 percent of
postmenopausal women [21]. No obvious etiology can be found in most cases.

The major *identifiable* causes of isolated hematuria are listed in Table 18-3. In adults,
prostatic disease; renal or ureteral calculi; trauma; malignancy of the prostate, bladder,
or kidney; and probably long-distance running are the most common [21,22]. If, however,
these conditions are excluded by the history, physical examination, and appropriate
radiologic tests, then mild glomerular diseases (such as IgA nephropathy) become more
prevalent, particularly in patients with gross hematuria [23].

The etiologic distribution is different in children. Glomerular disease, perineal irri-
tation or trauma, and hypercalciuria (with or without demonstrable calculi) appear to
be most common [8,24]. The role of hypercalciuria (defined as calcium excretion >4 mg/
kg/day) has only recently been appreciated. In one study of 83 children with isolated
hematuria, 23 had hypercalciuria, 17 had glomerular disease, and 38 of the remainder
were of unknown cause [24]. Furthermore, the majority of children with increased urinary calcium excretion had a positive family history of nephrolithiasis (versus only 15%

in the normocalciuric group) and two subsequently formed calcium stones. It is presumed that the hematuria results from crystals or microcalculi damaging the tubular or mucosal epithelia. Lowering urinary calcium excretion with a thiazide diuretic usually leads to resolution of the hematuria [24].

Diagnosis
The initial step in the evaluation of the patient with isolated hematuria is to distinguish glomerular from extraglomerular bleeding [2]. As described in Chap. 16, the finding of dysmorphic red cells, red cell casts, more than 500 mg of protein per day, or brown "Coca-Cola"-colored urine is suggestive of glomerular disease. In contrast, normal red cell morphology or the presence of blood clots favors an extraglomerular lesion. An interesting use of these principles can be seen with the hematuria associated with long-distance running. It had been assumed that bladder trauma was primarily responsible for this problem; however, almost all patients have dysmorphic red cells and up to 30 percent have red cell–casts and mild proteinuria, suggesting a glomerular origin [22]. How this might occur is not known.

In comparison to the urinary findings, the *magnitude* of the bleeding is usually not of prognostic or diagnostic importance. The presence of red or brown urine, for example, does not necessarily reflect heavy bleeding, since as little as 1 ml of blood per liter of urine is sufficient to produce a visible color change. Furthermore, most of the disorders in Table 18-3 can cause either gross or microscopic hematuria. There is, however, one exception to this general rule. The most common glomerular causes of isolated hematuria are IgA nephropathy, hereditary nephritis, and thin glomerular basement membrane disease [25,26]. Episodes of gross hematuria are common in the first two disorders (which may ultimately be associated with progressive renal failure, particularly hereditary nephritis in males) but are unusual in the benign thin membrane disease [25,26].

In addition to the urinalysis, the history and physical examination may be helpful by suggesting one of the conditions in Table 18-3. For example, rectal examination in men may reveal evidence of prostatic disease. In addition, a ureteral calculus should be excluded if the patient complains of unilateral flank pain; black patients should be tested for sickle cell trait or hemoglobin SC disease; polycystic kidney disease or hereditary nephritis should be considered if there is a positive family history of kidney disease; a focal glomerulonephritis (such as IgA nephropathy) should be suspected if there are episodes of gross hematuria following upper respiratory infections; and the urine should be cultured for *Mycobacterium tuberculosis* if there is concurrent dysuria and pyuria but a negative culture for common bacteria [2]. A 24-hour urine collection for calcium should also be obtained if no identifiable etiology appears to be present, even though the role of hypercalciuria as a cause of hematuria in adults remains to be defined.

In many patients, the initial evaluation does not lead to a definite diagnosis. This is in part related to the observation that the great majority of patients with isolated microscopic hematuria do not have any serious underlying disease [21]. It is therefore uncertain how often to proceed with intravenous pyelography (looking for stones, polycystic kidney disease, or a renal cell carcinoma) and, if it is negative, cystoscopic examination of the prostate (in men) and bladder. Many physicians would perform these tests in patients over the age of 55 because of the possibility of an underlying urinary tract malignancy, even though the frequency with which these disorders will be found is quite low [21]. Urinary cytology also may be helpful in this setting.

References

1. Dodge, WF, West, EF, Smith, EH, Bunce, H. Proteinuria and hematuria in school children: Epidemiology and early natural history. *J Pediatr* 88:327, 1976.
2. Rose, BD. *Pathophysiology of Renal Disease* (2nd ed). New York: McGraw-Hill, 1987.
3. Bohrer, MP, Baylis, C, Humes, HD, Glassock, RJ, Robertson, CR, Brenner, BM. Permselectivity of the glomerular capillary wall. Facilitated filtration of circulating polycations. *J Clin Invest* 61:72, 1978.
4. Bertolatus, JA, Abuyousef, M, Hunsicker, LG. Glomerular sieving of high molecular weight proteins in proteinuric rats. *Kidney Int* 31:257, 1987.

5. Myers, BD, Okarma, TB, Friedman, S, Bridges, C, Ross, J, Asseff, S, Deen WM. Mechanisms of proteinuria in human glomerulonephritis. *J Clin Invest* 70:732, 1982.
6. Portman, RJ, Kissane, JM, Robson, AM. Use of β_2-microglobulin to diagnose tubulointerstitial renal lesions in children. *Kidney Int.* 30:91, 1986.
7. Ginsberg, JM, Chang, BS, Matarese, RA, Garella, S. Use of single voided urine samples to estimate quantitative proteinuria. *N Engl J Med* 309:1543, 1983.
8. West, CD. Asymptomatic hematuria and proteinuria in children: Causes and appropriate diagnostic studies. *J Pediatr* 89:173, 1976.
9. Cameron, JS. Membranous nephropathy: The treatment dilemma. *Am J Kid Dis* 1:371, 1982.
10. Hardwicke, J, Squire, JR. The relationship between plasma albumin concentration and protein excretion in patients with proteinuria. *Clin Sci* 14:509, 1955.
11. Shemesh, O, Deen, WM, Brenner, BM, McNeely, E, Myers, BD. Effect of colloid volume expansion on glomerular barrier size-selectivity in humans. *Kidney Int* 29:916, 1986.
12. Robinson, RR. Isolated proteinuria in asymptomatic patients. *Kidney Int* 18:395, 1980.
13. Poortmans, JR. Postexercise proteinuria in humans: Facts and mechanisms. *J Am Med Assoc* 253:236, 1985.
14. Springberg, PD, Garrett, LE, Jr, Thompson, AL, Collins, NF, Lordon, RE, Robinson, RR. Fixed and reproducible orthostatic proteinuria: Results of a 20-year follow-up study. *Ann Intern Med* 97:516, 1982.
15. Rytand, D, Spretier, S. Prognosis in postural (orthostatic) proteinuria. Forty to fifty-year follow-up of six patients after diagnosis by Thomas Addis. *N Engl J Med* 305:618, 1981.
16. Brown, EA, Upadhyaya, K, Hayslett, JP, Kashgarian, M, Siegel, NS. The clinical course of mesangial proliferative glomerulonephritis. *Medicine* 58:195, 1979.
17. Carrie, BJ, Hilberman, M, Schroeder, JS, Myers, BD. Albuminuria and the permselective properties of the glomerulus in cardiac failure. *Kidney Int* 17:507, 1980.
18. Kannel, WB, Stampfer, MJ, Castelli, WP, Verter, J. The prognostic significance of proteinuria: The Framingham study. *Am Heart J* 108:1347, 1984.
19. Potter, EV, Lipschultz, SA, Abidh, S, Poon-King, T, Earle, DP. Twelve to seventeen-year follow-up of patients with poststreptococcal acute glomerulonephritis in Trinidad. *N Engl J Med* 307:725, 1982.
20. Froom, P, Ribak, J, Benbassat, J. Significance of microhaematuria in young adults. *Br Med J* 288:20, 1984.
21. Mohr, DN, Offord, KP, Owen, RA, Melton, J, III. Asymptomatic microhematuria and urologic disease. A population-based study. *J Am Med Assoc* 256:224, 1986.
22. Fassett, RG, Owen, JE, Fairley, J, Birch, DF, Fairley, KF. Urinary red-cell morphology during exercise. *Br Med J* 285:1455, 1982.
23. Copley, JB, Hasbargen, JA. "Idiopathic" hematuria. A prospective evaluation. *Arch Intern Med* 147:434, 1987.
24. Stapleton, FB, Roy, S, III, Noe, NH, Jenkins, G. Hypercalciuria in children with hematuria. *N Engl J Med* 310:1345, 1984.
25. Trachtman, H, Weiss, RA, Bennett, B, Griefer, I. Isolated hematuria in children: Indications for a renal biopsy. *Kidney Int* 25:94, 1984.
26. Tiebosch, ATMG, Wolters, J, Frederik, PFM, van der Wiel, TWN, Zeppenfeldt, E, van Breda Vriesman, PJC. Epidemiology of idiopathic glomerular diseases. A prospective study. *Kidney Int* 32:112, 1987.

IV. ACUTE RENAL FAILURE

19. DIFFERENTIAL DIAGNOSIS OF ACUTE RENAL FAILURE: PRERENAL DISEASE VERSUS ACUTE TUBULAR NECROSIS

Acute renal failure is a common clinical problem characterized by a relatively abrupt decline in renal function. This is manifested by a reduction in the glomerular filtration rate (GFR) (which produces an elevation in the plasma creatinine concentration) and often a decrease in urine volume.

The simplest definition of acute renal failure is a recent rise in the plasma creatinine concentration of at least 0.5 mg/dl if the baseline level is ≤3.0 mg/dl, or at least 1.0 mg/dl if the baseline level is >3.0 mg/dl. Although these increments in the plasma creatinine concentration are numerically small, they usually reflect large reductions in the GFR. A rise in the plasma creatinine concentration from 0.8 to 1.6 mg/dl, for example, can represent a fall in the GFR from 120 to 60 ml/min or less (see Chap. 17).

The many causes of acute renal failure, their associated urinary abnormalities, and a general approach to differential diagnosis are reviewed in Chap. 16. However, two conditions, *prerenal disease* (in which renal function is impaired by decreased renal perfusion, rather than intrinsic renal disease) and *acute tubular necrosis* (ATN) account for approximately 70 to 75 percent of cases. These disorders are particularly common when acute renal failure develops in the hospital, since the other causes (such as glomerulonephritis, vasculitis, or obstruction) most often begin prior to hospitalization.

As will be reviewed in the following chapters, both prerenal disease and ATN can occur in a variety of clinical settings. Differentiating between them may be difficult, however, since renal ischemia is the major cause of ATN. This distinction is important because volume repletion may restore renal function in prerenal disease but will be without benefit (and may induce peripheral or pulmonary edema) in ATN.

History and Physical Examination
The history and physical examination often reveal important diagnostic information, such as the identification of potential causes of either prerenal disease (true volume depletion, heart failure, or hepatic cirrhosis) or ATN (marked hypotension or the administration of an aminoglycoside or radiocontrast media). It is also possible, in hospitalized patients, to determine the day on which the plasma creatinine concentration began to rise. In this setting, either some renal insult occurred on that day (such as hypotension or a radiocontrast study) or the cumulative effect of some prior toxin first became apparent (as with aminoglycoside nephrotoxicity). In regard to the latter, the duration of drug usage is also important. Aminoglycosides, for example, gradually accumulate in the renal cortex and usually do not cause an elevation in the plasma creatinine concentration for at least 7 to 10 days. Thus, renal failure occurring within a few days of the onset of therapy is probably not due to the aminoglycoside alone.

The physical examination also may be helpful in selected cases. Decreased skin turgor, a low jugular venous pressure, and postural tachycardia or hypotension are signs of true volume depletion that can lead to prerenal disease and possibly to postischemic ATN. In contrast, peripheral or pulmonary edema or ascites suggests the presence of heart failure or hepatic cirrhosis.

Laboratory Tests
In most patients, laboratory tests are required to confirm or establish the cause of the acute renal failure (Table 19-1) [1,2]. It is important, when evaluating the different tests that have been used to differentiate prerenal disease from ATN, to define the "gold standard": the return of baseline renal function within 48 to 72 hours of increasing the effective circulating volume (by, for example, administering fluids or treating hypotension) is considered to reflect prerenal disease; in comparison, continued renal failure despite adequate fluid repletion is called ATN.

It is also important to note that the laboratory findings in Table 19-1 are most useful in *oliguric* patients (urine output ≤500 ml/day). Patients with *nonoliguric* ATN tend to have less severe tubular damage and there is likely to be more overlap with prerenal

Table 19-1. Laboratory findings in acute renal failure

Test	Favors prerenal disease	Favors ATN
BUN/P_{cr} ratio	> 20:1	10–15:1
Rise in P_{cr}	Variable rate of rise with downward fluctuations in some patients	Progressive increase of ≥ 0.5 mg/dl/day, particularly in oliguric patients
Urinalysis	Normal or near-normal; hyaline casts may be seen but are not abnormal	Many granular casts with renal tubular epithelial cells and epithelial cell casts; may be normal in nonoliguric patients
Urine osmolality	> 500 mosmol/kg	< 350 mosmol/kg
Urine sodium	< 20 meq/L	> 40 meq/L
Fractional excretion of sodium	< 1%	> 2%

Source: From Rose, BD. *Pathophysiology of Renal Disease* (2nd ed). New York: McGraw-Hill, 1987. P. 65.

disease [2,3]. This overlap is sufficiently common that many of the tests are helpful only at the extremes, when clearly high or low values are obtained.

BUN/P_{cr} Ratio
A decline in the GFR should elevate both the blood urea nitrogen (BUN) and the plasma creatinine concentration, maintaining a normal ratio between these parameters of 10–15:1 [4]. In prerenal disease, however, the compensatory increase in proximal sodium and water reabsorption promotes an elevation in passive urea reabsorption. The ensuing fall in urea excretion raises the BUN out of proportion to any reduction in the GFR thereby increasing the BUN/P_{cr} ratio to 20 : 1 or more [4]. Thus, a high ratio is suggestive of prerenal disease *in the absence* of some cause of increased urea production such as gastrointestinal bleeding, increased tissue breakdown, or high-dose corticosteroid therapy. A *normal ratio is less useful* since the expected rise in the BUN in prerenal disease may be prevented if protein intake is reduced (due, for example, to vomiting) or if urea synthesis is impaired by concurrent liver disease.

The time course of the rise in the plasma creatinine concentration also may be of diagnostic importance. The plasma creatinine concentration typically increases by 0.5 mg/dl or more per day in established ATN, particularly in oliguric patients. In comparison, the daily increment may be smaller, with occasional downward fluctuation in prerenal disease [5]. Transient improvements in renal perfusion are presumably responsible for the intermittent declines in the plasma creatinine concentration in the latter setting.

Urinalysis
The urinalysis is generally different in prerenal disease and ATN, usually being normal in the former but showing dark brown granular casts and free renal tubular epithelial cells and epithelial cell casts in the latter. Once again, however, there is more overlap with nonoliguric ATN, where the urinalysis may be near normal in 20 to 30 percent of cases.

Another potential source of confusion comes in patients who slowly evolve from prerenal disease into postischemic ATN. The urinalysis early in this interphase may begin to show granular casts indicative of some tubular damage; however, the urine sodium concentration and fractional excretion of sodium may still be low, and fluid repletion may still restore renal function [1].

The urinalysis may also be helpful in identifying an additional cause of acute renal failure that is often hospital-acquired, drug-induced acute interstitial nephritis (see Chap. 46). The urinary findings in this condition are different from those in ATN and typically include hematuria, pyuria (including eosinophiluria in some patients), and white cell casts. This is an important diagnosis to establish since treatment consists of discontinuation of the offending drug and the possible use of corticosteroids.

Urine Osmolality
The urine osmolality is, in theory, useful in differentiating prerenal disease from ATN [1,2]. Effective volume depletion is a potent stimulus to the release of antidiuretic hormone. This should result in a highly concentrated urine (above 500 mosmol/kg) when tubular function is intact. In ATN, however, renal ischemia primarily affects the medulla, leading to dysfunction of cells in both the thick ascending limb of the loop of Henle (the segment that is responsible for the generation of the countercurrent gradient) and the collecting tubules (the segments that respond to antidiuretic hormone) [6,7]. As a result, loss of concentrating ability is an early finding in ATN and the urine osmolality is generally below 400 mosmol/kg [2,8].

Despite these considerations, the urine osmolality is often not helpful in the diagnosis of acute renal failure. A value above 500 mosmol/kg is highly suggestive of prerenal disease; however, lower values (similar to those in ATN) can be seen in this disorder because patients with prerenal disease frequently have an associated concentrating defect. For example, renal ischemia can diminish loop of Henle function without producing overt tubular necrosis [9]. In addition, elderly patients or those with underlying renal disease frequently are unable to concentrate normally even in the presence of antidiuretic hormone [10].

Urine Sodium Concentration
The urine sodium concentration is another test that may be important diagnostically. Sodium retention is an appropriate response to prerenal disease, whereas tubular damage usually limits the efficiency of sodium reabsorption in ATN. As depicted in Fig. 19-1a, however, there is again considerable overlap: a urine sodium concentration above 40 meq/L usually indicates ATN while a value below 20 meq/L generally, but not always, reflects prerenal disease [2,8].

Part of the reason for this overlap is that the urine sodium concentration is affected by the degree of *water* as well as sodium reabsorption. If, for example, the tubules reabsorb almost all of the filtered water, then the urine sodium concentration in prerenal disease can be raised (by urinary concentration) above 20 meq/L even though there is also avid sodium retention. Conversely, decreased water reabsorption in ATN can lower the urine sodium concentration by dilution, despite an impairment in sodium transport. These potentially confusing effects of water handling can be partially eliminated by calculation of the fractional excretion of sodium (FE_{Na}), which is a direct measure of tubular sodium transport.

FRACTIONAL EXCRETION OF SODIUM.   The fractional excretion of sodium reflects the percent of the filtered sodium load that is excreted:

$$FE_{Na} (\%) = \frac{\text{quantity of sodium excreted}}{\text{quantity of sodium filtered}} \times 100$$

Sodium excretion is equal to the product of the urine sodium concentration and the urine volume; the quantity of sodium filtered is equal to the product of the plasma sodium concentration and the GFR (as estimated from the creatinine clearance, $U_{cr}V/P_{cr}$). Thus:

$$FE_{Na} (\%) = \frac{U_{Na} \times V \times 100}{P_{Na} \times (U_{cr}V/P_{cr})}$$

$$= \frac{U_{Na} \times P_{cr}}{P_{Na} \times U_{cr}} \times 100$$

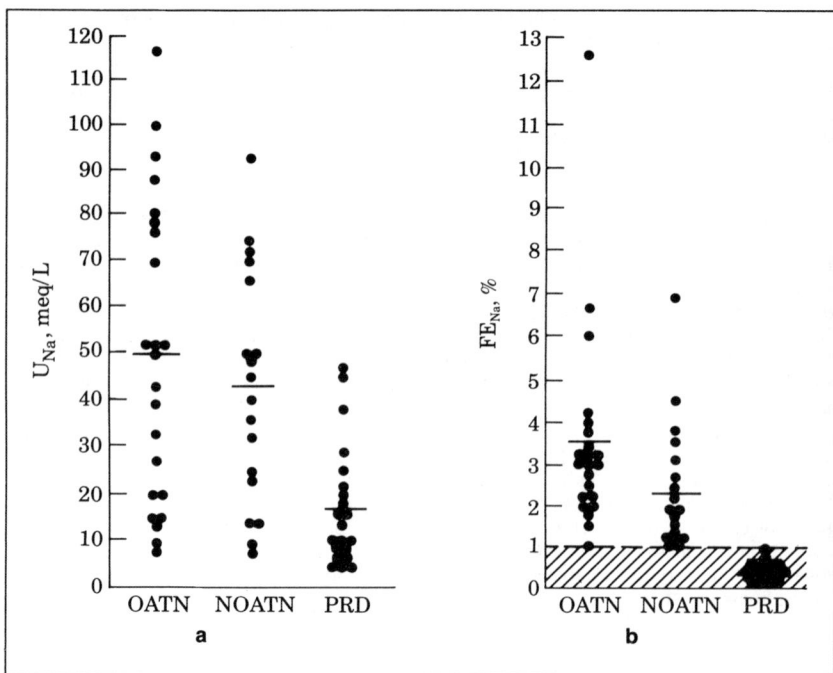

Fig. 19-1. The urine sodium concentration (a) and the fractional excretion of sodium (b) in 61 patients with oliguric or nonoliguric ATN (OATN and NOATN) or prerenal disease (PRD). The almost complete separation between ATN and prerenal disease with the fractional excretion of sodium in these patients has not been confirmed in other studies in which some overlap can occur. (Adapted from Espinel, CH, Gregory, AW. *Clin Nephrol* 13:73, 1980.)

As shown in Fig. 19-1b, the fractional excretion of sodium is more effective than the urine sodium concentration (or any other laboratory test) in distinguishing prerenal disease from ATN [1,2,5,8]. A value below 1 percent favors the former and above 2 percent favors the latter; there is some overlap between 1 and 2 percent [11].

Although the fractional excretion of sodium is very useful, it is now apparent that a variety of causes of acute renal failure other than prerenal disease can on occasion be associated with a value below 1 percent (Table 19-2) [1,11,12]. This can occur when ATN is superimposed on a chronic prerenal state (such as hepatic cirrhosis or heart failure) or when the GFR is reduced in the presence of *intact tubular function*. The latter situation can occur in acute glomerulonephritis or vasculitis, acute obstructive uropathy, or intratubular obstruction (with no or little tubular necrosis) due to hemoglobinuria or myoglobinuria [1].

A low fractional excretion of sodium can also be seen in some patients with ATN and no prior prerenal state. This is most likely to be found in *postischemic ATN when there is a lesser degree of tubular injury*: examples include approximately 10 percent of nonoliguric cases [2,11] and those evaluated within the first 2 days of the disease, near the interphase between prerenal disease and ATN [12].

VOLUME DEPLETION AND UNDERLYING RENAL DISEASE. An additional source of potential difficulty arises when volume depletion is superimposed on underlying renal disease. In this setting, the characteristic laboratory findings of prerenal disease may be absent, since chronic renal disease frequently impairs both sodium conservation and concentrating ability, and the urinalysis may be abnormal because of the underlying disease.

Table 19-2. Causes of acute renal failure in which the fractional excretion of sodium may be below 1 percent

Prerenal disease
ATN
   More likely in early or nonoliguric cases
   Superimposed on chronic prerenal state
      Hepatic cirrhosis
      Heart failure
      Severe burns
   Myoglobinuria or hemoglobinuria
   Radiocontrast media
   Sepsis
Acute glomerulonephritis or vasculitis
Acute obstructive uropathy
Acute interstitial nephritis

Source: From Rose, BD. *Pathophysiology of Renal Disease* (2nd ed). New York: McGraw-Hill, 1987. P. 69.

    Furthermore, a relatively small degree of volume depletion can produce a relatively large increase in the plasma creatinine concentration in such patients. For example, a patient with a baseline plasma creatinine concentration of 4 mg/dl may have a GFR of 20 ml/min or less. In this setting, a minor amount of volume loss can lower renal perfusion enough to reduce the GFR to 10 ml/min; this 50 percent decline in filtration will produce an approximate doubling of the plasma creatinine concentration to 8 mg/dl (see Chap. 17). Despite these impressive laboratory changes, there may not have been sufficient volume depletion to produce the characteristic physical findings such as decreased skin turgor, tachycardia, and a fall in blood pressure.

    Thus, the physician must be aware that hypovolemia (which may be subclinical) may be responsible for an otherwise unexplained and *reversible* acute deterioration in renal function in a patient with chronic renal insufficiency. This possibility can be confirmed by a return in the plasma creatinine concentration toward the baseline level after a cautious trial of fluid repletion.

Summary

There is as yet no single test that can clearly differentiate prerenal disease from ATN. This difficulty is in part related to the similarities between these disorders, since renal ischemia is the major cause of ATN. Thus, the proper approach to diagnosis relies on using all of the available information on history, physical examination, and laboratory testing. For example, granular casts in the urine sediment, a urine osmolality of 320 mosmol/kg, and a fractional excretion of sodium of 3.2 percent almost certainly reflects ATN. In contrast, prerenal disease is likely in a patient who is dehydrated from vomiting and has a normal urinalysis, a urine osmolality of 540 mosmol/kg, and a fractional excretion of sodium of 0.4 percent.

    It is also important to emphasize that the initial treatment of prerenal disease and postischemic ATN is similar: fluid repletion to restore normal perfusion and, if the patient is oliguric, the possible use of furosemide or mannitol to preserve renal function (see Chap. 24). As a result, establishing the exact diagnosis at the time of presentation may not be essential in the hypovolemic patient. Renal failure that persists or progresses after fluid administration is considered to reflect ATN.

References

1. Rose, BD. *Pathophysiology of Renal Disease* (2nd ed). New York: McGraw-Hill, 1987. Pp. 65-70.
2. Miller, TR, Anderson, RJ, Linas, SL, Henrich, WL, Berns, AS, Gabow, PA, Schrier,

RW. Urinary diagnostic indices in acute renal failure: A prospective study. *Ann Intern Med* 89:47, 1978.

3. Dixon, BS, Anderson, RJ. Nonoliguric acute renal failure. *Am J Kid Dis* 6:71, 1985.
4. Dossetor, JB. Creatininemia versus uremia. The relative significance of blood urea nitrogen and serum creatinine concentrations in azotemia. *Ann Intern Med* 65:1287, 1966.
5. Oken, DE. On the differential diagnosis of acute renal failure. *Am J Med* 71:916, 1981.
6. Brezis, M, Rosen, S, Silva, P, Epstein, FH. Renal ischemia. A new perspective. *Kidney Int* 26:375, 1984.
7. Hanley, MJ. Isolated nephron segments in a rabbit model of ischemic acute renal failure. *Am J Physiol* 239:F17, 1980.
8. Espinel, CH, Gregory, AW. Differential diagnosis of acute renal failure. *Clin Nephrol* 13:73, 1980.
9. Miller, PD, Krebs, RA, Neal, BJ, McIntyre, DO. Polyuric prerenal failure. *Arch Intern Med* 140:907, 1980.
10. Sporn, IN, Lancestremere, RG, Papper, S. Differential diagnosis of oliguria in aged patients. *N Engl J Med* 267:130, 1962.
11. Steiner, RW. Interpreting the fractional excretion of sodium. *Am J Med* 77:699, 1984.
12. Brosius, FC, Lau, K. Low fractional excretion of sodium in acute renal failure: Role of timing of the test and ischemia. *Am J Nephrol* 6:450, 1986.

20. PRERENAL DISEASE

Reduced renal perfusion is a common cause of renal failure. It occurs in two basic settings: when there is a generalized decline in tissue perfusion, as with true volume depletion or heart failure; or when there is selective renal ischemia, as with bilateral renal artery stenosis or, in some patients, the administration of a nonsteroidal anti-inflammatory drug (Table 20-1) [1].

Both hemodynamic and neurohumoral factors contribute to the decrease in the glomerular filtration rate (GFR) with hypovolemia. Systemic hypoperfusion is initially sensed by pressure (or stretch) receptors in the heart and in the arterial circulation (such as those in the carotid sinus and the afferent glomerular arteriole). The ensuing release of norepinephrine and angiotensin II leads to systemic and renal vasoconstriction; this response is in part appropriate in that it maintains the blood pressure and preserves perfusion to the heart and brain. However, the renal ischemia ultimately lowers the GFR, as manifested by a rise in the blood urea nitrogen (BUN) and plasma creatinine concentration.

It is important to appreciate that, despite marked edema, congestive heart failure and hepatic cirrhosis are also conditions in which effective tissue perfusion is reduced. The decrease in tissue perfusion in these disorders is initiated, respectively, by a fall in cardiac output and by systemic vasodilatation and ascites formation. Thus, increasingly severe cardiac or hepatic disease is associated with a progressive rise in the secretion of the three *"hypovolemic"* hormones—renin, norepinephrine, and antidiuretic hormone (ADH)—and with a subsequent fall in the GFR [2,3].

This chapter will review only true volume depletion and hypotension. The other causes of prerenal disease listed in Table 20-1 as well as the characteristic laboratory findings associated with this disorder are discussed in the appropriate chapters elsewhere in the book.

True Volume Depletion
The presence of one of the causes of true volume depletion is usually evident from the history. In addition, fluid loss severe enough to produce renal insufficiency should be

Table 20-1. Major causes of prerenal disease

True volume depletion
    Gastrointestinal losses (vomiting, diarrhea, tube drainage)
    Renal losses (diuretics, glucosuria)
    Skin or respiratory losses (insensible losses, sweat, burns)
    Third-space sequestration or bleeding (crush injury, acute pancreatitis, intestinal
        obstruction)
Hypotension
    Shock
    Posttreatment of marked hypertension
Edematous states
    Heart failure
    Hepatic cirrhosis and the hepatorenal syndrome
Selective renal ischemia
    Bilateral renal artery stenosis (the decline in glomerular filtration is frequently
        exacerbated by converting enzyme inhibition)
    Nonsteroidal anti-inflammatory drugs (primarily in patients with underlying
        hypovolemia and renal vasoconstriction)
    Calcium channel blockers (?)

associated with at least some of the characteristic physical findings including decreased skin turgor, dry mucous membranes, estimated jugular venous pressure below 5 cm H_2O, and postural tachycardia with or without hypotension. Those patients with the clinical syndrome of hypovolemic shock also have signs of marked hypoperfusion (due in part to intense peripheral vasoconstriction), such as cold, clammy extremities; cyanosis; agitation; confusion; and little or no urine output.

Concurrent abnormalities in electrolyte and acid-base balance also may be seen and may be of diagnostic importance when the history is not helpful. As an example, elderly patients with diminished mental status may become hypovolemic due to lack of replacement of insensible losses. This sequence *must lead to hypernatremia* since water is lost in excess of sodium. If, however, a normal plasma sodium concentration is found, then *sodium and water must have been lost in proportion,* and some source of sodium loss must be identified (such as concurrent diuretic therapy). More commonly, the plasma sodium concentration is normal or low in prerenal states; the combination of a reduced GFR and increased secretion of ADH promotes the retention of ingested or administered water, thereby favoring the development of hyponatremia.

Concurrent acid-base abnormalities also may be of diagnostic assistance. Metabolic alkalosis, for example, suggests either diuretic therapy or vomiting. In comparison, metabolic acidosis may be seen with diarrhea, diabetic ketoacidosis, or shock-induced lactic acidosis.

Treatment

Therapy is aimed at fluid repletion. The major questions that must be addressed are the *type* of fluid used and the *rate* at which it is given [1]. Excluding patients in shock, the *tonicity of the administered fluid is determined by the plasma sodium concentration.* Hypotonic fluids should be given if the patient is hypernatremic in an effort to also lower the plasma sodium concentration toward normal. The proper fluid may vary from dextrose in water to quarter- or half-isotonic saline, depending on whether there is pure water loss (as with insensible losses or diabetes insipidus) or both sodium and water loss. In contrast, isotonic or, if the plasma sodium concentration is below 110 to 115 meq/L, hypertonic saline is indicated in hyponatremic patients. Finally, either half-isotonic or isotonic saline can be used if the plasma sodium concentration is relatively normal. In addition, blood replacement may be required in patients with active bleeding or marked anemia.

The ionic composition of the administered fluid is also affected by other electrolyte abnormalities that may be present. For example, suppose a patient with severe diarrhea has the following laboratory findings:

$$\begin{aligned} \text{Plasma Na} &= 131 \text{ meq/L} \\ \text{K} &= 3.1 \text{ meq/L} \\ \text{Cl} &= 110 \text{ meq/L} \\ \text{HCO}_3 &= 10 \text{ meq/L} \\ \text{Arterial pH} &= 7.27 \end{aligned}$$

This patient has both metabolic acidosis and hypokalemia in addition to volume depletion. The plasma sodium concentration is somewhat low, indicating that a relatively isotonic fluid should be given. Thus, an appropriate replacement fluid would be half-isotonic saline to which 22 meq of sodium bicarbonate and 40 meq of potassium chloride have been added.

The rate at which this fluid is given depends on the patient's clinical state. As a general rule, 75 to 100 ml/hour is adequate in most adults. More-rapid fluid repletion may be deleterious in patients with underlying cardiac disease and is unnecessary in the absence of continued fluid loss, marked volume depletion (as with uncontrolled hyperglycemia), or shock*.

The adequacy of fluid repletion can be assessed from both the physical examination and monitoring of renal function. Increasing urine output and urinary sodium excretion, for example, are generally indicative of the restoration of euvolemia. Reversal of the azotemia and elevated plasma creatinine concentration take somewhat longer to achieve. Even when the GFR has returned to normal, a finite time period is still required for the retained urea and creatinine to be excreted.

HYPOVOLEMIC SHOCK.   Early and rapid therapy is required in hypovolemic shock to prevent tissue necrosis or the development of irreversible shock. In general, fluid is given as quickly as possible (up to 1–2 liters in the first hour) until tissue perfusion improves. The central venous or pulmonary capillary wedge pressure should be monitored during this period to prevent fluid overload. It is important to note, however, that the development of peripheral edema is not necessarily a sign of overexpansion, since it may result from dilutional hypoalbuminemia at a time when plasma volume depletion persists [4].

Blood, isotonic saline, and colloid-containing solutions have been used for fluid repletion in this setting. Blood transfusions are indicated if bleeding is the primary problem. The initial aim is to raise the hematocrit to about 35 percent; higher values are not required for adequate oxygen transport but can increase blood viscosity, possibly leading to stasis in the already impaired capillary circulation.

Isotonic saline (or Ringer's lactate) is generally the preferred plasma replacement fluid. Although colloid solutions were thought to be preferable because they might expand the plasma volume more effectively (by increasing the plasma oncotic pressure), controlled studies have failed to confirm this advantage in the absence of underlying hypoalbuminemia [5,6].

Intravenous infusion of pressor agents, such as dopamine or norepinephrine, have little role in the treatment of hypovolemic shock. These agents will not correct the fluid deficit and can, via vasoconstriction, exacerbate the tissue ischemia. In comparison, military antishock trousers may be beneficial; they can raise the systemic blood pressure both by increasing vascular resistance (by mechanical compression of the legs) and by translocation of fluid from the legs into the central (cardiopulmonary) circulation [4,7].

Hypotension

Hypotension can directly impair renal function by reducing the intraglomerular pressure, which is the main driving force for glomerular filtration. This can occur in two

---

*These recommendations often have to be modified in patients with marked hyponatremia or hypernatremia. In these settings, therapy is aimed at both fluid repletion and the restoration of normonatremia. However, the latter must be done at the correct rate, since rapid changes in the plasma sodium concentration can lead to neurologic complications such as central pontine myelinolysis or cerebral edema (see Chaps. 1 and 2).

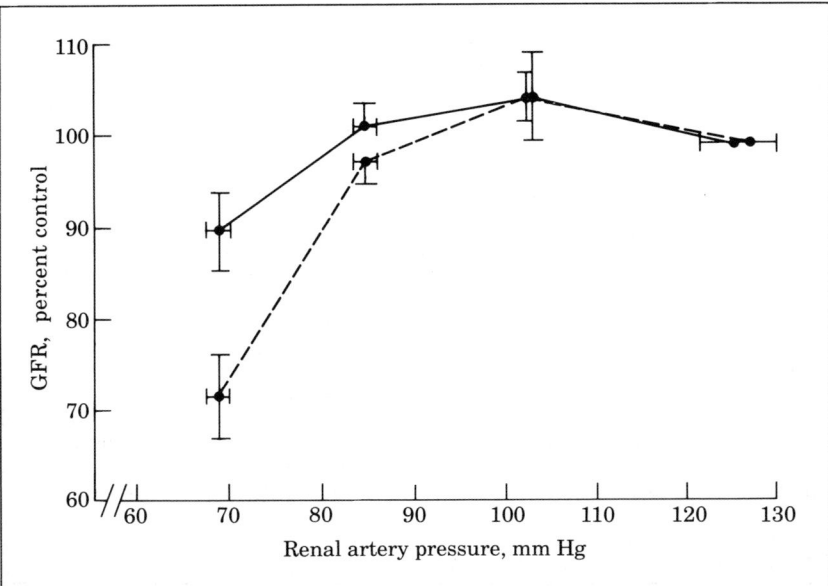

Fig. 20-1. Effect of reducing renal artery pressure on glomerular filtration rate (GFR) in normal dogs (solid lines) and dogs pretreated with an angiotensin II antagonist (dashed lines). The GFR is well maintained in the normals, but the autoregulatory response is substantially impaired in the absence of angiotensin II; this defect is more pronounced in volume-depleted dogs in which maintenance of the GFR has a greater angiotensin II-dependence. (From Hall, JE, Guyton, AC, Jackson, TE, Coleman, TG, Lohmeier, TE, Trippodo, NC. *Am J Physiol* 233:F366, 1977.)

major settings: disorders in which there is a marked fall in blood pressure (hypovolemia, sepsis, advanced cardiac disease, or the administration of interleukin-2 as immunotherapy for cancer [8]); and in the treatment of marked hypertension.

It is important to be aware, however, that the intraglomerular pressure and therefore glomerular filtration are initially maintained as the blood pressure first falls because of *autoregulation* (Fig. 20-1) [9]. This protective phenomenon, which is not restricted to the renal circulation, results from changes in arteriolar resistance. In theory, maintenance of the intraglomerular pressure in the face of hypotension could result from two mechanisms: dilation of the preglomerular afferent arteriole, which allows more of the systemic pressure to be transmitted to the glomerulus; or constriction of the efferent postglomerular arteriole, which raises the pressure behind the constriction. Studies in experimental animals suggest that both of these factors may be important: afferent dilation by a direct myogenic response and by tubuloglomerular feedback*; and efferent constriction via angiotensin II (Fig. 20-1) [9,10].

Observations in humans have indirectly confirmed the importance of angiotensin II in autoregulation. In bilateral renal artery stenosis (where the intrarenal pressure distal to the stenosis tends to be lower than systemic), the administration of a converting enzyme inhibitor can lead to acute renal failure that is presumably due to removal of the angiotensin II–mediated contribution to autoregulation [11]. A similar problem can

---

*Tubuloglomerular feedback refers to a process in which glomerular filtration is regulated by the cells of the macula densa in the early distal tubule [9]. A reduction in the GFR, for example, is associated with a concomitant reduction in flow to the macula densa; this change is sensed locally and, by an incompletely understood mechanism, leads to dilation of the afferent arteriole, which returns both the GFR and secondarily macula densa flow toward normal.

occur in patients with congestive heart failure who have a low systemic pressure; in this setting, the GFR may fall even though the converting enzyme inhibitor increases the cardiac output by lowering peripheral vascular resistance (see Chap. 22) [12].

Figure 20-1 also demonstrates that autoregulation is only effective over a limited range of blood pressure. Thus, *any antihypertensive agent can lead to a decline in glomerular filtration* in bilateral renal artery stenosis if the intrarenal pressure falls far enough (due, for example, to severe stenoses) [13]. In this setting, only correction of the stenoses by surgery or transluminal angioplasty will allow the blood pressure to fall while preserving glomerular filtration.

Acute renal failure can also occur with the rapid correction of chronic severe hypertension of any cause. In this condition, renal arteriolar hyperplasia is present, a change that is in part adaptive in that it has protected the glomerular capillaries from the elevated systemic pressure; similar findings are seen in the arterioles in other organs. The increase in thickness of these vessels, however, impairs their ability to dilate when the blood pressure is lowered toward normal. This can result in a decrease in tissue perfusion that, in the kidney, leads to a decline in the GFR and a subsequent elevation in the plasma creatinine concentration [14]. Fortunately, this response is transient, since continued control of the blood pressure permits arteriolar hyperplasia to regress and renal function to improve over a period of 1 to 3 months [14]. Antihypertensive medications do not have to be discontinued during this interval unless there has been an excessive fall in blood pressure or an unacceptably large rise in the plasma creatinine concentration.

References

1. Rose, BD. Pathophysiology of Renal Disease (2nd ed). New York: McGraw-Hill, 1987, Pp. 70-84.
2. Mettauer, B, Rouleau, J-L, Bichet, D, Juneau, C, Kortas, C, Barjon, J-N, de Champlain, J. Sodium and water excretion abnormalities in congestive heart failure. *Ann Intern Med* 105:161, 1986.
3. Perez-Ayuso, RM, Arroyo, N, Campos, J, Rimola, A, Gaya, J, Costa, J, Rivera, F, Rodes, J. Evidence that renal prostaglandins are involved in renal water metabolism in cirrhosis. *Kidney Int* 26:72, 1984.
4. Shine, KI, Kuhn, M, Young, LS, Tillisch, JH. Aspects of the management of shock. *Ann Intern Med* 93:723, 1980.
5. Moss, GS, Lowe, RJ, Jilek, J, Levine, HD. Colloid or crystalloid in the resuscitation of hemorrhagic shock: A controlled trial. *Surgery* 89:434, 1981.
6. Monafo, W. Expensive salt water. *Surgery* 89:525, 1981.
7. Kaback, KR, Sanders, AB, Meslin, HW. MAST suit update. *J Am Med Assoc* 252:2598, 1984.
8. Belldegrun, A, Webb, D, Austin, HA, III, Steinberg, SM, White, DE, Rosenberg, SA. Effects of interleukin-2 on renal function in patients receiving immunotherapy for advanced cancer. *Ann Intern Med* 106:817, 1987.
9. Rose, BD. *Clinical Physiology of Acid-Base and Electrolyte Disorders* (2nd ed). New York: McGraw-Hill, 1984. Pp. 66-69.
10. Schnermann, J, Briggs, JP, Weber, PC. Tubuloglomerular feedback, prostaglandins, and angiotensin in the autoregulation of glomerular filtration rate. *Kidney Int* 25:53, 1984.
11. Jackson, B, Mathews, PG, McGrath, BP, Johnston, CI. Angiotensin converting enzyme inhibition in renovascular hypertension: Frequency of reversible renal failure. *Lancet* 1:225, 1984.
12. Packer, M, Lee, WH, Medina, N, Yushak, M, Kessler, PD. Functional renal insufficiency during long-term therapy with captopril and enalapril in severe chronic heart failure. *Ann Intern Med* 106:346, 1987.
13. Textor, SC, Novick, AC, Tarazi, RC, Klimas, V, Vidt, DG, Pohl, M. Critical perfusion pressure for renal function in patients with bilateral atherosclerotic renal vascular disease. *Ann Intern Med* 102:308, 1985.
14. Mroczek, WJ, Davidov, MD, Gavrilovich, L, Finnerty, FA, Jr. The value of aggressive therapy in the hypertensive patient with azotemia. *Circulation* 40:893, 1969.

21. HEPATIC CIRRHOSIS AND THE HEPATORENAL SYNDROME

Hepatic cirrhosis is often associated with two major changes in renal function: sodium retention, which first becomes clinically evident as ascites; and a progressive decline in the glomerular filtration rate (GFR) that, in its later stages, is called the hepatorenal syndrome. Both humoral and hemodynamic factors play a primary role in the development of these problems.

Sodium Retention and Ascites

Abnormal sodium handling can be demonstrated early in the course of hepatic cirrhosis, prior to the presence of either ascites or peripheral edema. For example, many cirrhotic patients are less able to excrete a sodium load when compared to normals, even though the plasma volume increases, renal function is normal, and renin secretion is appropriately suppressed [1]. Similar findings can be demonstrated in experimental models of hepatic disease [2]. These observations suggest that at least the initial sodium retention represents an *overflow* phenomenon in which hepatic disease stimulates renal sodium reabsorption independent of any changes in systemic hemodynamics [2-4].

Studies in animal models of hepatic cirrhosis have shed some light on the mechanisms responsible for these alterations in sodium handling. The initial sodium retention appears to be related to the increase in *intrahepatic* pressure that results from fibrosis-induced postsinusoidal obstruction [2]. This intrahepatic hypertension may then activate a hepatorenal reflex that leads to an elevation in renal sympathetic nerve activity [5]. Increased renal sympathetic tone lowers renal perfusion and directly stimulates sodium reabsorption, both of which promote sodium retention and edema formation [5]. The elevated intrasinusoidal pressure then favors the intraperitoneal accumulation of this excess fluid as ascites.

By the time that ascites has become clinically apparent, however, a variety of additional changes have occurred that lead to decreased tissue perfusion or *underfilling* of the arterial circulation (rather than overflow) [3,4]. These include: (1) a further increase in intrasinusoidal pressure, which promotes fluid accumulation both in the peritoneum and in the dilated splanchnic venous system; (2) peripheral vasodilatation, due in part to the formation of arteriovenous fistulas (such as the spider angiomas on the skin); and (3) hypoalbuminemia, which promotes fluid movement out of the vascular space.

These changes slowly become more marked so that increasingly severe liver disease is associated with progressively enhanced secretion of the three "hypovolemic" hormones—renin, norepinephrine, and antidiuretic hormone (ADH)—and a very low rate of sodium excretion [6-8]. Furthermore, the cardiac output, which is elevated early in the disease due to flow through the arteriovenous fistulas*, often falls to a level that is below normal [9].

Fluid retention induced by underfilling can be seen as representing an *appropriate* attempt to enhance perfusion by expanding the plasma volume. Nevertheless, it is somewhat difficult to appreciate how the massively edematous patient with hepatic cirrhosis can be effectively hypovolemic. One indirect proof of the presence of volume depletion has come from studies in which cirrhotic patients are immersed to the neck in warm water. In this setting, the hydrostatic pressure of the water on the lower extremities results in the redistribution of intravascular fluid from the legs to the central cardiopulmonary circulation. This increase in venous return (which is roughly equivalent to an infusion of 2 liters of isotonic saline) raises the cardiac output, often resulting in a relatively marked natriuresis (in comparison to the very low baseline level of sodium excretion) and a reduction in the secretion of renin, norepinephrine, and ADH [8,10].

These findings indicate that acute volume expansion can reverse the sodium-retaining tendency of cirrhosis, thereby suggesting an important role for underlying hypoperfusion. There are, however, cirrhotic patients who do not respond to neck immersion; these patients tend to have a greater baseline degree of effective volume depletion as

---

*Blood flow through the fistulas is *ineffective,* since it bypasses the capillary circulation. Thus, the cardiac output is elevated at a time that capillary perfusion is probably reduced.

evidenced by higher vasoactive hormone levels, leading to enhanced renal vasoconstriction, which lowers both renal blood flow and glomerular filtration [8].

Diagnosis
The diagnosis of hepatic cirrhosis as the cause of ascites and, in some cases, peripheral edema is often easily made from the history and physical examination. However, right-sided heart failure can produce similar findings. These disorders can usually be differentiated at the bedside by estimation of the jugular venous pressure. The increase in venous pressure in hepatic cirrhosis is below the hepatic vein. As a result, the venous pressure above the liver in the external jugular vein is generally low or normal (< 7 cm of water), not elevated as in heart failure [11]. One exception to this general rule can occur in cirrhotic patients with tense ascites in whom upward pressure on the diaphragm raises the intrathoracic pressures. The central venous pressure, however, rapidly falls with relief of the intraabdominal tension by removal of a small amount of ascitic fluid [11].

Treatment
Therapy aimed at fluid removal in cirrhosis consists of bed rest, marked dietary sodium restriction, and, if necessary, the use of diuretics. Measurement of the urine sodium concentration may also be helpful in this setting by assessing the degree of dietary compliance. A value above 50 meq/L, for example, suggests that the patient is able to excrete some sodium and that the continued fluid retention is in part due to dietary indiscretion. In contrast, patients with severe hepatic cirrhosis often excrete less than 10 meq of sodium per day [12]; these patients also tend to retain water and become hyponatremic [8]. Both hyponatremia and marked sodium retention (urinary sodium excretion <10 meq/day) are poor prognostic findings because they reflect severe underlying hepatic disease: the mean duration of survival is less than 6 months in these patients in comparison to over 2 years in patients without these abnormalities [8,12].
    As reviewed in detail in Chap. 4, a number of relatively unique problems may arise with attempted fluid removal in the cirrhotic patient. Summarized briefly:

1. Spironolactone is often more effective than a loop diuretic in this setting [13], a paradoxical finding that may reflect decreased tubular secretion of loop diuretics into the tubular lumen in cirrhosis [14]. Spironolactone is unique in that it enters the tubular cell from the capillary side; it does not require entry into the tubular lumen and therefore there is no apparent resistance to its diuretic activity.
2. Spironolactone is also safer, since the development of hypokalemia and metabolic alkalosis with a loop or thiazide diuretic can lead to increased circulating ammonia levels and hepatic encephalopathy.
3. The rate of fluid removal *should not exceed 300 to 500 ml/day* in patients with *ascites but no peripheral edema* [15]. In any edematous patient treated with diuretics, the fluid lost in the urine initially comes from the plasma; the intravascular volume is then repleted by mobilization of the edema fluid, as the fall in venous pressure promotes fluid movement from the interstitium into the vascular space. This process is rate-unlimited in the cirrhotic patient who also has peripheral edema, since all of the peripheral capillaries can contribute to edema mobilization. In comparison, mobilization can only occur via the peritoneal capillaries in the patient who has only ascites; this process is relatively slow with a maximum rate that is usually less than 500 ml/day [15]. More rapid diuresis leads to plasma volume depletion, a decline in renal function, and possible precipitation of the hepatorenal syndrome [15].
4. Nonsteroidal anti-inflammatory drugs, which diminish the synthesis of vasodilator prostaglandins, should be avoided if possible. The ensuing renal vasoconstriction can lead to a decline in both the GFR and sodium excretion. One possible exception is sulindac, which appears to relatively spare renal prostaglandin synthesis and is therefore less likely to lead to deleterious changes in renal function [16].

USE OF PARACENTESIS.   Paracentesis (with the removal of 4–6 liters of ascitic fluid per day) is a possible alternative to diuretic therapy in patients with tense ascites [17]. When used with intravenous albumin replacement to maintain the plasma volume and diuretics to prevent recurrent edema formation, paracentesis can lead to much more rapid removal of the ascites, fewer fluid and electrolyte complications, and a shorter period of hospitalization, when compared to similar patients treated with diuretics [17].

Renal Dysfunction and Hepatorenal Syndrome

The increases in circulating norepinephrine and angiotensin II that promote sodium retention also lead to renal vasoconstriction, a change that contributes to a progressive fall in the GFR (Fig. 21-1) [7,8,18]. The relatively early decrease in glomerular filtration is easily missed, however, because there is often *little or no rise in the blood urea nitrogen (BUN) or plasma creatinine concentration*. Decreased hepatic production of urea limits the rise in BUN whereas malnutrition (which diminishes muscle mass) and perhaps decreased hepatic production of creatine (the precursor of creatinine) limit the rise in the plasma creatinine concentration [19]. The net effect is that up to one-half of cirrhotic patients with an apparently normal plasma creatinine concentration of 1.0 to 1.2 mg/dl have a reduced GFR (as measured by inulin clearance) that may be as low as 15 ml/min [19]. Calculation of the creatinine clearance from a 24-hour urine collection, although not a very accurate measure of the GFR (see Chap. 17), should be able to detect that a fall in filtration is present in this setting.

Pathogenesis

The progressive decline in renal function seen in hepatic cirrhosis is thought to be hemodynamically mediated, since tubular function is intact (as evidenced by the low urine sodium concentration and a normal urinalysis) [7,12] and the kidneys are histologically normal, having been successfully used for renal transplantation [20].

A possible explanation for the deterioration in renal function is a *neurohumoral imbalance* in which the level of renal vasoconstrictors is elevated at a time when renal vasodilator activity is diminished. As described above, intrahepatic hypertension and arterial underfilling lead to progressive increases in the activities of the sympathetic nervous and renin-angiotensin systems [5-8]. This tendency to renal ischemia is, at first, partially counteracted by enhanced production of vasodilator prostaglandins and kinins [7,21,22]. These important protective responses, however, become impaired with more severe hepatic disease as *both prostaglandin and kinin levels are diminished* [7,21,22]. These changes may reflect the importance of normal hepatic function in the production of prekallikrein (which, when activated to kallikrein, cleaves lysyl-bradykinin from kininogen) and in the conversion of linoleic acid to arachidonic acid (the precursor of prostaglandins) [7].

The response to insertion of a peritoneovenous shunt in patients with the hepatorenal syndrome is also compatible with this hemodynamic hypothesis. The ensuing volume expansion (as ascitic fluid is reinfused into the internal jugular vein) is associated with diminished release of renin [23] that may contribute to the improvement in the GFR [23,24]. The peritoneovenous shunt also may reduce intrahepatic pressure (via an unknown mechanism) [25,26], an effect that could decrease renal sympathetic neural tone [5].

Hepatorenal Syndrome

The hepatorenal syndrome represents the most advanced stage of these hemodynamic changes, being characterized by oliguria and a slowly progressive rise in the BUN and plasma creatinine concentration [27]. The latter may increase by as little as 0.1 mg/dl/day with intermittent periods of stabilization or even slight improvement. The onset of renal failure may be insidious or precipitated by an acute insult such as gastrointestinal bleeding or the excessive use of diuretics.

This disorder is most often seen with advanced alcoholic cirrhosis but can also occur with other hepatic diseases, including metastatic involvement of the liver or rarely uncomplicated acute viral hepatitis [27,28]. Hepatic encephalopathy, ascites, and biochemical abnormalities such as hyperbilirubinemia, hypoalbuminemia, and a prolonged prothrombin time are also commonly present.

One form of liver disease, *primary biliary cirrhosis* appears to be relatively protected from these alterations in renal function [29]. Sodium retention and ascites formation are late events, and the hepatorenal syndrome is unusual in this condition. These

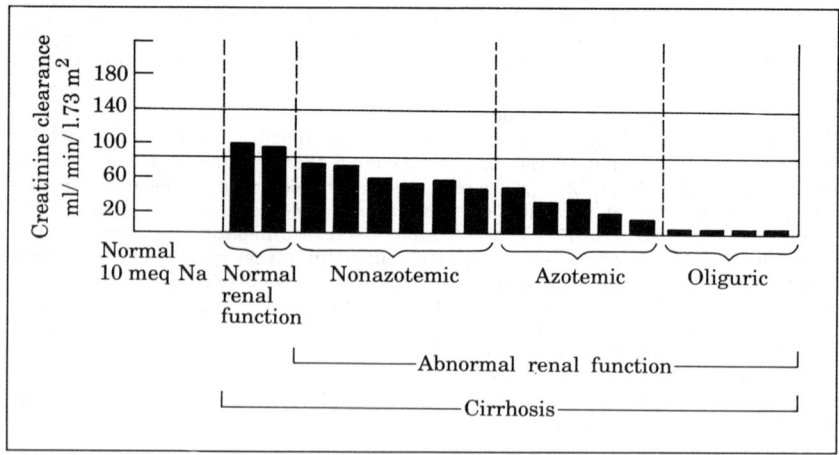

Fig. 21-1. The glomerular filtration rate, as estimated from the creatinine clearance, in normal subjects ingesting 10 meq of sodium per day and in cirrhotic patients of increasing severity. (Adapted from Epstein, M, Berk, DP, Hollenberg, NK, Adams, DF, Chalmers, TC, Abrams, HL, Merrill, JP. *Am J Med* 49:175, 1970.)

unique findings may be related to the natriuretic and renal vasodilator properties of retained bile salts [29].

DIAGNOSIS.   The diagnosis of the hepatorenal syndrome is one of exclusion, after other possible causes of acute renal failure have been excluded. Patients with hepatic cirrhosis, for example, may develop acute tubular necrosis following aminoglycoside therapy or an episode of sepsis or hypotension [30]. However, the history and urinary findings usually allow this disorder to be distinguished from the hepatorenal syndrome.

The major condition that can simulate the findings in the hepatorenal syndrome—normal urinalysis*, low urine sodium concentration, and fractional excretion of sodium—is superimposed volume depletion in a cirrhotic patient due to the use of diuretics or to gastrointestinal bleeding [15]. Thus, the diagnosis of the hepatorenal syndrome requires the proper clinical setting and no improvement in renal function following a trial of fluid repletion.

PROGNOSIS AND TREATMENT.   The prognosis in the hepatorenal syndrome is poor with many patients dying within weeks of the onset of renal failure [24]. Concurrent hepatic encephalopathy is common and death is usually due to a complication of the severe liver disease such as gastrointestinal bleeding. Recovery of renal function occurs only when there is improvement in hepatic function due to partial resolution of the primary disease or rarely to hepatic transplantation [27,28].

Initial therapy is supportive, including avoidance of nephrotoxins such as nonsteroidal anti-inflammatory drugs [16]. Attempts to increase the effective circulating volume with saline, fresh-frozen plasma, or dextran have only transiently improved renal function [9,25,27]. Another modality that might, in theory, be effective is lowering angiotensin II levels with a converting enzyme inhibitor in an effort to partially reverse the renal vasoconstriction. However, patients with the hepatorenal syndrome generally have a systolic blood pressure of 90 to 100 mm Hg [9], a relatively low level that is maintained in part by angiotensin II. Thus, decreasing angiotensin II effect can lead to a marked reduction in blood pressure of as much as 25 mm Hg [32].

*The urinalysis may be abnormal in some patients with the hepatorenal syndrome because hyperbilirubinemia alone can induce changes in the urine sediment similar to those in acute tubular necrosis: granular casts and free epithelial cells and epithelial cell casts [31]. Urinary sodium excretion, however, remains very low in this setting.

The major therapeutic modalities that have been shown to improve renal function in the hepatorenal syndrome are insertion of a peritoneovenous shunt, initially accompanied by loop diuretics to begin the diuresis, and performance of a side-to-side portasystemic shunt, which lowers the intrahepatic pressure and diminishes ascites formation [23,24,33].

The mechanism by which the peritoneovenous shunt works is not well understood. Volume expansion, due to reinfusion of the ascitic fluid, cannot be the entire explanation, since fluid administration alone does not produce any persistent benefit [9,25]. Thus, some other contributing factor appears to be necessary. There is evidence, for example, that the peritoneovenous shunt also reduces intraperitoneal and intrahepatic pressures [25,26]; the latter effect could, by diminishing a hepatorenal reflex, lower renal sympathetic nerve activity, thereby further enhancing renal perfusion [5].

Despite the ability of the peritoneovenous shunt to improve renal function and to relieve refractory ascites [23,24,33], its use is limited by the high incidence of potentially fatal complications. These include disseminated intravascular coagulation, due to entry into the blood stream of endotoxin or other procoagulant material in the ascitic fluid; infection of the shunt, which can lead to bacteremia; variceal bleeding, induced in part by the volume expansion and subsequent rise in portal venous pressure; and small bowel obstruction [33,34].

The net effect is that the perioperative mortality rate can reach 25 percent in patients with advanced hepatic failure [34]. It has been suggested that this morbidity can be somewhat diminished by intraoperative drainage of the ascites. This should minimize those problems directly related to acute and massive ascites reinfusion: volume overload, increased portal pressure, and disseminated intravascular coagulation [34].

In addition to these potential complications, there is little evidence that insertion of a peritoneovenous shunt increases patient survival [24], even though it often improves renal function [23,24]. This is not surprising in view of the severity of the liver disease, which is not affected by use of the shunt. Thus, the peritoneovenous shunt should be limited to those patients with the hepatorenal syndrome who have relatively stable hepatic function, are not encephalopathic, and have not had a recent variceal bleed.

References

1. Naccarato, R, Messa, P, D'Angelo, A, Fabris, A, Messa, M, Chiaramonte, M, Gregolin, C, Zanon, G. Renal handling of sodium and water in early chronic liver disease. *Gastroenterology* 81:205, 1981.
2. Unikowsky, B, Wexler, MJ, Levy, M. Dogs with experimental cirrhosis of the liver but without intrahepatic hypertension do not retain sodium or form ascites. *J Clin Invest* 72:1594, 1983.
3. Better, OS, Schrier, RW. Disturbed volume homeostasis in patients with cirrhosis of the liver. *Kidney Int* 23:303, 1983.
4. Rocco, VK, Ware, AJ. Cirrhotic ascites. Pathophysiology, diagnosis, and management. *Ann Intern Med* 105:572, 1986.
5. DiBona, GF. Renal neural activity in hepatorenal syndrome. *Kidney Int* 25:841, 1984.
6. Bichet, DG, VanPutten, MJ, Schrier, RW. Potential role of increased sympathetic activity in impaired sodium and water excretion in cirrhosis. *N Engl J Med* 307:1552, 1982.
7. Perez-Ayuso, RM, Arroyo, N, Campos, J, Rimola, A, Gaya, J, Costa, J, Rivera, F, Rodes, J. Evidence that renal prostaglandins are involved in renal water metabolism in cirrhosis. *Kidney Int* 26:72, 1984.
8. Nicholls, KM, Shapiro, MD, Groves, BS, Schrier, RW. Factors determining response to water immersion in non-excretor cirrhotic patients. *Kidney Int* 30:417, 1986.
9. Tristani, RE, Cohn, JN. Systemic and renal hemodynamics in oliguric hepatic failure: Effect of volume expansion. *J Clin Invest* 46:1894, 1967.
10. Bichet, DG, Groves, BM, Schrier, RW. Mechanisms of improvement of sodium and water excretion by immersion in decompensated cirrhotic patients. *Kidney Int* 24:788, 1983.
11. Guazzi, M, Polese, A, Magrini, F, Fiorentini, C, Olivar, MT. Negative influences of

ascites on the cardiac function of cirrhotic patients. *Am J Med* 59:165, 1975.
12. Arroyo, V, Bosch, J, Gaya-Beltran, J, Kravetz, D, Estrada, L, Rivera, R, Rodess, J. Plasma renin activity and urinary sodium excretion as prognostic indicators in nonazotemic cirrhosis with ascites. *Ann Intern Med* 94:198, 1981.
13. Perez-Ayuso, RM, Arroyo, V, Planas, R, Gaya, J, Bory, F, Rimola, A, Rivera, F, Rodes, J. Random comparative study of efficacy of furosemide vs spironolactone in nonazotemic cirrhosis with ascites: Relationship between the diuretic response and the activity of the renin-aldosterone system. *Gastroenterology* 84:961, 1983.
14. Pinzani, M, Daskalopoulos, G, Laffi, G, Gentilini, P, Zipser, RD. Altered furosemide pharmacokinetics in chronic alcoholic liver disease with ascites contributes to diuretic resistance. *Gastroenterology* 92:294, 1987.
15. Pockros, PJ, Reynolds, TB. Rapid diuresis in patients with ascites from chronic liver disease: The importance of peripheral edema. *Gastroenterology* 90:1827, 1986.
16. Laffi, G, Daskalopoulos, G, Kronborg, I, Hsueh, W, Gentilini, P, Zipser, RD. Effects of sulindac and ibuprofen in patients with cirrhosis and ascites. An explanation for the renal-sparing effect of sulindac. *Gastroenterology* 90:182, 1986.
17. Gines, P, Arroyo, V, Quintero, E, et al. Comparison of paracentesis and diuretics in the treatment of cirrhotics with tense ascites. Results of a randomized study. *Gastroenterology* 93:234, 1987.
18. Epstein, M, Berk, DP, Hollenberg, NK, Adams, DF, Chalmers, TC, Abrams, HL, Merrill, JP. Renal failure in patients with cirrhosis. *Am J Med* 49:175, 1970.
19. Papadakis, MA, Arieff, AI. Unpredictability of clinical evaluation of renal function in cirrhosis. Prospective study. *Am J Med* 82:945, 1987.
20. Koppel, MH, Coburn, JW, Mimes, MD, Goldstein, H, Boyle, JD, Rubini, ME. Transplantation of cadaveric kidneys from patients with the hepatorenal syndrome: Evidence for the functional nature of renal failure in advanced liver disease. *N Engl J Med* 280:1367, 1969.
21. Laffi, G, La Villa, G, Pinzani, M, Ciabbatoni, G, Patrignani, P, Mannelli, M, Cominelli, F, Gentilini, P. Altered renal and platelet arachidonic acid metabolism in cirrhosis. *Gastroenterology* 90:274, 1986.
22. Wong, PY, Talamo, RC, Williams, GH. Kallikrein-kinin and renin-angiotensin systems in functional renal failure of cirrhosis of the liver. *Gastroenterology* 73:1114, 1977.
23. Schroeder, ET, Anderson, GH, Smulyan, H. Effects of a portacaval or peritoneovenous shunt on renin in the hepatorenal syndrome. *Kidney Int* 15:54, 1979.
24. Linas, SL, Schaefer, JW, Moore, EE, Good, JT, Jr, Giansiracusa, R. Peritoneovenous shunt in the management of the hepatorenal syndrome. *Kidney Int* 30:736, 1986.
25. Cade, R, Wagemaker, H, Vogel, S, et al. Hepatorenal syndrome. Studies of the effect of vascular volume and intraperitoneal pressure on renal and hepatic function. *Am J Med* 82:427, 1987.
26. Greig, PD, Blendis, LM, Langer, B, Taylor, BR, Colapinto, RF. Renal and hemodynamic effects of the peritoneovenous shunt. II. Long-term effects. *Gastroenterology* 80:119, 1981.
27. Rose, BD. *Pathophysiology of Renal Disease* (2nd ed). New York: McGraw-Hill, 1987, Pp. 77-81.
28. Wilkinson, SP, Davies, MH, Portmann, B, Williams, R. Renal failure in otherwise uncomplicated acute viral hepatitis. *Br Med J* 2:338, 1978.
29. Better, OS. Renal and cardiovascular function in liver disease. *Kidney Int* 29:598, 1986.
30. Diamond, JR, Yoburn, DC. Nonoliguric acute renal failure associated with a low fractional excretion of sodium. *Ann Intern Med* 96:597, 1982.
31. Eknoyan, G. Renal disorders in hepatic failure (letter). *Br Med J* 2:670, 1974.
32. Schroeder, ET, Anderson, GH, Goldman, SH, Streeten, DHP. Effect of blockade of angiotensin II on blood pressure, renin, and aldosterone in cirrhosis. *Kidney Int* 9:511, 1976.
33. Epstein, M. Peritoneovenous shunt in the management of ascites and the hepatorenal syndrome. *Gastroenterology* 82:790, 1982.
34. Smadja, C, Franco, D. The LeVeen shunt in the elective treatment of ascites in cirrhosis. A prospective study of 140 patients. *Ann Surg* 201:488, 1985.

22. THE KIDNEY IN CONGESTIVE HEART FAILURE

From a renal viewpoint, congestive heart failure (CHF) is associated with two major changes: sodium retention early in the course of the disease, and a decline in renal perfusion and glomerular filtration rate as cardiac function worsens. Both neurohumoral factors and certain therapies may contribute to these problems [1].

Sodium Retention
Sodium retention in CHF is thought to occur initially as an adaptive response to a decline in cardiac output. This can be appreciated from the Frank-Starling relationship between the stroke volume and the left ventricular end-diastolic pressure (Fig. 22-1). If a previously normal subject develops mild heart disease, there will be an initial reduction in stroke volume, leading to a fall in cardiac output (line AB) and systemic blood pressure. The decrease in blood pressure then activates both the sympathetic nervous and renin-angiotensin systems [1].

At first, sympathetically mediated increases in heart rate and cardiac contractility can return the cardiac output to normal, at least at rest. However, enhanced renal sympathetic activity produces renal vasoconstriction and directly stimulates tubular sodium reabsorption, both of which diminish sodium excretion [2]. Thus, a usually mild limitation in the ability to excrete sodium can occur in cardiac disease even when the cardiac output is normal [2a]; this defect can, however, lead to sodium retention and edema if sodium intake is high [3].

With more advanced disease, however, the sympathetic effects on cardiac function are inadequate and sodium retention and plasma volume expansion are required to restore the cardiac output. As illustrated in line BC in Fig. 22-1, these changes lead to a rise in left ventricular filling pressure that, by enhancing the end-diastolic volume, increases cardiac contractility and cardiac output toward normal. At this point, the patient may be in a state of *compensated* heart failure in which the cardiac output is normal, sodium excretion matches intake, and the activity of the renin-angiotensin-aldosterone system returns toward normal [4].

This compensated state, however, usually applies only at rest. Patients with moderate CHF and a normal cardiac output at rest are often unable to increase the cardiac output adequately with exertion. This relative decrease in tissue perfusion can lead to reactivation of the above neurohumoral mechanisms, producing sodium retention and eventually edema [5]. In this setting, substantial improvement may result from limiting physical activity.

Severe CHF, in comparison, is associated with a persistent decline in cardiac output. As depicted in the lower curve in Fig. 22-1, a plateau may occur as increases in left ventricular filling pressure do not produce further elevations in stroke volume. Decreased cardiac compliance may play an important role in this setting; as a result, a small increase in volume, which will not substantially stretch the muscle fibers or therefore enhance stroke volume, will lead to a relatively large rise in intraventricular pressure (and possibly pulmonary edema).

The Downside of Neurohumoral Adaptation
Increasing cardiac dysfunction is associated with increasing release of the three *"hypovolemic"* hormones: norepinephrine, renin, and antidiuretic hormones [1,6,6a]. This adaptation is initially beneficial because of the elevations in cardiac contractility (by norepinephrine), vascular resistance (which prevents a fall in blood pressure), and plasma volume (which increases the intracardiac filling pressures)*.

---

*To some degree, these sodium-retaining forces may be counteracted by increased release of natriuretic hormones, such as atrial natriuretia peptide [6b] and renal prostaglandins [6]; the increase in atrial pressure and renal ischemia are the respective stimuli for the secretion of these agents. Their clinical importance is incompletely understood, although blocking prostaglandin synthesis with a nonsteroidal anti-inflammatory drug often leads to worsening renal function and more sodium retention (see the following) [6].

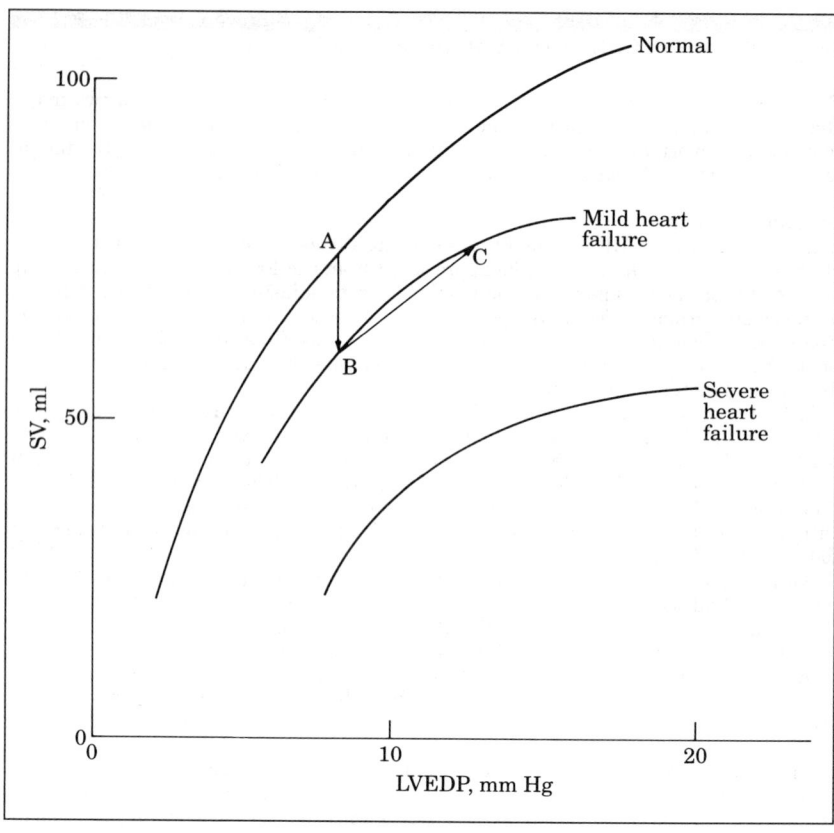

Fig. 22-1. Frank-Starling curves showing the relationship between stroke volume (SV) and left ventricular end-diastolic pressure (LVEDP) in normal subjects and in patients with heart failure. (Adapted from Cohn, JN. *Am J Med* 55:131, 1975.)

In the long-term, however, the vasoconstriction produced by these hormones is *maladaptive* since the failing heart has to pump against a higher resistance (i.e., cardiac afterload is increased). Thus, lowering the systemic vascular resistance with a converting enzyme inhibitor or the combination of hydralazine and isosorbide dinitrate has been shown in many patients to increase the cardiac output, to lead to symptomatic improvement, and to decrease the incidence of progressive cardiac dysfunction. Furthermore, these agents appear to *lower cardiovascular mortality* by 30 to 40 percent at 1 to 3 years [7,8].

Diagnosis
The diagnosis of CHF as the cause of peripheral or pulmonary edema, or both, is usually apparent from the history and physical findings. From a therapeutic viewpoint, however, it is important to distinguish between the two general forms of CHF: *systolic* dysfunction in which impaired contractility is the primary abnormality; and *diastolic* dysfunction in which decreased compliance of the ventricular wall limits diastolic filling and therefore forward output. The latter problem is most likely to occur with hypertensive and less often ischemic heart disease [9,10]. It can be diagnosed by measurement of the ejection fraction, which will be normal, not reduced as with systolic dysfunction.

Another laboratory test that may be prognostically helpful is measurement of the plasma sodium concentration; otherwise unexplained *hyponatremia appears to be a marker for advanced disease* [6,11]. This relationship to cardiac function is indirect. The fall in the plasma sodium concentration is due to water retention that is primarily induced by enhanced secretion of ADH. The stimulus to ADH release in this setting is decreased perfusion, similar to that for renin; thus, renin and ADH levels tend to rise in parallel with increasing cardiac dysfunction [6,11]. As a result, hyponatremia is also a poor prognostic sign, being associated with a shorter survival than seen in normonatremic patients [11].

Treatment
Therapy of CHF is aimed at removing the excess fluid with diuretics and at improving cardiac function. The manner by which the latter is achieved varies with the type of heart failure. Patients with reduced contractility (as evidenced by a diminished ejection fraction) are usually treated with digitalis if diuretic therapy does not lead to symptomatic relief [12]. In comparison, *inotropic therapy is not likely to be effective with diastolic dysfunction,* since contractility is normal. Diuretics or vasodilators should also be avoided in this setting, since they can lead to symptomatic hypotension by further limiting diastolic filling [10]. Optimal therapy is aimed at increasing ventricular compliance during diastole with the use of a calcium channel blocker or β-adrenergic blocker [9,10].

The stage at which vasodilator therapy is instituted remains to be defined. The administration of the converting enzyme inhibitor enalapril to patients who were symptomatic at rest (New York Heart Association (NYHA) functional class IV) lowered the 1-year mortality rate (when compared to placebo) from 63 to 47 percent [7]. Similarly, the administration of hydralazine and isosorbide dinitrate to less-severe patients who were symptomatic with exertion or at rest (NYHA functional class III or IV) reduced the 3-year mortality rate (when compared to placebo or use of the α_1-adrenergic blocker prazosin) from 47 to 36 percent [8]. These observations indicate that *neurohumorally mediated vasoconstriction plays a contributory role in the progressive myocardial dysfunction.* It is therefore possible that these agents might be beneficial if begun as soon as evidence of left ventricular dysfunction is identified, even in patients who respond well to diuretics and digitalis.

In general, converting enzyme inhibitors (which directly inhibit angiotensin II production) appear to be somewhat more effective than hydralazine and isosorbide dinitrate. These agents may, however, lead to symptomatic hypotension in a minority of patients. This problem can be minimized in patients with advanced disease* by using a lower initial dose (such as 2.5 mg of enalapril) [7] and perhaps by using captopril rather than enalapril, since the former has a shorter duration of action and therefore a shorter duration of vasodilation [13].

Another potential therapy for severe CHF involves the administration of newer oral inotropic agents, such as milrinone and β-adrenergic agonists [14]. The role of these modalities remains to be defined.

Renal Failure in CHF
Patients with CHF also may develop acute or chronic renal failure due to reduced tissue perfusion. The decline in renal function is associated with the characteristic findings of prerenal disease: an elevated ratio of the blood urea nitrogen (BUN) to the plasma creatinine concentration; a normal urinalysis; and a low urine sodium concentration (unless diuretics have recently been given).

Several different mechanisms can lead to renal failure in this setting, each of which requires somewhat different therapy (Table 22-1).

---

*One marker for severe cardiac dysfunction is hyponatremia [6,11]. In this setting, use of a converting enzyme inhibitor as an unloading agent has an additional advantage: it can raise the plasma sodium concentration toward normal, especially if given with a loop diuretic (see Chap. 1).

Table 22-1. Causes of renal failure in CHF

Cause	Treatment
Excessive diuretic use	Withhold diuretics temporarily Cautious fluid repletion, if indicated Vasodilator therapy
Nonsteroidal anti-inflammatory drug	Discontinue drug Trial of sulindac, if indicated
Converting enzyme inhibitor	Limit diuretic therapy Captopril rather than enalapril Switch to hydralazine-isosorbide dinitrate

Worsening cardiac function	Vasodilator therapy can be tried,
	  but improvement in plasma
	  creatinine concentration is
	  uncommon

Diuretics
The administration of diuretics leads to fluid loss and a reduction in intravascular pressure. This is a beneficial effect in that it allows pulmonary and peripheral edema to be mobilized, leading to marked symptomatic improvement [15]. However, the decline in left ventricular filling pressure often leads to a decrease in cardiac output (moving, for example, from point C to point B in Fig. 22-1) [15].

Although this fall in tissue perfusion is usually not clinically important, the BUN and plasma creatinine concentration do rise in some patients. Proper therapy at this time is to temporarily avoid further diuretic use and, if the patient has been excessively diuresed, to attempt cautious fluid repletion. If, however, edema persists, then vasodilator therapy is indicated in an effort to improve cardiac function.

Nonsteroidal Anti-inflammatory Drugs
Nonsteroidal anti-inflammatory drugs act primarily by diminishing the synthesis of prostaglandins. They can have important hemodynamic effects in CHF when prostaglandin synthesis is enhanced, namely, in those patients with elevated angiotensin II and norepinephrine levels in whom the kidney secretes vasodilator prostaglandins in an attempt to minimize the associated renal vasoconstriction. As described before, the presence of otherwise unexplained hyponatremia is a good marker for this hormonal pattern [6].

In these patients, the fall in vasodilator prostaglandin production induced by a nonsteroidal anti-inflammatory drug can lead to acute renal failure by two mechanisms: unopposed renal vasoconstriction by angiotensin II and norepinephrine; and a reduction in cardiac output, due to the associated rise in systemic vascular resistance (an effect that is opposite to the beneficial decrease in cardiac afterload induced by vasodilators) [6].

Proper therapy consists of discontinuing the nonsteroidal anti-inflammatory drug. If, however, there is a strong indication for the use of these agents, sulindac should be tried since it appears to be much less likely to impair renal prostaglandin synthesis (see Chap. 23) [16].

Converting Enzyme Inhibitors
Although they frequently increase the cardiac output and renal blood flow, converting enzyme inhibitors can lead to a rise in the plasma creatinine concentration in approximately 25 to 30 percent of patients with severe CHF [17,18]. This is most likely to occur

in those settings in which maintenance of the glomerular filtration rate is most dependent on angiotensin II: when there has been an excessive diuresis (with a left ventricular end-diastolic pressure below 15 mm Hg) or when the mean arterial pressure has fallen below 65 mm Hg [17].

In these settings, renal perfusion pressure and therefore the intraglomerular pressure tend to be reduced; maintenance of the intraglomerular pressure and therefore the glomerular filtration rate occurs via an autoregulatory response that consists, in part, of angiotensin II–mediated vasoconstriction of the efferent glomerular arteriole. A rise in the plasma creatinine concentration can ensue (as it also can in bilateral renal artery stenosis; see Chap. 14) when this protective effect of angiotensin II is withdrawn by use of a converting enzyme inhibitor [17].

Restoration of renal function can often be achieved by lowering the diuretic dose [17] and, if enalapril is being used, possibly switching to a shorter-acting agent such as captopril [13]. This is preferable to discontinuing the converting enzyme inhibitor, which can both improve cardiac function and prolong survival [7]. A final alternative is to use hydralazine and isosorbide dinitrate for unloading therapy [8]; these drugs do not interfere with angiotensin II production and are therefore more likely to allow stable renal function.

Worsening Cardiac Function

Worsening cardiac function is a final cause of progressive prerenal disease in CHF. In many patients, this diagnosis will be clinically apparent because of increasing cardiac symptoms or a recent myocardial infarction. In some cases, however, the evidence for a deterioration in myocardial function is somewhat masked. For example, an episode of severe coronary ischemia, without infarction, can lead to impaired cardiac contractility that persists for up to 3 to 5 days [19]. The generation of ozygen-free radicals during the period of ischemia may be responsible for the delayed recovery of cellular function in this setting (a phenomenon that has been called the "stunned" myocardium) [20].

In other patients, chronic ischemia can impair left ventricular function in the absence of chest pain or electrocardiographic changes [19]. This problem, which is in part adaptive by limiting myocardial oxygen requirements in the presence of diminished oxygen delivery, should be suspected in patients with ischemic heart disease in whom the severity of the heart failure is out of proportion to the apparent degree of cardiac damage. This is an important diagnosis to establish, since coronary revascularization can lead to improved cardiac function [19].

Even if it is established that declining renal function is due to progressive cardiac disease, medical therapy is usually ineffective in reversing this process. Although converting enzyme inhibition, for example, can increase the cardiac output, only 9 to 12 percent of patients have a concomitant reduction in the BUN or plasma creatinine concentration [17,18]. Furthermore, patients with a plasma creatinine concentration above 2.8 mg/dl are also unlikely to have a beneficial *cardiac* response to these agents [18].

Optimal therapy in this setting therefore is uncertain. These patients have severe disease and tend to be unresponsive to diuretics and to other vasodilator regimens [18]. The possible role of inotropic agents remains to be defined [14].

References

1. Dzau, VJ. Renal and circulatory mechanisms in congestive heart failure. *Kidney Int* 31:1402, 1987.
2. Moss, NG. Renal function and renal afferent and efferent nerve activity. *Am J Physiol* 243:F425, 1982.
2a. Hostetter, TH, Pfeffer, JM, Pfeffer, MA, Dworkin, LD, Braunwald, E, Brenner, BM. Cardiorenal hemodynamics and sodium excretion in rats with myocardial infarction. *Am J Physiol* 245:H98, 1983.
3. Braunwald, E, Plauth, WH, Morrow, AG. A method for the detection and quantification of impaired sodium excretion. *Circulation* 32:223, 1965.

4. Watkins, L, Jr, Burton, JA, Haber, E, Cant, JR, Smith, FW, Barger, AC. The renin-angiotensin-aldosterone system in congestive failure in conscious dogs. *J Clin Invest* 57:1606, 1976.

5. Millard, RW, Higgins, CB, Franklin, D, Vatner, SF. Regulation of the renal circulation during severe exercise in normal dogs and dogs with experimental heart failure. *Circ Res* 31:881, 1972.

6. Dzau, VJ, Packer, M, Lilly, LS, Swartz, SL, Hollenberg, NK, Williams, GH. Prostaglandins in severe congestive heart failure. *N Engl J Med* 310:347, 1984.

6a. Mettauer, B, Rouleau, J-L, Bichet, D, Juneau, C, Kortas, C, Barjon, J-N, de Champlain, J. Sodium and water excretion abnormalities in congestive heart failure. *Ann Intern Med* 105:161, 1986.

6b. Needleman, P, Greenwald, JE. Atriopeptin: A cardiac hormone intimately involved in fluid, electrolyte, and blood-pressure homeostasis. *N Engl J Med* 314:828, 1986.

7. The CONSENSUS Trial Study Group. Effects of enalapril on mortality in severe congestive heart failure: Results of the Cooperative North Scandinavia Enalapril Survival Study (CONSENSUS). *N Engl J Med* 316:1429, 1987.

8. Cohn, JN, Archibald, DG, Ziesche, S, et al. Effect of vasodilator therapy on mortality in chronic congestive heart failure: Results of a Veterans Administration Cooperative Study. *N Engl J Med* 314:1547, 1986.

9. Soufer, R, Wohlgelertner, D, Vita, NA, Amuchestegui, M, Sostman, HD, Berger, HJ, Zaret, BL. Intact systolic left ventricular function in clinical congestive heart failure. *Am J Cardiol* 55:1032, 1985.

10. Topol, EJ, Traill, TA, Fortuin, NJ. Hypertensive hypertrophic cardiomyopathy of the elderly. *N Engl J Med* 312:277, 1985.

11. Lee, WH, Packer, M. Prognostic importance of serum sodium concentration and its modification by converting-enzyme inhibition in patients with severe congestive heart failure. *Circulation* 73:257, 1986.

12. Lee, DC-S, Johnson, RA, Bingham, JB, Leahy, M, Dinsmore, RE, Goroll, AH, Newell, JB, Strauss, HW, Haber, E. Heart failure in outpatients: A randomized trial of digoxin versus placebo. *N Engl J Med* 306:699, 1982.

13. Packer, M, Lee, WH, Yushak, M, Medina, M. Comparison of captopril and enalapril in patients with severe chronic heart failure. *N Engl J Med* 315:847, 1986.

14. Colucci, WS, Wright, RF, Braunwald, E. New positive inotropic agents in the treatment of congestive heart failure: Mechanisms of action and recent clinical developments. *N Engl J Med* 314:290, 349, 1986.

15. Stampfer, M, Epstein, SE, Beiser, GD, Braunwald, E. Hemodynamic effects of diuresis at rest and during intense exercise in patients with impaired cardiac function. *Circulation* 37:900, 1968.

16. Laffi, G, Daskalopoulos, G, Kronberg, I, Hsueh, W, Gentilini, P, Zipser, RD. Effects of sulindac and ibuprofen in patients with cirrhosis and ascites. An explanation for the renal-sparing effect of sulindac. *Gastroenterology* 90:182, 1986.

17. Packer, M, Lee, WH, Medina, N, Yushak, M, Kessler, PD. Functional renal insufficiency during long-term therapy with captopril and enalapril in severe chronic heart failure. *Ann Intern Med* 106:346, 1987.

18. Packer, M, Lee, WH, Medina, N, Yushak, M. Influence of renal function on the hemodynamic and clinical responses to long-term captopril therapy in severe chronic heart failure. *Ann Intern Med* 104:147, 1986.

19. Braunwald, E, Rutherford, JD. Reversible ischemic left ventricular dysfunction: Evidence for the "hibernating myocardium". *J Am Coll Cardiol* 8:1467, 1986.

20. Charlat, ML, O'Neill, PG, Egan, JM, Abernethy, DR, Michael, LH, Myers, ML, Roberts, R, Bolli, R. Evidence for a pathogenetic role of xanthine oxidase in the "stunned" myocardium. *Am J Physiol* 252:H566, 1987.

23. NEPHROTOXICITY OF NONSTEROIDAL ANTI-INFLAMMATORY DRUGS

Nonsteroidal anti-inflammatory drugs (NSAIDs) are widely used in the treatment of rheumatologic disorders, acting primarily by diminishing the synthesis of prostaglandins. These agents generally produce no renal abnormalities because the basal rate of renal prostaglandin production is relatively low. There are, however, conditions in which prostaglandin synthesis is enhanced, primarily prostacyclin by the glomeruli and PGE_2 by the tubular and interstitial cells in the medulla [1,2]. This is most likely to occur with any of the prerenal states (see Chap. 20) that activate both the sympathetic nervous and renin-angiotensin systems. The ensuing release of norepinephrine and angiotensin II produces renal vasoconstriction, a reduction in renal perfusion, and diminished excretion of sodium, all in an appropriate attempt to restore perfusion of the critical organs (heart and brain) toward normal. These hormones, however, also stimulate prostaglandin production by the kidney, leading to several modulating effects, including vasodilation to minimize the degree of renal ischemia [1-3]. In this setting, the administration of a NSAID can limit this compensatory response leading to several possible complications, including acute renal failure, a rise in blood pressure in patients with hypertension, hyperkalemia, and possibly sodium and water retention (Table 23-1) [4-6].

In addition to these humoral effects, the NSAIDs also may be associated with a variety of toxic effects including acute interstitial nephritis or the nephrotic syndrome or both (see Chap. 49), papillary necrosis (see Chap. 49), and acute renal failure with suprofen [4,5,7]. The last problem is typically associated with flank pain and, since suprofen is additionally a uricosuric drug, may be due to intratubular obstruction by precipitated uric acid [7].

Acute Renal Failure
The increase in renal perfusion induced by vasodilator prostaglandins creates a situation in which the administration of a NSAID can diminish renal perfusion and secondarily the glomerular filtration rate. The conditions in which this problem has been described are listed in Table 23-2 [6]. Each of these disorders is associated with an increase in baseline renal prostaglandin synthesis, most often representing a compensatory response to renal vasoconstriction induced by angiotensin II and norepinephrine (as in true volume depletion, heart failure, or hepatic cirrhosis) or by hypercalcemia directly. The mechanism by which glomerular disease enhances prostaglandin release is not known, but these patients also may be sensitive to a NSAID [6,8,9]. In comparison, renal function is generally well maintained in patients with other forms of chronic renal disease [10].

The sensitivity to use of a NSAID in hypovolemic states is related to the intensity of the underlying renal vasoconstriction. For example, cirrhotic patients who excrete more than 10 meq of sodium per day generally have little or no decline in renal function as prostaglandin synthesis is diminished [11]. In comparison, patients with more marked sodium retention (and presumably higher levels of angiotensin II, norepinephrine, and renal prostaglandins) may have a relatively large reduction in the glomerular filtration rate after a NSAID (Fig. 23-1) [11]. This deleterious effect is usually rapidly reversible with discontinuation of the offending drug.

Patients taking triamterene, the potassium-sparing diuretic, appear to be particularly sensitive to the concurrent administration of a NSAID [12]. The mechanism by which this occurs is incompletely understood. Triamterene does lead to a substantial rise in renal prostaglandin production; this response, however, is not likely to be due to volume depletion since other, more potent diuretics (furosemide, hydrochlorothiazide) are not associated with the same risk of developing acute renal failure with the use of NSAIDs [12].

Is Sulindac Renal Prostaglandin Sparing?
Many studies suggest that one NSAID, *sulindac,* seems to relatively preserve renal prostaglandin synthesis (particularly prostacyclin production by the glomeruli) [1,8,11,13] and seems to be more likely to maintain renal function (Fig. 23-1) [1,8,11]. The mecha-

Table 23-1. Renal actions of the prostaglandins and possible complications with nonsteroidal anti-inflammatory drugs

Effect of prostaglandins	Possible drug complication
Maintain renal blood flow and glomerular filtration rate by ameliorating angiotensin II and norepinephrine-induced renal vasoconstriction	Acute renal failure in conditions associated with increased release of renal vasoconstrictors (Table 23-2)
Antagonize systemic vasoconstriction	May raise the blood pressure in hypertensive patients treated with a diuretic or β-adrenergic blocker
Increase the secretion of renin	Hyperkalemia due to hyporeninemic hypoaldosteronism, primarily in patients with renal insufficiency
May increase sodium excretion in states of effective volume depletion	May promote more intense sodium retention
Antagonize water-retaining effect of antidiuretic hormone (ADH)	May potentiate effect of ADH, possibly promoting the development of hyponatremia

Table 23-2. Conditions associated with NSAID-induced, hemodynamically mediated acute renal failure

True volume depletion (vomiting, diarrhea, diuretics)
Congestive heart failure
Hepatic cirrhosis
Nephrotic syndrome
Glomerulonephritis, including lupus nephritis
Hypercalcemia
Concurrent administration of triamterene

nism by which this occurs is not well understood; both renal metabolism of the active drug metabolite and sulindac being a somewhat weaker cyclooxygenase inhibitor have been proposed [1,11]. Regardless of the mechanism, sulindac can be used safely in most patients with one of the disorders in Table 23-2. Careful monitoring is still essential, however, because this protection is not absolute [14,15].

Renal prostaglandin production also appears to be spared by low-dose aspirin therapy [1]. This effect may be related to different rates of recovery of cyclooxygenase; this enzyme is irreversibly inactivated by aspirin in platelets but perhaps only transiently inhibited in the kidney.

Elevation in Blood Pressure
The decrease in vasodilator prostaglandins induced by NSAIDs can also lead to a 5 to 10 mm Hg rise in blood pressure in some treated patients with hypertension. This response again seems less likely to occur with sulindac [16,17].

This elevation in systemic vascular resistance can have an additional deleterious effect in patients with severe heart failure [18]. By increasing afterload, a NSAID can lead to a further reduction in cardiac contractility and therefore in cardiac output.

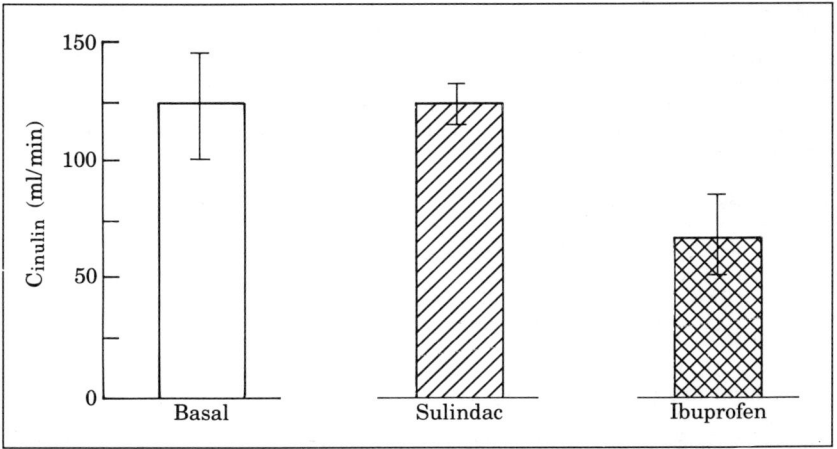

Fig. 23-1. Effect of sulindac and ibuprofen on the glomerular filtration rate (as estimated from the inulin clearance, C_{inulin} in five patients with hepatic cirrhosis and marked sodium retention (sodium excretion < 1 meq/day). The protective effect of sulindac was associated with a less marked inhibition of renal prostacyclin and PGE_2 synthesis. (Adapted from Laffi, G, Daskalopoulos, G, Kronberg, I, Hsueh, W, Gentilini, P, Zipser, RD. *Gastroenterology* 90:182, 1986. Reprinted with permission; copyright 1986 by the American Gastroenterological Association.)

Hyperkalemia
The stimulation of renin release by the baroreceptors in the afferent glomerular arteriole and by the macula densa cells in the early distal tubule is mediated in part by the local release of prostaglandins, particularly prostacyclin [19]. This response is inhibited by a NSAID, leading in some patients to hyporeninemic hypoaldosteronism (since angiotensin II is the major stimulus to aldosterone release) [20]. To the extent that prostaglandin inhibition also promotes sodium reabsorption in the thick ascending limb of the loop of Henle, the ensuing reduction in sodium and water delivery to the potassium secretory site in the cortical collecting tubule is another mechanism by which potassium excretion might be impaired. The net effect is that the plasma potassium concentration can rise by a mean of 0.2 meq/L in normals [21] and 0.6 meq/L in patients with renal insufficiency [10], with the occasional development of overt hyperkalemia in the latter setting [20].

Sodium Retention
Locally produced prostaglandins also may have a natriuretic effect, possibly decreasing sodium reabsorption in the thick ascending limb and the cortical collecting tubule [22]. Thus, prostaglandins may modulate the sodium-retaining as well as the renal vasoconstrictive effects of angiotensin II and norepinephrine in hypovolemic patients. As a result, a NSAID can promote further sodium retention both by reducing the glomerular filtration rate and by increasing tubular reabsorption [1,10]. These effects also limit the responsiveness of edematous patients to diuretic therapy [21,23,24]; it is likely that this problem is less prominent with sulindac.

Water Retention
Prostaglandins, primarily prostaglandin E_2 produced in the medulla, impair the ability of antidiuretic hormone (ADH) to increase water reabsorption. Multiple factors appear to contribute to this response, including reductions in ADH-induced generation of cyclic AMP and in medullary hypertonicity [25,26]; the latter is due in part to diminished

sodium reabsorption in the thick ascending limb, the primary factor normally responsible for the generation of the medullary osmotic gradient. These modulating influences, however, are removed by the administration of a NSAID, leading to a rise in urine osmolality above baseline that can exceed 200 mosmol/kg [27]. This limitation in the ability to excrete water may contribute to the development of hyponatremia in patients with elevated ADH levels due to volume depletion or to the syndrome of inappropriate ADH secretion.

References

1. Patrono, C, Dunn, MJ. The clinical significance of inhibition of renal prostaglandin synthesis. *Kidney Int* 32:1, 1987.
2. Stahl, RAK, Paravicini, M, Schollmeyer, P. Angiotensin II stimulation of prostaglandin E_2 and 6-keto-$F_{1\alpha}$I formation by isolated human glomeruli. *Kidney Int* 26:30, 1984.
3. Oliver, JA, Pinto, J, Sciacca, RR, Cannon, PJ. Increased renal secretion of norepinephrine and prostaglandin E_2 during sodium depletion in the dog. *J Clin Invest* 66:748, 1980.
4. Clive, DM, Stoff, JS. Renal syndromes associated with nonsteroidal antiinflammatory drugs. *N Engl J Med* 310:563, 1984.
5. Garella, S, Matarese, RA. Renal effects of prostaglandins and clinical adverse effects of nonsteroidal anti-inflammatory agents. *Medicine* 63:165, 1984.
6. Rose, BD. *Pathophysiology of Renal Disease* (2nd ed). New York: McGraw-Hill, 1987. Pp. 82-83.
7. Hart, D, Ward, M, Lifschitz, M. Suprofen-related nephrotoxicity. A distinct clinical syndrome. *Ann Intern Med* 106:235, 1987.
8. Cibattoni, G, Cinotti, GA, Pierucci, A, Simonetti, BM, Manzi, M, Pugliese, F, Barsotti, P, Pecci, G, Taggi, F, Patrono, C. Effects of sulindac and ibuprofen in patients with chronic glomerular disease. *N Engl J Med* 310:279, 1984.
9. Shemesh, O, Ross, JC, Deen, WM, Grant, GW, Myers, BD. Nature of the glomerular capillary injury in human membranous nephropathy. *J Clin Invest* 77:868, 1986.
10. Toto, RD, Anderson, SA, Brown-Cartwright, D, Kokko, JP, Brater, DC. Effects of acute and chronic dosing of NSAIDs in patients with renal insufficiency. *Kidney Int* 30:760, 1986.
11. Laffi, G. Daskalopoulos, G, Kronberg, I, Hsueh, W, Gentilini, P, Zipser, RD. Effects of sulindac and ibuprofen in patients with cirrhosis and ascites. An explanation for the renal-sparing effect of sulindac. *Gastroenterology* 90:182, 1986.
12. Favre, L, Glasson, P, Vallotton, MB. Reversible acute renal failure from combined triamterene and indomethacin. *Ann Intern Med* 96:317, 1982.
13. Roberts, DG, Gerber, JG, Barnes, JS, Zerbe, GO, Nies, AS. Sulindac is not renal sparing in man. *Clin Pharmacol Therap* 38:258, 1985.
14. Brater, DC, Anderson, S, Baird, B, Campbell, WB. Effects of ibuprofen, naproxen, and sulindac on renal prostaglandins in man. *Kidney Int* 27:66, 1985.
15. Brater, DC, Anderson, SA, Brown-Cartwright, D, Toto, RD. Effects of nonsteroidal antiinflammatory drugs on renal function in patients with renal insufficiency and in cirrhotics. *Am J Kid Dis* 8:351, 1986.
16. Puddey, IE, Beilin, EJ, Vandongen, R, Banks, R, Rouse, I. Differential effects of sulindac and indomethacin on blood pressure in treated essential hypertensive subjects. *Clin Sci* 69:327, 1985.
17. Wong, DG, Spence, JD, Lamki, L, Freeman, L, McDonald, JWD. Effect of nonsteroidal anti-inflammatory drugs on control of hypertension by β-blockers and diuretics. *Lancet* 1:997, 1986.
18. Dzau, VJ, Packer, M, Lilly, LS, Swartz, SL, Hollenberg, NK, Williams, GH. Prostaglandins in severe congestive heart failure. *N Engl J Med* 310:347, 1984.
19. Francisco, LL, Osborn, JL, DiBona, GF. Prostaglandins in renin release during sodium deprivation. *Am J Physiol* 243:F537, 1982.
20. Tan, SY, Shapiro, R, Franco, R, Stockard, H, Mulrow, PJ. Indomethacin-induced prostaglandin inhibition with hyperkalemia: Reversible cause of hyporeninemic hypoaldosteronism. *Ann Intern Med* 90:783, 1979.

21. Ruilope, LM, Robles, RG, Paya, C, Alcazar, JM, Miravalles, E, Sancho-Rof, J, Rodicio, J, Knox, FG, Romero, JC. Effects of long-term treatment with indomethacin on renal function. *Hypertension* 8:677, 1986.
22. Kokko, JP. Effect of prostaglandins on renal epithelial electrolyte transport. *Kidney Int* 19:791, 1981.
23. Brater, DC. Analysis of the effect of indomethacin on the response to furosemide in man: Effect of dose of furosemide. *J Pharmacol Exp Therap* 210:386, 1979.
24. Kirchner, KA. Indomethacin antagonizes furosemide's intratubular effects during loop segment microperfusion. *J Pharmacol Exp Therap* 243:881, 1987.
25. Stokes, JB. Integrated actions of renal medullary prostaglandins in the control of water excretion. *Am J Physiol* 240:F471, 1981.
26. Garcia-Perez, A, Smith, WL. Apical-basolateral membrane asymmetry in canine cortical collecting tubule cells. Bradykinin, arginine vasopressin, prostaglandin E_2 interrelationships. *J Clin Invest* 74:63, 1984.
27. Kramer, HJ, Glanzer, K. Dusing. R. Role of prostaglandins in the regulation of renal water excretion. *Kidney Int* 19:851, 1981.

24. ACUTE TUBULAR NECROSIS

Acute tubular necrosis (ATN) is, with prerenal disease, one of the two most common causes of acute renal failure. The characteristic tubular injury in this disorder represents a nonspecific response that can be seen with a variety of renal insults, particularly renal ischemia and exogenous or endogenous nephrotoxins (Table 24-1). The net effect is a rapid decline in renal function that, in many patients, requires a variable period of dialysis before spontaneous resolution occurs.

There are two major histologic changes in ATN: *tubular necrosis* with denuding of the epithelial cells and *occlusion of the tubular lumina* by casts and by cellular debris (including the brush border of the proximal tubular cells and Tamm-Horsfall mucoprotein released from damaged cells in the thick ascending limb of the loop of Henle) [1,2]. These changes are often patchy and seem relatively mild in relation to the severity of the renal failure. It is important to remember, however, that many nephrons drain into a single cortical collecting tubule. Thus, obstruction of a seemingly small number of collecting tubules can lead to marked renal dysfunction.

In addition to tubular obstruction, two other factors appear to contribute to the development of renal failure in ATN: *backleak of filtrate* across the damaged tubular epithelia; and a primary *reduction in glomerular filtration,* due both to arteriolar vasoconstriction and to mesangial contraction (the latter limits the surface area available for filtration) [1].

The data supporting the role of these factors and the mechanisms by which they might occur have come primarily from studies in experimental animals and are reviewed in refs. 1 and 3. It is presumed that they may also apply to humans. The following observations, for example, provide indirect evidence that backleak occurs in patients with postischemic ATN [4]. Both freely filtered inulin (molecular radius 14 Å) and larger dextrans (molecular radius 22–30 Å) were infused. Neither of these compounds typically undergoes tubular reabsorption. As a result, the renal clearance of inulin normally exceeds that of the larger and therefore less well filtered dextrans. This pattern is reversed in ATN, however, with dextrans having a greater clearance. The most likely explanation for these findings is that inulin is able to leak back across the damaged epithelia (and is therefore not excreted); the larger dextrans, in comparison, cannot as easily pass through the tubular cells.

Table 24-1. Major causes of acute tubular necrosis

Postischemia
  All causes of severe prerenal disease, particularly hypotension with surgery or
    sepsis
Nephrotoxins
  Aminoglycoside antibiotics
  Radiocontrast media
  Cisplatin
  Heme pigments
    Rhabdomyolysis—myoglobinuria
    Hemolysis—hemoglobinuria

Pathogenesis and Etiology

Postischemia

Almost any of the causes of severe prerenal disease can lead to ATN, particularly hypotension in the settings of surgery (primarily open heart surgery or abdominal aortic aneurysm repair), sepsis, or an obstetrical complication [1]. The association with major surgery, for example, is related in part to the hemodynamic changes that often occur in this setting. Preoperative fluid depletion, anesthesia, and intraoperative fluid losses can combine to lower the glomerular filtration rate (GFR) (by as much as 30–45%), the urine volume, and urinary sodium excretion [5,6]. Most patients are able to tolerate this transient renal ischemia without developing tubular injury. However, ATN may ensue if a further insult, such as hypotension, is added.

The development of postischemic tubular necrosis is related in part to the *balance between energy delivery to and energy consumption by the tubular cells.* Studies in experimental animals indicate that, although any nephron segment can be damaged, three segments are most susceptible to ischemic injury: the early proximal convoluted tubule, which has a limited capacity for anaerobic metabolism and is therefore highly sensitive to diminished oxygen delivery; and those segments in the outer medulla, the S_3 (or straight) segment of the proximal tubule and the thick ascending limb of the loop of Henle [7,8]. These actively transporting tubular cells in the outer medulla generally function in a borderline hypoxic environment, since *the normal outer medullary PO_2 is only 10 to 20 mm Hg* [7]. Thus, even a modest decrease in medullary perfusion puts these cells at risk of ischemic damage. Sloughing of the brush border from the proximal tubule and the release of Tamm-Horsfall mucoprotein from the loop of Henle can then lead to intratubular obstruction and acute renal failure.

The importance of the relation between energy delivery and energy requirement in the maintenance of cellular integrity also has possible therapeutic implications. Most of the oxygen used by the thick ascending limb, for example, is related to active sodium chloride reabsorption. Thus, inhibiting this transport process with a loop diuretic might protect these cells during a period of ischemia. Furosemide, for example, has been shown to minimize both cellular necrosis and the degree of renal dysfunction in experimental forms of ATN [7]; it is not clear, however, if a similar benefit is present in humans (see the following).

The *duration* of ischemia is another important factor in the development of ATN. In most patients, the renal failure phase lasts for 7 to 21 days after the ischemic episode. However, recovery may occur within 1 to 3 days when there is only a brief period of ischemia. Some patients undergoing abdominal aortic aneurysm surgery, for example, require clamping of the aorta above the renal arteries, leading to total cessation of renal perfusion for 15 to 80 minutes [6]. Two hours after the operation, the GFR is reduced and the urinary findings are typical of ATN: high urine sodium concentration and fractional excretion of sodium; and urine osmolality similar to that in the plasma (see Chap. 19). By 24 hours, these parameters begin to normalize and recovery is usually complete within 3 days. In comparison, patients with recurrent episodes of hypotension (as with persistent infection) may have continued tubular injury and persistent renal failure [3].

Aminoglycosides
Acute tubular necrosis is a relatively common complication of a prolonged course of aminoglycoside antibiotics, occurring in 5 to 15 percent of patients [9,10]. The nephrotoxicity of these agents is largely dependent on their preferential accumulation in the renal cortex. The aminoglycosides are freely filtered and then taken up by and stored in the proximal tubular cells. As late as 28 days after the drug is given to an experimental animal, for example, the concentration in the renal cortex still exceeds that in the plasma on day 1 [11]. In addition to these proximal effects, the aminoglycosides also affect other nephron segments, such as the collecting tubules. These more distal effects may account for the common findings of nonoliguric ATN due in part to ADH resistance and hypomagnesemia due to urinary magnesium wasting [1,12].

The number of cationic amino groups (NH_3^+) per molecule appears to correlate closely with clinical nephrotoxicity [13]. Thus, neomycin (6/molecule) produces the most renal damage and streptomycin (3) the least. Gentamicin, tobramycin, netilmicin (5), and amikacin (4) have intermediate toxicity.

The importance of molecular charge appears to be related to the binding of the cationic aminoglycoside to anionic phospholipid receptors in the luminal and subcellular membranes [13]. This interaction at the luminal membrane facilitates the movement of the drug from the lumen into the tubular cell. Within the cell, the drug accumulates within lysosomes, an effect that may be mediated by a similar charge interaction. Interference with lysosomal function or the release of lysosomal enzymes into the cytosol may then account for the cellular injury [13].

A variety of factors predispose to aminoglycoside-induced ATN. These include excess plasma levels, prolonged duration of therapy, increasing patient age (which is usually associated with a reduction in the GFR), and underlying volume depletion or hypotension [9,10]. The effect of volume depletion may reflect decreased perfusion to the tubular cells, making them more susceptible to the metabolic dysfunction induced by the aminoglycoside.

It has also been proposed that gentamicin is more nephrotoxic than tobramycin and that aminoglycoside nephrotoxicity is enhanced by the concurrent administration of cephalothin. There were, however, methodologic problems with these observations and more recent reports question whether there is any increased risk associated with gentamicin or the use of cephalothin [9]. Furthermore, even if the cephalothin effect is real, it does not appear to apply to at least some other cephalosporin-like drugs, such as cephazolin and moxalactam.

The renal damage associated with the aminoglycosides is cumulative, representing continued drug accumulation in the proximal tubular cells. The earliest manifestation is increased excretion of low-molecular-weight proteins (such as β_2-microglobulin), due to diminished proximal reabsorption. The first clinically detectable abnormality, however, is a rise in the plasma creatinine concentration that usually requires at least 7 days of therapy [10]. Furthermore, the development of renal insufficiency may be delayed in some patients until several days *after* the aminoglycoside has been discontinued; this effect presumably reflects the prolonged storage of the drug in the tubular cells.

PREVENTION.   Prevention of aminoglycoside-induced ATN is best achieved by careful monitoring of drug levels and avoidance, if possible, of prolonged administration. Periodic determination of the plasma creatinine concentration is also important to allow detection of early nephrotoxicity. Measurement of drug levels is required because there are no other satisfactory methods to optimize drug dosage. In particular, drug dosage must be diminished when the GFR is reduced, since urinary excretion is the major route of aminoglycoside elimination. However, use of the plasma creatinine concentration or the creatinine clearance often leads to an *overestimate* of the GFR that can mask the presence of underlying renal insufficiency. For example, both loss of muscle mass (a common event in older patients) and increased tubular creatinine secretion can prevent or minimize any rise in the plasma creatinine concentration despite a decline in the GFR (see Chap. 17).

Radiocontrast Media

In contrast to the delayed effect with aminoglycoside-induced ATN, the renal failure seen with radiocontrast media typically begins shortly after the procedure has been performed. This problem most commonly occurs with intravenous pyelography, arteriography, or contrast-enhanced CT scanning. Two major risk factors have been identified: *diabetes mellitus* and *renal insufficiency* [14–16]. The quantity of contrast administered and underlying effective volume depletion also appear to play an important role [16].

Patients with a plasma creatinine concentration below 1.5 mg/dl have less than a 1 to 2 percent chance of developing renal failure which, when it occurs, is usually mild. However, the incidence of acute renal failure rises substantially in diabetics with more-advanced underlying renal disease, reaching as high as 90 percent in diabetic nephropathy with a plasma creatinine concentration above 4.5 mg/dl [14]. Nondiabetics with severe primary renal disease are at less risk, especially if the dose of radiocontrast media is kept below 125 ml and multiple studies are avoided [16].

Radiocontrast media-induced nephrotoxicity also appears to be increased in those patients with multiple myeloma who excrete free light chains in the urine. An interaction between the contrast agent and the urinary light chains may promote the development of intratubular obstruction [17]. However, fluid restriction prior to the x-ray study may be of greater importance by promoting light-chain precipitation.

The mechanism by which radiocontrast media leads to acute renal failure is unclear. Direct tubular toxicity, renal vasoconstriction, and sludging of blood in the renal microcirculation all have been proposed. Regardless of the mechanism, the degree of injury appears to be relatively mild in comparison to other causes of ATN: the urine sodium concentration and fractional excretion of sodium are often low, similar to that seen in prerenal disease [18]; and the duration of renal failure is typically only 3 to 5 days, not 7 to 21 days [14]. Many patients are asymptomatic, and the transient decline in renal function will be missed if the plasma creatinine concentration is not measured.

PREVENTION.   The best method of preventing contrast-induced acute renal failure is to avoid the use of these agents in high-risk patients. For example, ultrasonography or CT scanning without contrast can often supply the same information as intravenous pyelography. If an arteriogram must be done, then *intraarterial* digital subtraction angiography is preferable, since this procedure markedly reduces the quantity of contrast that must be administered. There is also suggestive evidence that hydration with 250 ml of a 20% mannitol solution, given over 1 hour after the contrast study may be protective [18a].

Cisplatin

Cisplatin is an effective chemotherapeutic agent that is also a frequent nephrotoxin [19,20]. As with aminoglycosides, this toxic effect is cumulative. Approximately 25 to 35 percent of patients will develop a mild and partially reversible rise in the plasma creatinine concentration after the first course of therapy [20]. The incidence and severity of renal failure increases with continued drug administration, eventually becoming irreversible.

Cisplatin is a direct tubular toxin, which probably acts by interacting with nucleophilic sites on DNA [19]. It preferentially affects the S_3 (or straight) segment of the proximal tubule but can also affect the more distal nephron segments. In addition to renal failure, *hypomagnesemia* due to urinary magnesium wasting is a common problem in this disorder. Over one-half of patients may develop a fall in the plasma magnesium concentration that often persists for a prolonged period after cisplatin has been discontinued [21].

Cisplatin may also be associated with another form of acute renal failure when given with bleomycin: thrombotic microangiopathy, with the features of the hemolytic-uremic syndrome or thrombotic thrombocytopenic purpura [22]. The diagnosis of the latter disorder is suggested by the concurrent findings of microangiopathic hemolytic anemia and thrombocytopenia (see Chap. 43).

PREVENTION. The nephrotoxicity of cisplatin can probably be reduced by vigorous hydration (250 ml/hour of saline) and by giving the drug in a hypertonic saline solution (such as 250 ml of 3% saline) [19,22a]. The presence of a very high chloride concentration appears to minimize the formation of highly reactive and toxic cisplatin compounds and also to limit drug uptake by the tubular cells [19].

Heme Pigments
Acute renal failure can be induced by the urinary excretion of heme pigments, due either to myoglobinuria with rhabdomyolysis or, less commonly, hemoglobinuria with hemolysis. Neither myoglobin nor hemoglobin is directly nephrotoxic, as the decline in renal function appears to result from the combination of intratubular obstruction by precipitated pigment casts and renal vasoconstriction [1,23]. The latter can be due to several factors including volume depletion, secondary to fluid loss into the damaged muscle, or the release of vasoactive substances from muscle or red cell membranes. True tubular necrosis is uncommon, an observation that probably accounts for the frequent findings of a low urine sodium concentration and low fractional excretion of sodium [24].

Marked overproduction of either myoglobin or hemoglobin typically leads to red or brown urine, unless pigment excretion is limited because the GFR is very low or the plasma has been cleared of these substances by extrarenal metabolism [25]. These substances, however, usually have *different effects on the color of the plasma.* Hemoglobin is relatively poorly filtered, due both to its large size (molecular weight of the tetramer is 69,000) and to protein binding to haptoglobin; as a result, hemoglobinuria (due primarily to the filtration of the nonbound dimer) is always associated with hemoglobin accumulation in the plasma, which at least evanescently has a red color. In comparison, myoglobin is smaller (molecular weight 17,000) and not protein bound. Consequently, it is rapidly excreted, allowing the plasma to maintain its normal color unless renal failure prevents myoglobin excretion.

The most common causes of rhabdomyolysis are trauma (including ischemic muscle damage after a drug overdose), alcoholism, seizures, and exertional heat stroke, particularly in untrained subjects or those with sickle cell trait [25,26]. Hypokalemia also may play a contributory role, both by impairing cell metabolism and by limiting the normal hyperemic response to exercise [27]. Heat stroke in untrained men, for example, typically develops during the second week of exercise, the same time as the maximum potassium deficit (due mostly to marked sweat losses) [27].

Renal failure in rhabdomyolysis is typically associated with the triad of pigmented granular casts in the urine, a red to brown color of the urine supernatant, which is hemepositive, and a marked elevation in the plasma level of the muscle enzyme, creatine phosphokinase. Other cellular constituents also may be released in this setting, possibly resulting in hyperphosphatemia, hypocalcemia (due to calcium phosphate precipitation in damaged muscle), hyperkalemia, hyperuricemia, and a rapid increase in the plasma creatinine concentration out of proportion to the duration of renal failure [1,25].

PREVENTION. Producing a forced diuresis with mannitol, saline, and if necessary, a loop diuretic may minimize pigment nephrotoxicity, probably by washing out obstructing tubular casts. It has also been suggested that alkalinization of the urine by the administration of sodium bicarbonate may also be beneficial. There is some risk to this regimen, however, since alkalinization will also promote tissue calcium phosphate deposition in those patients who release large quantities of intracellular phosphate.

Clinical Presentation and Course
The decline in the GFR in ATN has a variable onset. It typically begins abruptly following a hypotensive episode, rhabdomyolysis, or the administration of radiocontrast media. In comparison, the onset is more insidious with aminoglycoside nephrotoxicity, with the plasma creatinine concentration beginning to rise slowly after 7 or more days of therapy. Some patients with marked prerenal disease also may have a gradual course with the urinary findings showing a gradual transition from prerenal indices (low urine sodium concentration and fractional excretion of sodium, normal urinalysis) to those typical of ATN (high fractional excretion of sodium and granular and epithelial cell casts in the urine; see Chap. 19).

Once renal failure begins, the blood urea nitrogen (BUN) and plasma creatinine concentration usually rise in daily increments of 10 to 25 mg/dl and 0.5 to 2.5 mg/dl, respectively. The rise in BUN, however, can reach 50 mg/dl per day or more in hypercatabolic patients; marked hyperkalemia is also more common in this setting.

Nonoliguric versus Oliguric ATN
The urine volume is variable in ATN, ranging from oliguria (< 500 ml/day) to normal or even above normal levels. The maintenance of a high urine output could, in theory, be due to one of two factors: a less-marked decline in the GFR than in oliguric patients or a lesser degree of tubular reabsorption. In most patients, the former seems to predominate as nonoliguric ATN is associated with evidence of less severe tubular damage [28,29]. When compared to oliguric patients, those who maintain their urine output tend to have a lower peak plasma creatinine concentration, a lower mortality rate, and a less frequent requirement for dialysis (28 versus 84% in one study) [28].

The better prognosis associated with nonoliguric ATN is primarily seen with spontaneous disease. In comparison, raising the urine output with a loop diuretic in *established* oliguric ATN does not appear to change the renal prognosis when compared to untreated patients [30]. This can be explained by the diuretic increasing the urine output from those few nephrons that are still functioning, rather than recruiting new functioning nephrons.

Diuretic and Recovery Phases
The mean duration of the renal failure phase in ATN is approximately 7 to 21 days. This general finding, however, does not apply to all patients. For example, a short, self-limited insult, as with suprarenal aortic clamping during aneurysm surgery or the administration of radiocontrast media, is associated with a decline in renal function that lasts only a few days [6,14]. On the other hand, patients with recurrent ischemic episodes or persistent infection may remain in renal failure for 3 to 6 months or more [3]. Infection may be deleterious by producing a prolonged hypercatabolic state that prevents the regeneration of tubular cells that is required for recovery to occur.

The period of renal failure is usually followed by the gradual recovery of renal function, characterized at first by a plateau in the plasma creatinine concentration and then a slow reduction most or all of the way toward the previous baseline value [1]. This elevation in the GFR is generally associated with a progressive rise in urine output (particularly in oliguric patients), which can initially average 50 to 100 percent per day. Studies in experimental animals suggest that recovery begins with the relief of tubular obstruction by the washout of casts and cellular debris and later by the return of normal tubular function [31]. Thus, the initial rise in urine output is often in part nonphysiologic, reflecting a persistent defect in tubular sodium and water reabsorption. As a result, maintenance of an adequate intake is required at this stage to prevent the development of volume depletion.

Treatment
Therapy in established ATN, other than correction of the underlying problem (such as discontinuation of an aminoglycoside), is largely supportive. In particular, attention must be paid to maintenance of fluid and electrolyte balance and of adequate nutrition. Despite optimal management, however, many patients will still require a transient period of dialysis. The major indications for dialysis are marked fluid overload or hyperkalemia, or the presence of uremic signs or symptoms, such as pericarditis, colitis, confusion, or bleeding in a patient with a prolonged bleeding time. The institution of *prophylactic* dialysis at a particular level of BUN or plasma creatinine concentration has not been shown to be of benefit as long as the BUN is <150 mg/dl [32].

It has also been suggested that the use of a high-calorie, low-protein, high-essential–amino acid diet may minimize protein breakdown and perhaps accelerate the recovery of renal function. This theory, however, has not been generally confirmed. Only those patients with multisystem abnormalities who are likely to be hypercatabolic appear to benefit from this regimen [1,33].

Even with the use of dialytic and dietary therapy, the mortality rate of all patients with ATN remains between 40 and 60 percent, with infection and the underlying disease (such as persistent postoperative hypotension) being the major causes of death [1,33,34]. This general statistic, however, is somewhat misleading because *survival is largely dependent on the patient's general health.* Mortality is very high in patients with persistent multisystem involvement such as abdominal infection, pneumonia, neurologic dysfunction, and circulatory instability [1,34]. In comparison, the prognosis is generally excellent with aminoglycoside- or radiocontrast-induced ATN if the patient is otherwise well.

Prevention of Postischemic ATN
In addition to fluid repletion and reversal of hypotension, mannitol, loop diuretics (such as furosemide), and dopamine have been given in an attempt to prevent postischemic ATN [1]. The use of these agents is based on several possible beneficial effects. They may, for example, preserve cellular integrity by diminishing active transport and therefore energy requirements in the loop of Henle (furosemide), by minimizing postischemic cell swelling (hypertonic mannitol), and by increasing renal perfusion (dopamine in low doses). The diuresis associated with mannitol and furosemide also may wash out obstructing tubular casts.

Both mannitol and furosemide have been shown to be effective in experimental models of postischemic ATN when given at the time of the ischemic insult [1,7,35]. It is unclear, however, how applicable these findings are in humans. Furosemide, for example, was not found to be beneficial in established ATN [30]; this is not surprising since the drug was administered well after the ischemic insult.

In comparison, there are a few studies in which mannitol, furosemide, or dopamine has been given to oliguric patients within the first 48 hours of the renal insult. Those patients who responded with an increase in urine output had a more rapid recovery of renal function, a less frequent requirement for dialysis, and were treated earlier (within 24 hours) than the nonresponders [36,37]. However, the responders also had evidence of less severe tubular injury (lower urine sodium concentration and higher urine output) and may have done well without specific therapy. Thus, these results do not offer definitive proof of benefit.

In another study, all patients undergoing open heart surgery were treated prophylactically with mannitol, furosemide, and dopamine *during and after the operation* [4]. Sixteen patients with ATN were identified. No conclusions could be reached about the prevention of acute renal failure, since there was no control group. Therapy did seem to be effective in maintaining an adequate urine output; all patients were nonoliguric, not oliguric as had been the experience prior to the use of this regimen. However, the nonoliguric ATN in this setting was not associated with the expected benign course [28,29] as 14 of 16 required dialysis. Thus, intensive therapy increased the output from the few functioning nephrons but did not appear to prevent nephron loss.

In summary, there is no definitive proof that mannitol, a loop diuretic, or dopamine protects against or ameliorates postischemic ATN. Nevertheless, these agents are relatively nontoxic and a short trial is reasonable in high-risk patients, such as those with postoperative oliguria not responsive to fluid repletion. These modalities are most likely to be effective if given within 24 hours of the onset of oliguria [36,37]. If they do produce an increase in urine output, the losses must be replaced to avoid further volume depletion and exacerbation of the renal ischemia.

The usual doses are 12.5 to 25.0 gm of mannitol and 80 to 320 mg of furosemide, given over 30 to 60 minutes. Dopamine (3–5 μg/kg/min) can then be added if a diuresis is not induced. Potential complications include fluid overload and hyperosmolality (due to retained hypertonic mannitol) and deafness (due to high-dose intravenous furosemide) [1]. As a result, the use of multiple doses or prolonged therapy should be avoided.

References

1. Rose, BD. *Pathophysiology of Renal Disease* (2nd ed). New York: McGraw-Hill, 1987. Pp. 84-104.
2. Solez, K, Morel-Maroger, L, Sraer, J-D. The morphology of "acute tubular necrosis" in man: Analysis of 57 renal biopsies and a comparison with the glycerol model. *Medicine* 58:362, 1979.

3. Myers, BD, Moran, SM. Hemodynamically mediated acute renal failure. *N Engl J Med* 314:97, 1986.

4. Myers, BD, Hilberman, M, Spencer, RJ, Jamison, RL. Glomerular and tubular function in non-oliguric acute renal failure. *Am J Med* 72:642 1982.

5. Barry, KG, Mazze, RI, Schwartz, FD. Prevention of surgical oliguria and renal hemodynamic suppression by sustained hydration. *N Engl J Med* 270:1373, 1964.

6. Myers, BD, Miller, D, Mehigan, JT, Olcott, C, IV, Golbetz, H. Robertson, CR, Spencer, R, Friedman, S. Nature of the renal injury following total renal ischemia in man. *J Clin Invest* 73:329, 1984.

7. Brezis, M, Rosen, S, Silva, P, Epstein, FH. Renal ischemia. A new perspective. *Kidney Int* 26:375, 1984.

8. Shanley, PF, Rosen, MD, Brezis, M, Silva, P, Epstein, FH, Rosen, S. Topography of focal proximal tubular necrosis after ischemia with reflow in the rat kidney. *Am J Pathol* 122:462, 1986.

9. Moore, RD, Smith, CR, Lipsky, JJ, Mellits, ED, Lietman, PS. Risk factors for nephrotoxicity in patients treated with aminoglycosides. *Ann Intern Med* 100:352, 1984.

10. Meyer, RD. Risk factors and comparisons of clinical nephrotoxicity of aminoglycosides. *Am J Med* 80 (suppl 6B):119, 1986.

11. Fabre, J, Rudhardt, M, Blanchard, P, Regamey, C. Persistence of sisomicin and gentamicin in renal cortex and medulla compared with other organs and serum of rats. *Kidney Int* 10:444, 1976.

12. Patel, R, Savage, A. Symptomatic hypomagnesemia associated with gentamicin therapy. *Nephron* 23:50, 1979.

13. Humes, WD. Aminoglycoside nephrotoxicity. *Kidney Int* 33:900, 1988.

14. Fang, LS-T. Contrast medium-induced acute renal failure. *Med Grand Rounds* 2:263, 1983.

15. vanZee, BE, Hoy, WE, Talley, TE, Jaenike, JR. Renal injury associated with intravenous pyelography in nondiabetic and diabetic subjects. *Ann Intern Med* 89:51, 1978.

16. Taliercio, CP, Vlietstra, RE, Fisher, LD, Burnett, JC. Risk for renal function with cardiac angiography. *Ann Intern Med* 104:510, 1986.

17. Holland, MD, Galla, JH, Sanders, PW, Luke, RG. Effect of urinary pH and diatrizoate on Bence Jones protein nephrotoxicity in the rat. *Kidney Int* 27:46, 1985.

18. Fang, LS-T, Sirota, RA, Ebert, TH, Lichtenstein, NS. Low fractional excretion of sodium with contrast media-induced acute renal failure. *Arch Intern Med* 140: 531, 1980.

18a. Anto, HR, Chou, S-Y., Porush, JG, Shapiro, WB. Infusion intravenous pyelography and renal function. Effects of hypertonic mannitol in patients with chronic renal insufficiency. *Arch Intern Med* 141:1652, 1981.

19. Ries, F, Klastersky, J. Nephrotoxicity induced by cancer chemotherapy with special emphasis on cisplatin toxicity. *Am J Kid Dis* 8:368, 1986.

20. Madias, NE, Harrington, JT. Platinum nephrotoxicity. *Am J Med* 65:307, 1978.

21. Schilsky, RL, Anderson, T. Hypomagnesemia and renal magnesium wasting in patients receiving cisplatin. *Ann Intern Med* 90:929, 1979.

22. Jackson, AM, Rose, BD, Graff, LG, Jacobs, JB, Schwartz, JH, Strauss, GM, Yang, JPS, Rudnick, MR, Elfenbein, IB, Narins, RG. Thrombotic microangiopathy and renal failure associated with antineoplastic chemotherapy. *Ann Intern Med* 101:41, 1984.

22a. Ozols, RF, Corden, BJ, Jacob, J, Wesley, MN, Ostchega, Y, Young, RC. High-dose cisplatin in hypertonic saline. *Ann Intern Med* 100:19, 1984.

23. Schrier, RW, Henderson, HS, Tisher, CC, Tannen, RL. Nephropathy associated with heat stress and exercise. *Ann Intern Med* 67:356, 1967.

24. Corwin, HL, Screiber, MJ, Fang, LS-T, Low fractional excretion of sodium. Occurrence with hemoglobinuric- and myoglobinuric-induced acute renal failure. *Arch Intern Med* 144:981, 1984.

25. Gabow, PA, Kaehny, WD, Kelleher, SP. The spectrum of rhabdomyolysis. *Medicine* 61:141, 1982.

26. Honda, N. Acute renal failure and rhabdomyolysis. *Kidney Int* 23:888, 1983.

27. Knochel, JP. Neuromuscular manifestations of electrolyte disorders. *Am J Med* 72:521, 1982.
28. Anderson, RJ, Linas, SL, Berns, AS, Henrich, WL, Miller, TR, Gabow, PA, Schrier, RW. Non-oliguric acute renal failure. *N Engl J Med* 296:1134, 1977.
29. Dixon, BS, Anderson, RJ. Nonoliguric acute renal failure. *Am J Kid Dis* 6:71, 1985.
30. Brown, CB, Ogg, CS, Cameron, JS. High dose frusemide in acute renal failure. *Clin Nephrol* 15:90, 1981.
31. Finn, WF, Chevalier, RL. Recovery from postischemic acute renal failure in the rat. *Kidney Int* 16:113, 1979.
32. Gillum, DM, Kelleher, SP, Dillingham, MA, et al. The role of intensive dialysis in acute renal failure. *Clin Nephrol* 25:249, 1986.
33. McMurray, SD, Luft, FC, Maxwell, DR, Hamburger, RJ, Futty, D, Szwed, JJ, Lavalle, KH, Kleit, SA. Prevailing patterns and predictor variables in patients with acute tubular necrosis. *Arch Intern Med* 138:950, 1978.
34. Lange, HW, Aeppli, DM, Brown, DC. Survival of patients with acute renal failure requiring dialysis after open heart surgery: Early prognostic indicators. *Am Heart J* 113:1138, 1987.
35. Hanley, MJ, Davidson, K. Prior mannitol and furosemide infusion in a model of ischemic acute renal failure. *Am J Physiol* 241:F556, 1981.
36. Luke, RG, Briggs, JD, Allison, MEM, Kennedy, AC. Factors determining response to mannitol in acute renal failure. *Am J Med Sci* 259:168, 1970.
37. Graziani, G, Cantaluppi, A, Casati, S, Citterio, A, Scalamonga, A, Aroldi, A, Silenzio, R, Branacaccio, D, Ponticelli, C. Dopamine and frusemide in oliguric acute renal failure. *Nephron* 37:39, 1984.

V. GLOMERULAR DISEASES

25. DIFFERENTIAL DIAGNOSIS OF GLOMERULAR DISEASE

The following chapters will discuss the individual causes of glomerular disease. Although many of these disorders are diagnosed primarily by renal biopsy, the urinalysis, physical findings, and the patient's age frequently allow the differential diagnosis to be narrowed to only a few conditions.

Urinary Findings

In general, glomerular disease can produce three different patterns of urinary abnormalities: nephrotic, nephritic, and chronic (Table 25-1) [1]. These patterns, particularly the first two, are important because they tend to be caused by different glomerular disorders (Table 25-2).

Nephrotic Sediment

A *nephrotic* sediment is characterized primarily by heavy proteinuria (usually > 2.5 gm/day) and lipiduria. Although mild microscopic hematuria may also be present, marked hematuria and cellular casts are not typically seen. The diseases associated with these findings have increased glomerular permeability due to damage to the glomerular basement membrane; however, cell proliferation, leukocyte infiltration, and necrosis are typically absent and it is this *lack of inflammatory change* that is responsible for the relatively benign urine sediment. The general absence of inflammation in the glomeruli can be illustrated by the fact that none of the nephrotic disorders listed in Table 25-2 are called glomerulo*nephritis,* other than the infrequent patient seen during the late recovery stage of postinfectious glomerulonephritis.

It is important to note that a nonglomerular disease, such as benign nephrosclerosis, can also lead to nephrotic range proteinuria [2]. This generally occurs in older patients with a long history of hypertension in whom renal insufficiency is already present. These patients, however, do not typically demonstrate the other findings of the nephrotic syndrome such as hypoalbuminemia and edema, probably because the glomerular damage is relatively mild[1]. Similar findings can also be seen with the secondary focal glomerulosclerosis induced by hemodynamic injury, as occurs with chronic pyelonephritis or unilateral renal agenesis (see Chap. 56).

Nephritic Sediment

A nephritic sediment is characterized by hematuria, pyuria, cellular and granular casts, and a variable degree of proteinuria. The nephrotic syndrome may occur in this setting, but the active sediment distinguishes these disorders from those with a pure nephrotic sediment. These urinary changes usually correlate with more marked abnormalities on renal biopsy such as cell proliferation, leukocyte infiltration, crescent formation, or areas of necrosis.

FOCAL VERSUS DIFFUSE. The nephritic disorders can often be subdivided further on clinical grounds into conditions associated with focal or diffuse[2] involvement since focal diseases tend to produce less severe abnormalities (Table 25-3). Thus, a patient with focal glomerulonephritis frequently presents with asymptomatic microscopic hematuria or proteinuria, or both, or an episode of gross hematuria. As a result, these conditions

---

[1]The degree of proteinuria, which is partially dependent on the plasma albumin concentration, is not necessarily predictive of the severity of the glomerular leak. Consider, for example, two patients with 5 gm of proteinuria per day, one with a plasma albumin concentration of 2.2 gm/dl and one with a near-normal value of 3.7 gm/dl as is often seen with nephrosclerosis. The former patient is hypoalbuminemic in part because he or she has a much greater increase in glomerular permeability. This could be demonstrated by the marked rise in protein excretion that would occur if the plasma albumin concentration were raised toward normal by an albumin infusion [3].

[2]In pathologic terms, focal disease means that less than 50 percent of the glomeruli are affected on light microscopy whereas more widespread involvement is called diffuse disease. The clinical distinction of focal versus diffuse in Table 25-2 generally, but not always, correlates with these histologic definitions.

Table 25-1. Urinalysis in various types of glomerular disease

Nephrotic	Nephritic	Chronic
Heavy proteinuria	Red and white cells	Less proteinuria and
Free fat droplets	Red cell casts	hematuria
Oval fat bodies	Variable proteinuria; may reach	Broad waxy casts
Fatty casts	nephrotic range	Granular casts
Variable hematuria	Frequent white cell and granular casts	

Source: Adapted from Schreiner, GE. *Arch Intern Med* 99:356, 1957. Copyright 1957, American Medical Association.

Table 25-3. Signs of focal and diffuse glomerulonephritis

Abnormality	Focal	Diffuse
Decreased GFR	Absent or mild	Usually present, may be severe
Hypertension	Unusual	Common
Edema	Unusual	Common
Nephrotic syndrome	Unusual	May occur

Table 25-4. Glomerular versus extraglomerular bleeding

Urinary finding	Glomerular	Extraglomerular
Red cell casts	May be present	Absent
Red cell morphology	Dysmorphic	Uniform
Proteinuria (> 500 mg/day)	May be present	Absent
Clots	Absent	May be present
Color	May be red or brown	May be red

must be differentiated from nonglomerular disorders that can produce similar findings, such as hematuria due to polycystic kidney disease, calculi, or prostatic disease. It is, therefore, important to be aware of the findings that can distinguish glomerular from extraglomerular bleeding (Table 25-4). Red cell casts, proteinuria, and dysmorphic red cells (which appear fragmented with blebs and budding) all favor a glomerular origin. The last finding is presumably due to mechanical injury as the red cells pass through rents in the damaged glomerular basement membrane [4]. In contrast, the red cells have a relatively uniform circular shape with extraglomerular lesions.

Hematuria (as little as 1 ml/L of urine) can also result in a visible change in urine color. With glomerular disease, the combination of prolonged transit time through the nephron and an acid urine pH can result in the formation of methemoglobin, which has a smoky brown ("Coca-Cola") color. In comparison, contact time is reduced with extraglomerular bleeding and only a pink or red color will be seen. (Red to brown urine also may be found in other disorders such as hemoglobinuria or myoglobinuria; in these conditions, however, it is the color of the supernatant, not the sediment, that is changed).

The more severe manifestations of glomerular disease—renal insufficiency, hypertension, edema, and the nephrotic syndrome—primarily occur with diffuse glomerulonephritis or vasculitis (Table 25-2). One disease that can be confused with diffuse glomerulonephritis is acute, usually drug-induced, interstitial nephritis (see Chap. 46). Acute renal failure with hematuria, pyuria (and occasional eosinophiluria), and white cell casts are typical manifestations of the latter condition, but marked proteinuria and red cell casts are generally absent. One interesting exception is the nephrotoxicity that may

Table 25-2. Major causes of glomerular disease according to urinary findings and age

Urinalysis	Age		
	< 15 years	15–40 years	> 40 years
Nephrotic pattern	Minimal change disease Focal glomerulosclerosis	Focal glomerulosclerosis Minimal change disease Membranous nephropathy (including SLE) Diabetes mellitus Preeclampsia Postinfectious glomerulonephritis (late stage)	Membranous nephropathy Diabetes mellitus Minimal change disease Primary amyloidosis Benign nephrosclerosis Postinfectious glomerulonephritis (late stage)
Nephritic pattern Focal disease	Benign hematuria IgA nephropathy Henoch-Schönlein purpura Mild postinfectious glomerulonephritis Hereditary nephritis	IgA nephropathy SLE Hereditary nephritis	IgA nephropathy
Diffuse disease	Postinfectious glomerulonephritis Membranoproliferative glomerulonephritis	SLE Membranoproliferative glomerulonephritis Rapidly progressive glomerulonephritis Postinfectious glomerulonephritis	Rapidly progressive glomerulonephritis Vasculitis Postinfectious glomerulonephritis

Source: From Rose, BD. *Pathophysiology of Renal Disease* (2nd ed). New York: McGraw-Hill, 1987, P. 167.

be seen with nonsteroidal anti-inflammatory drugs, particularly fenoprofen [5]. In this setting, interstitial nephritis is commonly accompanied by the nephrotic syndrome due to minimal change disease. The interstitial infiltrate is primarily composed of thymus-derived lymphocytes (T cells); these cells could also be responsible for the proteinuria by the release of a lymphokine that could lead to alterations in the glomerular basement membrane.

Chronic Sediment
Progressive chronic glomerular disease is characterized by replacement of the acute inflammatory changes by scarring. As a result, the urinalysis typically becomes less abnormal: the degree of proteinuria tends to fall due to the decline in the glomerular filtration rate (GFR); hematuria, pyuria, and cellular casts become less prominent; and broad waxy ("renal failure") casts may be seen. In some cases, the urinary findings become so nonspecific that it is difficult to be certain that the patient has a primary glomerular disease.

Age
Although most glomerular diseases can occur in any age group, many of these disorders are more prevalent in certain age groups. For example, benign hematuria is primarily a disease of children, systemic lupus erythematosus (SLE) of 15- to 40-year-old women, and primary amyloidosis of adults over the age of 40 to 50. As a result, the clinical differential diagnosis can frequently be narrowed further when the patient's age is considered along with the findings in the urinalysis and physical examination (Table 25-2).

Identifying the most likely diagnoses can also allow appropriate laboratory tests to be obtained in an effort to establish the presence of an underlying systemic disease. Included in this group are throat culture and anti-DNAase B titer in poststreptococcal glomerulonephritis, blood cultures in bacterial endocarditis, plasma glucose concentration in diabetes mellitus, antinuclear antibodies and DNA binding in SLE, and immunoelectrophoresis of the serum and urine to look for a paraprotein in primary amyloidosis. Measurement of plasma complement levels may also be helpful since hypocomplementemia occurs with many of the diffuse nephritic disorders, such as SLE, postinfectious glomerulonephritis, membranoproliferative glomerulonephritis, and the vasculitis associated with mixed cryoglobulinemia.

Clinical Examples
The use of the approach presented above can be illustrated by the following case histories.

CASE HISTORY
A 21-year-old woman presents with pedal and periorbital edema for 3 weeks. She denies gross hematuria, a recent upper respiratory infection, arthralgias, or skin rash. She has no history of diabetes mellitus and is not pregnant.

The physical examination is normal except for 4 + pedal edema; her blood pressure is 130/90. Laboratory tests reveal: BUN 26 mg/dl, P_{cr} 1.3 mg/dl, plasma albumin concentration 2.4 g/dl, and a negative antinuclear antibody titer. The urinalysis shows 4 + proteinuria, oval fat bodies, free fat droplets, 20 to 25 red cells per high power field, and occasional red cell casts; 24-hour urinary protein excretion is 6.2 gm.

COMMENT: This woman has the nephrotic syndrome but a *nephritic* sediment. These findings plus edema, renal insufficiency, and mild hypertension suggest the presence of diffuse glomerulonephritis. In this age group, SLE, membranoproliferative glomerulonephritis, and less often anti-glomerular basement membrane (GBM) antibody disease are the most likely diagnoses. The lack of systemic symptoms or antinuclear antibodies makes SLE improbable; similarly, the absence of pulmonary hemorrhage and severe renal insufficiency are unusual in anti-GBM antibody disease. Thus, membranoproliferative glomerulonephritis seems to be the leading diagnosis; this was confirmed by renal biopsy.

CASE HISTORY
A 53-year-old man is found to have microscopic hematuria when a urinalysis is performed as part of a yearly examination. Previous urinalyses have been unremarkable and he has no history or symptoms suggestive of renal disease or a systemic disorder.

The physical examination is normal with a blood pressure of 125/80. Pertinent laboratory tests reveal a P_{cr} of 0.9 mg/dl (unchanged from prior values) and a normal plasma albumin concentration. The urinalysis reveals no proteinuria (by dipstick), 10 red cells per high power field (most of which are dysmorphic), and occasional red cell casts. Twenty-four hour urine reveals only 84 mg of protein (normal < 150 mg).

COMMENT: The minimal urinary findings are compatible with a focal glomerulonephritis, which is most likely due to IgA nephropathy (Table 25-2). A renal biopsy, however, is probably not indicated since there is no proved therapy for this disorder and the patient has none of the signs suggestive of progressive disease such as proteinuria, an elevated P_{cr}, or hypertension. Therefore, only periodic follow-up is indicated in this patient who may well have benign disease with an excellent long-term prognosis.

Collection of a 24-hour urine is not unreasonable in this setting because of the relative lack of sensitivity of the dipstick. Unless the urine is very concentrated, the dipstick does not become positive until protein excretion is substantially elevated at 400 to 500 mg/day.

References

1. Rose, BD. *Pathophysiology of Renal Disease* (2nd ed.). New York: McGraw-Hill, 1987. Pp. 164-167.
2. Mujais, SK, Emmanouel, DS, Kasinath, BS, Spargo, BH. Marked proteinuria in hypertensive nephrosclerosis. *Am J Nephrol* 5:190, 1985.
3. Shemesh, O, Deen, WM, Brenner, BM, McNeely, E, Myers, BD. Effect of colloid volume expansion on glomerular barrier size-selectivity in humans. *Kidney Int* 29:916, 1986.
4. Fairley, KF, Birch, DF. A simple method for identifying glomerular bleeding. *Kidney Int* 21:105, 1982.
5. Clive, DM, Stoff, JS. Renal syndromes associated with nonsteroidal antiinflammatory drugs. *N Engl J Med* 310:563, 1984.

26. MANIFESTATIONS OF THE NEPHROTIC SYNDROME

The nephrotic syndrome (in which protein excretion usually exceeds 3.5 gm/day) is associated with a variety of renal and extrarenal manifestations (Table 26-1). A reduction in the glomerular filtration rate (GFR), for example, may occur because of damage to the glomeruli by the primary disease, thereby reducing the surface area available for filtration [1]. The mechanisms responsible for the other abnormalities, however, are frequently not as well understood; as a result, important clinical issues remain incompletely resolved.

Proteinuria

Glomerular diseases cause proteinuria by increasing the permeability of the glomerular basement membrane (GBM) to macromolecules such as albumin. The two major factors that normally limit the filtration of albumin and other large proteins are illustrated by the experiment in Fig. 26-1: (1) the GBM is *size-selective* as indicated by the progressive reduction in filtration as molecular size increases; and (2) the GBM is *charge-selective* as indicated by the greater filtration of neutral and cationic compounds than anionic compounds of the same molecular size. Negatively charged proteoglycans (especially heparan sulfate) within the GBM are thought to comprise most of the charge barrier that minimizes the filtration of anionic albumin [2,3].

Studies in both animals and humans indicate that proteinuria can result from impairment of both the size and charge barriers of the GBM [3,4]. In some disorders such as membranous nephropathy, infusion of neutral dextrans of different sizes (as in Fig. 26-1) reveals increased filtration of normally nonfiltered larger dextrans; this finding points to the existence of unusually large "pores" within the GBM [4]. A different ab-

Table 26-1. Manifestations of the nephrotic syndrome

Decreased GFR
Proteinuria
Hypoalbuminemia
Edema
Hypertension
Hyperlipidemia
Thromboembolic events
Other
    Vitamin D deficiency
    Infection
    Iron deficiency (rare)

normality is present in minimal change disease. In this disorder, the filtration of neutral dextrans is actually reduced (due to diminished surface area available for filtration); the proteinuria is entirely due to impairment of the charge barrier as evidenced by a *selective increase in the filtration of anionic dextrans* [5]. This change may result from primary damage to the glomerular epithelial cells, leading to diminished synthesis of anionic compounds such as heparan sulfate [2,5].

The charge barrier has another important role in immune-mediated glomerular diseases: it is a major determinant of the *site of immune complex formation* [6]. Anionic antigens are unable to cross the GBM, leading to predominantly mesangial deposits. Only cationic antigens in experimental animals are able to pass through the GBM and produce deposits in the subepithelial space (similar to those seen in membranous nephropathy; see Chap. 29) [6].

In addition to the increment in glomerular permeability, the degree of proteinuria is also influenced by the GFR and the plasma albumin concentration. As a result, a decline in the GFR with progressive disease or marked hypoalbuminemia can lead to a reduction in protein excretion, occasionally to less than nephrotic levels.

Daily protein excretion is usually measured by a 24-hour urine collection. However, serial monitoring of the degree of proteinuria can be estimated more simply by measuring the protein-creatinine ratio (mg/mg) in a random daytime urine specimen [7]. This ratio correlates closely with total protein excretion in gm/day/1.73 m^2 body surface area. For example, a ratio of 2 : 1 represents protein excretion of approximately 2 gm/day/1.73 m^2.

Hypoalbuminemia

The mechanism by which hypoalbuminemia occurs is incompletely understood. The liver normally has the capacity to increase albumin synthesis by as much as 30 gm/day, a quantity that usually markedly exceeds the degree of urinary protein loss. As an example, patients on continuous ambulatory peritoneal dialysis lose between 4 and 5 gm of albumin per day in the dialysate but do not become hypoalbuminemic because of enhanced hepatic albumin production [8]. In comparison, a nephrotic patient with equivalent urinary losses may be markedly hypoalbuminemic as the adaptive hepatic response does not seem to be present [8]. Why this occurs is not known. Nevertheless, the variability in the hepatic response probably accounts at least in part for the lack of correlation between the degree of proteinuria and the fall in the plasma albumin concentration.

Edema

Two factors have traditionally been thought to be responsible for the sodium retention that leads to nephrotic edema: intrarenal changes such as a fall in the GFR which, by slowing flow through the tubules, would promote sodium reabsorption; and "underfilling" of the vascular tree as hypoalbuminemia promotes the movement of fluid from the

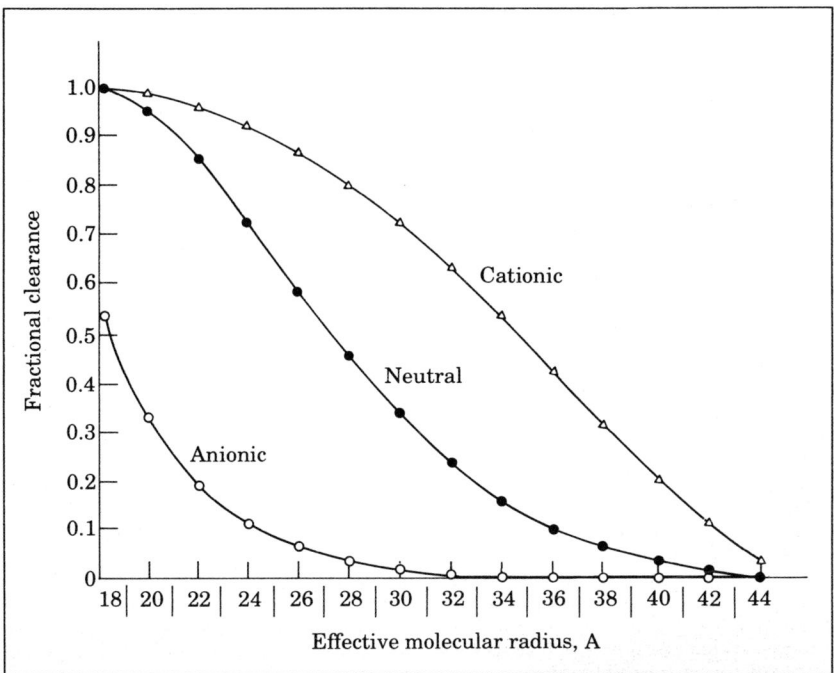

Fig. 26-1. Fractional clearances (the ratio of the filtration of a substance to that of inulin, which is freely filtered) of anionic, neutral, and cationic dextrans as a function of effective molecular radius. Both molecular size and charge are important determinants of filtration as smaller, neutral, or cationic compounds are more easily filtered. As a reference, the effective molecular radius of albumin is about 36 Å. (From Bohrer, MP, Baylis, C, Humes, HD, Glassock, RJ, Robertson, CR, Brenner, BM. *J Clin Invest* 61:72, 1978, by copyright permission of the American Society for Clinical Investigation.)

vascular space into the interstitium [9]. It has been presumed that the fall in plasma oncotic pressure associated with hypoalbuminemia favors the movement of fluid out of the vascular space into the interstitium; the ensuing plasma volume depletion would then promote compensatory renal sodium retention. If, however, there were a *parallel reduction* in the interstitial oncotic pressure (due both to less protein crossing the capillary wall and to washout of interstitial proteins by enhanced lymphatic flow), there would be no change in the oncotic pressure gradient and therefore no tendency to edema. Recent studies in both experimental animals and humans suggest that *hypoalbuminemia does not directly cause edema* until the plasma albumin concentration is below 2 gm/dl [10-13]; thus, nephrotic edema is most often due to an intrarenal defect that directly promotes sodium retention [10,13,14]. As an example, serial observations have been made in patients with minimal change disease undergoing corticosteroid-induced remission. In this setting, improvement in the glomerular lesion leads to enhanced sodium excretion and partial resolution of the edema, *prior* to any rise in the plasma albumin concentration [13].

These findings have important implications for the use of diuretics to treat nephrotic edema. Since the plasma volume is typically normal, relief of the edema with diuretics does not usually produce volume depletion or a rise in the P_{cr} [11], unless there is excessive fluid removal or the patient has marked hypoalbuminemia (below 2 gm/dl).

Hypertension

Hypertension is a relatively frequent complication of glomerular disease. In most patients with acute disease, the elevation in blood pressure is primarily due to volume expansion, with the level of vasoconstrictors (such as angiotensin II) being relatively low [15]. As a result, removal of the excess fluid with diuretics or dialysis lowers the blood pressure, frequently into the normal range.

The primary role of hypervolemia (manifested by peripheral edema on physical examination) may be of diagnostic importance. In a patient with apparent acute glomerular disease (by history and urinalysis), the finding of marked hypertension without edema suggests a different diagnosis: renin-mediated hypertension due to a vascular disease such as systemic vasculitis [16].

Additional factors appear to contribute in patients with chronic glomerular disease. Increased activity of both the renin-angiotensin system (probably due to regional ischemia induced by scarring) and the sympathetic nervous system (via an unknown mechanism) may be important in this setting [17].

Hyperlipidemia

Elevations in the plasma concentrations of cholesterol, triglycerides, and phospholipids are common in nephrotic patients, most often being associated with type IIa, IIb, or V pattern on lipoprotein electrophoresis [18]. Diminished levels of "cardioprotective" high-density lipoprotein cholesterol also may be present, due in part to loss of this protein in the urine [19].

Increased hepatic production of very low density lipoproteins, some of which are then converted to low-density lipoproteins (the major carrier of plasma cholesterol), seems to be the primary abnormality [20]. It has been suggested that the low plasma oncotic pressure directly stimulates lipoprotein production by the hepatocyte [21]. This hypothesis is supported by the observations that (1) the degree of hypercholesterolemia is inversely related to the fall in plasma oncotic pressure [21], and (2) raising the plasma oncotic pressure toward normal with an infusion of albumin rapidly lowers the plasma cholesterol level toward normal [22].

In view of the increasing evidence that hypercholesterolemia is a major risk factor for coronary heart disease [23], it might be expected that patients with persistent nephrotic syndrome would develop accelerated atherosclerosis. This hypothesis is as yet unproved [24]. Nevertheless, it seems prudent to institute a low-saturated fat diet and to consider the use of hypolipidemic agents such as colestipol or, if proven safe, lovastatin which can lower plasma cholesterol level by 20 to 30% or more and appear to be well tolerated [25].

Thromboembolic Events

Patients with the nephrotic syndrome have an increased incidence of arterial and venous thromboemboli, particularly deep vein and renal vein thrombosis (RVT) [26]. Between 10 to 40 percent of patients may be affected, although it is uncertain how this hypercoagulable state occurs [26,27]. A variety of abnormalities has been described, including a low plasma concentration of antithrombin III (an endogenous anticoagulant that may be lost in the urine since it is approximately the same size as albumin), an elevated plasma fibrinogen level, and increased activation of platelets. No single abnormality, however, appears to predict which patients are at risk; the initial suggestion that antithrombin III deficiency was of primary importance does not appear to apply in many patients [26,27].

Renal vein thrombosis (which is an unusual problem in nonnephrotics) may be unilateral or bilateral and may extend into the inferior vena cava. Some patients present with the signs and symptoms of renal infarction, such as flank pain, hematuria, an elevated plasma lactate dehydrogenase (LDH) level, and an increase in renal size on radiographic study. However, RVT has an *insidious onset* in most cases and *produces no symptoms referable to the kidney* [26,28]. In this setting, the only clinical clue to the possible presence of RVT is a pulmonary embolus.

RVT can occur with any form of the nephrotic syndrome but, for unknown reasons, seems to be *most common in membranous nephropathy.* Some prospective studies suggest that as many as 25 to 50 percent of patients with this disorder develop RVT, although a lower incidence has been found elsewhere [26-28].

The diagnosis of RVT is established by an inferior vena cavagram and selective renal venography. The question that remains unanswered, however, is when these tests should be performed in the asymptomatic patient who, if RVT is present, may be at increased risk of pulmonary embolism [26,28]. Some investigators recommend prospective renal venography in those patients with membranous nephropathy and heavy proteinuria, who appear to be at greatest risk. Although this may seem prudent, it is important to emphasize two potential problems with this approach: (1) no study has as yet compared the risk of undiagnosed and untreated RVT to the risk of long-term anticoagulation; and (2) patients with an initially negative radiographic study can still develop RVT at a later time [26].

Treatment of RVT (or other thrombotic event) consists of anticoagulation with heparin and then warfarin. This regimen should minimize the frequency of new thrombi or pulmonary emboli and may promote recanalization of the existing thrombus. Warfarin should probably be continued for as long as the patient remains nephrotic, since the hypercoagulable state persists. Surgical thrombectomy is generally not indicated. There may, however, be a role for fibrinolytic therapy in patients with acute RVT and acute renal failure [29].

Other

Proteins in addition to albumin also are lost in the urine in the nephrotic syndrome. These include thyroxine (bound to both thyroxine-binding prealbumin and to globulins), 25-hydroxyvitamin D (calcidiol, which is primarily bound to a circulating globulin that is normally not filtered), IgG, factors B and D of the alternate complement pathway, and transferrin-bound iron [30]. Although the loss of thyroxine is usually not sufficient to impair net thyroid function [31], the other changes may be important. For example, signs of vitamin D deficiency, such as impaired calcium absorption, a fall in the plasma concentration of ionized calcium, osteomalacia, and secondary hyperparathyroidism, all may occur [32]. An increased incidence of infection (perhaps due in part to the loss of IgG and factors B and D) and rarely refractory iron deficiency anemia (due to hypotransferrinemia) also may occur in selected patients [30]. Each of these changes is reversed with remission of the nephrotic syndrome.

References

1. Kaizu, K, Marsh, D, Zipser, R, Glassock, RJ. Role of prostaglandins and angiotensin II in experimental glomerulonephritis. *Kidney Int* 28:629, 1985.
2. Mahan, JD, Sisson-Ross, S, Vernier, RL. Glomerular basement membrane anionic charge site changes early in aminonucleoside nephrosis. *Am J Pathol* 125:393, 1986.
3. Kaysen, GA, Myers, BD, Couser, WG, Rabkin, R, Felts, JM. Mechanisms and consequences of proteinuria. *Lab Invest* 54:479, 1986.
4. Myers, BD, Okarma, TB, Friedman, S, Bridges, C, Ross, J, Asseff, S, Deen, WM. Mechanisms of proteinuria in human glomerulonephritis. *J Clin Invest* 70:732, 1982.
5. Carrie, BJ, Salyer, WR, Myers, BD. Minimal change nephropathy: An electrochemical disorder of the glomerular membrane. *Am J Med* 70:262, 1981.
6. Border, WA, Ward, HJ, Kamil, ES, Cohen, AH. Induction of membranous nephropathy in rabbits by administration of an exogenous cationic antigen. *J Clin Invest* 69:451, 1982.
7. Ginsberg, JM, Chang, RS, Matarese, RA, Garella, S. Use of single voided urine samples to estimate quantitative proteinuria. *N Engl J Med* 309:1543, 1983.
8. Kaysen, GA, Schoenfeld, PY. Albumin homeostasis in patients undergoing continuous ambulatory peritoneal dialysis. *Kidney Int* 25:107, 1984.
9. Meltzer, JI, Keim, HJ, Laragh, JH, Sealey, JE, Jan, K-M, Chien, S. Nephrotic syn-

drome: Vasoconstriction and hypervolemic types indicated by renin-sodium profiling. *Ann Intern Med* 91:688, 1979.

10. Kaysen, GA, Paukert, TT, Menke, DJ, Couser, WG, Humphreys, MH. Plasma volume expansion is necessary for edema formation in the rat with Heymann nephritis. *Am J Physiol* 248:F247, 1985.

11. Koomans, HA, Braam, B, Geers, AB, Roos, JC, Dorhout Mees, EJ. The importance of plasma protein for blood volume and blood pressure homeostasis. *Kidney Int* 30:730, 1986.

12. Manning, RD, Jr, Guyton, AC. Effects of hypoproteinemia on fluid volumes and arterial pressure. *Am J Physiol* 245:H284, 1983.

13. Brown, EA, Markandu, N, Sagnella, GA, Jones, BE, MacGregor, GA. Sodium retention in nephrotic syndrome is due to an intrarenal defect: Evidence from steroid-induced remission. *Nephron* 39:290, 1985.

14. Ichikawa, I, Rennke, HG, Hoyer, JR, Badr, KF, Schor, N, Troy, JL, Lechene, CP, Brenner, BM. Role for intrarenal mechanisms in the impaired salt excretion of experimental nephrotic syndrome. *J Clin Invest* 71:91, 1983.

15. Rodriguez-Iturbe, B, Baggio, B, Colina-Chourio, J, Favaro, S, Garcia, R, Sussana, F, Castillo, L, Borsatti, A. Studies on the renin-aldosterone system in the acute nephritic syndrome. *Kidney Int* 19:445, 1981.

16. Stockigt, JR, Topliss, DJ, Hewett, MJ. High-renin hypertension in necrotizing vasculitis. *N Engl J Med* 300:1218, 1979.

17. Acosta, JH. Hypertension in chronic renal disease. *Kidney Int* 22:702, 1982.

18. Goldberg, ACK, Eliaschewitz, FG, Quintao, ECR, Origin of hypercholesterolemia in chronic experimental nephrotic syndrome. *Kidney Int* 12:23, 1977.

19. Short, CD, Durrington, PN, Mallick, NP, Hunt, LP, Tetlow, L, Ishola, M. Serum and urinary high density lipoproteins in glomerular disease with proteinuria. *Kidney Int* 29:1224, 1986.

20. Marsh, JB, Sparks, CE. Hepatic secretion of lipoproteins in the rat and the effect of experimental nephrosis. *J Clin Invest* 64:1229, 1979.

21. Appel, GB, Blum, CB, Chien, C, Kunis, CL, Appel, AS. The hyperlipidemia of the nephrotic syndrome: Relation to plasma albumin concentration, oncotic pressure, and viscosity. *N Engl J Med* 312:1544, 1985.

22. Baxter, JH, Goodman, HC, Allen, JC. Effects of infusions of serum albumin on serum lipids and lipoproteins in nephrosis. *J Clin Invest* 40:490, 1961.

23. The Lipid Research Clinics Coronary Primary Prevention Trial Results. II. The relationship of reduction in incidence of coronary heart disease to cholesterol lowering. *J Am Med Assoc* 251:365, 1984.

24. Mallick, NP, Short, CD. The nephrotic syndrome and ischemic heart disease. *Nephron* 27:54, 1981.

25. Vega, GL, Grundy, SM. Lovastatin therapy in nephrotic hyperlipidemia: Effects on lipoprotein metabolism. *Kidney Int* 33:1160, 1988.

26. Llach, F: Hypercoagulability, renal vein thrombosis, and other thrombotic complications of the nephrotic syndrome. *Kidney Int* 28:429, 1985.

27. Robert, A, Olmer, M, Sampol, J, Gugliotta, J-E, Casanova, P. Clinical correlation between hypercoagulability and thromboembolic phenomena. *Kidney Int* 31:830, 1987.

28. Wagoner, RD, Stanton, AW, Holley, KE, Winter, CS. Renal vein thrombosis in idiopathic membranous glomerulopathy and nephrotic syndrome: Incidence and significance. *Kidney Int* 23:368, 1983.

29. Burrow, CW, Walker, WG, Bell, WR, Gatewood, OB. Streptokinase salvage of renal function after renal vein thrombosis. *Ann Intern Med* 100:237, 1984.

30. Rose, BD. *Pathophysiology of Renal Disease* (2nd ed.). New York: McGraw-Hill, 1987, P. 263.

31. Afrasiabi, MA, Vaziri, ND, Gwinup, G, Mays, DM, Barton, CH, Ness, RL, Valenta, LJ. Thyroid function studies in the nephrotic syndrome. *Ann Intern Med* 90:335, 1979.

32. Maluche, HH, Goldstein, DA, Massry, SG. Osteomalacia and hyperparathyroid bone disease in patients with nephrotic syndrome. *J Clin Invest* 63:494, 1979.

27. MINIMAL CHANGE DISEASE

Minimal change disease (MCD) is the most common cause of the nephrotic syndrome in children, accounting for over 90 percent of cases under the age of 10 and more than 50 percent in older children. It is not generally appreciated, however, that this disorder is also responsible for as many as 20 to 30 percent of cases in adults of all ages [1].

The term *minimal change* (or *nil*) disease is derived from the findings on light microscopy, which are either normal or reveal only focal areas of mild mesangial hypercellularity. Immunofluorescence studies are usually negative for immunoglobulins or complement, although scattered deposits of IgM or C3 may occasionally be seen. These findings are thought to represent nonspecific trapping in the abnormally permeable glomerular capillary wall [2]. The *diagnostic* histologic change in MCD is widespread fusion of the epithelial cell foot processes on electron microscopy (Fig. 27-1). This abnormality returns to normal with spontaneous or corticosteroid-induced remission of the disease.

Etiology and Pathogenesis

Although MCD is usually idiopathic, a specific cause can be identified in selected patients (Table 27-1) [3]. Malignancies, for example, appear to account for approximately 10 percent of cases in adults, most often due to lymphoma (particularly Hodgkin's disease) or leukemia* [4,5]. Both the lymphoma and the nephrotic syndrome typically present either simultaneously or within a few months of each other. In comparison, late development of the nephrotic syndrome (more than 12 months after diagnosis of the lymphoma) is more often due to secondary amyloidosis.

The course of the nephrotic syndrome generally parallels that of the lymphoma: effective treatment of the latter (with surgery, radiation, or chemotherapy) results in remission of the proteinuria; relapse of the lymphoma may then lead to recurrence of the glomerular lesion.

Nonsteroidal anti-inflammatory drugs (particularly fenoprofen and other proprionic acid derivatives) may be associated with the unusual combination of MCD and renal failure due to acute interstitial nephritis. The latter is characterized by hematuria, pyuria, and a prominent interstitial infiltrate on renal biopsy [6]. Similar findings can also rarely occur with recombinant leukocyte interferon, ampicillin, or rifampin [3].

The mechanism by which the disorders in Table 27-1 produce MCD is not known. It has been proposed that there may be an acquired and reversible *abnormality in T cell function,* with the release of a toxic lymphokine being responsible for the glomerular damage. In at least some patients, for example, the release of soluble immune response suppressor from suppressor T cells parallels the course of the proteinuria, being elevated when the disease is active and rapidly falling with corticosteroid-induced remission [6a]. The associations of MCD with Hodgkin's disease (in which T-cell function is abnormal) and with nonsteroidal anti-inflammatory drugs (in which the interstitial infiltrate is composed mostly of T cells) are also compatible with an important role for T cells [6]. However, the nature of the signal that leads to T-cell activation remains unclear [6a].

It is also thought that the target of attack is the *glomerular epithelial cell.* This cell is responsible for synthesis of the negatively charged proteoglycans (particularly heparan sulfate) and sialoproteins that are present in the glomerular basement membrane and coat the epithelial cell foot processes [7]. Reduced production of these compounds due to epithelial cell injury could account for both of the characteristic findings in MCD: fusion of the foot processes (which are normally separated by electrostatic repulsion by the anionic proteins) [8] and proteinuria due to loss of the anionic charge barrier that normally limits the filtration of albumin (see Chap. 26) [9].

---

*A variety of other glomerular lesions can also be seen with neoplasia, including membranous nephropathy (particularly with solid tumors), focal glomerulosclerosis, and a proliferative glomerulonephritis [4,5].

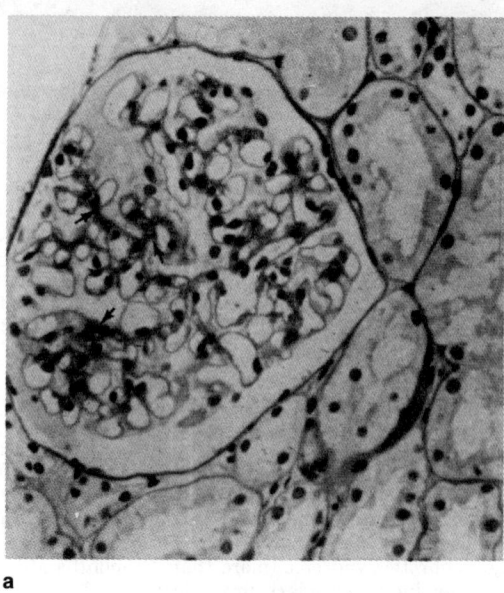

Fig. 27-1. Histology of normal glomeruli and those in minimal change disease. (a) Light microscopy of a normal glomerulus, with open capillary loops, thin glomerular basement membranes, and mesangial areas in the center of the lobules (arrows). Similar findings are typically present in minimal change disease, although some mesangial hypercellularity may be seen. (b) Electron microscopy of a normal glomerulus depicting the three layers of the glomerular capillary wall: fenestrated endothelial cell, basement membrane, and epithelial cell with foot processes. The foot processes are separated by slit pores, which are closed by a thin membrane, the slit diaphragm. (c) Electron microscopy showing the characteristic lesion in minimal change disease, diffuse fusion of the foot processes (arrow). The basement membrane is normal and, in contrast to many other glomerulopathies, no immune deposits are seen (From BD Rose, *Pathophysiology of Renal Disease* (2nd ed.). New York: McGraw-Hill, 1987.).

Table 27-1. Causes of minimal change disease

Idiopathic
Malignancy, particularly Hodgkin's disease
Drugs
Nonsteroidal anti-inflammatory drugs
Lithium
Gold
Recombinant leukocyte interferon
Ampicillin
Rifampin
IgA nephropathy (see Chap. 32)

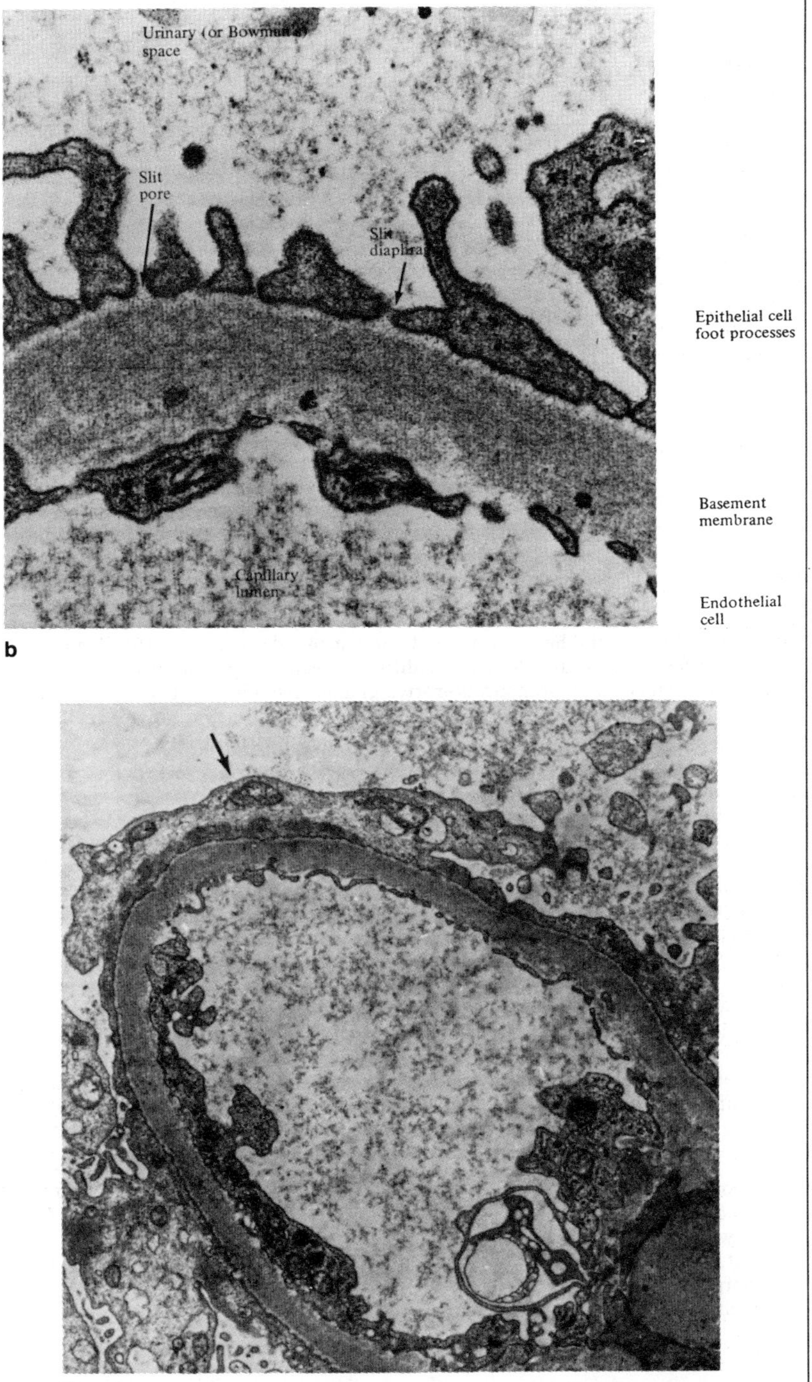

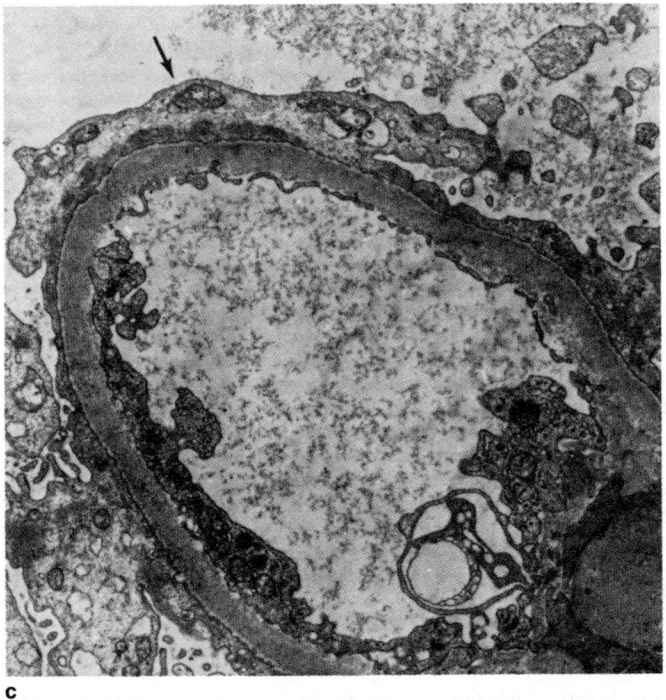

Fig. 27-1. (continued)

Clinical Presentation and Diagnosis

Patients with MCD usually present with edema, proteinuria, and the chemical findings of the nephrotic syndrome [1,10]. The onset of the disease is typically acute and often follows a viral upper respiratory infection; this probably represents a host response following activation of the immune system since no specific pathogenic virus appears to be involved [11]. The degree of fluid retention is variable, occasionally resulting in ascites as well as pedal and periorbital edema. Hypertension and microscopic hematuria occur in about 20 to 30 percent of children [10] but are somewhat more prevalent in adults [1]. The urine sediment, other than the red cells, is generally benign, characteristic of the nephrotic disorders (see Chap. 25).

The glomerular filtration rate (GFR) is usually normal or only mildly reduced in children; however, moderate-to-severe renal failure can occur in adults, primarily in patients over the age of 60 [1]. The mechanism by which this occurs is uncertain but three factors are thought to play a role in selected patients: a decrease in the surface area available for filtration due to foot process fusion*; severe interstitial edema in the kidney, producing tubular collapse; and aggressive diuretic therapy, leading to reduced renal perfusion [12-14]. Regardless of the mechanism, renal function improves with treatment of the primary disease.

The clinical and laboratory findings do not distinguish MCD from the other causes of the idiopathic nephrotic syndrome (membranous nephropathy and focal glomerulosclerosis). Thus, the diagnosis is established by renal biopsy in adults. In children, however, the marked prevalence of MCD usually results in the empiric administration of corticosteroids. A renal biopsy is performed only if the proteinuria persists after 8 weeks. Even in these corticosteroid-resistant patients, MCD still accounts for 50 percent of cases under the age of 6 but only about 4 percent in older children [15]. The remaining cases have focal glomerulosclerosis (or diffuse mesangial proliferation that may be a related disorder) or membranoproliferative glomerulonephritis [15]. The last disorder typically presents with an active nephritic urine sediment (containing red cells and cellular and granular casts) and is infrequently confused with MCD.

Course and Therapy

If untreated, patients with MCD typically remain edematous and are at risk of developing extrarenal complications such as thromboembolic events and infection (see Chap. 26). Fortunately, corticosteroids usually correct the glomerular lesion and are the therapy of choice in MCD. In children, for example, the use of prednisone has lowered the mortality rate from as high as 35 percent to less than 2 percent [16]. The absolute benefit has been somewhat harder to define in adults. Controlled studies indicate that most adults remit spontaneously within 4 years [1,17]. However, the earlier remission of proteinuria induced by prednisone markedly reduces the risk of thrombotic events, infection, and acute renal failure, a *benefit that outweighs the risks of prednisone therapy* [1].

A variety of corticosteroid regimens have been used to treat MCD. A standard daily regimen in children consists of 60 mg/m^2 (in 3 divided doses) for 4 weeks, followed by 40 mg/m^2 as a single morning dose on alternate days for 4 more weeks. In comparison, adults are given 1 mg/kg/day (in divided doses) until a remission is induced, followed by tapering of the dose over a total treatment period of 8 weeks [1].

The results of corticosteroid therapy can be summarized as follows:

1. Approximately 95 percent of children will undergo complete remission of proteinuria and edema: 70 percent within 2 weeks, 90 percent within 4 weeks, and 100 percent by 8 weeks [15].
2. Adults tend to respond somewhat less often and more slowly [1]. Roughly 80 percent undergo a complete remission and another 13 percent will have a partial remission (defined as loss of edema with persistent proteinuria of 300 mg–3 gm/day). Further-

---

*This decrease in permeability does not preclude the development of proteinuria, since loss of the anionic barrier to the filtration of macromolecules allows the filtration of normally nonfiltered compounds such as albumin [9].

more, the remission may not occur until as late as 16 weeks after the onset of prednisone therapy.
3. Only about 20 percent of responders are initially cured of their disease, with the remainder having one or more relapses [1,18]. Those who relapse infrequently can be retreated with short courses of prednisone. Approximately 40 to 50 percent of children (particularly if under the age of 7) and 20 percent of adults, however, are *frequent relapsers,* with proteinuria recurring while the prednisone is being tapered or shortly after therapy has been discontinued [1,18]. These patients can be treated either with long-term, low-dose, alternate-day prednisone therapy or with a 2-month course of cytotoxic therapy with cyclophosphamide or chlorambucil after prednisone-induced remission.

Cytotoxic therapy has been extremely effective in this setting: only 20 to 50 percent of patients have a relapse at 4 to 7 years [1,19,20]. Furthermore, the associated corticosteroid sparing prevents the inhibitory steroid effect on growth in children and allows catch-up growth to occur [20]. These benefits, however, must be weighed against the potential risks associated with cytotoxic therapy: bone marrow suppression, infection, gonadal fibrosis, alopecia, late neoplasia, and, with cyclophosphamide, hemorrhagic cystitis [3]. These complications can usually be prevented or minimized by careful monitoring and by limiting the course of therapy to 8 weeks. Nevertheless, it seems reasonable to limit the use of these agents to those frequent relapsers who cannot be maintained in remission with low-dose alternate-day prednisone (such as 10 mg every other day for 9–12 months) or who show signs of corticosteroid toxicity [20]. Therapy with azathioprine is another alternative. Although usually better tolerated than the other cytotoxic agents, azathioprine also tends to be less effective; long-term treatment of 6 to 12 months or more is required to induce a remission [21].
4. Those few patients who have no or only a partial response to prednisone also tend to remit with cytotoxic therapy [1,3]. Late relapses may occur in this setting but are now typically responsive to prednisone. Patients who remain resistant may respond to an 8-week course of cyclosporine [22].
5. Occasional frequent relapsers develop secondary corticosteroid resistance; biopsy at this time may show focal glomerulosclerosis, suggesting evolution of MCD into a more serious disorder* [23]. Cytotoxic therapy may induce a new remission, but some patients develop progressive renal failure.

In summary, MCD is a curable disease in almost all patients, although there is a variable requirement for prednisone and possibly cytotoxic therapy. In adults, for example, only about 5 percent of patients are still nephrotic at 5 to 10 years [1]. This is most likely to occur in patients over the age of 45 who initially present with evidence of renal insufficiency. Cure is also the general rule in children. Relapses are uncommon above the age of 20, but some patients have intermittent relapses into adulthood [20,25].

References

1. Nolasco, F, Cameron, JS, Heywood, EF, Hicks, J, Ogg, C, Williams, DG. Adult-onset minimal change nephrotic syndrome: A long-term follow-up. *Kidney Int* 29:1215, 1986.
2. Ji-Yun, Y, Melvin, T, Sibley, R, Michael, AF. No evidence for a specific role of IgM in mesangial proliferation in idiopathic nephrotic syndrome. *Kidney Int* 25:100, 1984.
3. Rose, BD. *Pathophysiology of Renal Disease* (2nd ed.). New York: McGraw-Hill, 1987, Pp 187-196.
4. Alpers, CE, Cotran, RS. Neoplasia and glomerular injury. *Kidney Int* 30:465, 1986.

*Focal glomerulosclerosis may also be present on renal biopsy in up to one-half of corticosteroid responsive, frequent relapsers who appear to have MCD [24]. This finding suggests that MCD and focal glomerulosclerosis may be related diseases (see Chap. 28). Its significance is uncertain, since the patients with sclerotic lesions continue to behave as if they have MCD, responding to cyclophosphamide and having normal renal function at 11 to 14 year follow-up [24].

5. Dabbs, DJ, Morel-Maroger Striker, L, Mignon, F, Striker, G. Glomerular lesions in lymphomas and leukemias. *Am J Med* 80:63, 1986.
6. Finkelstein, A, Fraley, DS, Stachura, I, Feldman, HA, Gandy, DR, Bourke, E. Fenoprofen nephropathy: Lipoid nephrosis and interstitial nephritis. A possible T-lymphocyte disorder. *Am J Med* 72:81, 1982.
6a. Schnaper, HW, Aune, TM. Steroid-sensitive mechanism of soluble immune response suppressor production in steroid-responsive nephrotic syndrome. *J Clin Invest* 79:257, 1987.
7. Sawada, H, Stukenbrok, H, Kerjaschki, D, Farquhar, MG. Epithelial polyanion (podocalyxin) is found on but not the soles of the foot processes of the glomerular epithelium. *Am J Pathol* 125:309, 1986.
8. Seiler, MW, Rennke, HG, Venkatachalam, MA, Cotran, RS. Pathogenesis of polycation-induced alterations ("fusion") of glomerular epithelium. *Lab Invest* 36:48, 1977.
9. Carrie, BJ, Salyer, WR, Myers, BD. Minimal change nephropathy: An electrochemical disorder of the glomerular membrane. *Am J Med* 70:262, 1981.
10. A Report of the International Study of Kidney Disease in Children. Nephrotic syndrome in children: Prediction of histopathology from clinical and laboratory characteristics at time of diagnosis. *Kidney Int* 13:159, 1978.
11. MacDonald, NE, Wolfish, N, McLaine, P, Phipps, R, Rossier, E. Role of respiratory viruses in exacerbations of primary nephrotic syndrome. *J Pediatr* 108:379, 1986.
12. Bohman, S-O, Jaremko, G, Bohlin, A-B, Berg, U. Foot process fusion and glomerular filtration rate in minimal change nephrotic syndrome. *Kidney Int* 25:696, 1984.
13. Lowenstein, J, Schacht, RG, Baldwin, DS. Renal failure in minimal change nephrotic syndrome. *Am J Med* 70:227, 1981.
14. Meltzer, JI, Keim, HJ, Laragh, JH, Sealey, JE, Jan, K-M, Chien, S. Nephrotic syndrome: Vasoconstriction and hypervolemic types indicated by renin-sodium profiling. *Ann Intern Med* 91:688, 1979.
15. A Report of the International Study of Kidney Disease in Children. The primary nephrotic syndrome in children. Identification of patients with minimal change nephrotic syndrome from initial response to prednisone. *J Pediatr* 98:561, 1981.
16. A Report of the International Study of Kidney Disease in Children. Minimal change nephrotic syndrome in children. Deaths during the first 5 to 15 years observation. *Pediatrics* 73:497, 1984.
17. Black, DAK, Rose, G, Brewer, DB. Controlled trial of prednisone in adult patients with the nephrotic syndrome. *Br Med J* 3:421, 1970.
18. A Report of the International Study of Kidney Disease in Children. Early identification of frequent relapsers among children with minimal change nephrotic syndrome. *J Pediatr* 101:514, 1982.
19. Arbeitgemeinschaft fur Padiatrische Nephrologie. Effect of cytotoxic drugs in frequently relapsing nephrotic syndrome with and without steroid dependence. *N Engl J Med* 306:451, 1982.
20. Berns, JS, Gaudio, KM, Krassner, LS, Anderson, FP, Durante, D, McDonald, BM, Siegel, NJ. Steroid-responsive nephrotic syndrome of childhood: A long-term study of clinical course, histopathology, efficacy of cyclophosphamide therapy, and effects on growth. *Am J Kid Dis* 9:108, 1987.
21. Cade, R, Mars, D, Privette, M, Thompson, R, Croker, B, Peterson, J, Campbell, K. Effect of long-term azathioprine administration in adults with minimal change glomerulonephritis and nephrotic syndrome resistant to corticosteroids. *Arch Intern Med* 146:737, 1986.
22. Tejani, A, Butt, K, Trachtman, H, et al. Cyclosporine A induced remission of relapsing nephrotic syndrome in children. *Kidney Int* 33:729, 1988.
23. A Report of the International Study of Kidney Disease in Children. Primary nephrotic syndrome in children: Clinical significance of histopathologic variants of minimal change and of diffuse mesangial hypercellularity. *Kidney Int* 20:765, 1981.
24. Siegel, NJ, Gaudio, KM, Krassner, LS, McDonald, BM, Anderson, FP, Kashgarian, M. Steroid-dependent nephrotic syndrome in children: Histopathology and relapses after cyclophosphamide treatment. *Kidney Int* 19:474, 1981.
25. Thrompeter, RS, Lloyd, WB, Hicks, J, White, RHR, Cameron, JS. Long-term outcome for children with minimal-change nephrotic syndrome. *Lancet* 1:368, 1985.

28. FOCAL GLOMERULOSCLEROSIS

Focal glomerulosclerosis (FGS) is the third most common form of the idiopathic nephrotic syndrome, after membranous nephropathy and minimal change disease. It accounts for approximately 10 to 15 percent of cases in both children and adults, most often occurring before the age of 50.

The characteristic pathologic change in FGS is the presence in some, but not all glomeruli (hence the term focal) of segmental areas of mesangial sclerosis (Fig. 28-1). This is usually accompanied by collapse of the adjacent capillary loops due in part to eosinophilic, hyaline deposits that are thought to represent the insudation of plasma proteins into the abnormally permeable glomerular wall. Only a few glomeruli, particularly those in the deep cortical or juxtamedullary region, may show these changes initially. With time, however, the sclerotic process typically becomes more widespread.

In all other respects, the *histologic findings in FGS simulate those in minimal change disease:* light microscopy is either normal or reveals mild mesangial hypercellularity in nonsclerotic glomeruli; immunofluorescence is negative for immunoglobulins and complement (except for nonspecific deposition of IgM and C3 in sclerotic areas); and electron microscopy shows diffuse fusion of the epithelial cell foot processes, indicating that most glomeruli are actually involved. As a result of the similarity to minimal change disease, careful examination of the renal biopsy specimen to find an affected glomerulus is often essential to distinguish between these two disorders. One clue that may be helpful is the presence of areas of tubular atrophy and interstitial infiltrate and fibrosis; these changes are presumably secondary to glomerular injury and suggest FGS even if no sclerotic lesions can be identified.

It is important to emphasize that segmental sclerotic lesions are not specific for idiopathic FGS. Similar changes can be seen during the healing phase of focal or poststreptococcal glomerulonephritis or with hemodynamically mediated injury due to intraglomerular hypertension (see Chap. 56). In these disorders, however, foot process fusion on electron microscopy is usually limited to the sclerotic areas (not diffuse as in idiopathic FGS), and the clinical findings of the nephrotic syndrome (such as hypoalbuminemia and edema) are generally absent.

Etiology and Pathogenesis

Although most cases of FGS are idiopathic, an identifiable cause is occasionally present (Table 28-1) [1]. The nephrotic syndrome, for example, can develop in up to 10 to 20 percent of patients with the acquired immune deficiency syndrome (AIDS) [2,3], less often in homosexuals than in other high-risk groups [3]. Renal biopsy generally reveals focal glomerulosclerosis or mesangial proliferation (which may be a precursor of FGS). Intracellular inclusions are often present, suggesting a possible viral etiology [3a]. In comparison, an exogenous toxin may play a primary role in the FGS seen in intravenous heroin abusers* [3a,4]. Genetic factors may also be important since FGS in this setting occurs almost exclusively in black patients [4].

A different mechanism may be involved in the infrequent development of FGS in patients with massive obesity. These patients frequently have an elevated GFR and hemodynamic factors may be responsible for the glomerular injury [6].

It has been proposed that the primary event in idiopathic FGS is *damage to the glomerular epithelial cell* [7]. As described in the preceding chapter, a similar mechanism is thought to play an important role in minimal change disease, due perhaps to the release of a toxic lymphokine. Thus, it is useful to summarize the experimental and clinical similarities between these two disorders:

1. The histologic changes are identical (particularly diffuse foot process fusion) except for the scattered sclerotic·lesions in FGS. The proteinuria in both disorders is also due to loss of the anionic charge barrier rather than increased pore size [8].

---

*Other glomerular lesions can also occur in intravenous drug users, particularly secondary amyloidosis in patients with chronic, suppurative subcutaneous infections [5].

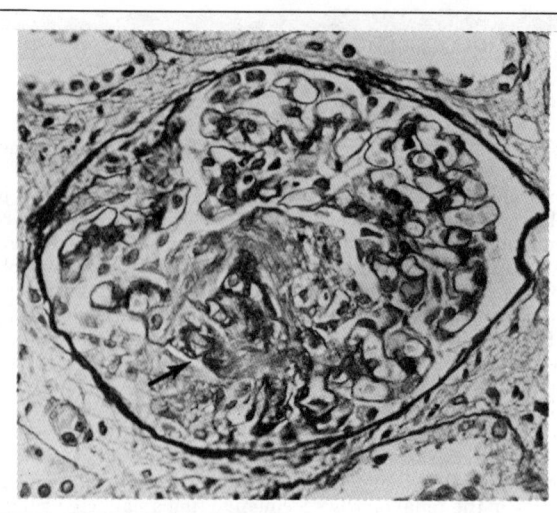

Fig. 28-1. Light microscopy in focal glomerulosclerosis. The characteristic change is segmental mesangial sclerosis with collapse of the capillary loops (arrow). The remainder of this glomerulus is normal although mild mesangial hypercellularity may occasionally be seen (From BD Rose, *Pathophysiology of Renal Disease* (2nd ed.). New York: McGraw-Hill, 1987.).

Table 28-1. Causes of focal glomerulosclerosis

Idiopathic
Including progression from minimal change disease
Acquired immune deficiency syndrome (AIDS)
Heroin abuse
Malignancy
Massive obesity
Chronic transplant rejection

2. The administration of the epithelial cell toxin puromycin to experimental animals results in dose-dependent glomerular injury: minimal change disease with a low dose or FGS with a higher dose [9].

3. Some patients with biopsy-proved minimal change disease progress to FGS [10]. Other patients with a steroid-responsive, frequently relapsing course typical of minimal change disease have FGS when finally biopsied [11].

In summary, at least some cases of FGS appear to represent either a similar but more-severe form of minimal change disease or possibly a consequence of recurrent protein-uria (due to mesangial overloading) in relapsing minimal change disease. Many patients, however, behave in a different fashion from minimal change disease, being corticosteroid resistant from the outset and progressing to end-stage renal failure relatively quickly [12,13]. It is not clear if this represents a different or merely a more severe form of FGS.

Clinical Presentation and Diagnosis

Most patients with idiopathic FGS present with the clinical and chemical findings of the nephrotic syndrome, although some patients have only nonnephrotic proteinuria [12-14]. In some cases, a precipitating factor such as an upper respiratory infection occurs prior to the onset of the disease; it is not clear if or how this might induce glomerular damage. Hypertension, hematuria, and an elevated plasma creatinine concentration are present initially in one-third to one-half of cases. In those patients with preceding minimal change disease, the onset of corticosteroid resistance is the primary clue suggesting progression to FGS [10].

The diagnosis of FGS is made by renal biopsy. In children in whom minimal change disease is particularly common, this procedure is usually performed only if there has been no response to an 8-week course of corticosteroid therapy. This regimen will not detect those cases of FGS that remit after a course of prednisone; these patients, however, appear to have a relatively benign prognosis as long as they remain corticosteroid responsive [11].

Course and Treatment

FGS has, in the past, been considered to have a uniformly poor prognosis, with most patients being unresponsive to immunosuppressive therapy and with renal failure developing over a variable period of 1 to 20 years [13]. Severe nephrotic syndrome (more than 10 gm of proteinuria per day), hypertension, and FGS secondary to AIDS are more likely to be associated with progressive disease [13a,14a]. In comparison, the course tends to be more indolent in patients with nonnephrotic proteinuria [14,14a].

It is now clear, however, that up to 40 percent of children and adults behave similarly to minimal change disease, with complete remission of proteinuria following a course of prednisone therapy [11,12,14a]. Furthermore, these corticosteroid-responsive patients appear to have a relatively good 5- to 10-year prognosis, with progression to end-stage renal disease being unusual during this time period [11,12,14a].

Some responsive patients develop relapsing proteinuria when the prednisone is discontinued. In this setting, as in minimal change disease, an 8-week course of cyclophosphamide can lead to a prolonged remission [11]. Cyclophosphamide may also be effective in initially responsive patients who develop secondary corticosteroid resistance [11,15]. However, repeated or prolonged courses of cyclophosphamide should be avoided because of the risks of gonadal fibrosis and late neoplasia.

In comparison, progressive disease is relatively common in those patients who are resistant to prednisone from the outset [12,14a]. In this setting, cyclophosphamide can induce complete or partial remission of proteinuria in some patients [16]. Once again, progression to end-stage renal disease is less frequent than in patients who have no response [16].

A final form of therapy that may prove to be effective consists of the use of meclofenamate (and probably most other nonsteroidal anti-inflammatory drugs). As many as one-half of patients respond with a marked reduction (50–75%) in proteinuria, a rise in the plasma albumin concentration, a fall in the plasma cholesterol concentration, and a mild rise in the P_{cr} that tends to be self-limited and stable [17]. These changes may be mediated hemodynamically as the reduction in vasodilator prostaglandin synthesis leads to renal vasoconstriction and a fall in intraglomerular pressure. The latter change could also minimize hemodynamic injury and might delay the rate of disease progression [17]. It is also possible that other measures aimed at lowering the intraglomerular pressure, such as a low-protein diet and antihypertensive therapy with a converting enzyme inhibitor (see Chap. 56), might be effective in patients resistant to immunosuppressive therapy.

Those patients who progress to end-stage renal disease are generally young and good candidates for renal transplantation. However, approximately 20 to 30 percent will develop recurrent disease in the transplant, with proteinuria typically reappearing within 1 month [18,19]. These findings suggest the presence of a circulating toxin (perhaps a lymphokine) directed against the glomerulus. Recurrent FGS leads to loss of the graft in one-third to one-half of these patients, particularly those whose initial disease led to renal failure within 3 years [18,19].

References

1. Rose, BD. *Pathophysiology of Renal Disease* (2nd ed.). New York: McGraw-Hill, 1987, Pp. 196-200.
2. Rao, TKS, Filippone, EJ, Nicastri, AD, Landesman, SH, Frank, E, Chen, CK, Friedman, EA. Associated focal and segmental glomerulosclerosis in the acquired immune deficiency syndrome. *N Engl J Med* 310:669, 1984.
3. Pardo, V, Menesses, R, Ossa, L, Jaffe, DJ, Strauss, J, Roth, D, Bourgoignie, JJ. AIDS-related glomerulopathy: Occurrence in specific high-risk groups. *Kidney Int* 31:1167, 1987.
3a. Chander, P, Soni, A, Suri, A, Bhagwat, R, Yoo, J, Treser, G. Renal ultrastructural markers in AIDS-associated nephropathy. *Am J Pathol* 126:513, 1987.
4. Cunningham, EE, Zielezny, MA, Venuto, RC. Heroin-associated nephropathy. A nationwide problem. *J Am Med Assoc* 250:2935, 1983.
5. Dubrow, A, Mittman, N, Ghali, V, Flamenbaum, W. The changing spectrum of heroin-associated nephropathy. *Am J Kid Dis* 5:36, 1985.
6. Kasiske, BL, Crosson, JT. Renal disease in patients with massive obesity. *Arch Intern Med* 146:1105, 1986.
7. Schwartz, MM, Lewis, EJ. Focal glomerulosclerosis: The cellular lesion. *Kidney Int* 28:968, 1985.
8. Winetz, JA, Robertson, CR, Golbetz, HV, Carrie, BJ, Salyer, WR, Myers, BD. The nature of the glomerular injury in minimal change and focal sclerosing glomerulopathies. *Am J Kid Dis* 1:91, 1981.
9. Diamond, JR, Karnovsky, MJ. Focal and segmental glomerulosclerosis following a single intravenous dose of puromycin aminonucleoside. *Am J Pathol* 122:481, 1986.
10. A Report of the Southwest Pediatric Nephrology Group. Focal segmental glomerulosclerosis in children with idiopathic nephrotic syndrome. *Kidney Int* 27:442, 1985.
11. Siegel, NJ, Gaudio, KM, Krassner, LS, McDonald, BM, Anderson, FP, Kashgarian, M. Steroid-dependent nephrotic syndrome in children: Histopathology and relapses after cyclophosphamide treatment. *Kidney Int* 19:454, 1981.
12. Korbet, SM, Schwartz, MM, Lewis, EJ. The prognosis of focal segmental glomerulosclerosis of adulthood. *Medicine* 65:304, 1986.
13. Jenis, EH, Teichman, S, Briggs, WA, Sandler, P, Hollerman, CE, Calcagno, PL, Kneiser, MR, Jensen, GE, Valeski, JE. Focal segmental glomerulosclerosis. *Am J Med* 57:695, 1974.
13a. Rao, TKS, Friedman, EA, Nicastri, AD. The types of renal disease in the acquired immune deficiency syndrome. *N Engl J Med* 316:1062, 1987.
14. Velosa, JA, Holley, KE, Torres, VE, Offord, KP. Significance of proteinuria on the outcome of renal function in patients with focal segmental glomerulosclerosis. *Mayo Clin Proc* 58:568, 1983.
14a. Pei, Y, Cattran, D, Delmore, T, Katz, A, Lang, A, Rance, P. Evidence suggesting under-treatment in adults with idiopathic focal segmental glomerulosclerosis. Regional Glomerulonephritis Registry Study. *Am J Med* 82:938, 1987.
15. Tejani, A, Nicastri, AD, Sen, D, Chen, CK, Phadke, K, Adamson, O, Butt, KMH. Longterm evaluation of children with nephrotic syndrome and focal segmental glomerular sclerosis. *Nephron* 35:225, 1983.
16. Geary, DF, Farine, M, Thorner, P, Baumal, R. Response to cyclophosphamide in steroid-resistant focal segmental glomerulosclerosis. *Clin Nephrol* 22:109, 1984.
17. Velosa, JA, Torres, VE. Benefits and risks of nonsteroidal antiinflammatory drugs in steroid-resistant nephrotic syndrome. *Am J Kid Dis* 8:345, 1986.
18. Lewis, EJ, Recurrent focal sclerosis after renal transplantation. *Kidney Int* 22:315, 1982.
19. Striegel, JE, Sibley, RK, Fryd, DS, Mauer, SM. Recurrence of focal segmental sclerosis in children following renal transplantation. *Kidney Int* 30 (suppl):S-44, 1986.

29. MEMBRANOUS NEPHROPATHY

Membranous nephropathy (MN) is the most common cause of the idiopathic nephrotic syndrome in adults, accounting for up to 50 percent of cases. As with many other glomerular diseases, MN is defined by its histologic characteristics (Fig. 29-1) [1]. On light microscopy, the glomeruli may be relatively normal with mild or early disease but generally show diffuse thickening of the glomerular basement membranes (GBM), hence the name *membranous,* with little or no increase in cellularity. The diagnosis is confirmed by immunofluorescent microscopy (which reveals prominent IgG and C3 deposition along the capillary walls) and by electron microscopy (which demonstrates immune deposits in the subepithelial space). In many patients, the basement membrane eventually grows between the deposits (leading to the characteristic appearance of spikes) and occasionally around the deposits, resulting in their incorporation into the GBM [1].

Etiology and Pathogenesis
Most cases of MN are idiopathic. It is possible, however, to identify an underlying disorder or antigen in approximately one-third of patients (Table 29-1). Among the most common are *tumors, systemic lupus erythematosus,* and *medications* such as gold and penicillamine. It is estimated, for example, that approximately 10 percent of cases of nephrotic syndrome in adults are associated with a malignancy [2,3]. Although many different histologic patterns may be seen, the most common are MN with solid tumors and minimal change disease with lymphomas, particularly Hodgkin's disease. Evidence supporting a pathogenetic role for the tumor includes remission of the nephrotic syndrome following removal of the tumor, the identification of tumor antigens in the glomeruli, and the elution of antibodies from the glomeruli that react with the underlying malignancy.

In the majority of patients, the tumor has already been diagnosed or is clinically apparent at the time of onset of the nephrotic syndrome. It is estimated that only about 15 percent of tumor-related MN or 1.5 percent of all adults with MN have an occult malignancy. As a result, an extensive evaluation for underlying tumor is not routinely indicated in the absence of suspicious signs or symptoms such as weight loss, unexplained anemia, or heme-positive stools.

MN accounts for about 10 to 20 percent of cases of lupus nephritis [4]. Some of these patients, however, have few if any extrarenal or serologic signs of SLE at the time of presentation with the nephrotic syndrome [5]. Nevertheless, there may be findings on electron microscopy that suggest underlying lupus, such as concurrent subendothelial or tubular basement membrane deposits or tubuloreticular structures in the glomerular endothelial cells (see Chap. 36) [6].

MN is also a relatively common complication of therapy with certain drugs. In patients with rheumatoid arthritis, for example, MN may occur in as many as 1 to 3 percent of patients treated with parenteral gold (the incidence may be substantially lower with oral gold) and 7 percent of patients treated with penicillamine [7,8]. Penicillamine appears to be less nephrotoxic when used to treat Wilson's disease. The reason for this difference is uncertain but may be related to an increased predisposition of all patients with rheumatoid arthritis to develop MN [1].

The pathogenesis of the immune deposition in MN is incompletely understood. It appears, however, that the traditional theory that intact circulating immune complexes are deposited in the kidney is not applicable to MN. Considering the relative impermeability of the GBM to macromolecules, passage of large intact complexes across the GBM into the subepithelial space would be difficult. This problem appears to be overcome by two additional factors. First, the formation of immune complexes may occur by an *in situ* mechanism in which *free* antigen is first deposited in the glomeruli followed at a later time by *free* antibody [9]. Continued antigen and antibody deposition would then allow growth of the immune complex lattice.

Second, experimental models suggest that only *cationic* antigens are able to deposit in the subepithelial space, since they are not restricted by the anionic charge barrier in

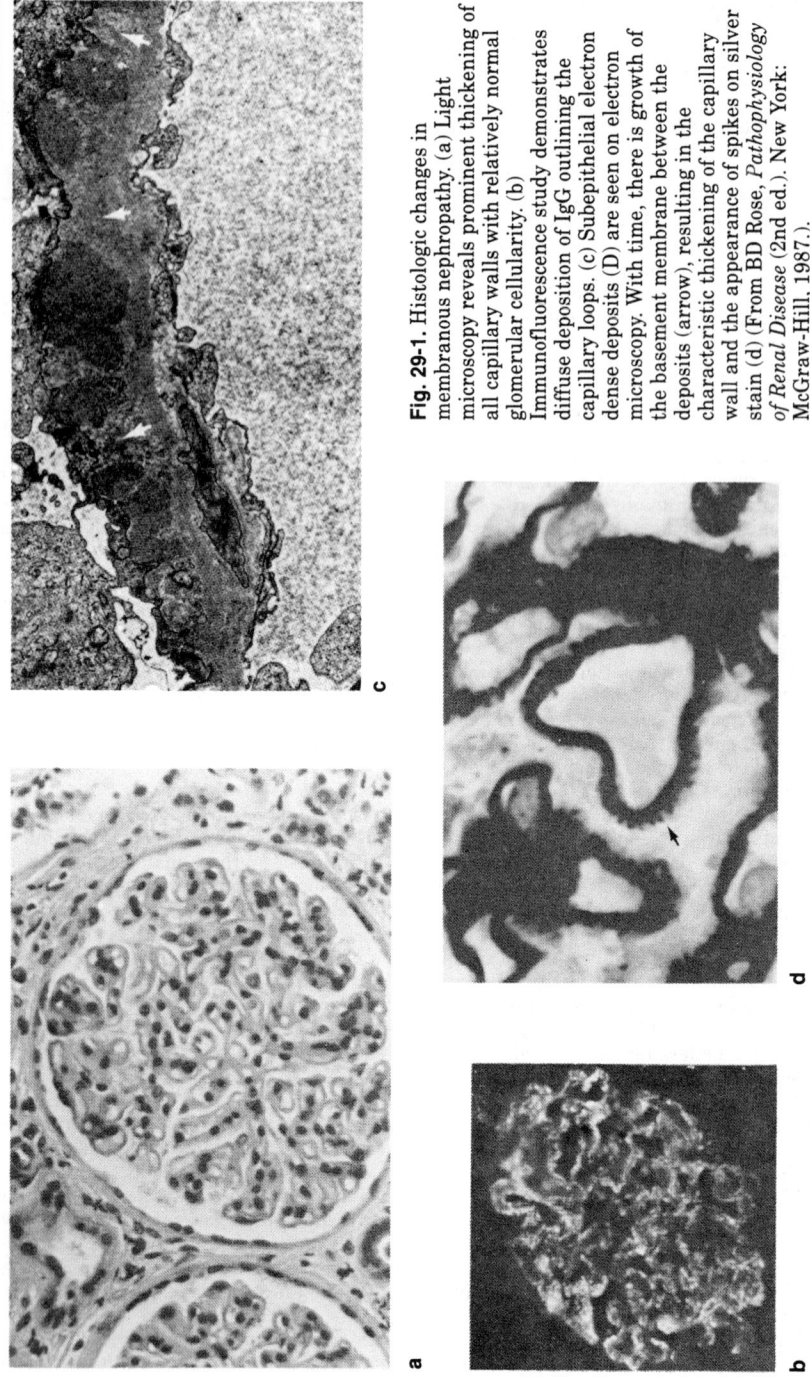

Fig. 29-1. Histologic changes in membranous nephropathy. (a) Light microscopy reveals prominent thickening of all capillary walls with relatively normal glomerular cellularity. (b) Immunofluorescence study demonstrates diffuse deposition of IgG outlining the capillary loops. (c) Subepithelial electron dense deposits (D) are seen on electron microscopy. With time, there is growth of the basement membrane between the deposits (arrow), resulting in the characteristic thickening of the capillary wall and the appearance of spikes on silver stain (d) (From BD Rose, *Pathophysiology of Renal Disease* (2nd ed.). New York: McGraw-Hill, 1987.).

Table 29-1. Major antigens and disorders associated with membranous nephropathy

Endogenous antigens
   DNA (in SLE)
   Tumors
   Thyroglobulin
   ? Renal tubular epithelial antigen

Exogenous antigens
   Medications
      Gold
      Penicillamine
      Captopril
      Mercury
   Infections
      Hepatitis B virus
      Syphilis—secondary or congenital
      Quartan malaria

Antigen or inciting agent unidentified
   Idiopathic
   Rheumatoid arthritis
   Sickle cell disease
   Sarcoidosis
   Chronic transplant rejection

Source: From Rose, BD. *Pathophysiology of Renal Disease* (2nd ed). New York: McGraw-Hill, 1987. P. 184.

the GBM [10]. Once these deposits are large enough, activation of the complement system is then responsible for the membrane damage that leads to proteinuria [11].

Clinical Presentation and Course

Most patients with MN present with edema and nephrotic range proteinuria [12,13]. About 15 to 25 percent of patients, however, will have only nonnephrotic proteinuria (<2.5–3.0 gm/day). Other findings that may be present at the time of diagnosis include hypertension (25–40%) and hematuria (40–60%). The plasma complement levels are normal except for patients with SLE or hepatitis B infection [1].

The course of MN is variable. Recovery is the rule when MN is due to drugs or treatable infection. With gold nephropathy, for example, cessation of therapy leads to complete resolution of proteinuria, usually within the first year but occasionally taking as long as 3 years [13a]. In comparison, the prognosis is much worse in patients with an underlying malignancy, most of whom die from their tumor.

The natural history is variable in idiopathic MN. At 5- to 10-year follow-up in untreated adults, approximately 20 to 25 percent will have progressed to end-stage renal failure, 20 to 25 percent will be in remission, and the remainder will have persistent proteinuria or the nephrotic syndrome [12,13].

It is possible, however, to identify subgroups with differing prognoses. The outlook is *more benign in children, women, and patients with nonnephrotic proteinuria,* less than 10 percent of whom will have progressive disease over 5 to 10 years [12,13]. On the other hand, men with nephrotic syndrome are at greatest risk of developing renal failure (about 50%), particularly if they present with an elevated P_{cr}.

The course of MN also may be complicated by the development of renal vein thrombosis in up to 25 to 50 percent of cases. This problem is most often asymptomatic and discovered only if the patient is prospectively evaluated with a renal venogram or if the patient has a pulmonary embolus (see Chap. 26).

Treatment

The evaluation of therapy in idiopathic MN is somewhat difficult because of the relatively frequent spontaneous remissions and the generally slow rate of progression in

Table 29-2. Results of clinical trials in membranous nephropathy

Regimen	Control	Treated
ALTERNATE-DAY PREDNISONE [14]		
Doubling of P_{cr} by 2.5 years	11/38	2/34
Persistent remission of proteinuria	7/38	12/34
PREDNISONE PLUS CHLORAMBUCIL [15]		
50% rise in P_{cr} by 2 years	10/35	0/38
Persistent remission of proteinuria	10/35	26/38
Number with complete remission	2/35	15/38
MECLOFENAMATE* [16]		
In 17 of 30 patients who responded		
P_{cr}	1.5	1.6
Proteinuria, gm/day	13	4.1
Plasma albumin, gm/dl	1.9	3.0
Plasma cholesterol, mg/dl	413	346

*Approximately one-half of patients in the meclofenamate study had membranous nephropathy; almost all of the remaining patients had focal glomerulosclerosis. The results from this study are limited to the responders, with the laboratory findings compared before (Control) and after (Treated) the institution of meclofenamate.

those who ultimately develop renal failure. Three modalities have been evaluated (only the first two in controlled studies): corticosteroids alone, corticosteroids with chlorambucil (or cyclophosphamide), and nonsteroidal anti-inflammatory drugs.

Several uncontrolled and controlled trials have suggested a benefit from therapy with prednisone. The results of the best of these studies are presented in Table 29-2. Patients either received no therapy or alternate-day prednisone (2 mg/kg up to a maximum of 120 mg every other day) for 2 to 3 months [14]. Prednisone appeared to improve the long-term prognosis (2 of 34 having a doubling of the P_{cr} versus 11 of 38 in the control group) but did not significantly affect the degree of proteinuria.

More impressive results have been obtained with an unusual 6-month regimen consisting of corticosteroids in months 1, 3, and 5 (1 gm of methylprednisolone intravenously for 3 days, followed by 0.5 mg/kg/day of oral prednisone) and chlorambucil in months 2, 4, and 6 (0.2 mg/kg/day) [15]. None of the 38 treated patients had an elevation in the P_{cr} at 2 years; this stability in renal function appeared to be maintained at 4 years. Furthermore, complete or partial remission of proteinuria occurred in 15 and 11 of 38 patients, respectively; these remissions, which were frequently associated with regression or disappearance of immune deposits on repeat renal biopsy, were sustained in about two-thirds of cases. These results were significantly better than those in the untreated control group (Table 29-2). Side effects with chlorambucil were generally minor. Although this drug can be carcinogenic, the duration of therapy and the total dose administered are well below that received by patients described in the literature who appear to have developed a malignancy following chlorambucil therapy [15].

Chronic low-dose cyclophosphamide (1.5 mg/kg/day for 18–24 months) also appears to produce similar beneficial results [16]. Loss of proteinuria and stabilization of renal function can be induced with this regimen even in paients who already have mild-to-moderate renal insufficiency (plasma creatinine concentration 1.5–3.0 mg/dl).

Despite these impressive results, the potential toxicity of prednisone and particularly chlorambucil and cyclophosphamide makes definite recommendations difficult. It may be preferable, for example, to initially withhold immunosuppressive therapy in those patients likely to do well: children or women (in whom edema can be easily controlled) and patients with nonnephrotic proteinuria (< 2.5 gm/day) [1,12,13]. Men with nephrotic-range proteinuria, on the other hand, should probably be given a trial of alternate-day prednisone. The addition of chlorambucil or cyclophosphamide should be considered in those patients who have an elevated P_{cr} at baseline, who progress despite a course of prednisone, or who have severe nephrotic syndrome (marked edema and hyperlipidemia), since these agents seem to be more effective than prednisone alone in reducing the degree of proteinuria (Table 29-2).

An additional form of therapy that has been evaluated in preliminary trials is the use of nonsteroidal anti-inflammatory drugs. Only meclofenamate and indomethacin have been used thus far, although other agents that inhibit renal prostaglandin synthesis may be equally effective. These drugs can, in up to one-half of patients, substantially reduce protein excretion, raise the plasma albumin concentration, and lower the plasma cholesterol level (Table 29-2) [17,18]. In some patients, there is also a self-limited and reversible fall in the glomerular filtration rate of about 20 to 25 percent [18]. These changes in renal function are presumably a consequence of renal vasoconstriction due to the reduction in synthesis of vasodilator prostaglandins. To the degree that the intraglomerular pressure also declines in this setting [18], it is possible that nonsteroidal anti-inflammatory drugs could slow the rate of disease progression by minimizing hemodynamic injury (see Chap. 56) [17].

At present, however, the risk/benefit ratio of the nonsteroidal anti-inflammatory drugs is uncertain. As a result, their use should probably be limited to patients with severe nephrosis in whom lowering protein excretion might lead to considerable clinical improvement.

Finally, those patients who develop progressive renal insufficiency despite the above modalities should be given a trial of antihypertensive therapy (preferably with a converting enzyme inhibitor) in an attempt to prevent the damage induced by compensatory intraglomerular hypertension (see Chap. 56). Dietary protein restriction can also be used in this setting, although its safety in proteinuric, hypoalbuminemic patients is unproved. Preliminary short-term studies have demonstrated that limiting protein intake often leads to decreased proteinuria (perhaps due to a decline in intraglomerular pressure) and no change in either the plasma albumin concentration or the total albumin pool [19]. These findings suggest that protein restriction may not lead to negative nitrogen balance in nephrotic patients, although long-term studies are clearly required.

References

1. Rose, BD. *Pathophysiology of Renal Disease* (2nd ed.). New York: McGraw-Hill, 1987. Pp 181-187.
2. Eagen, JW, Lewis, EJ. Glomerulopathies of neoplasia. *Kidney Int* 11:297, 1977.
3. Alpers, CE, Cotran, RS. Neoplasia and glomerular injury. *Kidney Int* 30:465, 1986.
4. Baldwin, DS, Gluck, MC, Lowenstein, J, Gallo, GR. Lupus nephritis: Clinical course as related to morphologic forms and their transitions. *Am J Med* 62:12, 1977.
5. Adu, D, Williams, DG, Taube, D, Vilches, AR, Turner, DR, Cameron, JS, Ogg, CS. Late onset systemic lupus erythematosus and lupus-like disease in patients with apparent idiopathic glomerulonephritis. *Q J Med* 52:471, 1983.
6. Jeanette, JC, Iskandar, SS, Dalldorf, FG. Pathologic differentiation between lupus and nonlupus membranous glomerulopathy. *Kidney Int* 24:377, 1983.
7. Katz, WA, Blodgett, RC, Pietrysko, RG. Proteinuria in gold-treated rheumatoid arthritis. *Ann Intern Med* 101:176, 1984.
8. Hall, CL, Jawad, S, Harrison, PR, et al. Natural course of penicillamine nephropathy: A long-term study of 33 patients. *Br Med J* 296:1083, 1988.
9. Couser, WG, Salant, DJ. In situ immune complex formation and glomerular injury. *Kidney Int* 17:1, 1980.
10. Couser, WG. Mechanisms of glomerular injury in immune complex disease. *Kidney Int* 28:569, 1985.
11. Couser, WG, Baker, PJ, Adler, S. Complement and the direct mediation of glomerular injury: A new perspective. *Kidney Int* 28:879, 1985.
12. Mallick, NP, Short, CD, Manos, J. Clinical membranous nephropathy. *Nephron* 34:209, 1983.
13. Davison, AM, Cameron, JS, Kerr, DNS, Ogg, CS, Wilkinson, RW. The natural history of renal function in untreated idiopathic membranous glomerulonephritis in adults. *Clin Nephrol* 22:61, 1984.

13a. Hall, CL, Fothergill, NJ, Blackwell, MM, et al. The natural history of gold nephropathy: Long term study of 21 patients. *Br Med J* 295:745, 1987.
14. Collaborative Study of the Adult Idiopathic Nephrotic Syndrome. A controlled study of short-term prednisone treatment in adults with membranous nephropathy. *N Engl J Med* 301:1301, 1979.
15. Ponticelli, C. Prognosis and treatment of membranous nephropathy. *Kidney Int* 29:927, 1986.
16. West, ML, Jindal, KK, Bear, RA, Goldstein, MB. Controlled trial of cyclophosphamide in patients with membranous glomerulonephritis. *Kidney Int* 32:579, 1987.
17. Velosa, JA, Torres, VE. Benefits and risks of nonsteroidal antiinflammatory drugs in steroid-resistant nephrotic syndrome. *Am J Kid Dis* 8:345, 1986.
18. Shemesh, O, Ross, JC, Deen, WM, Grant, GW, Myers, BD. Nature of the glomerular capillary injury in human membranous glomerulopathy. *J Clin Invest* 77:868, 1986.
19. Kaysen, GA, Gambertoglio, J, Jiminez, I, Jones, H, Hutchinson, FN. Effect of dietary protein intake on albumin homeostasis in nephrotic patients. *Kidney Int* 29:572, 1986.

30. DIABETIC NEPHROPATHY

Glomerular disease is a common complication of diabetes mellitus, leading to renal failure in 30 to 35 percent of insulin-dependent (IDDM or type 1) and about 6 percent of noninsulin-dependent (NIDDM or type 2) patients. The more benign course in NIDDM is not universal, however. As an example, progressive renal disease is common in the Pima Indians [1]; it is not clear whether this increase in susceptibility is due to genetic factors or to less-effective control of hyperglycemia and hypertension.

The primary glomerular changes in diabetic nephropathy are diffuse and nodular glomerulosclerosis (Fig. 30-1) [2]. The diffuse lesion is manifested on light and electron microscopy by a widespread increase in mesangial matrix (which represents basement membrane–like material). This process ultimately involves the glomerular basement membrane (GBM), leading to up to a 5- to 10-fold increase in its width.

Nodule formation (the Kimmelstiel-Wilson lesion) occurs at a later stage of the disease. The nodules are hyaline, acellular masses of varying size that seem to reflect extension of the diffuse process from the mesangium into the capillary wall. Progression of the diffuse and nodular changes leads to compression and narrowing of the capillary loops and an eventual decline in glomerular filtration.

The nodular lesions are considered to be pathognomonic of diabetic nephropathy, although somewhat similar lesions can be seen on light microscopy in light-chain deposition disease (see Chap. 31). Another change that is highly suggestive of diabetes is the presence of hyaline deposits in the afferent and particularly the efferent glomerular arterioles. The latter finding, for example, is often the first sign of recurrent disease in the kidney transplant [3].

Immunofluorescent microscopy often reveals linear deposition of IgG, similar to that seen in anti-GBM antibody disease [4]. However, circulating anti-GBM antibodies are absent and the immunoglobulin deposition appears to reflect nonspecific adsorption onto the highly permeable glomerular capillary wall. Concurrent linear deposition of albumin is often seen and is consistent with this hypothesis.

Pathogenesis

An increasing body of evidence suggests that hyperglycemia is responsible for the microvascular complications of diabetes mellitus, rather than a separate inherited vascular abnormality. For example, patients with secondary (or acquired) diabetes mellitus due to toxin exposure or pancreatic disease can develop the same vascular lesions (proteinuria, retinopathy, and thickening of the muscle capillary basement membranes) that are seen in primary IDDM [5]. Also compatible with a central role for hyperglycemia is

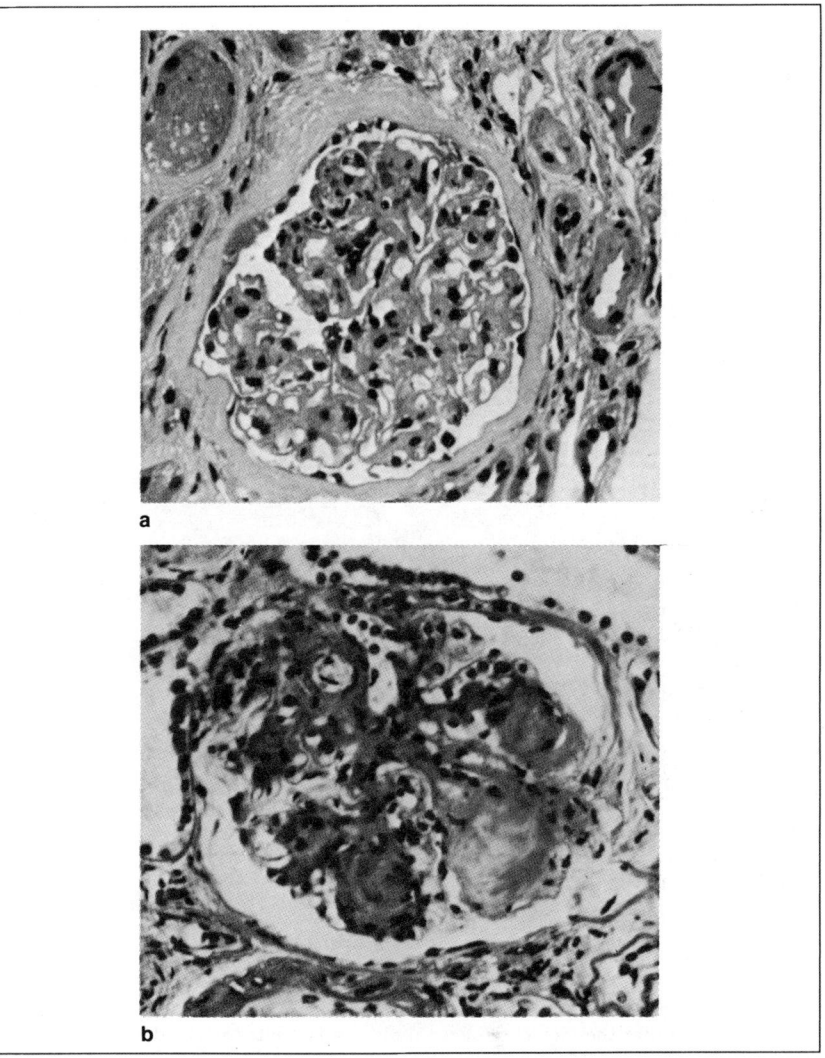

Fig. 30-1. Pathologic changes in diabetic nephropathy. (a) Diffuse glomerulosclerosis occurs first and is manifested on light microscopy by an increase in mesangial matrix (or basement membrane-like material) and by thickening of the glomerular capillary wall. Subintimal hyaline thickening of the arterioles may also be found (arrow). (b) Nodular glomerulosclerosis develops later and is associated with hyaline, acellular masses extending out of the mesangium into the capillary wall. (c) Electron microscopy demonstrates marked thickening of the glomerular basement membrane (BM) (approximately 5–10 times normal) and increased mesangial matrix (M) (From BD Rose, *Pathophysiology of Renal Disease* (2nd ed.). New York: McGraw-Hill, 1987.).

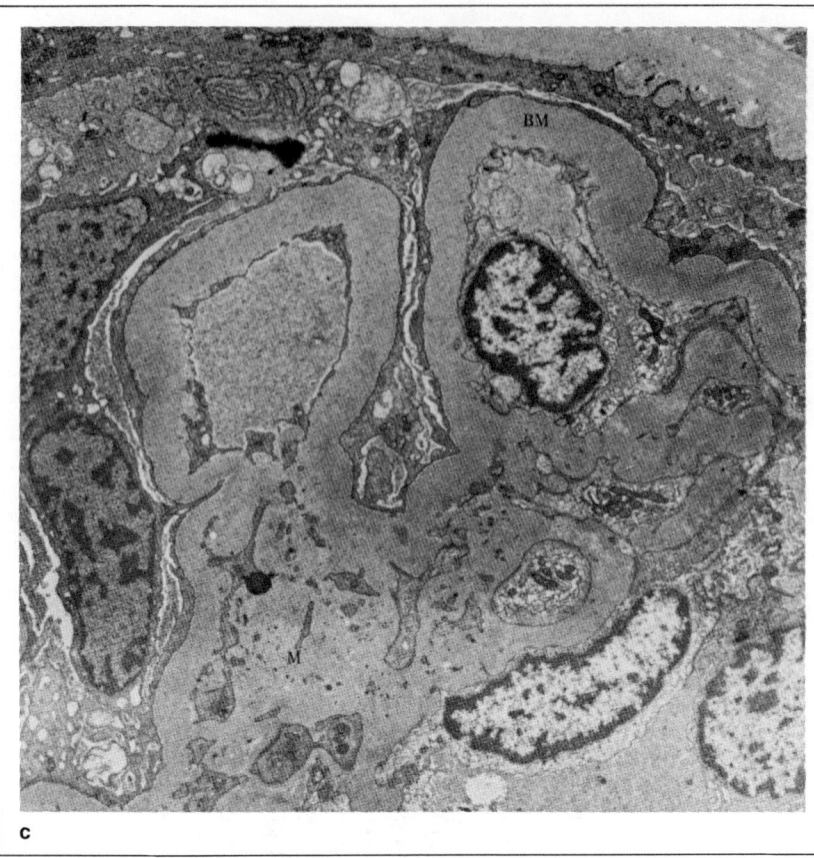

Fig. 30-1. (continued)

the observation that the incidence of renal disease is related to the degree of glycemic control [6,7].

There is, however, a wide variability in the degree of microvascular disease in primary diabetes. In particular, only about one-third of patients with IDDM are at risk of developing diabetic nephropathy, which usually becomes clinically apparent within 25 years of the onset of the disease [7]. Thus, factors other than hyperglycemia alone (such as hypertension or genetic susceptibility to metabolic or hemodynamic injury) must also play a contributory role.

Two major and not mutually exclusive theories have been proposed to explain how hyperglycemia leads to glomerulosclerosis [2]. According to the first, *metabolic* factors are of primary importance. For example, glycosylation of mesangial and basement membrane proteins (similar to that which occurs with hemoglobin) may promote trapping of circulating macromolecules in the glomerular capillary wall, possibly leading to mesangial hyperplasia and enhanced production of basement membrane–like material. Abnormal cellular function due to a hyperglycemia-induced decline in myo-inositol uptake also may play an important role [8].

The second theory proposes a primary role for a hyperglycemia-induced *alteration in renal hemodynamics* [2,9]. There is often a 25 to 50 percent elevation in the glomerular filtration rate (GFR) in both experimental animals and many patients early in the course of IDDM. This effect appears to be mediated by renal vasodilatation and a subsequent rise in intraglomerular pressure. According to the hemodynamic hypothesis, the glomeruli are unable to tolerate this intraglomerular hypertension, leading to endothelial injury and progressive glomerulosclerosis (see Chap. 28). In experimental diabetes, for example, lowering the glomerular pressure toward normal with dietary protein restriction or administration of a converting enzyme inhibitor *almost completely prevents glomerular injury even in the absence of glycemic control* [10,11].

A variety of preliminary observations suggest that similar hemodynamic changes may be important in human diabetic nephropathy. For example, diabetic patients who develop renal disease are more likely to have had a higher initial GFR (above 150 ml/min), a higher initial systemic blood presure (although still within the normal range), and a history of hypertension in one or both parents [6,12]. Furthermore, those therapies that are protective in animals also may be beneficial in humans. Both dietary protein restriction and converting enzyme inhibition can decrease the degree of proteinuria [13,14] and, in initial preliminary studies, may slow the rate of decline in the GFR [15,16].

The early renal vasodilation and glomerular hyperfiltration can be reversed by return of the plasma glucose concentration toward normal [17]. It is unclear, however, how hyperglycemia produces these changes in renal hemodynamics as a variety of factors have been implicated [2]. These include increased surface area available for filtration due to the rise in production of basement membrane–like material, enhanced production of vasodilator prostaglandins or reduced secretion of or response to the vasoconstrictor angiotensin II, a volume expansion–induced stimulation of the release of atrial natriuretic peptide, and possible intrarenal factors [2,18,19]. How these changes might occur is not well understood.

Clinical Presentation and Course

The renal disease in IDDM follows a relatively characteristic course [20]. Mesangial expansion and basement membrane thickening begin within the first few years; however, clinical evidence of these changes is masked by the initially elevated GFR (which prevents a rise in the plasma creatinine concentration) and by the relative insensitivity of the urinary dipstick for protein (which does not become positive until protein excretion exceeds 300 to 400 mg/day [upper limit of normal is 150 mg/day]).

These problems with early detection can be overcome by testing for the presence of *microalbuminuria* [20-23]. The normal rate of albumin excretion is less than 15 μg/min on a resting specimen or 20 mg/day on a 24-hour collection; this low rate of excretion can be detected by a sensitive radioimmunoassay for albumin. Early diabetic nephropathy can elevate albumin excretion above the normal range at a time when total protein excretion is not yet elevated.

Documenting the presence of microalbuminuria is important because it is both indicative of glomerular damage and *highly predictive of the subsequent development of clinically evident disease.* In two studies of patients with IDDM followed for 7 to 14 years, progressive renal disease (as first evidenced by an increase in protein excretion to a level that is detectable by the dipstick) occurred in 19 of 22 (86%) with initial microalbuminuria versus only 2 of 84 (2.5%) without this abnormality [21,22]. Patients with microalbuminuria also tended to have at baseline a higher GFR and systolic blood pressure (both of which are compatible with an important role for hemodynamic factors in diabetic nephropathy) [12,20] and were more likely to subsequently develop progressive retinopathy [21].

Clinically detectable proteinuria (by dipstick) usually occurs within 15 to 25 years after the onset of IDDM [7,20]. It is typically associated with advanced glomerulosclerosis even though the plasma creatinine concentration may at first be within the normal range. This apparently paradoxical finding is a reflection of the initial 25 to 50 percent elevation in the GFR that is often present in these patients. As a result, marked glomerular injury must be present before the filtration rate falls below the normal range.

The discovery of proteinuria usually heralds a progressive downhill course characterized by increasing protein excretion (which reaches the nephrotic range in up to 40% of cases), hypertension, and eventual renal failure. In general, the GFR falls 10 to 15 ml/min/year, leading to end-stage renal disease within 3 to 10 years [6,20].

NIDDM

The course of the nephropathy is generally more indolent in NIDDM [24]. Although microalbuminuria is the first sign of glomerular disease in this setting, only about 22 percent progress to clinically evident renal disease within 9 years [20,23] versus over 80 percent in IDDM [20–22]. The glomerular filtration rate may remain stable for many years after onset of detectable proteinuria; less than 10 percent of patients develop the nephrotic syndrome [24].

The relatively benign renal course in many patients with NIDDM is in part age-dependent. If all diabetics are considered, the incidence of renal failure is related to the age of onset of the diabetes: roughly 40 percent if below 20 (most of whom have IDDM), 9 percent between 20 and 40, less than 3 percent over 40 (most of whom have NIDDM) [24]. Aging may limit the degree of hyperglycemia-induced renal vasodilation and therefore the degree of intraglomerular hypertension that seems to contribute to the glomerular injury. The observation that glomerular hyperfiltration cannot usually be demonstrated in NIDDM [20] is compatible with this hypothesis.

The likelihood of developing diabetic nephropathy is also increased in patients with poor glycemic control [7], which could explain the relatively severe renal course seen in some patients with NIDDM, such as the Pima indians [1], although genetic factors may also be important.

Diagnosis

Presence of diabetic nephropathy is usually suggested by a long history of diabetes, increasing proteinuria with a benign sediment, slowly progressive renal failure, and usually concurrent evidence of retinal involvement. Other glomerular diseases can also occur in diabetic patients, including membranous nephropathy, minimal change disease, and proliferative glomerulonephritis [25]. Clues suggesting nondiabetic renal disease include persistent hematuria (particularly if accompanied by red cell casts), known duration of diabetes of less than 10 years, and, in IDDM, the nephrotic syndrome with a persistently normal plasma creatinine concentration, since heavy proteinuria is typically a late finding in diabetic nephropathy, occurring when renal insufficiency is already present [25].

Acute renal failure is unusual in uncomplicated diabetic nephropathy. Other renal diseases can lead to an acute decline in renal function in diabetic patients, such as prerenal disease due to the use of diuretics, a reaction to radiocontrast media, and urinary tract obstruction due to papillary necrosis.

Treatment

Optimal therapy varies with the stage of the disease, particularly the efficacy of restoring normoglycemia with an intensive insulin regimen. Early in the course, lowering the plasma glucose concentration can reverse the initial glomerular hyperfiltration [17]. Insulin is somewhat less effective once microalbuminuria is present, when some glomerulosclerosis is already present. Intensive insulin therapy in this setting is associated with stabilization or reduction of the degree of proteinuria, versus a common increase in protein excretion in patients treated with a conventional regimen [26], a difference that is not apparent until 2 years of relative normoglycemia. Strict control of the plasma glucose concentration is usually *ineffective in preserving renal function* once proteinuria is clinically detectable by dipstick [27]. At this time, daily protein excretion exceeds 300 to 400 mg/day and marked glomerulosclerosis is typically present [20].

Lack of efficacy of insulin in relatively advanced disease probably reflects the importance of hemodynamic factors (particularly intraglomerular hypertension) in producing further glomerular injury. In this setting, restricting dietary protein intake (to 0.6 g/kg per day) [15] or lowering systemic blood pressure with a converting enzyme inhibitor [16] or other antihypertensive agents [28] may slow the rate of decline in the glomerular filtration rate, possibly by decreasing intraglomerular pressure [10,11].

Diuretics (in addition to a converting enzyme inhibitor) may be particularly important for blood pressure control, since volume expansion is thought to play an important role in hypertension associated with diabetic renal disease [29]. Both renal insufficiency and enhanced activity of the sodium-glucose cotransporter in the proximal tubule (due to hyperglycemia-induced increase in filtered glucose load) may promote sodium retention.

It is at present unknown if these hemodynamic therapies will be beneficial if initiated earlier in the course of the disease. Considering the poor long-term renal prognosis associated with microalbuminuria, for example, it may not be unreasonable to avoid excess protein intake and to lower the systemic blood pressure with a converting enzyme inhibitor in this setting, even in patients who are normotensive. These modalities have been shown to diminish protein excretion in early renal disease [13,14], although their effects on preservation of the GFR have not been determined.

Experimental studies in a possible animal model of NIDDM suggest that the frequently associated hyperlipidemia may be another factor contributing to glomerular injury, perhaps by inducing endothelial damage [30]. Lowering plasma lipids with drug therapy in this setting was associated with a marked diminution in glomerulosclerosis, in the absence of any change in glycemic control. The applicability of these intriguing findings to human disease remains to be proved, although hypolipidemic therapy is often indicated for a different reason: to diminish the risk of atherosclerotic cardiovascular disease.

References

1. Kunzelman, CL, Nelson, RG, Knowles, WC, Pettitt, DJ. Proteinuria determines prognosis in type 2 (non-insulin-dependent) diabetes (abstract). *Kidney Int* 33:197, 1988.
2. Rose, BD. *Pathophysiology of Renal Disease* (2nd ed). New York: McGraw-Hill, 1987. Pp. 200-208.
3. Mauer, SM, Barbosa, J, Vernier, RL, Kjellstrand, CM, Buselmeier, TJ, Simmons, RL, Najarian, JS, Goetz, FC. Development of diabetic vascular lesions in normal kidney transplanted into patients with diabetes mellitus. *N Engl J Med* 295:916, 1976.
4. Westberg, NG, Michael, AF. Immunohistopathology of diabetic glomerulosclerosis. *Diabetes* 21:163, 1972.
5. Feingold, KR, Lee, TH, Chung, MY, Siperstein, MD. Muscle capillary basement membrane width in patients with vacor-induced diabetes mellitus. *J Clin Invest* 78:102, 1986.
6. Krowlewski, AS, Canessa, M, Warram, JH, et al. Predisposition to hypertension and susceptibility to renal disease in insulin-dependent diabetes mellitus. *N Engl J Med* 318:140, 1988.
7. Krowlewski, AS, Warram, JH, Rand, LI, Kahn, CR. Epidemiologic approach to the etiology of type I diabetes mellitus and its complications. *N Engl J Med* 317:1390, 1987.
8. Greene, DA, Lattimer, SA, Sima, AAF. Sorbitol, phosphoinositides, and sodium-potassium ATPase in the pathogenesis of diabetic complications *N Engl J Med* 316:599, 1987.
9. Hostetter, TH, Rennke, HG, Brenner, BM. The case for intrarenal hypertension in the initiation and progression of diabetic and other glomerulopathies. *Am J Med* 72:375, 1982.
10. Zatz, R, Meyer, TW, Rennke, HG, Brenner, BM. Predominance of hemodynamic rather than metabolic factors in the pathogenesis of diabetic nephropathy. *Proc Natl Acad Sci USA* 82:5963, 1985.
11. Zatz, R, Dunn, BR, Anderson, S, Rennke, HG, Brenner, BM. Prevention of diabetic glomerulopathy by pharmacological amelioration of glomerular capillary hypertension. *J Clin Invest* 77:1925, 1986.
12. Mogensen, CE. Early glomerular hyperfiltration in insulin-dependent diabetics and late nephropathy. *Scand J Clin Lab Invest* 46:201, 1986.

13. Cohen, D, Dodds, R, Viberti, G. Effect of protein restriction in insulin dependent diabetics at risk of nephropathy. *Br Med J* 294:795, 1987.
14. Hommel, E, Parving, H-H, Mathiesen, E, Eldsberg, B, Damkjaer Nielsen, M, Giese, J. Effect of captopril on kidney function in insulin-dependent diabetic patients with nephropathy. *Br Med J* 293:467, 1986.
15. Evanoff, GV, Thompson, CS, Brown, J, Weinman, EJ. The effect of dietary protein restriction in the progression of diabetic nephropathy. A 12-month follow-up. *Arch Intern Med* 147:492, 1987.
16. Bjorck, S, Nyberg, G, Mulec, H, Granerus, G, Herlitz, H, Aurell, M. Beneficial effects of angiotensin converting enzyme inhibition on renal function in patients with diabetic nephropathy. *Br Med J* 293:471, 1986.
17. Wiseman, MJ, Saunders, AJ, Keen, H, Viberti, G-C. Effect of blood glucose control on increased glomerular filtration rate and kidney size in insulin-dependent diabetics. *N Engl J Med* 312:617, 1985.
18. Ortola, FV, Ballerman, BJ, Anderson, S, Brenner, BM. Glomerular hyperfiltration in diabetic rats is associated with high circulating atrial natriuretic peptide (ANP) levels and reversed by specific ANP antiserum infusion (abstract). *Abstracts, Second World Congress on Biologically Active Atrial Peptides,* New York, 1987, P. 196.
19. Woods, LL, Mizelle, HL, Hall, JE. Control of renal hemodynamics in hyperglycemia: Possible role of tubuloglomerular feedback. *Am J Physiol* 252:F65, 1987.
20. Mogensen, CE. Microalbuminuria as a predictor of clinical diabetic nephropathy. *Kidney Int.* 31:673, 1987.
21. Mogensen, CE, Christiansen, CK. Predicting diabetic nephropathy in insulin-dependent patients. *N Engl J Med* 311:89, 1984.
22. Viberti, G-C, Jarrett, RJ, Mahmud, U, Hill, RD, Argyropoulos, A, Keen, H. Microalbuminuria as a predictor of clinical nephropathy in insulin-dependent diabetes mellitus. *Lancet* 1:1430, 1982.
23. Mogensen, CE. Microalbuminuria predicts clinical proteinuria and early mortality in maturity-onset diabetes. *N Engl J Med* 310:356, 1984.
24. Fabre, J, Balant, LP, Dayer, PG, Fox, HM, Vernet, AT. The kidney in maturity onset diabetes: A clinical study of 510 patients. *Kidney Int* 21:730, 1982.
25. Kasinath, BS, Mujais, SK, Spargo, BH, Katz, AI. Nondiabetic renal disease in patients with diabetes mellitus. *Am J Med* 75:613, 1983.
26. Feldt-Rasmussen, B, Mathiesen, ER, Deckert, T. Effect of two years of strict metabolic control on progression of incipient nephropathy in insulin-dependent diabetes. *Lancet* 2:1300, 1986.
27. Bending, JJ, Viberti, G-C, Watkins, PJ, Keen, H. Intermittent clinical proteinuria and renal function in diabetes: Evolution and effect of glycemic control *Br Med J* 292:83, 1986.
28. Parving, H-H, Andersen, AR, Smidt, UM, Homel, E, Mathiessen, ER, Svendsen, PA. Effect of antihypertensive treatment on kidney function in diabetic nephropathy. *Br Med J* 294:1443, 1987.
29. Lipson, LG. Special problems in treatment of hypertension in the patient with diabetes mellitus. *Arch Intern Med* 144:1829, 1984.
30. O'Donnell, MP, Cleary, MP, Keane, WF. Treatment of hyperlipidemia reduces glomerular injury in obese Zucker rats. *Kidney Int* 33:667, 1988.

31. AMYLOIDOSIS AND LIGHT-CHAIN DEPOSITION DISEASE

Renal involvement occurs in over 90 percent of patients with either primary or secondary amyloidosis [1-3]. The primary form, which now accounts for the great majority of cases, is a plasma cell dyscrasia that may progress to multiple myeloma in some patients. It is a disease of adults, almost always occurring in patients over the age of 40

[1]. In comparison, secondary amyloidosis results from chronic inflammatory disorders and can occur at any age.

The primary pathologic abnormality on light microscopy with either form of amyloidosis is the diffuse glomerular deposition of amorphous hyaline material, initially in the mesangium and then in the capillary loops (Fig. 31-1A). Eventually, nodule formation can occur, similar to that in diabetic nephropathy. Amyloid deposits may also be seen in the arterioles, small arteries, and the tubular basement membranes.

The diagnosis of amyloidosis, although suggested on light microscopy, can be confirmed by the use of special stains or by electron microscopy. As examples, thioflavine-T produces an intense yellow-green fluorescence while Congo red leads to green birefringence when viewed under polarized light. These stains, however, can on occasion yield misleading results; consequently, the most diagnostic finding is the demonstration of characteristic amyloid fibrils on electron microscopy (Fig. 31-1B).

Immunofluorescent microscopy, in comparison, is generally negative in secondary amyloidosis but may be weakly positive for monoclonal lambda or kappa light chains in the primary form. These findings are consistent with the lack of a role for immunoglobulin or complement deposition in these disorders.

Etiology and Pathogenesis

Primary Amyloidosis
The fibrils in primary amyloidosis consist of fragments of the variable portions of monoclonal light chains [2]. Although this disorder is associated with the proliferation of a single clone of plasma cells, most patients do not demonstrate the malignant characteristics of multiple myeloma. Conversely, most patients with myeloma do not develop amyloidosis despite the overproduction of light chains. This finding suggests that additional factors must also be important. The light chains, for example, must be able to be taken up by macrophages where they are catabolized to preamyloid fragments. These fragments must then have the biochemical properties that allow them to form amyloid fibrils. This may explain why *lambda* light chains are much more likely to produce amyloidosis than kappa light chains [4].

LIGHT-CHAIN DEPOSITION DISEASE. Light-chain deposition disease is similar pathogenetically to primary amyloidosis except that the light chains, which are most often of the *kappa* type, are unable to form amyloid fibrils [5]. As a result, nodules may be seen in the glomeruli but electron microscopy reveals granular rather than fibrillar material along both the glomerular and tubular basement membranes [5,6]. In some cases, this material may be dense enough to suggest type 2 membranoproliferative glomerulonephritis (see Chap. 35). However, immunofluorescent microscopy is usually diagnostic, being strongly positive for the monoclonal light chain. This difference from primary amyloidosis is related to the portion of the light chain that is typically deposited. The *variable* region of the light chain is involved in the primary amyloidosis, leading to relatively weak staining with anti-kappa or anti-lambda–light-chain antisera; in comparison, at least part of the *constant* region is present in light-chain deposition disease, accounting for the positive immunofluorescent findings [5,6].

It is also important to note that patients with either of these conditions do not develop intratubular light-chain precipitation similar to that seen in multiple myeloma [2,5,7]. One possible explanation is that the light-chain fragments in amyloidosis or light-chain deposition disease are less likely to promote intratubular obstruction than the intact light chains excreted in multiple myeloma [2]. In addition, the degree to which the monoclonal light chain is filtered may also be important [7]. For example, polymeric or negatively charged light chains are less able to cross the size- and charge-selective barriers of the glomerular capillary wall. They would, therefore, tend to accumulate in the plasma, thereby promoting tissue deposition.

Secondary Amyloidosis
Secondary amyloidosis has been associated with a variety of chronic inflammatory diseases including rheumatoid arthritis, osteomyelitis, bronchiectasis, chronic skin or decubitus ulcer infections in intravenous drug abusers or paraplegics, some neoplasms

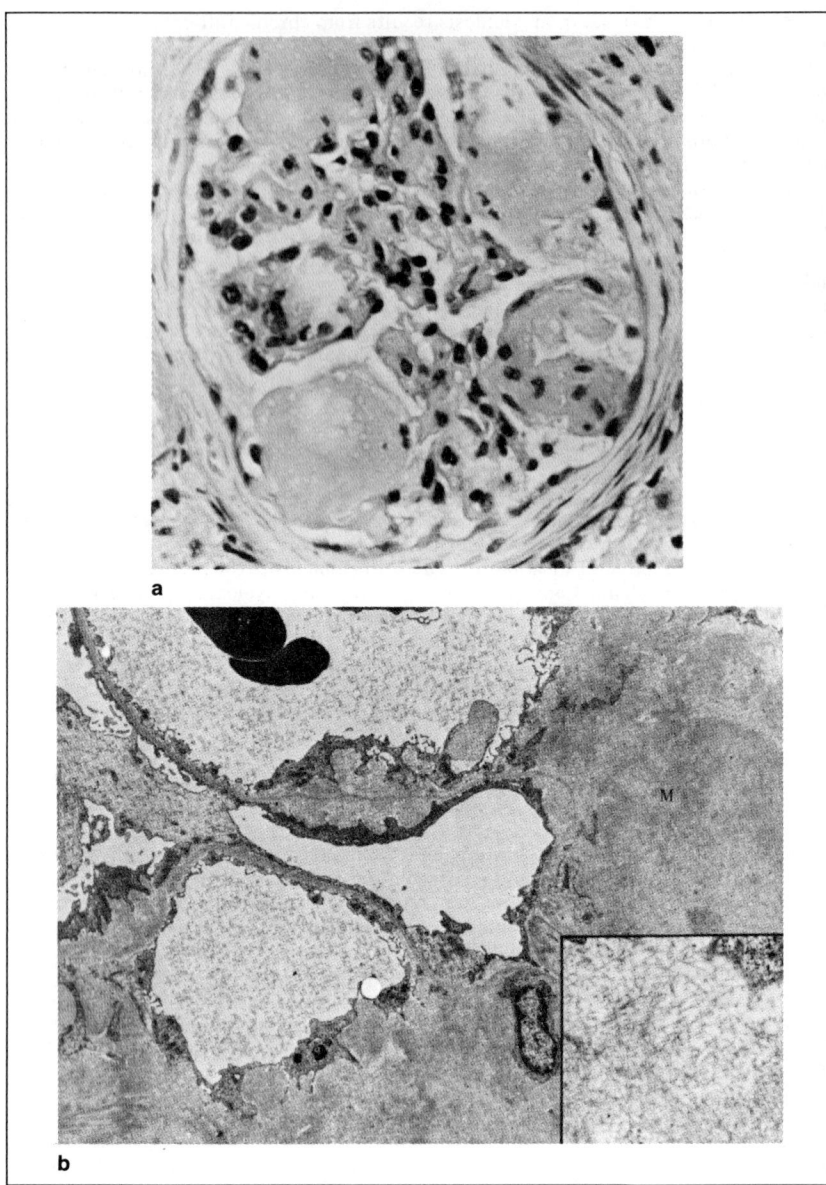

Fig. 31-1. Histologic findings in renal amyloidosis. (a) Light microscopy reveals diffuse deposition of amorphous hyaline material that can lead to nodules resembling those in diabetic glomerulosclerosis. (b) Definitive confirmation is made by electron microscopy, which demonstrates widening of the mesangium (M) and then the subendothelial space by the characteristic amyloid fibrils (inset) (From BD Rose, *Pathophysiology of Renal Disease* (2nd ed.). New York: McGraw-Hill, 1987.).

(particularly renal cell carcinoma and Hodgkin's disease), and familial Mediterranean fever [3]. In these disorders, it is thought that activated macrophages release a soluble factor (perhaps interleukin-1) that stimulates the production by hepatocytes of serum amyloid A, an acute phase reactant similar to C-reactive protein. This protein is in part taken up by circulating monocytes/macrophages, where it is cleaved to a smaller fragment called AA protein (molecular weight 5000–8000), which is the major component of the deposited amyloid fibrils [2].

It is at present unclear why only some patients with one of the above inflammatory conditions develop secondary amyloidosis. Genetic differences either in AA degradation or in the amyloidogenic potential of this protein may be important in selected cases [8].

Clinical Presentation

Patients with renal amyloidosis typically present with proteinuria and edema, often accompanied by nonspecific systemic symptoms such as fatigue and weight loss [1,2]. In addition, the history and physical examination may reveal one of the disorders associated with secondary amyloidosis or findings induced by systemic amyloid deposition such as hepatomegaly, splenomegaly, macroglossia, congestive heart failure, or the carpal tunnel syndrome. However, *clinically apparent* extrarenal involvement is frequently absent and therefore lack of the above findings does not exclude the diagnosis of amyloidosis [9].

Proteinuria occurs in almost all patients with renal amyloidosis and is often in the nephrotic range [9]. This is typically accompanied by a benign urine sediment and a plasma creatinine concentration that is elevated in up to one-half of patients [1,5,9]. An uncommon exception to these characteristic renal findings is seen in patients in whom the amyloid deposits are primarily limited to the blood vessels, resulting in narrowing of the vascular lumen. In this setting, proteinuria is minimal or absent, with renal insufficiency being due to glomerular ischemia [10].

Another important abnormality in patients with primary amyloidosis or light-chain deposition disease is the presence of a monoclonal paraprotein in the plasma (as an M spike on protein electrophoresis) or urine (as monoclonal light chains) in over 85 percent of cases [1,5]. In addition, malignant transformation into multiple myeloma occurs in about 20 percent of patients and may be manifested by hypercalcemia or lytic bone lesions.

Diagnosis

Although suggested by one or more of the aforementioned findings, the diagnosis of amyloidosis can be made only by the demonstration of tissue deposits of amyloid fibrils. Kidney or liver biopsy is positive in over 90 percent of cases; however, the diagnosis can often be made less invasively by biopsy of abdominal fat pad (85%), rectum (50–80%), gingiva (60%), or skin (50%) [1,3,11]. In comparison, light-chain deposition disease (with granular not fibrillar deposits) can be diagnosed only by renal biopsy [5].

Course and Treatment

The prognosis and therapy are dependent on the form of amyloidosis that is present. Patients with *primary* amyloidosis, for example, do relatively poorly with mean survival rates ranging from as low as 4 months with concurrent multiple myeloma to 12 to 15 months with primary amyloidosis alone [1]. Cardiac or renal failure, infection, and progression of the myeloma are the major causes of death. The nephropathy usually progresses slowly to renal failure if the patient survives long enough [1,5]. The heavy proteinuria typically persists even with advanced renal failure, a reflection of the marked increase in glomerular permeability to macromolecules in this disorder.

The combination of prednisone and melphalan (as used in uncomplicated multiple myeloma) is the major therapeutic modality that has been tried in primary amyloidosis and light-chain deposition disease [1,5]. A reduction in proteinuria has been noted in up to 50 percent of treated patients [12]; the importance of this response is uncertain, however, since it may be associated with a further increase in renal amyloid deposition on repeat renal biopsy [13].

The effect of therapy on patient survival is also unclear, since few well-randomized studies are available. There is suggestive, but by no means conclusive, evidence that colchicine (which, in a dose of 0.6 mg twice a day, may diminish amyloid protein synthesis) may prolong mean survival by up to 11 months [14] and that prednisone and melphalan may be more effective than colchicine alone [12].

The course of *secondary* amyloidosis, in comparison, is directly dependent on the ability to control the underlying inflammatory disease, since plasma levels of serum amyloid A appear to roughly correlate with the severity of the clinical manifestations of amyloid deposition [15]. This can perhaps be best exemplified by the use of colchicine (in a dose of 1–2 gm/day) in the treatment of familial Mediterranean fever [16]. In this condition, colchicine markedly reduces the frequency of attacks of abdominal pain, substantially diminishes the incidence of clinical renal disease (including prevention of recurrent amyloidosis in the kidney transplant), and can stabilize the glomerular filtration rate in patients with moderate (nonnephrotic proteinuria) but not advanced renal involvement. Similarly, control of inflammation can lead to stabilization or improvement in renal function and gradual resolution of the amyloid deposits in other causes of secondary amyloidosis [17].

There is, however, no proved therapy to prevent amyloid formation if the underlying inflammatory disease cannot be effectively treated. The positive response to colchicine in familial Mediterranean fever may be related to decreased neutrophilic chemotaxis or phagocytosis, thereby decreasing the peritoneal inflammatory process, rather than to a direct impairment in serum amyloid A release [18]. Thus, this agent may not be effective in other forms of secondary amyloidosis. Both colchicine and dimethylsulfoxide (which may cause dissolution of amyloid fibrils) have been tried in selected, uncontrolled cases with some possible benefit [19]. Their role, however, remains to be defined.

References

1. Kyle, RA, Greipp, PR. Amyloidosis (AL). Clinical and laboratory features in 229 cases. *Mayo Clin Proc* 58:665, 1983.
2. Glenner, GG. Amyloid deposits and amyloidosis. The β-fibrilloses. *N Engl J Med* 302:1283, 1333, 1980.
3. Rose, BD. *Pathophysiology of Renal Disease* (2nd ed). New York: McGraw-Hill, 1987. Pp. 208-214.
4. Solomon, A, Fragione, B, Franklin, EC. Bence Jones proteins and light chains of immunoglobulins. Preferential association of the V_{AVI} subgroup of human light chains with amyloidosis AL (λ). *J Clin Invest* 70:453, 1982.
5. Ganeval, D, Noel, L-H, Preud'Homme, J-L, Droz, D, Grunfeld, J-P. Light chain deposition disease: Its relation with AL-type amyloidosis. *Kidney Int* 26:1, 1984.
6. Noel, L-H, Droz, D, Ganeval, D, Grunfeld, J-P. Renal granular monoclonal light chain deposits: Morphological aspects in 11 cases. *Clin Nephrol* 21:263, 1984.
7. Hill, GS, Morel-Maroger, L. Mery, J-P, Brouet, JC, Mignon, F. Renal lesions in multiple myeloma *Am J Kid Dis* 2:423, 1983.
8. Lavie, G, Zucker-Franklin, D, Franklin, EC. Degradation of serum amyloid A protein by surface-associated enzymes of human blood monocytes. *J Exp Med* 148:1020, 1978.
9. Triger, DR, Joekes, AM. Renal amyloidosis -- a fourteen year follow-up. *Q J Med* 42:15, 1972.
10. Falck, HM, Tornroth, T, Wegelius, O. Predominantly vascular amyloid deposition in the kidney in patients with minimal or no proteinuria. *Clin Nephrol* 19:137, 1983.
11. Dustan, MA, Skinner, M, Shirahama, T, Cohen, AS. Diagnosis of amyloidosis by abdominal fat pad aspiration. Analysis of four years' experience. *Am J Med* 82:412, 1987.
12. Kyle, RA, Greipp, PR, Garton, JP, Gertz, MA. Primary systemic amyloidosis. Comparison of melphalan/prednisone versus colchicine. *Am J Med* 79:708, 1985.
13. Kyle, RA, Wagoner, RD, Holley, KE. Primary systemic amyloidosis: Resolution of the nephrotic syndrome with melphalan and prednisone. *Arch Intern Med* 142:1445, 1982.
14. Cohen, AS, Rubinow, A, Anderson, JJ, Skinner, M, Mason, JH. Libbey, C, Kayne, H. Survival of patients with primary (AL) amyloidosis. Colchicine-treated cases from

1976 to 1983 compared with cases seen in previous years (1961 to 1973). *Am J Med* 82:1182, 1987.

5. Falck, HM, Maury, CPJ, Teppo, A-M, Wegelius, O. Persistently high serum amyloid A protein and C-reactive protein levels correlate with rapid progression of secondary amyloidosis. *Br Med J* 286:1391, 1983.

6. Zemer, D, Pras, M, Sohar, E, Modan, M, Cabili, S, Gafni, J. Colchicine in the prevention and treatment of the amyloidosis of familial Mediterranean fever. *N Engl J Med* 314:1001, 1986.

7. Dirkman, SH, Kahn, T, Gribetz, D, Churg, J. Resolution of renal amyloidosis. *Am J Med* 63:430, 1977.

8. Matzner, Y, Brzezinski, A. C5a-inhibitor deficiency in peritoneal fluids from patients with familial Mediterranean fever. *N Engl J Med* 311:287, 1984.

9. Scheinberg, MA, Pernambuco, JC, Benson, MD. DMSO and colchicine in amyloid disease. *Ann Rheum Dis* 43:421, 1984.

32. IgA NEPHROPATHY

IgA nephropathy is probably the most common cause of glomerulonephritis, particularly in patients presenting with asymptomatic microscopic hematuria or with recurrent episodes of gross hematuria. In one study, for example, up to 60 percent of such adults had IgA nephropathy [1].

This disorder is characterized histologically by IgA deposition in the mesangium [2,3]. As a result, immunofluorescence is required to establish the diagnosis, demonstrating IgA, C3, and, to a lesser degree, IgG and IgM deposition in the mesangium (Fig. 32-1). Prominent mesangial IgA deposition is seen in only two other disorders: Henoch-Schönlein purpura, which is histologically indistinguishable from IgA nephropathy; and lupus nephritis, in which IgG is the primary immunoglobulin that is deposited.

Light microscopy is less specific, usually revealing mild-to-moderate increases in mesangial cellularity and matrix involving some or all of the glomeruli. In the later stages of the disease, these changes lead to glomerular sclerosis. Electron microscopy typically demonstrates glomerular dense deposits in the mesangium and occasionally in the subendothelial or subepithelial space.

Etiology and Pathogenesis

IgA nephropathy is most often idiopathic; it may, however, be seen in a variety of other disorders (Table 32-1) [4]. These associations shed some light on how this disorder might occur. As examples, intestinal and pulmonary diseases can lead to increased mucosal IgA production, and hepatic cirrhosis can impair the removal of circulating IgA-containing immune complexes by the Kupffer cells [4,5]. The latter defect could explain why glomerular IgA deposition is relatively common (but often clinically silent) in many patients with advanced liver disease [6].

A number of experimental and clinical observations have increased our understanding of the possible pathogenetic mechanisms involved in this disorder [4,5]:

1. Most patients seem to have a specific abnormality in IgA regulation. This may be manifested by an elevated plasma IgA level (in up to one-half of cases), concurrent IgA deposition in dermal capillaries of normal skin, circulating IgA-containing immune complexes that roughly parallel the activity of the disease, and an increased number of circulating IgA-specific B and T cells following an upper respiratory infection, a response that is not seen in normals [5,7]. Thus, an *exaggerated mucosal IgA response* to an infectious agent may initiate clinically evident disease. It has been observed, for example, that tonsillar lymphocytes from patients with IgA nephropathy have a higher-than-normal percentage of cells producing polymeric IgA [8]. It is unclear how this occurs; it is possible that either primary B-cell activation or a deficiency of IgA-specific suppressor T cells plays a major role.

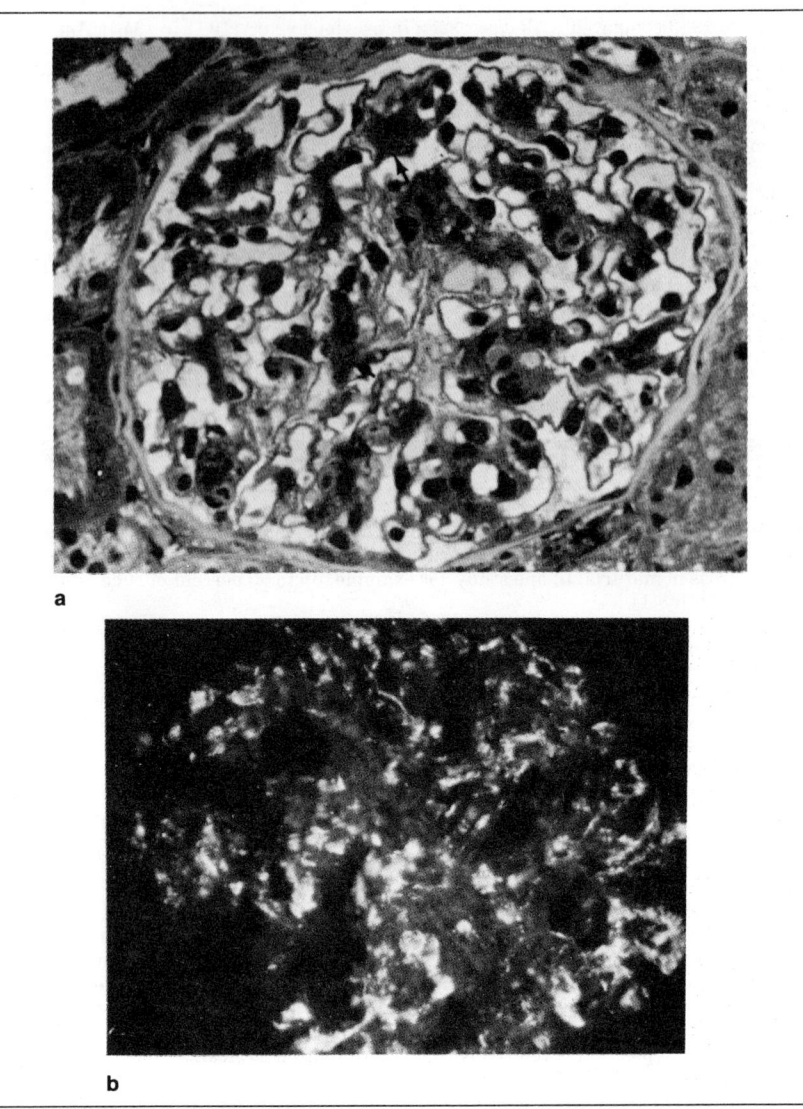

a

b

Fig. 32-1. Histologic changes in IgA nephropathy. (a) Light microscopy shows prominence of the mesangial areas with increased cellularity and matrix (arrows). The capillary loops and basement membrane are typically normal. (b) Immunofluorescent microscopy is diagnostic, demonstrating prominent mesangial IgA deposits. These mesangial deposits can also be seen by electron microscopy (not shown) (From BD Rose, *Pathophysiology of Renal Disease* (2nd ed.). New York: McGraw-Hill, 1987.).

Table 32-1. Causes of IgA nephropathy

Idiopathic, may be familial
Hepatic cirrhosis
Dermatitis herpetiformis and gluten enteropathy
Seronegative arthritis, especially ankylosing spondylitis
Pulmonary diseases
Oat-cell carcinoma
Disseminated tuberculosis
Mycosis fungoides

Oral antigens, leading to activation of intestinal IgA production, also may be important in certain patients [5,9]. As an example, IgA nephropathy is occasionally associated with overt gluten enteropathy. In addition, some patients without gastrointestinal symptoms have circulating IgA-antigliadin antibodies and mucosal atrophy on intestinal biopsy. Institution of a gluten-free diet in this setting has led to disappearance of the circulating antibodies and resolution of the urinary abnormalities [9].

2. These abnormalities in IgA regulation also can be demonstrated in some asymptomatic parents and siblings [10]. This observation suggests an important genetic or common environmental role in determining susceptibility to this disorder.

3. IgA-containing immune complexes appear to have a particular propensity to deposit in the glomeruli [5,11], perhaps because they are more difficult to clear both from the circulation and from tissue sites once they are deposited. Most antigen-antibody complexes bind C1, thereby activating the classic complement pathway. This leads to the formation of C3b which, via attachment to C3b receptors on erythrocytes, facilitates removal of the complexes and subsequent delivery to their site of elimination in the reticuloendothelial system [12]. IgA, however, can activate the alternate complement pathway but does not bind C1, an effect that could eliminate binding to and removal by erythrocytes [11].

4. Once IgA is deposited in the kidney, it is likely that glomerular damage is mediated by the terminal complement components (C5b-C9), which have been called the membrane attack complex [13]. It is possible that the codeposited IgG and IgM contribute to this process, since these immunoglobulins are more effective activators of the complement pathway than IgA [13a].

Clinical Presentation and Course

The major modes of presentation are similar to those in other focal glomerulonephritides (see Chap. 25): single or recurrent episodes of macroscopic hematuria or the incidental finding of hematuria and proteinuria (usually < 1 gm/day) on a routine urinalysis [2,3]. The GFR, blood pressure, and complement levels are typically normal. Some patients with gross hematuria, however, develop transient acute renal failure (without edema or hypertension) that appears to be due primarily to red cell obstruction of the tubules [14].

The episodes of macroscopic hematuria may be recurrent, typically occurring 1 to 3 days after an upper respiratory infection (versus 7–21 days with poststreptococcal glomerulonephritis) or, less commonly, after gastroenteritis. The gross bleeding lasts only a few days, although microscopic hematuria generally persists.

Less frequently, IgA nephropathy presents with the nephrotic syndrome or with a picture similar to diffuse glomerulonephritis. In the latter setting, hypertension and renal insufficiency accompany the urinary abnormalities, and more severe glomerular involvement, often with crescents, is found on renal biopsy [2,3].

The prognosis in IgA nephropathy is frequently good, although the microscopic hematuria or episodes of gross hematuria may persist for many years. It is important to emphasize, however, that *a stable and normal plasma creatinine concentration does not necessarily mean stable disease.* Both compensatory hyperfiltration in less-affected nephrons and increased tubular secretion of creatinine can initially mask disease progression in this setting (see Chap. 17). Thus, serial monitoring for other signs of continued disease activity, such as hypertension or increasing proteinuria, is essential. For example, a patient with a stable plasma creatinine concentration of 1 mg/dl, persistent hematuria, and red cell casts, but increasing proteinuria from 400 to 1200 mg/day is likely to have progressive glomerular damage.

IgA nephropathy, however, is not always a benign condition. End-stage renal disease occurs in approximately 10 percent of patients at 10 years and 20 percent at 20 years [2,3]. In addition, another 20 to 30 percent may have some decline in renal function by 20 years. As with other glomerulopathies, relatively bad prognostic signs include proteinuria exceeding 1 gm/day, hypertension, persistent renal insufficiency, and, on biopsy, glomerulosclerosis, tubulointerstitial scarring, or crescent formation that may be associated with rapid progression to renal failure [2,3,15].

Recent studies suggest important heterogeneity in patients with IgA nephropathy who have the nephrotic syndrome. This usually occurs in the setting of advanced or progressive glomerular damage [3,16]. A subgroup of nephrotic patients, however, has a normal plasma creatinine concentration, little or no hematuria, and relatively mild mesangial proliferation on renal biopsy. These patients often *behave clinically as if they have minimal change disease,* with remission of the proteinuria after a course of corticosteroid therapy, followed in some by frequent relapses [16,17].

Diagnosis

IgA nephropathy should be suspected in patients presenting with either macroscopic or microscopic hematuria and proteinuria. The absence of hypocomplementemia, the lack of evidence of an antecedent streptococcal infection, and a usually negative family history of renal disease tend to exclude other disorders that can present in a similar fashion such as poststreptococcal or membranoproliferative glomerulonephritis or hereditary nephritis. Similarly, the absence of purpura, arthritis, and abdominal pain rules out Henoch-Schönlein purpura, a multisystem condition associated with the same histologic findings in the kidney as IgA nephropathy.

However, IgA nephropathy cannot be differentiated on clinical grounds from other mild glomerulopathies presenting with hematuria and no or mild proteinuria. Included in this group are disorders characterized by mesangial proliferation plus a variety of immunofluorescent and electron microscopic findings such as IgG or IgM deposits in the mesangium, thinning of the glomerular basement membranes, or focal deposits of C3 in the glomeruli or blood vesels; each of these conditions is associated with a benign prognosis [18,19]. In addition, some biopsies will be normal, indicating either minimal glomerular disease or nonglomerular bleeding [18].

Thus, a renal biopsy should be performed only when it seems likely that a progressive glomerular disease might be present (as with proteinuria above 1 gm/day, hypertension, or renal insufficiency). A patient who has glomerular hematuria with only 10 red cells per high power field, no proteinuria, and a plasma creatinine concentration of 0.9 mg/dl probably has a benign disorder as long as there is no worsening of these findings. As a result, the patient can be followed and biopsy deferred. It has been suggested that IgA nephropathy can be diagnosed indirectly in this setting by demonstrating the deposition of IgA in dermal capillaries of normal skin. This test, however, is not very sensitive or specific and tells nothing of disease severity [20].

Treatment

There has been no treatment that has been proved to alter the course of IgA nephropathy, as both prednisone and cytotoxic agents have been generally ineffective [2,3,17]. However, that subset of patients with *heavy proteinuria, often little or no hematuria, and only mild glomerular lesions* appears to respond well to corticosteroid therapy, with remission of proteinuria and no progressive renal failure [16,17]. Those patients with frequent relapses when the prednisone is discontinued can be effectively treated with a short course of cyclophosphamide (similar to that used in minimal change disease).

It is possible that *hemodynamic factors* may contribute to the glomerular damage in those patients with progressive renal insufficiency. As a result, an attempt at lowering the intraglomerular pressure with a converting enzyme inhibitor or dietary protein restriction, or both, is probably warranted (see Chap. 56).

Recurrent IgA nephropathy occurs in up to 50 percent of patients receiving a renal transplant, despite antirejection therapy with prednisone and azathioprine [21]. However, loss of the allograft due to recurrent disease is unusual, apparently occurring more commonly with living related donor than with cadaver transplants [21]. This finding suggests the importance of genetic factors in determining the severity of injury induced by IgA deposition.

References

1. Petersson, E, von Bonsdorff, M, Tornroth, T, Lindholm, H. Nephritis among young Finnish men. *Clin Nephrol* 22:217, 1984.
2. Rodicio, JL. Idiopathic IgA nephropathy. *Kidney Int* 25:717, 1984.
3. Nicholls, KM, Fairley, KF, Dowling, JP, Kincaid-Smith, P. The clinical course of mesangial IgA associated nephropathy in adults. *Q J Med* 53:227, 1984.
4. Rose, BD. *Pathophysiology of Renal Disease* (2nd ed.). New York: McGraw-Hill, 1987. Pp. 215-219.
5. Rifai, A. Experimental models for IgA-associated nephritis. *Kidney Int* 31:1, 1987.
6. Newell, GC. Cirrhotic glomerulonephritis: Incidence, morphology, clinical features, and pathogenesis. *Am J Kid Dis* 9:183, 1987.
7. Feehally, J, Beattie, TJ, Brenchley, PEC, Coupes, BM, Mallick, NP, Postlethwaite, RJ. Sequential study of the IgA system in relapsing IgA nephropathy. *Kidney Int* 30:924, 1986.
8. Bene, MC, Faure, G, Hurault de Ligny, B, Kessler, M, Duheille, J. Immunoglobulin A nephropathy. Quantitative immunohisto-morphometry of the tonsillar plasma cells: Evidence on inversion of the immunoglobulin A versus immunoglobulin G secreting cell balance. *J Clin Invest* 71:1342, 1983.
9. Fornasieri, A, Sinico, RA, Maldifassi, P, Bernasconi, P, Vegni, M, D'Amico, G. IgA-antigliadin antibodies in IgA mesangial nephropathy (Berger's disease). *Br Med J* 295:78, 1987.
10. Waldo, F, Beischel, L, West, CD. IgA synthesis by lymphocytes from patients with IgA nephropathy and their relatives. *Kidney Int* 29:1229, 1986.
11. Waxman, FJ, Hebert, LA, Cosio, FG, Smead, WL, VanAman, ME, Taguiam, JM, Birmingham, DJ. Differential binding of immunoglobulin A and immunoglobulin G1 immune complexes to primate erythrocytes in vitro. Immunoglobulin A immune complexes bind less well to erythrocytes and are preferentially deposited in glomeruli. *J Clin Invest* 77:82, 1986.
12. Schifferli, JA, Ng, YC, Peters, DK. The role of complement and its receptors in the elimination of immune complexes. *N Engl J Med* 315:488, 1986.
13. Rauterberg, EW, Lieberknecht, H-M, Wingen, A-M, Ritz, E. Complement membrane attack (MAC) in idiopathic IgA-glomerulonephritis. *Kidney Int* 31:820, 1987.
13a. Emancipator, SN, Ovary, Z. Lamm, ME. The role of mesangial complement in the hematuria of experimental IgA nephropathy. *Lab Invest* 57:269, 1987.
14. Praga, M, Gutierrez-Millet, V, Navas, JJ, Ruilope, LM, Morales, JM, Alcazar, JM, Bello, I, Rodicio, JL. Acute worsening of renal function during episodes of macroscopic hematuria in IgA nephropathy. *Kidney Int* 28:69, 1985.
15. D'Amico, G, Minetti, L, Ponticelli, C, Fellini, G, Ferrario, F, Barbiano de Belgioioso, G, Imbasciati, E, Ragni, A, Bertoli, S, Fogazzi, G: Prognostic indicators in idiopathic IgA mesangial nephropathy. *Q J Med* 59:363, 1986.
16. Mustonen, J, Pasternack, A, Rantala, A. The nephrotic syndrome in IgA glomerulonephritis: Response to corticosteroid therapy. *Clin Nephrol* 20:172, 1983.
17. Lai, KN, Lai, FM, Ho, CP, Chan, KW. Corticosteroid therapy in IgA nephropathy with nephrotic syndrome: A long-term controlled trial *Clin Nephrol* 26:174, 1986.
18. Trachtman, H, Weiss, RA, Bennett, B, Greifer, I. Isolated hematuria in children: Indications for a renal biopsy. *Kidney Int* 25:94, 1984.
19. Migone, L, Olivetti, G, Allegri, L, Dall'Aglio, P. Mesangioproliferative glomerulonephritis. *Clin Nephrol* 13:219, 1980.

20. Hasbargen, JA, Copley, JB. Utility of skin biopsy in the diagnosis of IgA nephropathy. *Am J Kid Dis* 6:100, 1985.
21. Bachman, U, Biava, C, Amend. W, Feduska, N, Melzer, J. Salvatierra, O, Vincenti, F. The clinical course of IgA-nephropathy and Henoch-Schönlein purpura following renal transplantation. *Transplantation* 42:511, 1980.

33. HEREDITARY NEPHRITIS

Heriditary nephritis (or Alport's syndrome) is a progressive form of glomerular disease (at least in males) that is often accompanied by hearing loss and lenticular abnormalities [1]. The earliest histologic changes in the kidney in this disorder are present on electron microscopy, which initially reveals thinning of the glomerular basement membrane (GBM) [2]. This finding is not pathognomonic, since it also occurs in some cases of familial benign hematuria in which glomerular damage and renal failure do not occur [3]. With time, however, the changes in hereditary nephritis become more diagnostic, particularly the development of progressive longitudinal splitting of the glomerular and occasionally the tubular basement membranes, producing a characteristic laminated appearance (Fig. 33-1).

The number of glomeruli showing splitting of the GBM is both age- and sex-dependent. In males, this change can usually be demonstrated in 30 percent of glomeruli by age 10 but more than 90 percent by age 30 [2]. Thus, early renal biopsy in a young boy could, by sampling error, be nondiagnostic. In comparison, less than 30 percent of glomeruli are typically affected in females, who generally follow a benign course with no or only slowly progressive glomerular damage [1].

Light microscopy also demonstrates increasing, although nonspecific, glomerular changes. Focal increases in mesangial cellularity eventually progress to glomerular sclerosis. These abnormalities are accompanied by an interstitial infiltrate that characteristically includes foam cells (large cells of uncertain origin with foamy, lipid-containing cytoplasm). Immunofluorescent microscopy is usually negative for immunoglobulins and complement except for the occasional nonspecific deposition of IgG and C3 in sclerotic areas.

Pathogenesis and Inheritance

An unusual observation that has helped to elucidate the possible pathogenesis of hereditary nephritis is that the GBM in most males and some females *does not bind anti-GBM antibodies* from patients with Goodpasture's syndrome* [4,5]. The GBM does, however, bind antibodies derived from rabbits who are immunized with human GBM [4]. These findings suggest that hereditary nephritis is frequently associated with the *absence of a normal GBM antigen* against which antibodies are directed in Goodpasture's syndrome. This antigen, which appears to be part of the noncollagenous domain of type IV collagen, is also missing from the basement membranes of other tissues, including the lens, eye, and organ of Corti in the ear [5,6], suggesting that both the renal and extrarenal manifestations of hereditary nephritis may be due to a basement membrane defect.

It is not clear, however, how a GBM abnormality leads to glomerular sclerosis and renal failure. One possibility is that hemodynamic factors play an important role in the glomerular injury (see Chap. 56). Although the glomerular pressure and flow are initially "normal," they may be too high for the weakened, thin GBM in this disorder. This can lead to cycles of damage and then repair that are manifested by the laminations in the GBM.

Three modes of inheritance have been reported in different kindreds with hereditary

---

*This test is performed by incubating the patient's kidney with serum containing anti-GBM antibodies. The presence or absence of binding can then be detected by adding fluorescein-labelled antibodies directed against human IgG.

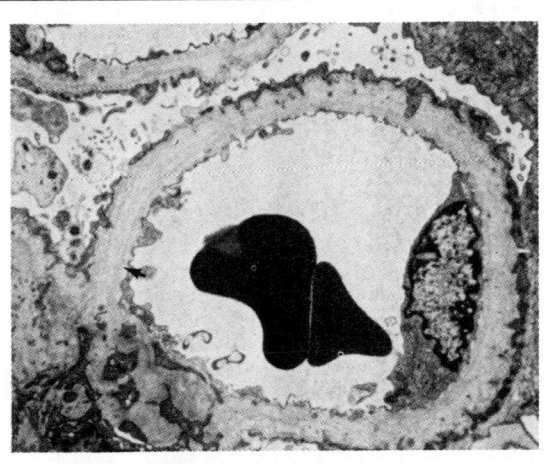

Fig. 33-1. Electron microscopy in hereditary nephritis reveals the characteristic split or laminated appearance of the glomerular basement membrane (arrow) (From BD Rose, *Pathophysiology of Renal Disease* (2nd ed.). New York: McGraw-Hill, 1987.).

nephritis: X-linked dominant; autosomal dominant, which may preferentially segregate with the X chromosome; and, less commonly, autosomal recessive [7]. In most families, the disease is not transmitted from affected fathers to their sons. This finding could be explained by either of the first two mechanisms, since the father would pass on only the unaffected Y chromosome. X-linked inheritance could also account, by the Lyon hypothesis, for the more benign course in females. Since only one X chromosome is active per cell, roughly one-half of the cells will be normal in females, thereby minimizing the clinical manifestations of the disease.

A minority of patients with classic histologic and clinical manifestations of hereditary nephritis have no family history of renal disease [8]. It is presumed that these cases represent new mutations of the gene(s) responsible for the characteristic basement membrane abnormalities.

Clinical Presentation and Course

The most common abnormalities in hereditary nephritis are renal disease (which can occur alone), sensorineural hearing loss (primarily high-tone), and eye changes such as anterior lenticonus, cataracts, and whitish perimacular lesions in the retina [1]. Other disturbances that can be seen in some kindreds include peripheral neuropathy, retinitis pigmentosa, and platelet dysfunction.

The initial renal manifestations are similar to those in the other forms of focal glomerulonephritis: recurrent episodes of gross hematuria or microscopic hematuria with or without mild proteinuria [1]. The blood pressure, plasma creatinine concentration, and plasma complement level are usually normal at the time of presentation. Hematuria begins early in boys (often before the age of 5); it may not be discovered, however, until adulthood unless the patient is prospectively examined because of a positive family history. Similarly, hearing loss can begin in childhood but does not become clinically apparent for many years. There is no necesary relationship between the degrees of renal disease and hearing impairment.

Males are characteristically affected more frequently, earlier, and more severely than females [1]. Renal disease in males is usually progressive, ultimately leading to increasing proteinuria, hypertension, and end-stage renal disease between the ages of 16 and 35. The course of the renal disease is more indolent in some families with renal failure being delayed until the age of 45 to 60. Despite this interfamilial variability, the age at which renal failure is seen is relatively uniform within a given kindred. Hearing loss is also typically progressive, frequently leading to deafness.

In comparison, affected females are often asymptomatic carriers who have only microscopic hematuria. Uremia and hearing loss are much less common than in males; when they occur, their onset is usually delayed until 45 years of age or above. There are exceptions, however, since females can develop end-stage renal disease before the age of 25 in some families [9].

Diagnosis and Treatment

The diagnosis of hereditary nephritis can often be made from the personal and family history of the renal and extrarenal manifestations of the disease. Familial hematuria alone is insufficient, however, since some families have a *benign* renal prognosis with different glomerular lesions, including thinning (but not splitting) of the GBM and C3 deposition in the glomeruli or blood vessels [3]. A renal biopsy is indicated only if there is no documented family history [8] or the presentation is very atypical.

There is no proved therapy that will alter the course of hereditary nephritis. In view of the primary GBM abnormality, however, lowering the intraglomerular pressure by restricting dietary protein intake or by antihypertensive therapy with a converting enzyme inhibitor might be beneficial (see Chap. 56). The efficacy of these modalities is at present unproved and their use should be limited to patients at high risk, such as males with hypertension, proteinuria, an already elevated plasma creatinine concentration, or a family history of the early development of renal failure.

Dialysis or transplantation can be used in those patients who progress to end-stage renal disease. Although recurrent disease does not develop in the transplant (since the donor GBM is normal), some patients are at risk of developing de novo anti-GBM antibody disease due to exposure to previously unseen GBM antigen(s) [4,10,11]. This unique problem may occur in up to 15 percent of patients [10]; it can lead to loss of the transplant due to crescentic glomerulonephritis [11] but is often not associated with any significant decline in transplant function [10]. Thus, the possibility of anti-GBM antibody disease should not preclude renal transplantation in this disorder.

References

1. Grunfeld, J-P, The clinical spectrum of hereditary nephritis. *Kidney Int* 27:83, 1985.
2. Rumpelt, H-J. Hereditary nephropathy (Alport's syndrome): Correlation of clinical data with glomerular basement membrane alterations. *Clin Nephrol* 13:203, 1980.
3. Trachtman, H, Weiss, RA, Bennett, B, Greifer, I. Isolated hematuria in children: Indications for a renal biopsy. *Kidney Int* 25:94, 1984.
4. McCoy, RC, Johnson, HK, Stone, WJ, Wilson, CB. Absence of nephritogenic GBM antigen(s) in some patients with hereditary nephritis. *Kidney Int* 21:642, 1982.
5. Savage, COS, Pusey, CD, Kershaw, MJ, Cashman, SJ, Harrison, P, Hartley, B, Turner, DR, Cameron, JS, Evans, DJ, Lockwood, CM. The Goodpasture antigen in Alport's syndrome: Studies with a monoclonal antibody. *Kidney Int* 30:107, 1986.
6. Kashtan, C, Fish, AJ, Kleppel, M, Yoshioka, K, Michael, AF. Nephritogenic antigen determinant in epidermal and renal basement membranes of kindreds with Alport-type familial nephritis. *J Clin Invest* 78:1035, 1986.
7. Feingold, J, Bois, E, Chompret, A, Broyer, M, Gubler, M-C, Grunfeld, J-P. Genetic heterogeneity of Alport's syndrome. *Kidney Int* 27:672, 1985.
8. Yoshikawa, N, Matsuyama, S, Ito, H, et al. Nonfamilial hematuria associated with glomerular basement membrane alterations characteristic of hereditary nephritis: Comparison with hereditary nephritis. *J Pediatr* 111:519, 1987.
9. Grunfeld, J-P, Noel, L-H, Hafez, S, Droz, D. Renal prognosis in women with hereditary nephritis. *Clin Nephrol* 23:267, 1985.
10. Querin, S, Noel, L-H, Grunfeld, J-P, Droz, D, Mahieu, P, Berger, J, Kreis, H. Linear glomerular IgG fixation in renal allografts: Incidence and significance in Alport's syndrome. *Clin Nephrol* 25:134, 1986.
11. Milliner, D, Pierides, AM, Holley, KE. Renal transplantation in Alport's syndrome. Anti-glomerular basement membrane glomerulonephritis in the allograft. *Mayo Clin Proc* 57:35, 1982.

34. POSTINFECTIOUS GLOMERULONEPHRITIS

A variety of bacterial, viral, and parasitic infections can lead to a proliferative glomerulonephritis [1-3]. Many of these infections produce only mild glomerular lesions that are typically manifested by transient, asymptomatic hematuria and proteinuria. Two disorders, however, are often associated with clinically important glomerular disease: poststreptococcal glomerulonephritis and bacterial endocarditis.

Poststreptococcal Glomerulonephritis

The pathologic changes in poststreptococcal glomerulonephritis vary with the severity of the disease. For example, only minimal-to-moderate mesangial cell proliferation may be found in patients with mild, frequently subclinical disease [4]. In comparison, patients with clinically evident disease have the more characteristic findings of *marked glomerular hypercellularity* due to proliferation of mesangial and endothelial cells and to the infiltration of circulating neutrophils and macrophages. The net effect is narrowing or closure of many of the capillary lumens (Fig. 34-1A). Crescent formation and areas of necrosis may also be seen in selected cases.

These changes on light microscopy, although suggestive, are not specific for poststreptococcal glomerulonephritis. Electron microscopy may, however, be relatively diagnostic, revealing mesangial deposits and characteristic subepithelial "humps" (Fig. 34-1B). These immune deposits can also be detected by immunofluorescent microscopy that demonstrates IgG and C3 along the glomerular capillary wall.

Pathogenesis

With rare exceptions, poststreptococcal glomerulonephritis follows infection only with *group A, β-hemolytic* streptococci. Furthermore, only some of these strains appear to be capable of producing glomerular disease, particularly type 12 with pharyngitis and type 49 with impetigo [5,6].

The mechanism by which certain streptococcal strains lead to glomerular disease is unknown. One possibility is that the nephritogenic strains have a unique antigen that can be identified both in circulating immune complexes and in the glomeruli [7]. Furthermore, this antigen may be cationic [8], an important characteristic that would promote both antigen binding to negatively charged heparan sulfate residues in the glomerular basement membrane (GBM) and subsequent antigen movement across the GBM into the subepithelial space. Experimental studies suggest that only cationic antigens are able to form subepithelial deposits as are found in poststreptococcal glomerulonephritis (see p. 197) [9].

An alternate hypothesis proposes that nephritogenic streptococci produce neuraminidase, an enzyme that can alter endogenous IgG, making it antigenic. As a result, anti-IgG antibodies are formed and IgG–anti-IgG complexes (detectable as rheumatoid factor) could be deposited in the kidney [10]. In support of this theory is the observation that elevated rheumatoid factor titers first appear 10 or more days after infection, the same time as the onset of the renal disease.

Clinical Presentation

Poststreptococcal glomerulonephritis usually follows an episode of either pharyngitis or impetigo (pyoderma) in children or less often in adults. This can occur in sporadic cases or during an epidemic. Even within an epidemic, the incidence of glomerulonephritis is only about 5 to 10 percent with pharyngitis and 25 percent with skin infections [5,6]. These findings suggest that host factors, such as the nature and intensity of the immune response, contribute to the susceptibility to glomerular involvement.

The latent period between the onset of infection and clinical evidence of renal disease is variable, averaging 10 days with pharyngitis and 21 days with impetigo [11]. In comparison, a latent period of 5 days or less suggests a viral-activated disorder such as IgA nephropathy.

The typical presenting symptoms of poststreptococcal glomerulonephritis include the acute onset of gross hematuria ("Coca-Cola"–colored urine), oliguria, edema, and bilat-

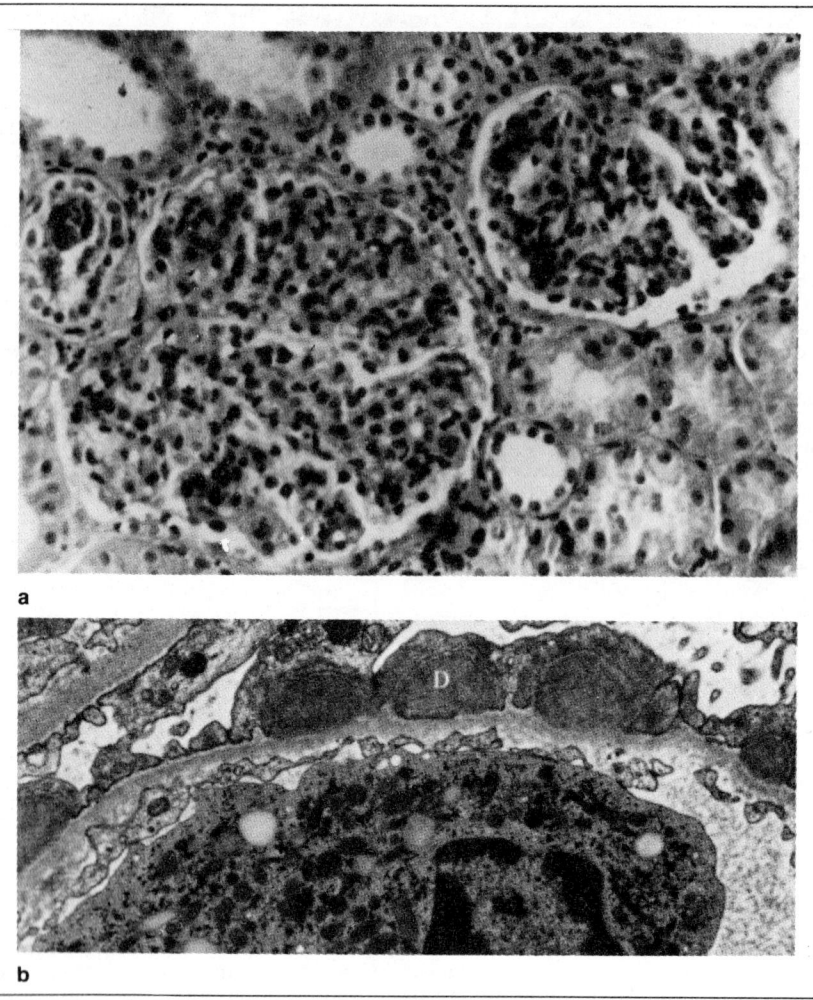

Fig. 34-1. Histologic findings in poststreptococcal glomerulonephritis. (a) Light microscopy shows diffuse mesangial and endothelial cell proliferation with neutrophilic infiltration. The net effect is narrowing or closure of most of the capillary lumens and enlargement of the glomerular tuft so that Bowman's space is almost obliterated. (b) Electron microscopy demonstrates the characteristic hump-shaped deposits (D) sitting on the subepithelial aspect of the glomerular basement membrane. A neutrophil is present in the capillary lumen (From BD Rose, *Pathophysiology of Renal Disease* (2nd ed.). New York: McGraw-Hill, 1987.).

eral flank pain due to stretching of the renal capsule [5]. Hypertension and congestive heart failure also may be seen, both of which are primarily due to sodium and water retention induced by the low glomerular filtration rate [12].

The initial laboratory data usually reveal a variable elevation in the plasma creatinine concentration and an abnormal urinalysis characterized by hematuria, proteinuria, and red cell and other casts. Pyuria is also frequently prominent (more than in other glomerular diseases) and presumably reflects neutrophilic infiltration of the glomeruli.

Hypocomplementemia, as evidenced by a low plasma C3 level, occurs during the first week in up to 90 percent of cases. Elevated rheumatoid factor titers and circulating cryoglobulins are also found in most patients [10]; why these autoantibodies are produced is not well understood.

In addition to this classic presentation, prospective evaluation of group A, β-hemolytic streptococcal infections has revealed that subclinical disease is common both in infected patients (up to 20% of whom may be affected) and in family members [4,6]. This occult syndrome is characterized clinically by microscopic hematuria, mild proteinuria, or hypocomplementemia, or a combination of these, and by mild mesangial changes on renal biopsy.

Diagnosis

The diagnosis of poststreptococcal glomerulonephritis is suggested by the history, urinary findings, and hypocomplementemia. Evidence of a recent streptococcal infection is best obtained from serologic tests, since throat or skin culture may be negative, especially if antimicrobials have already been administered. The plasma antistreptolysin O (ASO) titer is elevated in approximately 75 to 80 percent of patients with pharyngitis, but only 50 percent of those with impetigo, perhaps due to inactivation of this antigen by skin lipids [11]. Thus, measurement of other antistreptococcal antibodies, such as anti-DNAase B and antihyaluronidase, is often required to document a recent streptococcal infection [11].

The differential diagnosis includes other causes of acute glomerulonephritis, including membranoproliferative glomerulonephritis, IgA nephropathy, rapidly progressive glomerulonephritis, and lupus nephritis. Clues suggestive of poststreptococcal glomerulonephritis are the history, positive serologic tests, and improvement in renal function that usually begins within 1 to 2 weeks [13]. Establishing the diagnosis of poststreptococcal glomerulonephritis on clinical grounds is important because *renal biopsy is not necessary* in this disorder in which spontaneous recovery is the rule.

Treatment and Prognosis

Treatment of poststreptococcal glomerulonephritis is essentially supportive, since there is no specific therapy for the renal disease. Penicillin (in nonallergic patients) should be administered to control the local symptoms and to prevent spread of the infection to close contacts. Antimicrobial therapy, however, does not appear to prevent the development of glomerulonephritis, with the possible exception of very early therapy (within 36 hours) [14]. This finding suggests that the pathogenetic events in the development of poststreptococcal glomerulonephritis occur very early even though clinical disease is not apparent for 7 to 21 days.

Treatment should also be directed toward removal of excess fluid in edematous patients. This can usually be achieved with loop diuretics, leading to loss of edema and to correction of hypertension.

Spontaneous recovery of renal function occurs in almost all patients, even those with advanced renal insufficiency [13,15]. With current supportive therapy, death or irreversible renal failure during the initial episode probably occurs in less than 1 percent of children and perhaps a slightly higher percentage of adults [16]. In general, a diuresis begins within 1 week, and the plasma creatinine concentration returns to normal by 3 to 4 weeks [13]. This is associated with resolution of the histologic changes as evidenced by a marked reduction in the number of deposits, the neutrophilic infiltration, and the cellular proliferation [17].

The urinary changes tend to disappear more slowly. Hematuria usually resolves within 6 weeks; proteinuria also tends to fall during recovery from the acute episode, but a mild increase in protein excretion is still present in 15 percent of cases at 3 years and 2 percent at 7 to 10 years [18]. Resolution is slower in those patients with initially marked proteinuria; nephrotic range proteinuria, for example, may persist for 6 months or more. This problem is most likely to occur when there are a large number of subepithelial deposits (as in Fig. 34-1B) [18a]. The persistent elevation in protein excretion in this setting may reflect delayed healing of the initial injury or some degree of irreversible, probably complement-mediated glomerular damage, as also occurs with subepithelial deposits in membranous nephropathy (see Chap. 29).

Although most patients have apparently complete recovery from the acute episode, the *long-term prognosis is not necessarily benign*. Some patients develop hypertension, proteinuria (with a benign urine sediment), and renal insufficiency as long as 10 to 40 years after the initial illness [16,19,20]. These late problems are associated with glomerular and vascular sclerosis on renal biopsy and are thought to represent hemodynamically mediated injury [19]. According to this hypothesis, some glomeruli are irreversibly damaged during the episode of acute glomerulonephritis but the total glomerular filtration rate stays within the normal range because of compensatory hyperfiltration in the remaining, less-affected glomeruli. This adaptive response is mediated in part by a rise in intraglomerular pressure that, over a period of many years, can lead to glomerulosclerosis (see Chap. 56).

The frequency with which late renal disease occurs is not known, but it is probably well below the initial estimates of 50 percent [18,20]. Nevertheless, periodic monitoring is required after the acute episode. Lowering the intraglomerular pressure with dietary protein restriction or a converting enzyme inhibitor may be beneficial in those patients who develop late evidence of progressive disease.

Bacterial Endocarditis

A similar form of postinfectious glomerulonephritis can occur with bacterial endocarditis or an infected ventriculoatrial shunt [2,21,22]. Although a variety of organisms may be involved, the most common are *Staphylococcus aureus* in acute bacterial endocarditis, *Streptococcus viridans* in subacute bacterial endocarditis, and *Staphylococcus epidermidis* with an infected shunt.

The pathologic findings in these disorders are often similar to those in poststreptococcal glomerulonephritis. In comparison to the latter disorder, however, the duration of antigenemia is often prolonged with endocarditis or shunt nephritis due to delays in diagnosis and treatment. As a result, more prominent immune complex deposition may occur with mesangial and subendothelial deposits occurring as well as subepithelial humps. These changes can lead to thickening of the glomerular capillary wall and a light microscopic picture similar to that in membranoproliferative glomerulonephritis (see Chap. 35).

The clinical manifestations of the renal disease are similar to those in poststreptococcal glomerulonephritis. The nephrotic syndrome is unusual in endocarditis but may occur in up to 30 percent of patients with shunt nephritis [22]. The plasma C3, C4, and C2 levels are diminished in both conditions, suggesting that complement activation has occurred by the classic pathway.

The diagnosis of either of these disorders is usually suggested by the history (including the presence of a ventriculoatrial shunt), physical examination, positive blood cultures, and abnormal urinalysis. However, glomerulonephritis must be differentiated from a drug-induced acute interstitial nephritis and, in endocarditis, from infected or sterile renal emboli. The presence of embolic disease, which can occur as late as several months after bacteriologic cure, should be suspected if there is unilateral flank pain or evidence of other systemic emboli; the diagnosis can be confirmed by demonstrating focal perfusion defects on a radionuclide scan.

Distinction of interstitial nephritis from glomerulonephritis is made primarily by the timing of the disease. Glomerular involvement is typically near or at its peak of severity just before the institution of antimicrobial therapy. In contrast, acute interstitial nephritis is a late event, usually requiring 10 or more days of drug treatment [23]. Eosinophilia, eosinophiluria, and recurrence of fever are also suggestive of this disorder (see Chap. 46).

The severity of the renal disease is primarily related to the duration of infection prior to the institution of appropriate antimicrobial therapy. In general, control of the infection (including removal of an infected shunt) leads to rapid resolution of the glomerular disease with return of renal function to or near the patient's previous baseline [21,22]. However, irreversible renal failure has occurred in selected patients with severe acute disease (initial plasma creatinine concentration above 4 mg/dl), particularly if there has been a long delay in the administration of antimicrobials [21].

References

1. Wilson, CB, Dixon, FJ. Renal response to immunologic injury. In Brenner, BM, Rector, FC, Jr (Eds.), *The Kidney* (3rd ed.). Philadelphia: Saunders, 1986. Pp. 840-843.
2. Rose, BD. *Pathophysiology of Renal Disease* (2nd ed). New York: McGraw-Hill, 1987. Pp. 222-230.
3. Smith, MC, Cooke, JH, Zimmerman, CM, Bird, JJ, Feaster, BL, Morrison, RE, Reimann, BEF. Asymptomatic glomerulonephritis after nonstreptococcal upper respiratory infections. *Ann Intern Med* 91:967, 1969.
4. Sagel, I, Treser, G, Ty, A, Yoshizawa, N, Kleinberger, H, Yuceoglu, AM, Wasserman, E, Lange, K. Occurrence and nature of glomerular lesions after group A streptococci infections in children. *Ann Intern Med* 79:492, 1973.
5. Stetson, CA, Rammelkamp, CH, Jr, Krause, RM, Kohen, RJ, Perry, WD. Epidemic acute nephritis: Studies on etiology, natural history, and prevention. *Medicine* 34:431, 1955.
6. Anthony, BF, Kaplan, EL, Wannamaker, LW, Briese, FW, Chapman, SS. Attack rates of acute nephritis after type 49 streptococcal infection of the skin and of the respiratory tract. *J Clin Invest* 48:1697, 1969.
7. Friedman, J, Van de Rijn, I, Ohkuni, H, Fischetti, VA, Zabriskie, JB. Immunological studies of poststreptococcal sequelae. Evidence for presence of streptococcal antigens in circulating immune complexes. *J Clin Invest* 74:1027, 1984.
8. Vogt, A, Batsford, S, Rodriguez-Iturbe, B, Garcia, R. Cationic antigens in poststreptococcal glomerulonephritis. *Clin Nephrol* 20:271, 1983.
9. Vogt, A. New aspects of the pathogenesis of immune complex glomerulonephritis: Formation of subepithelial deposits. *Clin Nephrol* 21:15, 1984.
10. McIntosh, RM, Garcia, R, Rubio, L, Rabideau, D, Allen, JE, Carr, RI, Rodriguez-Iturbe, B. Evidence for an autologous immune complex pathogenic mechanism in acute poststreptococcal glomerulonephritis. *Kidney Int* 14:501, 1978.
11. Rodriguez-Iturbe, B. Epidemic poststreptococcal glomerulonephritis. *Kidney Int* 25:129, 1984.
12. Rodriguez-Iturbe, B, Baggio, B, Colina-Chourio, J, Favaro, S, Garcia, R, Sussana, F, Castillo, L, Borsatti, A. Studies on the renin-aldosterone system in the acute nephritic syndrome. *Kidney Int* 19:445, 1981.
13. Lewy, JE, Salinas-Madrigal, L, Herdson, PB, Pirani, CL, Metcoff, J. Clinico-pathologic correlations in acute poststreptococcal glomerulonephritis: A correlation between renal functions, morphologic damage, and clinical course of 46 children with acute poststreptococcal glomerulonephritis. *Medicine* 50:453, 1971.
14. Weinstein, L, LeFrock, J. Does antimicrobial therapy of streptococcal pharyngitis or pyoderma alter the risk of glomerulonephritis? *J Infect Dis* 124:229, 1971.
15. Ferrario, F, Kourilsky, O, Morel-Maroger, L. Acute endocapillary glomerulonephritis in adults: A histologic and clinical comparison between patients with and without acute renal failure. *Clin Nephrol* 19:17, 1983.
16. Baldwin, DS. Postreptococcal glomerulonephritis. *Am J Med* 62:1, 1977.
17. Tornroth, T. The fate of subepithelial deposits in acute poststreptococcal glomerulonephritis. *Lab Invest* 35:461, 1976.
18. Potter, EV, Lipschultz, SA, Abidh, S, Poon-King, T, Earle, DP. Twelve to seventeen-year follow-up of patients with poststreptococcal acute glomerulonephritis in Trinidad. *N Engl J Med* 307:725, 1982.
18a. Sorger, K. Gessler, U, Hubner, FK, Kohler, H, Ulbing, H, Schulz, W, Thoenes, GH, Thoenes, W. Follow-up studies of three subtypes of acute postinfectious glomerulonephritis ascertained by renal biopsy. *Clin Nephrol* 27:111, 1987.

19. Baldwin, DS. Chronic glomerulonephritis: Nonimmunologic mechanisms of progressive glomerular damage. *Kidney Int* 21:109, 1982.
20. Lien, JWK, Mathew, TH, Meadows, R. Acute poststreptococcal glomerulonephritis in adults: A long-term study. *Q J Med* 48:99, 1979.
21. Neugarten, J, Baldwin, DS. Glomerulonephritis in bacterial endocarditis. *Am J Med* 77:297, 1984.
22. Arze, RS, Rashid, H, Morley, R, Ward, MK, Kerr, DNS. Shunt nephritis: Report of two cases and review of the literature. *Clin Nephrol* 19:48, 1983.
23. Nolan, CM, Abernathy, RS. Nephropathy associated with methicillin therapy: Prevalence and determinants in patients with staphylococcal bacteremia. *Arch Intern Med* 137:997, 1977.

35. MEMBRANOPROLIFERATIVE GLOMERULONEPHRITIS

Membranoproliferative glomerulonephritis (MPGN) is an uncommon cause of glomerular disease in both children and adults [1-3]. It primarily occurs between the ages of 8 and 30 but can affect patients of any age.

The name of this disorder is derived from the characteristic changes seen on light microscopy: diffuse mesangial hypercellularity (often leading to a lobular appearance of the glomerular tuft) and thickening of the basement membrane due to interposition of the mesangial cell cytoplasm between the basement membrane and the endothelial cell (Fig. 35-1). These changes are also associated with the deposition of new basement membrane–like material between the mesangial and endothelial cells, leading to a double-contour or tram-track appearance of the glomerular capillary wall.

Two major forms of idiopathic MPGN have been described that have different electron microscopic changes and mechanisms of complement activation [2,3]. Type 1 is charaterized by discrete mesangial and subendothelial deposits on electron microscopy*, similar to those seen in diffuse proliferative lupus nephritis; in comparison, type 2 is also called *dense deposit disease* because of the continuous, dense, ribbonlike deposits along the basement membranes of the glomeruli, tubules, and Bowman's capsule (Fig. 35-2). Immunofluorescent microscopy in the latter disorder is positive for C3 but is generally negative for immunoglobulins.

Both types 1 and 2 are usually associated with persistent hypocomplementemia [1,2]. In type 1, complement activation (perhaps initiated by immune complexes) occurs by the *classic* pathway. The plasma complement levels tend to be moderately reduced and may be normal in some patients. In comparison, marked hypocomplementemia due to activation of the *alternate* complement pathway occurs in type 2 [2]. Furthermore, the fall in complement levels appears to result primarily from enhanced peripheral catabolism, rather than deposition in the glomeruli. A circulating IgG, called *C3 nephritic factor* (C3NeF), appears to play an important role in this process [2,5]. This immunoglobulin is a conformational autoantibody that is directed against and binds to C3bBb, the *C3 convertase* of the alternate pathway that normally cleaves C3 into C3a and C3b [5]. C3NeF protects C3bBb from enzymatic inactivation, thereby permitting continued C3 breakdown.

The origin and clinical importance of C3NeF is uncertain; disease activity does not correlate with either complement or C3NeF levels and progressive renal damage can occur in patients who are persistently normocomplementemic [3].

---

*A third form of MPGN has also been described in which subepithelial, as well as mesangial and subendothelial, deposits are found. Recent studies, however, suggest that this disorder is probably a variant of type 1 MPGN [4].

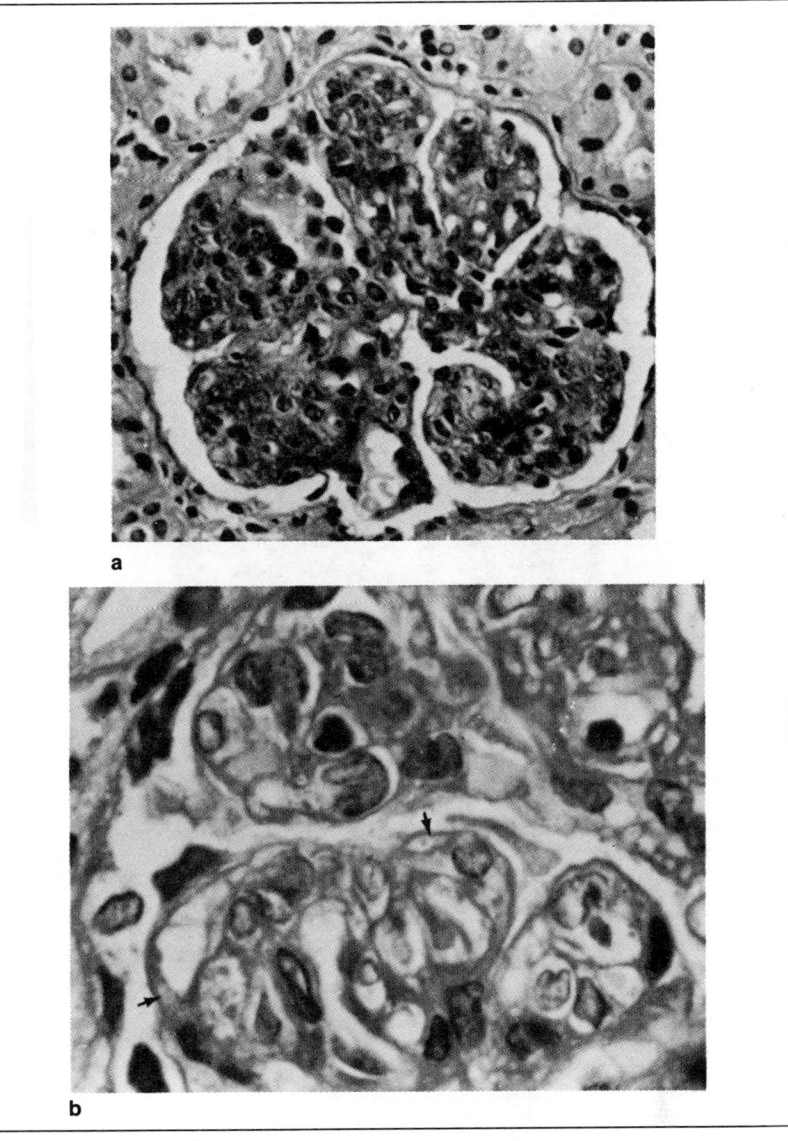

Fig. 35-1. Histologic findings in membranoproliferative glomerulonephritis. (a) Light microscopy typically shows increased cellularity, basement membrane thickening, and a lobular appearance of the glomerular tuft. (b) Higher power also reveals splitting of the glomerular basement membrane, resulting in a double contour or tram-track appearance of the capillary wall (arrows). (c) Electron microscopy demonstrates that widening of the basement membrane is primarily due to growth of the mesangial cell cytoplasm between the basement membrane (BM) and the endothelium (En). New basement membrane-like material is then formed between the interposed mesangium and the endothelial cell (arrow), leading to the characteristic double contour (From BD Rose, *Pathophysiology of Renal Disease* (2nd ed.). New York: McGraw-Hill, 1987.).

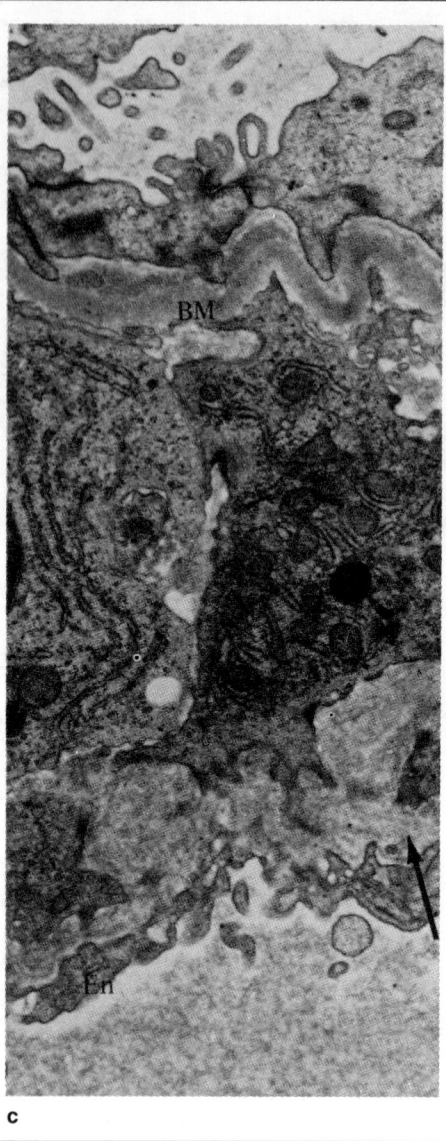

Fig. 35-1. (continued)

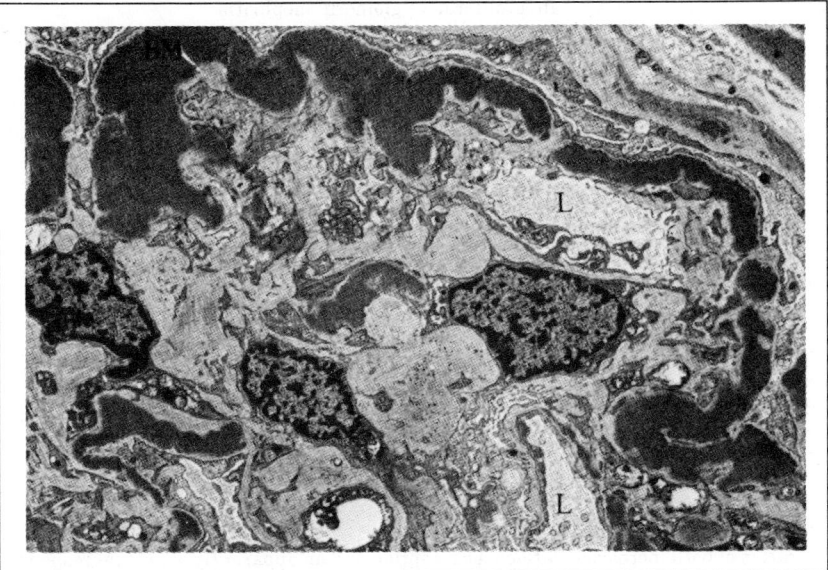

Fig. 35-2. Electron microscopy in type 2 membranoproliferative glomerulonephritis (MPGN) reveals dense, continuous ribbonlike deposits along the glomerular basement membrane (BM). Similar deposits can be found in the basement membranes of the tubules and Bowman's capsule. The tubular lumen (L) is markedly narrowed.

Etiology and Pathogenesis

Although MPGN is often idiopathic, a variety of underlying diseases have been associated with this disorder (Table 35-1) [3]. This finding may be in part a reflection of the nonspecific nature of the membranoproliferative changes in the glomeruli. For example, the electron microscopic findings in type 1 MPGN (mesangial and subendothelial deposits) suggest deposition of circulating immune complexes. It is not surprising, therefore, that MPGN can occur in those conditions in which immune complexes are continuously being formed, such as bacterial endocarditis or an infected ventriculoatrial shunt, chronic hepatitis B virus infection, and visceral abscesses.

The etiology of idiopathic type 1 MPGN is less clear. An intriguing observation is that IgG3 (one of four subclasses of IgG) appears to be the only or the predominant immunoglobulin deposited in the glomeruli (a pattern that is not seen in other forms of glomerulonephritis) [6]. These findings suggest a possible viral etiology, since IgG3 is the primary antiviral IgG.

The cause of the ribbonlike deposits in type 2 MPGN is also unknown. Immune complexes may not be important in this disorder, since immunoglobulins are frequently absent on immunofluorescent microscopy, and the deposits on electron microscopy do not have the characteristic discrete appearance typically seen with immune complex–mediated conditions. The rapid recurrence of type 2 MPGN in almost all patients who receive a renal transplant suggests the presence of a circulating factor that directly damages the renal basement membranes [7]. However, immune mechanisms may be involved in at least some patients as evidenced by the elution of melanoma antigen and antimelanoma antibody from the glomeruli of a patient with type 2 MPGN and malignant melanoma [8].

Regardless of the initial mechanism of glomerular damage, secondary platelet activation may be an important mediator of the inflammatory changes in MPGN. The dem-

Table 35-1. Causes of membranoproliferative glomerulonephritis

Idiopathic
Hepatitis B virus
Bacterial endocarditis or an infected ventriculoatrial shunt
Visceral abscesses
Complement deficient states
Partial lipodystrophy (only with type 2)
Chronic lymphocytic leukemia
Heroin or pentazocine abuse
Mixed cryoglobulinemia
Malignant melanoma
α_1-antitrypsin deficiency
Chlorpropamide
Schistosomiasis
Chronic transplant rejection

onstration of both increased platelet consumption and an apparently beneficial response to therapy with antiplatelet agents is consistent with this possibility [9].

Clinical Presentation and Diagnosis
Patients with MPGN may present in one of four ways: (1) an acute nephritic syndrome similar to that in poststreptococcal glomerulonephritis—macroscopic or microscopic hematuria, edema, and hypertension; (2) recurrent episodes of gross hematuria (similar to IgA nephropathy); (3) the incidental discovery of hematuria and proteinuria on a routine urinalysis; or (4) the insidious onset of edema due to nephrotic syndrome [1-3]. The first two modes of presentation often are preceded by an upper respiratory infection, a finding that is compatible with a viral etiology.

The blood urea nitrogen (BUN) and plasma creatinine concentration are usually normal or only mildly elevated when the patient is first seen; however, advanced renal failure may occur in those patients with an acute nephritic syndrome. The urinalysis typically reveals hematuria, cellular and granular casts, and proteinuria that is in the nephrotic range in over one-half of patients.

The different modes of presentation mean that MPGN can simulate either focal or diffuse glomerulonephritis (see Chap. 25). The differential diagnosis, therefore, can include IgA nephropathy, rapidly progressive or poststreptococcal glomerulonephritis, and lupus nephritis (assuming that no underlying cause of MPGN can be identified [Table 35-1]). The major clinical clue suggesting idiopathic MPGN is *hypocomplementemia*, occurring in the absence of the clinical and serologic abnormalities of lupus and in the absence of evidence of a recent streptococcal infection. The diagnosis, however, must be confirmed by renal biopsy.

Course
Most patients with idiopathic MPGN eventually progress to end-stage renal disease [1-3]. The course is usually prolonged: the glomerular filtration rate may be relatively stable for the first few years but about one-half of patients will have renal failure by 10 years. Bad prognostic findings include type 2 disease, early renal insufficiency (particularly if crescents are seen on renal biopsy), hypertension, and persistent nephrotic syndrome.

Some patients, however, follow a relatively benign course. These patients are more likely to present with asymptomatic hematuria and proteinuria and to have focal, rather than diffuse, glomerular involvement [10].

Treatment
A variety of different therapeutic regimens have been used in MPGN with somewhat conflicting results [3]. Two modalities, however, appear to be effective in at least some patients: long-term, alternate-day *corticosteroids,* and *antiplatelet agents.*

The use of corticosteroids has been primarily evaluated in children. In a large uncontrolled study, for example, prednisone was administered in a dose of 2 mg/kg to a maximum of 80 mg every other day for 1 year, followed by slow tapering to a maintenance dose of 20 mg every other day that was continued for 3 to 10 years [1]. In most patients, this regimen was associated with stable renal function and, on repeat renal biopsy, decreased cellular proliferation but some glomerulosclerosis. At 15 years, only 10 percent had progressed to end-stage renal disease as compared to 50 percent or more in historical controls. Type 1 MPGN seemed to have a better response.

The effectiveness of long-term prednisone has been better evaluated by a controlled trial performed by the International Study of Kidney Disease in Children [11]. In type 1 MPGN, the children treated with prednisone had a substantially lower incidence of progressive renal insufficiency (5 versus 43%). This benefit, however, was offset in many patients by corticosteroid toxicity, particularly marked exacerbation of hypertension, possibly leading to seizures.

Some controlled trials also suggest that the progressive nature of MPGN can be slowed by the use of antiplatelet agents* [9,12]. In one study, for example, the use of aspirin (975 mg/day) and dipyridamole (225 mg/day) for 1 year reversed the common increase in platelet consumption, substantially slowed the rate of decline in glomerular filtration rate (1.3 versus 19.6 ml/min/1.73 m^2/year in the control group), and reduced the incidence of progression to renal failure (14 versus 47% at 3–5 years) [9]. Warfarin has been added to dipyridamole in two other studies; this combination should probably be avoided since it is associated with a high incidence (up to 40%) of bleeding complications [12,13].

In summary, the optimal treatment of idiopathic MPGN is at present uncertain. Therapy can probably be withheld in those patients who appear to be at low risk for progressive disease, for example, those with a normal plasma creatinine concentration, normal blood pressure, nonnephrotic proteinuria, and focal glomerular changes on renal biopsy [2,10].

In comparison, treatment is probably warranted in most other patients with MPGN in view of the progressive course that is typically seen. Children, especially those with type 1 disease, can be tried on the alternate-day prednisone regimen [1,11]. Careful monitoring of the blood pressure is essential in this setting, since marked hypertension can be induced. Children who fail on prednisone and adults can be given a trial of aspirin and dipyridamole [9,12]. It should be emphasized that the plasma creatinine concentration is often stable for several years in patients with untreated MPGN. Thus, monitoring of the urinalysis is also important since decreases in protein excretion and in the activity of the urinary sediment are frequently the earliest clinical signs of a beneficial response to therapy.

Dialysis or transplantation can be used in patients who develop end-stage renal failure. There is, however, a high incidence of recurrent disease in the transplanted kidney, averaging 30 percent in type 1 and almost 90 percent in type 2 MPGN [7,14]. Fortunately, most cases are asymptomatic and loss of the transplant due to recurrent MPGN occurs in only about 10 percent of cases [14]. This is most likely to occur in those patients whose initial disease progressed to renal failure within a few years. Delaying transplantation for 1 year may be beneficial in this setting by allowing the activity of the underlying disorder to diminish.

---

*Although two studies have been positive, a third found no benefit from anticoagulant therapy at 2 years [13]. The cause of these disparate results is uncertain; one possibility is that the follow-up was too short in the last trial, although this remains unproved.

References

1. West, CD. Childhood membranoproliferative glomerulonephritis: An approach to management. *Kidney Int* 29:1077, 1986.
2. Cameron, JS, Turner, DR, Heaton, J, Williams, DG, Ogg, CS, Chantler, C, Haycock, GB, Hicks, J. Idiopathic mesangiocapillary glomerulonephritis and alpha₁-antitrypsin deficiency in children and adults and long-term prognosis. *Am J Med* 74:175, 1983.
3. Rose, BD. *Pathophysiology of Renal Disease* (2nd ed). New York: McGraw-Hill, 1987. Pp. 230-237.
4. Jackson, EC, McAdams, AJ, Strike, CF, Forristal, J, Welch, TR, West, CD. Differences between MPGN types I and III in clinical presentation, glomerular morphology, and complement perturbation. *Am J Kid Dis* 9:115, 1987.
5. Daha, MR, Austen, KF, Fearon, DT. Heterogeneity, polypeptide chain composition, and antigenic reactivity of C3 nephritic factor. *J Immunol* 120:1389, 1978.
6. Bannister, KM, Howarth, GS, Clarkson, AR, Woodroffe, AJ. Glomerular IgG subclass distribution in human glomerulonephritis. *Clin Nephrol* 19:161, 1982.
7. Galle, P, Mahieu, P. Electron dense alterations of kidney basement membranes: A renal lesion specific of a systemic disease. *Am J Med* 58:749, 1975.
8. Olson, JL, Philips, TM, Lewis, MG, Solez, K. Malignant melanoma with renal dense deposits containing tumor antigens. *Clin Nephrol* 12:74, 1979.
9. Donadio, JV, Jr. Anderson, CF, Mitchell, JC, III, Holley, KE, Ilstrup, DM, Fuster, V, Cheesbro, JH. Membranoproliferative glomerulonephritis. A prospective clinical trial of platelet inhibitor therapy. *N Engl J Med* 310:1421, 1984.
10. Strife, CF, McAdams, AJ, West, CD. Membranoproliferative glomerulonephritis characterized by focal, segmental proliferative lesions. *Clin Nephrol* 18:9, 1982.
11. A Report of the International Study of Kidney Disease in Children. Alternate day steriod therapy in membranoproliferative glomerulonephritis: A randomized controlled trial (abstract). *Kidney Int* 21:150, 1982.
12. Zimmerman, S, W, Moorthy, AV, Dreher, WH, Friedman, A, Varanasi, U. Prospective trial of warfarin and dipyridamole in patients with membranoproliferative glomerulonephritis. *Am J Med* 75:920, 1983.
13. Cattran, DC, Cardella, CJ, Roscoe, JM, Charron, RC, Rance, PC, Ritchie, SM, Corey, PN. Results of a controlled drug trial in membranoproliferative glomerulonephritis. *Kidney Int* 27:436, 1985.
14. Cameron, JS. Glomerulonephritis in renal transplants. *Transplantation* 34:237, 1982.

36. LUPUS NEPHRITIS

Renal involvement is common in systemic lupus erythematosus (SLE). An abnormal urinalysis with or without an elevated plasma creatinine concentration is present in approximately 50 percent of patients at the time of diagnosis and eventually develops in up to 75 percent of cases. However, focal or diffuse proliferative glomerulonephritis may be seen in many of those patients who have no urinary abnormalities [1], raising the total incidence of renal involvement to approximately 90 percent. It is of interest that, at 5- to 10-year follow-up, many of these patients with histologic but not clinical disease continue to behave as if they have no renal damage.

Four distinct forms of glomerular involvement have been identified in SLE: *mesangial, focal* or *diffuse proliferative* (focal disease is arbitrarily considered to be present if fewer than 50% of glomeruli are affected on light microscopy), and *membranous* (Fig. 36-1) [2,3]. Although they have different histologic and clinical characteristics (Table 36-1), these disorders cannot be considered to be strictly separate since 15 to 40 percent of patients change from one form to another [2,4]. This evolution is not surprising be-

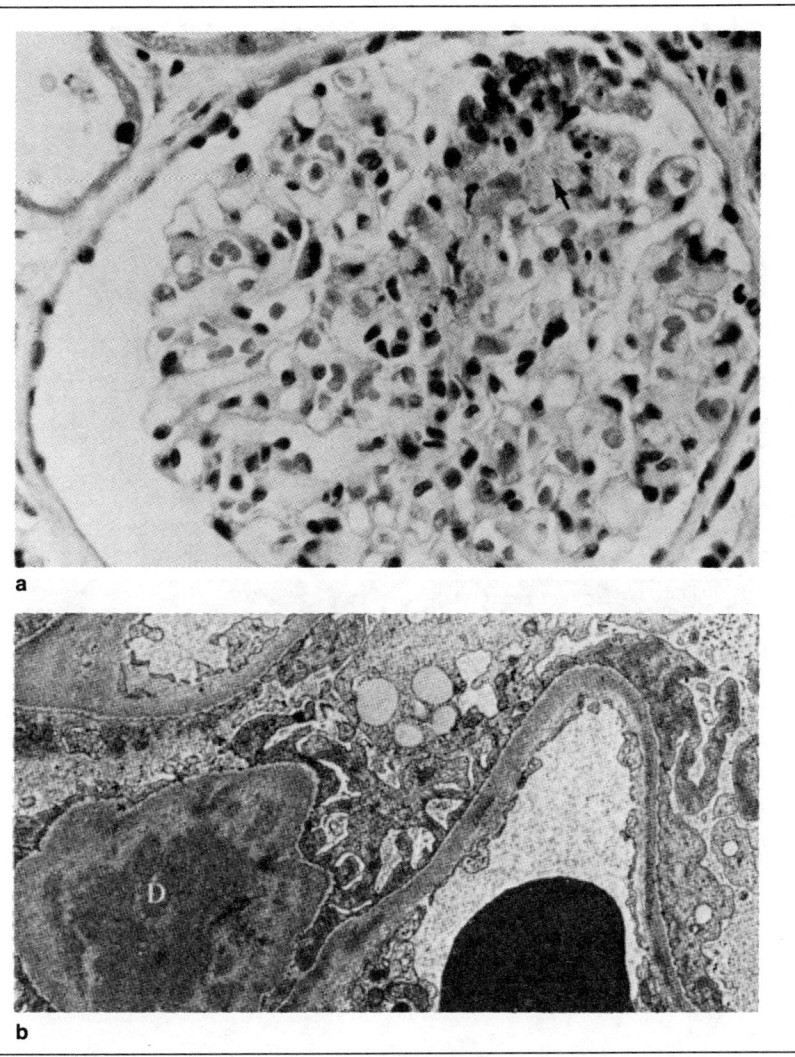

Fig. 36-1. Major histologic changes in lupus glomerulonephritis. (a) Light microscopy in mesangial or mild focal proliferative disease shows segmental areas of cellular proliferation. On electron microscopy, these findings are accompanied by dense deposits (D) limited to the mesangium (b) or extending into the subendothelial space (c) in mesangial and proliferative lupus, respectively. (d) Light microscopy in the diffuse proliferative form demonstrates more severe changes characterized by hypercellularity, basement, membrane thickening with wire-loop formation (arrow) due to marked immune complex deposition [as in (c)], and enlargement of the glomerular tuft filling Bowman's space. (e) All of the forms of lupus nephritis are frequently associated with intraendothelial, tubuloreticular particles (arrow) that are thought to represent aggregates of interferon. The histologic findings in membranous lupus are similar to those in idiopathic membranous nephropathy (see Chap. 29). (From Rose, BD. *Pathophysiology of Renal Disease* [2nd ed.]. New York: McGraw-Hill, 1987.)

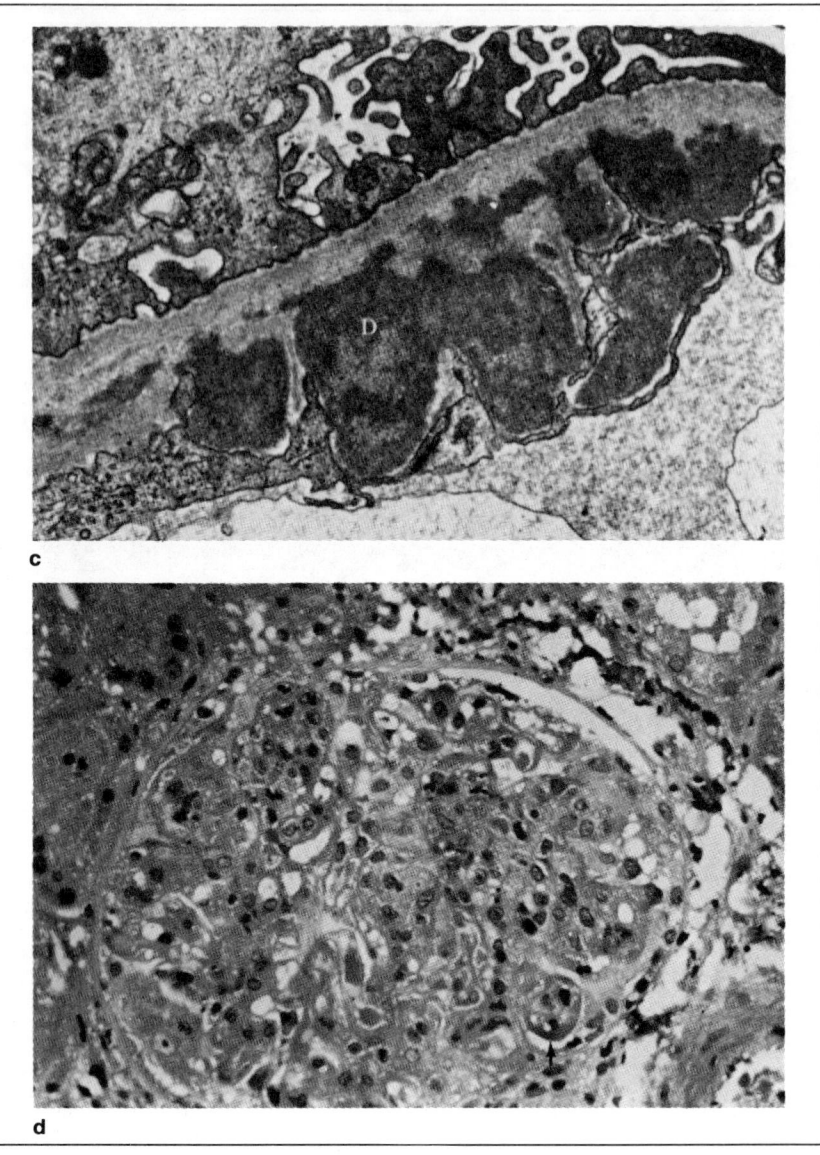

Fig. 36-1. (continued)

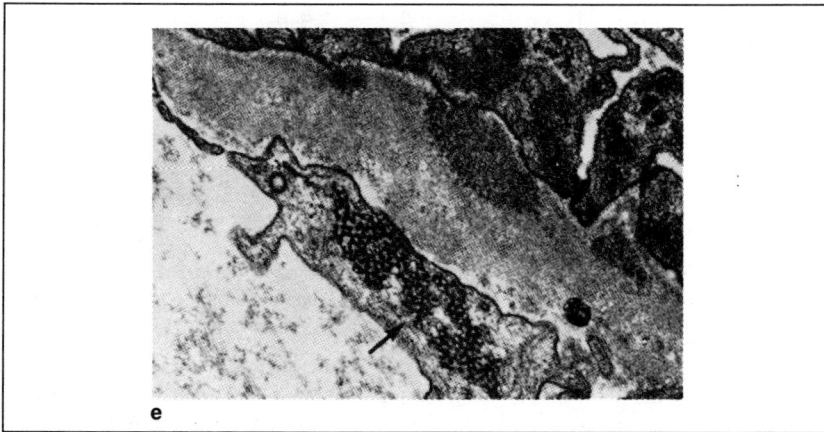

e

Fig. 36-1. (continued)

cause the different types of lupus nephritis represent *nonspecific responses to immuno-logic injury,* replicating the histologic patterns seen in other glomerulopathies. For ex-ample, diffuse proliferative and membranous lupus nephritis are histologically similar to membranoproliferative glomerulonephritis (type 1) and idiopathic membranous ne-phropathy, respectively.

Pathogenesis
Autoantibody formation is a central event in SLE and it is thought that the deposition of DNA–anti-DNA complexes, with the subsequent activation of complement, is respon-sible for the glomerular injury [3,5]. The observation that DNA has a high affinity for binding to basement membranes may explain its propensity for glomerular deposition [6].

In addition, the quantity of antigen and the intensity of the antibody response appear to be important determinants of the pattern of glomerular injury that is seen [3]. Im-mune complexes are initially deposited in the mesangium, producing a disease that is limited to that area (mesangial lupus). If, however, the quantity of the complexes formed exceeds the capacity of the mesangium, there is expansion of the deposits into the ad-jacent sub*endothelial* space (Fig. 36-1C), leading to focal or diffuse proliferative lupus nephritis.

The pathogenesis of membranous lupus appears to be somewhat different. Experi-mental studies of membranous nephropathy (in which deposits are formed across the glomerular basement membrane in the sub*epithelial* space) indicate that (1) cationic antigens are most likely to cross the negatively charged basement membrane and that (2) free antigen and free antibody are deposited at different times (the in situ mechanism of complex formation), rather than as an intact complex [7]. There is suggestive evidence that these principles apply to humans: Patients with membranous lupus tend to form fewer antibodies (the ANA titer may initially be negative in 20–50 % of cases) and to have fewer circulating intact complexes than patients with proliferative lupus nephritis [3,8].

Drug-Induced Lupus
A lupuslike syndrome may be induced by a variety of drugs. This is most likely to occur with hydralazine and procainamide, drugs that are metabolized by hepatic acetylation [3]. It may also be seen with other agents including isoniazid, quinidine, penicillamine, β-adrenergic blockers, and methyldopa [3]. Studies with hydralazine and procainamide suggest that the autoantibodies are primarily directed against nuclear histones or a drug-histone complex, not against DNA as in idiopathic lupus [9].

Table 36-1. Characteristics of different types of lupus glomerular disease

	Mesangial	Focal proliferative	Diffuse proliferative	Membranous
Approximate incidence, % of patients	10–20	10–20	40–60	10–20
Light microscopy	Normal, or mild, mesangial proliferation	Focal segmental mesangial and endothelial proliferation. Areas of necrosis may also be seen.	Diffuse proliferative and necrotizing lesions. "Wire-loop" changes and crescents may be found.	Diffuse basement membrane thickening as in other forms of membranous nephropathy
Immunofluorescence	IgG, C3, and sometimes IgA, IgM in granular pattern in mesangial areas even if LM is normal	Diffuse mesangial and occasionally capillary wall granular deposition of IgG, C3, C4, and less commonly IgM, IgA	Diffuse granular staining throughout glomeruli for IgG, C3, C4, IgM, and occasionally IgA	Diffuse granular deposition in capillary walls of IgG, C3, and less commonly IgA
Electron microscopy (intraendothelial viruslike particles seen in all forms)	Deposits only in mesangium	Deposits in mesangium and in subendothelial and subepithelial areas	Deposits in all sites, larger and more numerous than focal form, especially mesangial and subendothelial	Subepithelial and occasionally mesangial deposits

Clinical presentation	No clinical abnormalities in some. Others have mild proteinuria or hematuria, or both. Nephrotic syndrome, hypertension, and renal insufficiency absent	Proteinuria and hematuria in almost all. Nephrotic syndrome, mild renal insufficiency, hypertension uncommon but may occur	Proteinuria, hematuria in all. Nephrotic syndrome, hypertension, renal insufficiency common and may be severe	Proteinuria in all. Nephrotic syndrome initially in 50%, eventually in 90%. Microscopic hematuria and hypertension may occur. Mild renal insufficiency may be present at onset
Renal prognosis	Excellent unless patient develops diffuse proliferative or membranous forms	Renal insufficiency does not develop unless there is transition to diffuse proliferative glomerulonephritis	If untreated, common progression to end-stage renal failure in 2–4 years. Commonly associated with severe extrarenal lupus. With remission, may develop mesangial or membranous forms	May see slow progression to renal failure in patients with persistent nephrotic syndrome. Remission in one-third. May rarely develop diffuse proliferative form
Treatment for renal disease	None required	None required unless chronic changes or transition to diffuse proliferative form	Prednisone and add cyclophosphamide or azathioprine if chronic changes or progressive increase in P_{cr}. Pulse methylprednisolone for severe acute disease	Probably none if normal renal function. Prednisone with cytotoxic agents if progressive disease or severe nephrosis

Source: From Rose, BD. *Pathophysiology of Renal Disease* (2nd ed). New York: McGraw-Hill, 1987. P. 238.

Risk factors favoring the development of drug-induced lupus include increasing dose, female sex, slow hepatic acetylation, and the HLA-DR4 genotype [10,11]. In one study, for example, lupus developed in 19 percent of women taking 200 mg of hydralazine per day, but 13 of 13 with the HLA-DR4 genotype [11]. Even lower doses may not be safe as clinical disease can occur in up to 5 percent of slow acetylators taking only 100 mg/day [10]. Furthermore, the incidence of asymptomatic autoantibody formation is even higher than that of symptomatic disease, reaching 50 to 80 percent with procainamide in slow acetylators [12].

Clinical Presentation
Patients with SLE, 90 percent of whom are female, typically present with systemic symptoms and signs such as arthralgias, fatigue, malar rash, and pleuritis. Renal disease usually becomes evident within the first year but is occasionally delayed for 3 years or more.

The clinical abnormalities associated with lupus nephritis are typically related to the severity and nature of the histologic changes [2,13]. Patients with the proliferative forms, for example, present with findings characteristic of a *nephritic* disorder (see Chap. 25). Thus, mesangial lupus is usually manifested by asymptomatic microscopic hematuria, red cell casts, or mild proteinuria, or a combination of these; the plasma creatinine concentration, however, is normal. Similar mild findings may be seen with focal proliferative disease, but some patients develop hypertension, a mild elevation in the plasma creatinine concentration, or the nephrotic syndrome. These signs tend to be even more common in diffuse proliferative lupus: the sediment is often very active, containing red and white cells, red cell and other cellular, granular, and fatty casts; the nephrotic syndrome is often present; and hypertension and renal insufficiency of varying severity are common.

In comparison, patients with membranous nephropathy tend to have renal findings similar to other *nephrotic* disorders. Heavy proteinuria and lipiduria are typically present, but the urine sediment tends to be normal or near-normal (with only mild microscopic hematuria), and the plasma creatinine concentration is usually not elevated at the time of presentation [3,14].

Clinically important renal disease is uncommon in drug-induced lupus. However, exceptions do occur as some patients have evidence of a focal or diffuse proliferative glomerulonephritis [15].

Diagnosis
The clinical diagnosis of SLE is usually based on the characteristic multisystem involvement and serologic abnormalities: an elevated ANA titer, circulating antibodies to native (double-stranded) DNA, and low plasma C4 and C3 levels, indicative of activation of the classic complement pathway due, presumably, to immune complex deposition [13]. In comparison, anti-DNA antibodies and hypocomplementemia are unusual in drug-induced lupus [3].

Measurement of the individual complement components may also be indicated in patients with a family history of SLE or other autoimmune disease because *complement deficient states can increase the susceptibility to SLE*. C2 deficiency, for example, may be associated with SLE or other immune complex disease in up to 50 percent of cases [16]. This finding is related to the important role of complement in immune complex removal from the circulation. Activation of the classic complement pathway by circulating complexes leads to the formation of C3b, which attaches to specific receptors on erythrocytes; the erythrocytes then carry the complexes to their site of elimination in the reticuloendothelial system [16]. Complex clearance would therefore be impaired with deficiency of one of the early complement components (C1,C4,C2), thereby promoting deposition in the glomeruli.

An infrequent diagnostic problem arises when patients present with renal disease but no extrarenal or serologic manifestations of SLE. This almost always occurs with membranous lupus [17], which, as described above, is associated in some patients with a

Table 36-2. Treatment of lupus nephritis

Type	Treatment
Mesangial	No specific therapy
Focal proliferative, mild	No specific therapy
Membranous	No specific therapy
Diffuse proliferative*	
Chronic changes	
Few or none	Prednisone
Moderate	Cyclophosphamide (or azathioprine) plus prednisone
Advanced	Control of systemic blood pressure and dietary protein restriction
Acute renal failure	Initiate therapy with pulse methylprednisolone

*The recommendations for diffuse proliferative lupus also apply to those patients with the focal proliferative or membranous forms who have evidence of progressive disease.

lower rate of antibody formation, a negative ANA titer, and normal complement levels [8,13,14]. Even in this setting, however, there are often pathologic findings that suggest the presence of lupus rather than idiopathic membranous nephropathy. These include subendothelial as well as subepithelial deposits, tubular basement membrane deposits*, and tubuloreticular structures (which may represent interferon aggregates) within the endothelial cells (Fig. 36-1) [3].

In most patients, however, renal biopsy is not necessary to confirm the diagnosis of SLE. Rather, biopsy is usually performed to assess the severity of the glomerular disease, because this is an important determinant of the appropriate therapeutic regimen.

Treatment

Many patients with SLE are treated with nonsteroidal anti-inflammatory drugs (including aspirin) or corticosteroids, or both, for control of extrarenal symptoms. The necessity for specific therapy directed against the kidney disease varies with the type of lupus nephritis that is present (Table 36-2) [2,3,18-21]. Mesangial lupus, for example, follows a benign course requiring no treatment. Periodic monitoring, however, is important because transformation to focal or diffuse proliferative glomerulonephritis may occur if the degree of immune complex deposition overwhelms the capacity of the mesangium [2,4].

The renal prognosis is also relatively good in membranous nephropathy [2,14]. Partial or complete remissions in proteinuria may occur, and most patients maintain a normal or near-normal plasma creatinine concentration for 5 or more years. However, some patients develop progressive glomerulosclerosis or transform into the diffuse proliferative form [2,14]. Therapy with a cytotoxic agent and prednisone (see the following) may be beneficial in these settings [18,19].

Focal proliferative glomerulonephritis also tends to have a benign long-term prognosis with no requirement for specific therapy. However, 20 to 30 percent of patients develop progressive renal dysfunction, usually with evidence of transformation into the diffuse

*Tubulointerstitial disease is often seen in SLE and may be mediated in part by tubular complex deposition. This almost always occurs in patients with underlying glomerular disease but has rarely been described as the sole manifestation of lupus nephritis [3]. This condition should be suspected in the patient who presents with renal insufficiency but a relatively normal urinalysis (which is indicative of the lack of glomerular injury).

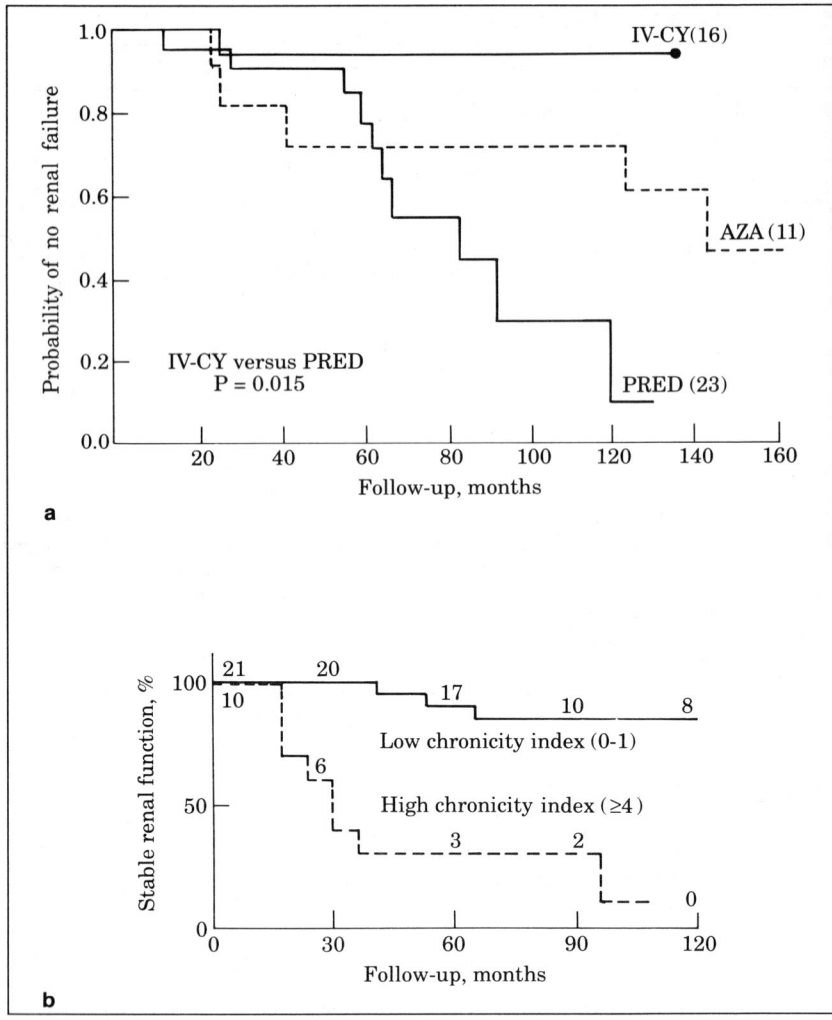

Fig. 36-2. The effect of therapy and the prognostic importance of the severity of "chronic" scarring changes (as defined in text) in patients with diffuse proliferative lupus nephritis. (a) The probability of high-risk patients (those with an important degree of scarring on renal biopsy) not progressing to end-stage renal failure versus time following treatment with intravenous boluses of cyclophosphamide (IV-CY), oral azathioprine (AZA), or oral prednisone alone (PRED). The numbers in parentheses represent the number of patients in each group. A significant improvement occurred in patients treated with cyclophosphamide. (b) The likelihood of having stable renal function (defined as < a twofold rise in the plasma creatinine concentration) versus time according to the degree of chronic changes. Patients with few or no chronic changes had a relatively benign course; those with advanced scarring had a bad prognosis regardless of therapy. An important benefit from the addition of cyclophosphamide occurred only in patients with intermediate chronicity as shown in (a). (Adapted from Steinberg, AD. *Kidney Int* 30:769, 1986, reprinted by permission from Kidney International; and Carette, S, Klippel, JH, Decker, JL, Austin, HA, Plotz, PH, Steinberg, AD, Balow, JE. *Ann Intern Med* 99:1, 1983.)

form [2,4]. This should not be surprising since the distinction of focal from diffuse disease is arbitrary (< or > 50 % of glomeruli involved on light microscopy, respectively).

Diffuse proliferative glomerulonephritis is the most serious form of renal disease in SLE with frequent progression to end-stage renal failure. The optimal therapy of this disorder* remains uncertain. Although some patients respond to prednisone alone (1mg/kg/day with tapering to an alternate-day dose once improvement has occurred), continued glomerular injury and corticosteroid toxicity are major problems. Recent studies, particularly those from the National Institutes of Health, suggest that the addition of a cytotoxic agent (such as cyclophosphamide or azathioprine) substantially enhances renal survival [18-21]. As depicted in Fig. 36-2A, for example, the probability of avoiding renal failure in high-risk patients at 10 to 12 years is over 90 percent with cyclophosphamide, 60 percent with azathioprine, but under 20 percent with prednisone alone. Furthermore, repeat renal biopsy reveals progressive tubular and glomerular scarring only in the prednisone group [19]. These differences in renal survival, however, do not become apparent for more than 5 years after the initiation of therapy; this finding may explain why some earlier studies with shorter periods of follow-up did not demonstrate an advantage of cytotoxic therapy.

The reason for the apparently greater efficacy of cyclophosphamide is incompletely understood. One possibility is that cyclophosphamide is a more potent immunosuppressive agent. An alternative explanation is that prednisone, via its hemodynamic effects, directly promotes glomerular injury. High doses of prednisone lead to renal vasodilation and, at least in experimental animals, an elevation in glomerular capillary pressure. This intraglomerular hypertension can exacerbate experimental renal disease (see Chap. 56) [22] and could have a similar long-term effect in lupus nephritis.

However, the beneficial effect of cyclophosphamide must be weighed against its considerable potential toxicity. Problems such as bone marrow suppression, infection, alopecia, gonadal fibrosis, hemorrhagic cystitis, and late neoplasia (especially cancer of the bladder) all may occur [3,18]. These possible complications often limit patient acceptance, even though the total risk appears small with no demonstrable increase in extrarenal mortality [21]. Net toxicity can also be minimized by treating only those patients who are likely to benefit from cyclophosphamide and by then administering the drug in the safest manner.

The nature of the changes on renal biopsy appears to be the best method of identifying cyclophosphamide-responsive patients. Of greatest importance is the degree of *irreversible "chronic" changes,* such as glomerular scarring, fibrous crescents, tubular atrophy, and interstitial fibrosis [18,19]. Patients with few or no chronic changes seem to be at low risk for progressive glomerular injury and generally respond well to prednisone alone (Fig. 36-2B). On the other hand, patients with marked scarring already have advanced disease that does not usually respond to any form of immunosuppressive therapy. In this setting, the risks of aggressive treatment outweigh the potential benefits. Thus, therapy should probably be limited to control of systemic hypertension (preferably with a converting enzyme inhibitor) and dietary protein restriction to minimize the role of secondary hemodynamic injury (see Chap. 56).

Those patients with *intermediate chronicity* (some but not marked scarring) seem to represent the subgroup most likely to benefit from the addition of cyclophosphamide Fig. 36-2A) [18-20]. The presence of some scarring presumably identifies patients with progressive disease, the severity of which is not yet severe enough to preclude benefit from aggressive immunosuppressive therapy.

Cyclophosphamide is usually administered with low-dose prednisone (0.5 mg/kg/day) which is rapidly tapered to an alternate-day dose. Patient compliance can be improved and at least some of the complications associated with cyclophosphamide minimized by administering the drug in monthly boluses (0.5–1.0 gm/m² of body surface area), rather than in the more common daily oral dose of 2.5 mg/kg/day [18,20]. The intravenous regimen results in up to a two-thirds reduction in total drug dosage per month. It also markedly diminishes the incidence of hemorrhagic cystitis (since the bladder is exposed

---

*The treatment regimen described for diffuse proliferative lupus nephritis also applies to patients with progressive focal proliferative or membranous disease.

to toxic metabolites for only 1 day/month), but it is not known if similar protection is offered against late neoplasia.

The optimal duration of cyclophosphamide therapy is also uncertain. The current recommendation is to give 6 to 8 monthly boluses, followed by maintenance therapy every 3 months for 1 to 3 years [20]. A possibly safer alternative is to use cyclophosphamide for 3 to 6 months to induce a remission of the renal disease (as evidenced by decreased cells and casts in the urine sediment, improvement in and stabilization of the plasma creatinine concentration, and usually return of the plasma C3 level and DNA-binding titer toward the normal range); the patient can then be switched to oral azathioprine (2 mg/kg/day), which has fewer long-term adverse effects. Azathioprine can also be used in patients who refuse (because of the potential complications) or cannot tolerate cyclophosphamide.

More aggressive initial therapy is often required in patients with severe disease who develop acute renal failure. Such patients often have high levels of circulating immune complexes and evidence of an arteritis on renal biopsy [23]. Conventional oral doses of prednisone may be ineffective in this setting and a response to cyclophosphamide is not seen for 1 to 2 weeks. However, beginning therapy with intravenous pulse corticosteroids (250–1000 mg of methylprednisolone given over 30 minutes daily for 3 days) has been effective in controlling the renal and extrarenal manifestations in many patients [23]. This response can then be maintained with cyclophosphamide and prednisone.

End-Stage Renal Disease

Despite the above therapies, 20 to 30 percent of patients will still progress to renal failure. An interesting finding in this setting is the common *complete or partial reversal of the extrarenal and serologic manifestations of the disease* [24]. Furthermore, the lupus remains inactive following dialysis or transplantation and recurrent nephritis in the transplanted kidney is rare [24-26]. Why this occurs is not understood. Although the uremia-induced decrease in immune responsiveness may contribute, reversal of uremia by transplantation does not typically lead to reactivation of the disease. However, recurrent symptoms may occur in selected cases after a remission of 12 months or more [26].

Pregnancy

A final factor that can affect the course of women with lupus nephritis is pregnancy [27,28]. This is associated with an increased risk of fetal loss and exacerbation of the renal and extrarenal abnormalities in 25 to 45 percent of pregnancies. Worsening of the lupus is most often seen in the first 8 weeks after delivery but can occur at any time during the pregnancy. This risk can be minimized if pregnancy is delayed until the disease can be made inactive (if possible) for at least 6 months. It has also been suggested that increasing the corticosteroid dose for 4 to 5 days after delivery can diminish the incidence of postpartum flares [28].

References

1. Leehey, DJ, Katz, AI, Azaran, AH, Aronson, AJ, Spargo, BH. Silent diffuse lupus nephritis: Long-term follow-up. *Am J Kid Dis* 2 (suppl 1):188, 1982.
2. Baldwin, DS, Gluck, MC, Lowenstein, J, Gallo, G. Lupus nephritis: Clinical course as related to morphologic forms and their transitions. *Am J Med* 62:12, 1977.
3. Rose, BD. *Pathophysiology of Renal Disease* (2nd ed). New York: McGraw-Hill, 1987. Pp. 237-253.
4. Lee, HS, Mujais, SK, Kasinath, BS, Spargo, BH, Katz, AI. Course of renal pathology in patients with systemic lupus erythematosus. *Am J Med* 77:612, 1984.
5. Winfield, JB, Faiferman, I, Koffler, D. Avidity of anti-DNA antibodies in serum and IgG glomerular eluates from patients with systemic lupus erythematosus: Association of high avidity antinative DNA antibody with glomerulonephritis. *J Clin Invest* 59:90, 1977.
6. Izui, S, Lambert, PH, Miescher, PA. In vitro demonstration of a particular affinity of glomerular basement membrane and collagen for DNA: A possible basis for the for-

mation of DNA-anti-DNA complexes in systemic lupus erythematosus. *J Exp Med* 144:428, 1976.

7. Couser, WG. Mechanisms of glomerular injury in immune-complex disease. *Kidney Int* 28:569, 1985.

8. Wener, MH, Mannik, M, Schwartz, MM, Lewis, EJ. Relationship between renal pathology and the size of circulating immune complexes in patients with systemic lupus erythematosus. *Medicine* 66:85, 1987.

9. Tan, EM, Portanova, JP. The role of histones as nuclear-autoantigens in drug-related lupus erythematosus. *Arth Rheum* 24:1064, 1981.

10. Cameron, HA, Ramsay, LE. The lupus syndrome induced by hydralazine: A common complication with low dose treatment. *Br Med J* 289:410, 1984.

11. Batchelor, JR, Welsh, KI, Tinoco, RM, Dollery, CT, Hughes, GRV, Bernstein, R, Ryan, P, Naish, PF, Aber, GM, Bing, RF, Russell, GI. Hydralazine-induced systemic lupus erythematosus: Influence of HLA-DR and sex on susceptibility. *Lancet* 1:1107, 1980.

12. Lahita, JR, Kluger, J, Drayer, DE, Koffler, D, Reidenberg, MM. Antibodies to nuclear antigens in patients treated with procainamide or acetylprocainamide. *N Engl J Med* 301:1382, 1979.

13. Appel, GB, Silva, FG, Pirani, CL, Meltzer, JI, Estes, D. Renal involvement in systemic lupus erythematosus: A study of 56 patients emphasizing histologic classification. *Medicine* 57:371, 1978.

14. Donadio, JV, Jr, Burgess, JH, Holley, KE. Membranous lupus nephropathy: A clinicopathologic study. *Medicine* 56:527, 1977.

15. Bjorck, S, Svalander, C, Westberg, G. Hydralazine-associated glomerulonephritis. *Acta Med Scand* 218:261, 1985.

16. Schifferli, JA, Ng, YC, Peters, DK. The role of complement and its receptors in the elimination of immune complexes. *N Engl J Med* 315:488, 1986.

17. Adu, D, Williams, DG, Taube, D, Vilches, AR, Turner, DR, Cameron, JS, Ogg, CS. Late onset systemic lupus erythematosus and lupus-like disease in patients with apparent idiopathic glomerulonephritis. *Q J Med* 52:471, 1983.

18. Austin, HA, III, Klippel, JH, Balow, JE, le Riche, NGH, Steinberg, AD, Plotz, PH, Decker, JL. Therapy of lupus nephritis. Controlled trial of prednisone and cytotoxic drugs. *N Engl J Med* 314:614, 1986.

19. Balow, JE, Austin, HA, III, Muenz, LR, Joyce, KM, Antonovych, TT, Klippel, JH, Steinberg, AD, Plotz, PH, Decker, JL. Effect of treatment on the evolution of the renal abnormalities in lupus nephritis. *N Engl J Med* 311:491, 1984.

20. Steinberg, AD. The treatment of lupus nephritis. *Kidney Int* 30:769, 1986.

21. Felson, DT, Anderson, J. Evidence for the superiority of immunosuppressive drugs and prednisone over prednisone alone in lupus nephritis. Results of a pooled analysis. *N Engl J Med* 311:1528, 1984.

22. Garcia, DL, Anderson, S, Rennke, HG, Brenner, BM. Chronic steroid therapy amplifies glomerular injury in rats with reduced renal mass (abstract). *Clin Res* 32(2):697a, 1986.

23. Kimberly, RP, Lockshin, MD, Sherman, RL, McDougal, JS, Inman, RD, Christian, CL. High-dose intravenous methylprednisolone pulse therapy in systemic lupus erythematosus. *Am J Med* 70:817, 1981.

24. Coplon, NS, Diskin, CJ, Petersen, J, Swenson, RS. The long-term clinical course of systemic lupus erythematosus in end-stage renal disease. *N Engl J Med* 308:186, 1983.

25. Correia, P, Cameron, JS, Ogg, CS, Williams, DG, Bewick, M, Hicks, JA. End-stage renal failure in systemic lupus erythematosus with nephritis. *Clin Nephrol* 22:293, 1984.

26. Amend, WJC, Jr, Vincenti, F, Feduska, NJ, Salvatierra, O, Jr, Johnston, WH, Jackson, J, Tilney, N, Garovoy, M, Burwell, EL. Recurrent systemic lupus erythematosus involving renal allografts. *Ann Intern Med* 94:444, 1981.

27. Hayslett, JP. Effect of pregnancy in patients with SLE. *Am J Kid Dis* 2(suppl 1):223, 1982.

28. Jungers, P, Dougados, M, Pelissier, C, Kuttenn, F, Tron, F, Lesaure, P, Bach, J-F. Lupus nephropathy and pregnancy. Report of 104 cases in 36 patients. *Arch Intern Med* 142:771, 1982.

37. RAPIDLY PROGRESSIVE GLOMERULONEPHRITIS

Rapidly progressive glomerulonephritis (RPGN) is characterized morphologically by crescent formation involving more than 50 percent of the glomeruli (Fig. 37-1) and clinically by progression to end-stage renal disease in most untreated patients within weeks to months. From an etiologic viewpoint, however, crescent formation is nonspecific, potentially occurring with almost any form of proliferative glomerulonephritis or vasculitis. It may also occur as an idiopathic disorder or in association with circulating antibodies directed against the glomerular basement membrane (GBM). Only the last disorders will be discussed in this chapter.

Pathogenesis and Etiology
The primary event in RPGN appears to be damage to the GBM that is severe enough to allow the entry of fibrin or fibrinogen into Bowman's space [1]. This appears to lead to the infiltration of circulating macrophages in an attempt to phagocytose the extravascular fibrin. The macrophages may then promote crescent formation both by comprising most of the cells of the crescent and by the release of monokines that promote epithelial cell proliferation and subsequent enlargement of the crescent [2,3]. Both immunofluorescent and electron microscopy reveal fibrin within the crescents.

This relatively nonspecific response to glomerular injury explains why crescents may be seen in so many different disorders. As a result, immunofluorescent and electron microscopy are very important in establishing the correct diagnosis. For example, the demonstration of mesangial IgA or subepithelial hump-shaped deposits are indicative of underlying IgA nephropathy and poststreptococcal glomerulonephritis, respectively.

In addition, three different idiopathic forms of RPGN have been described; anti-GBM antibody disease, immune complex glomerulonephritis, and nonantibody RPGN.

Anti-GBM Antibody Disease
Anti-GBM antibody disease is characterized by circulating anti-GBM antibodies that deposit in the glomeruli, leading on immunofluorescent microscopy to the *linear deposition* of IgG and less often C3 along the GBM (Fig. 37-2). Linear deposition of IgG may also be found along the basement membranes of the tubules and along the alveolar capillaries, possibly leading to tubulointerstitial damage and pulmonary hemorrhage (the combination of anti-GBM antibody disease and pulmonary bleeding is called Goodpasture's syndrome).

The source of these antibodies is uncertain [1]. IgG eluted from the lung or kidney binds to either of these organs but not to other tissues. It is not clear, however, whether pulmonary or renal damage is the primary event, leading to basement membrane antigens being exposed to the circulation or being made immunogenic. Studies in humans suggest that both of these possibilities may occur. For example, *alveolar injury* is likely to be the initial event in those patients in whom influenza or smoke inhalation precede the onset of the disease. On the other hand, a *renal origin* probably is present when anti-GBM antibody disease develops in the transplanted kidney of selected patients with hereditary nephritis. The latter disorder is often characterized by absence of the Goodpasture antigen* (see Chap. 33); thus, the transplant contains a normal antigen that is now "seen" for the first time and apparently recognized as foreign. The observation that the presence of pulmonary hemorrhage correlates closely with a history of smoking is also compatible with a primary role for renal damage [5]: circulating antibodies appear to have access to the alveolar basement membrane only when there is an increase in lung permeability [5a]. This requirement could also explain the association of pulmonary hemorrhage with hydrocarbon vapor exposure [5a].

---

*The antigen against which anti-GBM antibodies are directed may be an epitope of the noncollagenous domain of type IV collagen [4].

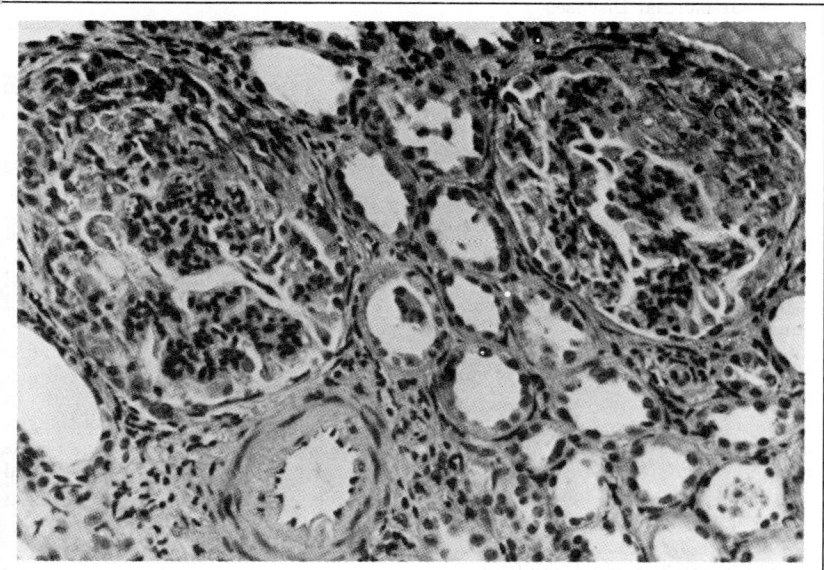

Fig. 37-1. Light microscopy in rapidly progressive glomerulonephritis shows cellular crescents (C) filling Bowman's space and encircling and compressing the capillary tufts. (From Rose, BD. *Pathophysiology of Renal Disease* [2nd ed.]. New York: McGraw-Hill, 1987.)

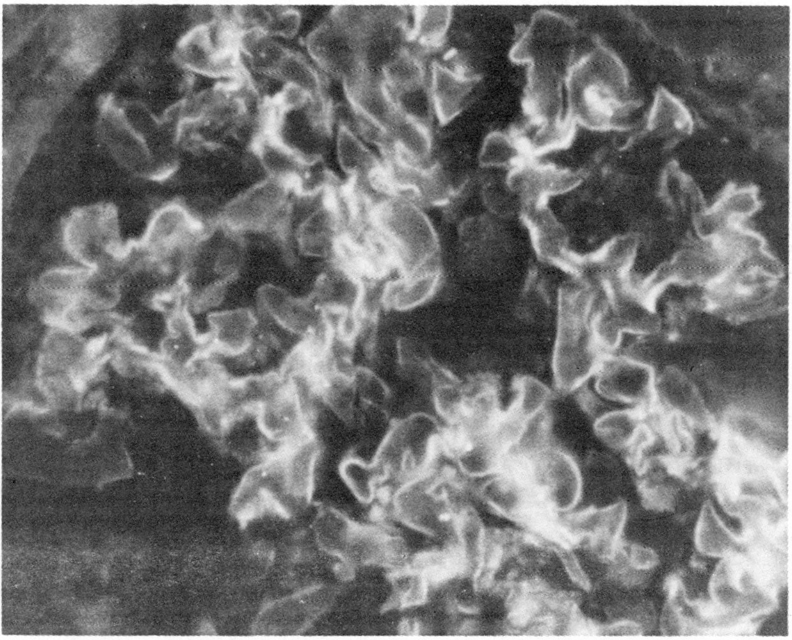

Fig. 37-2. Immunofluorescent microscopy in anti-GBM antibody disease reveals linear deposition of IgG. (From Rose, BD. *Pathophysiology of Renal Disease* [2nd ed.]. New York: McGraw-Hill, 1987.)

Immune Complex Deposition

RPGN may be associated with the deposition of discrete immune deposits in the glomeruli. The inciting antigen in this setting is usually unknown although penicillamine, syphilis, and possibly malignancies have been implicated in isolated cases [1,6,7].

Nonantibody RPGN

Up to 40 percent of patients with idiopathic RPGN have no immune deposits on either immunofluorescent or electron microscopy [8]. Two hypotheses have been proposed to explain the glomerular damage in this setting: underlying vasculitis (in which renal vascular involvement may be focal and easily missed on renal biopsy) and cell-mediated immunity [9,10]. The observation that some patients with apparently idiopathic nonantibody RPGN months later develop biopsy-proved Wegener's granulomatosis is indicative of the potential importance of vasculitis in this disorder [10a]. A role for cell-mediated immunity is as yet unproved in humans, although it has been demonstrated in some animal models of glomerular disease [10,11]. Lymphocytic infiltration of the glomeruli is not present in human RPGN; it is possible, however, that activated T cells against glomerular-bound antigen are only found early in the disease, prior to renal biopsy. These cells could release lymphokines that damage the glomeruli both directly and by promoting the accumulation of macrophages [11].

Clinical Presentation and Diagnosis

Idiopathic RPGN primarily affects adults (mean age about 50 years) with a slight male predominance [8,12]. Goodpasture's syndrome (anti-GBM antibody disease with pulmonary hemorrhage) represents an exception in that 75 to 80 percent of patients are men who are usually 20 to 30 years of age [12]. Although RPGN can occur in children, it is typically due to an identifiable underlying disease such as poststreptococcal glomerulonephritis, Henoch-Schönlein purpura, or membranoproliferative glomerulonephritis.

RPGN usually has an insidious onset [8,12]. A preceding upper respiratory or viral infection is present in many patients; this is followed over a period of weeks to months by nonspecific symptoms that are due to uremia or fluid retention including malaise, weakness, anorexia, edema, and eventually oliguria or anuria. Occasional patients, however, have an abrupt onset, similar to that in poststreptococcal glomerulonephritis in which the patient may present with macroscopic hematuria, decreased urine output, and edema.

Hemoptysis and dyspnea are characteristic of Goodpasture's syndrome and generally precede or occur simultaneously with the onset of the renal disease. The pulmonary hemorrhage and subsequent iron sequestration in the lung can lead to bilateral pulmonary infiltrates on chest x ray and to iron deficiency and an anemia that is out of proportion to the severity of the renal failure. These problems are not, however, specific for Goodpasture's syndrome, since pulmonary hemorrhage can also occur with the other forms of RPGN due to systemic vasculitis, fluid overload, or a uremia-induced increase in pulmonary capillary permeability [13].

Renal insufficiency is present at the time of presentation in almost all patients with RPGN, with the plasma creatinine concentration frequently exceeding 5 mg/dl [8,12,14]. The urinalysis typically reveals hematuria, red cell and other casts, and proteinuria that is usually not in the nephrotic range, presumably due to the very low GFR.

The presence of RPGN should be suspected in any patient presenting with acute oliguric or anuric renal failure and a nephritic sediment. These findings are, however, not diagnostic since they may also be seen with other forms of diffuse glomerulonephritis (such as lupus nephritis or poststreptococcal glomerulonephritis), vasculitis, or acute interstitial nephritis. Thus, renal biopsy is usually indicated unless there are signs, symptoms, or laboratory findings suggestive of a systemic disease. For example, renal biopsy is not required if there is evidence of a recent streptococcal infection or bacterial endocarditis, since postinfectious glomerulonephritis typically improves spontaneously with appropriate medical therapy (see Chap. 34).

If idiopathic RPGN is considered likely on clinical grounds, a rapid diagnosis of anti-GBM antibody disease can occasionally be made by testing for circulating anti-GBM antibodies with indirect immunofluorescence. This test involves incubation of the patient's serum with normal renal tissue; fluorescein-labelled antihuman IgG antibodies are then added to see if IgG deposition has occurred. A positive test is diagnostic of anti-GBM antibody disease, but up to 40 percent of patients have a falsely negative result. Thus, a negative test does not exclude the diagnosis. Radioimmunoassay (the results of which take much longer to obtain) is much more sensitive and is the preferred method for sequential monitoring of anti-GBM antibody titers.

Renal biopsy, if indicated, should not be delayed in patients suspected of having RPGN since *early diagnosis is essential* to allow therapy to be initiated before irreversible renal failure has occurred. It should be noted that linear deposition of IgG on immunofluorescent microscopy (Fig. 37-2) is not diagnostic of anti-GBM antibody disease. A similar finding can occur in other glomerular disorders, particularly diabetic nephropathy [15]. In this setting, however, neither crescents nor circulating anti-GBM antibodies are found and the immunofluorescent findings appear to reflect nonspecific protein adsorption onto the abnormally permeable glomerular capillary wall.

Prognosis

The renal prognosis of untreated RPGN is poor. It has been estimated that 70 to 80 percent of patients with this disorder and over 90 percent of those who are oliguric or anuric will require dialysis within weeks to months [12,16]. There are, however, exceptions to this general rule. Some patients, for example, have a slowly progressive course over a period of months to several years [17]. These patients tend to have less severe lesions on renal biopsy with crescents being found in less than 50 percent of the glomeruli and many of the crescents being segmental, rather than encircling the glomerular tuft.

One other setting in which the course is more benign is poststreptococcal glomerulonephritis where spontaneous recovery to normal or near-normal renal function is common [18]. These patients may, however, lose enough functioning nephrons during the acute episode to be susceptible to progressive hemodynamically mediated glomerulosclerosis over a period of many years (see Chap. 34).

The prognosis and likelihood of a positive response to treatment is *primarily related to the severity of the disease at the time at which therapy is initiated* [12,14,16]. A plasma creatinine concentration above 7 to 8 mg/dl is a bad prognostic sign, particularly in anti-GBM antibody disease in which *recovery of renal function is unusual* [19]. In comparison, prevention of end-stage renal disease is common in the latter disorder if the pretreatment plasma creatinine concentration is below 5 mg/dl [19].

The prognosis for recovery of renal function is somewhat better in those forms of secondary RPGN for which effective therapy of the underlying disorder is available such as vasculitis and systemic lupus erythematosus [16,20]. Even those patients who require dialysis initially may recover enough renal function to allow dialysis to be discontinued [20].

Treatment

In general, oral prednisone given alone or in combination with azathioprine or cyclophosphamide has little effect on the course of idiopathic RPGN [21]. Anticoagulant and antiplatelet therapy have also been tried in view of the central role of fibrin in crescent formation. These agents have had some success in selected patients but their toxicity limits their general use in this disorder [22]. There are, however, two modalities that may lead to a dramatic improvement in both renal function and many of the histologic changes: *pulse methylprednisolone* and *plasmapheresis* [1,2].

Pulse therapy consists of the intravenous administration (over 30 minutes) of 1 gm of methylprednisolone daily for 3 to 5 days followed by oral prednisone in conventional doses of 1 mg/kg/day. More than one-half of patients with idiopathic immune complex or nonantibody RPGN have responded to this regimen with, in some studies, a mean reduction in the plasma creatinine concentration from 10.6 to 2.2 mg/dl [23,24]. Nonresponders are more likely to have irreversible changes such as fibrosis of the crescents or of the glomerular tufts [24]. In comparison, the glomerular injury in anti-GBM antibody disease does not appear to respond to pulse steroid therapy [23].

Although pulse therapy is generally well tolerated, sudden cardiac arrest or a marked elevation in blood pressure has been reported in selected cases [25,26]. As a result, "minipulses" of 250 mg of methylprednisolone have been tried and been found to be as effective in some disorders, such as acute transplant rejection. There is little clinical experience with this regimen in RPGN; nevertheless, it may be advisable from a safety viewpoint to begin with the lower corticosteroid dose.

The mechanism by which high-dose methylprednisolone acts is uncertain. The excess steroid, which is derived from cholesterol, may intercalate into the lipid bilayer of cell membranes, leading to a reduction in inflammatory cell function [27]. Cyclophosphamide is usually not given with pulse therapy, except for patients with nonantibody RPGN who have signs or symptoms suggestive of a systemic vasculitis [1,2].

Plasmapheresis has also been found to be effective in RPGN [16,21,28]. In those patients who respond, renal function begins to improve within 10 days. This modality presumably acts by removing free antibody, intact immune complexes, and mediators of inflammation such as fibrinogen and complement. The fall in circulating immune complexes also may have an important secondary effect: previously saturated Fc receptors in the reticuloendothelial system become unblocked, permitting removal of newly formed complexes [29].

The optimal frequency and duration of plasmapheresis is uncertain. A reasonable plan is to perform 3- to 4-liter daily exchanges for 4 to 6 days and then to assess the clinical and laboratory response. This regimen should remove most of the initially present extra-cellular immunoglobulin; prednisone and cyclophosphamide must also be given to minimize new antibody formation.

With the exception of anti-GBM antibody disease, it appears that pulse therapy and plasmapheresis are equally effective in RPGN. As a result, it seems reasonable to begin with high-dose methylprednisolone since it is less toxic (cyclophosphamide is not required), simpler (vascular access and plasma exchange are not needed), and less expensive. Plasmapheresis can then be added if no improvement is seen within 2 weeks or if progression continues after 1 week.

Those patients who respond should, once their renal function is stable, be slowly tapered to a low maintenance dose of prednisone (15–20 mg every other day) that should be continued for 6 to 9 months. The improvement in renal function often persists for many years although drug-responsive relapses may occur as late as 2 to 4 years after remission has been induced [30].

Anti-GBM Antibody Disease

The above recommendations must be amended in several important ways in patients with anti-GBM antibody disease. First, treatment for the kidney disease should generally be instituted only if the plasma creatinine concentration is less than 7 to 8 mg/dl, since recovery of renal function is rare with more advanced renal failure, particularly in oliguric patients already requiring dialysis [19,20]. The early preservation of renal function is especially important because this disorder tends to be self-limited; circulating anti-GBM antibodies (as assessed by radioimmunoassay) typically disappear spontaneously within 6 to 12 months [31] or after as few as 8 weeks with combined plasmapheresis and immunosuppression [19]. Thus, permanent remission is likely after 12 months, although late relapses have rarely been seen as late as 5 years after apparent resolution of the disease [32].

Second, *plasmapheresis* is the treatment of choice in this disorder*, to prevent both progressive renal failure and, in patients with lung involvement, potentially life-threatening pulmonary hemorrhage [2,19,28,33]; pulse methylprednisolone is usually without effect on the glomerular disease [23] although it can improve the pulmonary disease.

---

*The proper therapy is less clear in patients who have only mild, noncrescentic renal disease with relatively normal renal function [1]. Spontaneous remission can occur in this setting although some patients will eventually progress to crescentic disease. Thus, careful monitoring is essential if it is elected to withhold plasmapheresis because of an apparently benign course.

The patient should be reassessed clinically and serologically after the first 4- to 6-day course of therapy. Further plasmapheresis may be unnecessary if the pulmonary and renal manifestations have improved and the plasma anti-GBM antibody titers are markedly reduced. The patient is then maintained on prednisone and cyclophosphamide for 9 to 12 months*. In patients who are doing well, it may be desirable to switch from cyclophosphamide to the less-toxic azathioprine at 3 to 4 months [19]. Infections should be treated as quickly as possible since they can lead to exacerbation of the renal and pulmonary disease, usually without elevation in anti-GBM antibody levels [34]. How this occurs is not known.

Finally, anti-GBM antibody disease presents a special problem in those patients who progress to end-stage renal failure and are considered for renal transplantation. Early transplantation can lead to recurrent anti-GBM–antibody-mediated glomerulonephritis in the transplant [35]. This can be almost completely prevented if transplantation is delayed for 9 to 12 months, after anti-GBM antibody production has ceased.

References

1. Rose, BD. *Pathophysiology of Renal Disease* (2nd ed). New York: McGraw-Hill, 1987. Pp. 254–262.
2. Salant, DJ. Immunopathogenesis of crescentic glomerulonephritis and lung purpura. *Kidney Int* 32:408, 1987.
3. Magil, AB. Histogenesis of glomerular crescents. Immunohistochemical demonstration of cytokeratin in crescent cells. *Am J Pathol* 120:222, 1985.
4. Kefalides, NA. The Goodpasture antigen and basement membranes: The search must go on. *Lab Invest* 56:1, 1987.
5. Donaghy, M, Rees, AJ. Cigarette smoking and lung hemorrhage in glomerulonephritis caused by antibodies to glomerular basement membrane. *Lancet* 2:1390, 1983.
5a. Yamomoto, T, Wilson, CB. Binding of anti-basement membrane antibody to alveolar basement membrane after intratracheal gasoline instillation in rabbits. *Am J Pathol* 126:497, 1987.
6. Walker, PD, Deeves, EC, Sahba, G, Wallin, JD, O'Neill, WM, Jr. Rapidly progressive glomerulonephritis in a patient with syphilis. Identification of antitreponemal antibody and treponemal antigen in renal tissue. *Am J Med* 76:1106, 1984.
7. Alpers, CE, Cotran, RS. Neoplasia and glomerular injury. *Kidney Int* 30:465, 1986.
8. Stilmant, MM, Bolton, WK, Sturgill, BC, Schmitt, GW, Couser, WG. Crescentic glomerulonephritis without immune deposits: Clinicopathologic features. *Kidney Int* 15:184, 1979.
9. Serra, A, Cameron, JS, Turner, DR, Hartley, B, Ogg, CS, Neild, GH, Williams, DG, Taube, D, Brown, CB, Hicks, JA. Vasculitis affecting the kidney: Presentation, histopathology, and long-term outcome. *Q J Med* 53:181, 1984.
10. Bolton, WK, Tucker, FL, Sturgill, BC. New avian model of experimental glomerulonephritis consistent with mediation by cellular immunity. *J Clin Invest* 73:1263, 1984.
10a. Woodworth, TG, Abuelo, JG, Austin, HA, III, Esparaza, A. Severe glomerulonephritis with late emergence of classic Wegener's granulomatosis. Report of 4 cases and review of the literature. *Medicine* 66:181, 1987.
11. Tipping, PG, Neale, TJ, Holdsworth, SR. T lymphocyte participation in antibody-induced experimental glomerulonephritis. *Kidney Int* 27:530, 1985.
12. Beirne, GJ, Wagnild, JP, Zimmerman, SW, Macken, PD, Burkholder, PM. Idiopathic crescentic glomerulonephritis. *Medicine* 56:349, 1977.
13. Boyce, NW, Holdsworth, SR. Pulmonary manifestations of the clinical syndrome of acute glomerulonephritis and pulmonary hemorrhage. *Am J Kid Dis* 8:31, 1986.
14. Heilman, RL, Offord, KP, Holley, KE, Velosa, JA. Analysis of risk factors for patient and renal survival in crescentic glomerulonephritis. *Am J Kid Dis* 9:98, 1987.

*Therapy may, however, be discontinued as soon as 3 months if anti-GBM antibodies have disappeared [19].

15. Westberg, NG, Michael, AF. Immunohistopathology of diabetic glomerulosclerosis. *Diabetes* 21:163, 1972.
16. Heaf, JG, Jorgensen, F, Nielsen, LP. Treatment and prognosis of extracapillary glomerulonephritis. *Nephron* 35:217, 1983.
17. Baldwin, DS, Neugarten, J, Feiner, HD, Gluck M, Spinowitz, B. The existence of a protracted course in crescentic glomerulonephritis. *Kidney Int* 31:790, 1987.
18. A Report of the Southwest Pediatric Nephrology Study Group. A clinico-pathologic study of crescentic glomerulonephritis in 50 children. *Kidney Int* 27:450, 1985.
19. Savage, COS, Pusey, CD, Bowman, C, Rees, AJ. Antiglomerular basement membrane antibody-mediated disease in the British Isles 1980–4. *Br Med J* 292:301, 1986.
20. Hind, CRK, Lockwood, CM, Peters, DK, Paraskevakou, H, Evans, DJ, Rees, AJ. Prognosis after immunosuppression of patients with crescentic glomerulonephritis requiring dialysis. *Lancet* 1:263, 1983.
21. Couser, WG. Idiopathic rapidly progressive glomerulonephritis. *Am J Nephrol* 2:57, 1982.
22. Border, WA. Anticoagulants are of little value in the treatment of renal disease. *Am J Kid Dis* 3:308, 1984.
23. Bolton, WK, Couser, WG. Intravenous pulse methylprednisolone therapy of acute crescentic rapidly progressive glomerulonephritis. *Am J Med* 66:495, 1979.
24. O'Neill, WM, Etheridge, WB, Bloomer, HA. High-dose corticosteroids. *Arch Intern Med* 139:514, 1979.
25. Bocanegra, TS, Castaneda, MO, Espinoza, LR, Vasey, FB, Germain, BF. Sudden death after methylprednisolone pulse therapy. *Ann Intern Med* 95:122, 1981.
26. Warren, DJ, Smith, RS. High-dose prednisolone. *Lancet* 1:594, 1983.
27. Jacobs, HS. Pulse steroids in hematologic diseases. *Hosp Pract* 20(8):87, 1985.
28. Kincaid-Smith, P, D'Apice, AJF. Plasmapheresis in rapidly progressive glomerulonephritis. *Am J Med* 65:564, 1978.
29. Lockwood, CM, Worlledge, S, Nicholas, A, Cotton, C, Peters, DK. Reversal of impaired splenic function in patients with nephritis or vasculitis (or both) by plasma exchange. *N Engl J Med* 300:524, 1979.
30. Bruns, FJ, Adler, S, Segel, DP, Fraley, DS. Long-term follow-up of aggressively treated rapidly progressive glomerulonephritis (abstract). *Kidney Int* 29:181, 1986.
31. Briggs, WA, Johnson, JP, Teichman, S, Yaeger, HC, Wilson, CB. Antiglomerular basement membrane antibody-mediated glomerulonephritis and Goodpasture's syndrome. *Medicine* 58:348, 1979.
32. Dahlberg, PJ, Kurtz, SB, Donadio, JV, Jr, Holley, KE, Velosa, JA, Williams, DE, Wilson, CB. Recurrent Goodpasture's syndrome. *Mayo Clin Proc* 53:533, 1978.
33. Rosenblatt, SG, Knight, W, Bannayan, GA, Wilson, CB, Stein, JH. Treatment of Goodpasture's syndrome with plasmapheresis: A case report and review of the literature. *Am J Med* 66:689, 1979.
34. Rees, AJ, Lockwood, CM, Peters, DK. Enhanced allergic tissue injury in Goodpasture's syndrome by intercurrent bacterial infection. *Br Med J* 2:723, 1977.
35. Wilson, CB, Dixon, FJ. Antiglomerular basement membrane antibody induced glomerulonephritis. *Kidney Int* 3:74, 1973.

VI. VASCULAR DISEASES

38. CLASSIFICATION OF SYSTEMIC VASCULITIS

The classification of systemic vasculitis has been difficult in part because the etiologies of the various disorders and their pathogeneses are poorly defined. The most frequently used scheme differentiates the renal vasculitides according to the size and site of vascular involvement (Table 38-1) [1,2]. Distinguishing between these disorders is important because of their differing courses and responses to therapy.

Wegener's granulomatosis and the *polyarteritis group* have many similarities. They cause vascular damage in multiple organs, but usually spare the skin. Glomerular injury in these disorders is primarily ischemic and is notable for an absence of immune deposits in most patients. Renal insufficiency is commonly observed prior to treatment but often can be arrested or improved by early immunosuppressive therapy with cyclophosphamide and prednisone.

In contrast, the *hypersensitivity vasculitides* are almost always associated with skin involvement, typically manifested by palpable purpura. Furthermore, renal biopsy usually reveals the glomerular deposition of immune complexes and complement; prominent mesangial IgA deposits, for example, are seen in Henoch-Schönlein purpura. Spontaneous recovery from the renal disease commonly occurs and, in contrast to the above disorders, a beneficial effect of immunosuppressive treatment has been difficult to demonstrate.

References

1. Black, RM. Vascular diseases of the kidney. In Rose, BD, *Pathophysiology of Renal Disease* (2nd ed). New York: McGraw-Hill, 1987. Pp. 297-318.
2. Balow, JE. Renal vasculitis. *Kidney Int* 27:954, 1985.

Table 38-1. Systemic vasculitis involving the kidney

Characteristic	Wegener's granulomatosis	Polyarteritis	Hypersensitivity vasculitis
Subtypes		Classic polyarteritis nodosa, microscopic polyarteritis, Churg-Strauss syndrome, overlap syndrome	Henoch-Schönlein purpura, mixed cryoglobulinemia, serum sickness
Vessels affected	Small- and medium-sized arteries, with granuloma formation in the respiratory tract	Small- and medium-sized arteries and occasionally arterioles	Small vessels, particularly post-capillary venules
Primary sites of involvement	Upper and lower respiratory tracts and kidneys	Any system may be affected, including kidneys, peripheral nerves, and heart	Prominent skin purpura and renal disease
Type of glomerular disease	Necrotizing glomerulonephritis with no demonstrable immune deposits	Necrotizing glomerulonephritis with no demonstrable immune deposits	Proliferative glomerulonephritis with immune complex deposition
Course and treatment	Fatal if untreated; cyclophosphamide is most effective initial therapy	Fatal if untreated; prednisone in mild cases, cyclophosphamide if severe or resistant to prednisone	Spontaneous recovery is common; cyclophosphamide and prednisone if severe renal disease

39. WEGENER'S GRANULOMATOSIS

Wegener's granulomatosis (WG) is an uncommon, but distinct, vasculitic syndrome that classically affects the upper and lower respiratory tracts and the kidneys, although virtually any organ system can be affected [1,2]. A necrotizing *granulomatous* vasculitis is almost always found in lesions in the nasopharynx, paranasal sinuses, or the lungs. Vascular involvement is also present in the kidneys; the primary histologic finding at this site, however, is a necrotizing glomerulonephritis (Fig. 39-1), often with crescent formation. Granulomas are infrequently seen on renal biopsy.

The pathogenesis of WG is poorly understood. Many observations suggest a central role for the deposition of antigen-antibody complexes in the vessel wall, with the subsequent activation of complement and the release of soluble mediators of immune injury [1,2]. The recent detection of antibodies directed against neutrophilic cytoplasmic antigens in this disorder supports this hypothesis [3]. These autoantibodies may be directed against an epitope on the enzyme alkaline phosphatase, which is also present in the endothelial cells in small arteries and, to a lesser degree, capillaries. Although the pathogenetic role of these antibodies remains to be proved, their plasma levels correlate with disease activity and they do not seem to be present in other conditions, except for the microscopic form of polyarteritis (see Chap. 40) [3].

Immunofluorescent staining of the renal vessels usually does not reveal the presence of immune complexes; this finding, however, does not preclude a pathogenetic role for antigen-antibody deposition since the immune complexes may be rapidly removed from the vessel walls. Alternatively, the presence of granulomas could indicate that cell-mediated immunity is of primary importance.

Clinical Presentation

Wegener's granulomatosis most commonly develops in middle-aged adults, but the presenting symptoms are often nonspecific (Table 39-1) [2]. For example, patients may complain of fever, anorexia, fatigue, or weight loss, symptoms that may be misdiagnosed as being due to infection, cancer, another connective tissue disease, or even depression. Symptoms referable to the respiratory system, such as sinus pain, chest pain, or hemoptysis, are more specific for WG.

The physical examination may be normal or may reveal various findings depending on the pattern of organ involvement (Table 39-1). A careful examination of the sinuses and nasopharynx is essential, since vasculitic (and easily biopsied) lesions in these areas may be found even in asymptomatic patients.

Clinically evident renal involvement is also commonly present at the time of diagnosis, although it usually follows the onset of extrarenal disease. The urinalysis at this time typically reveals hematuria (often with red cell casts) and proteinuria. In addition, the plasma creatinine concentration is often elevated, indicating substantial renal damage.

A "limited" form of WG has been described in which there is respiratory but not renal involvement. Most of these patients, however, will ultimately develop classic WG [4], but the pulmonary manifestations may be present for years before the renal disease becomes apparent. The reverse pattern may also occur as some patients present with acute glomerulonephritis and then develop characteristic pulmonary lesions [5]. In the absence of initial respiratory tract involvement, these patients will be considered to have idiopathic necrotizing glomerulonephritis [6] or possibly the microscopic form of polyarteritis. As described before, the latter disorder seems to be associated with the same antineutrophilic antibodies as in WG, suggesting that they may be related conditions [3].

The laboratory findings in WG are nondiagnostic and may include anemia, leukocytosis, and an elevated erythrocyte sedimentation rate. Complement levels are generally normal, and antinuclear antibodies are not detected. The chest x ray typically reveals solitary or multiple pulmonary nodules, which may undergo central necrosis. Radiologic examination of the nasal sinuses also may be abnormal in patients with sinus involvement.

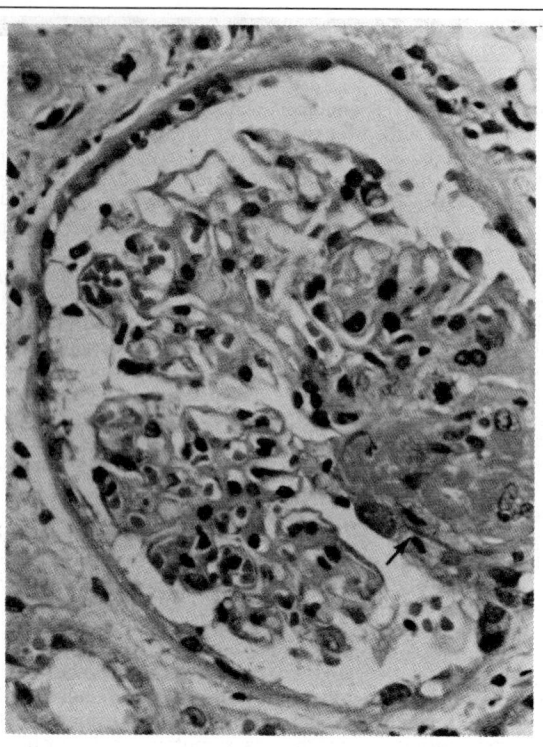

Fig. 39-1. Light microscopy in Wegener's granulomatosis typically reveals segmental areas of glomerular necrosis (arrow). This change affects a variable number of glomeruli and may be accompanied by crescent formation. Vascular inflammation and necrosis may be seen in some patients, but granulomas are uncommon. Immunofluorescent staining is usually negative and immune deposits are generally not seen by electron microscopy. (From Rose, BD. *Pathophysiology of Renal Disease* [2nd ed.]. New York: McGraw-Hill, 1987.)

Table 39-1. Organ involvement in Wegener's granulomatosis

Organ system	% involvement	Typical features
Lungs	95	Nodular cavitary infiltrates
Paranasal sinuses	90	Pansinusitis often with bacterial superinfection
Kidneys	85	Focal, segmental necrotizing glomerulonephritis
Nasopharynx	75	Mucosal ulcers, saddle nose deformity
Eyes	60	Uveitis, conjunctivitis
Joints	50	Polyarthralgias
Skin	40	Necrotic lesions with ulceration
Nervous system	20	Mononeuritis multiplex
Heart	15	Coronary vasculitis, pericarditis

Source: Adapted from Fauci, AS, Haynes, BR, Katz, P. *Ann Intern Med* 89:660, 1978.

Diagnosis

The presence of WG is often suggested from the clinical and laboratory findings; however, confirmation of the diagnosis requires a biopsy of tissue from an affected organ. The nasopharynx should be carefully examined, since this area can be biopsied with little risk to the patient. In the absence of nasopharyngeal lesions, a renal biopsy is usually required since this procedure is less invasive and generally better tolerated than an open lung biopsy.

The renal findings are usually not pathognomonic of WG, however, since granulomas are typically absent and a focal, segmental necrotizing glomerulonephritis with negative immunofluorescent staining may also be seen in polyarteritis or as an idiopathic disorder in which renal (or extrarenal) vasculitis cannot be identified [6,7]. However, the concurrent presence of upper or lower respiratory tract disease is highly suggestive of WG.

Prognosis and Treatment

The prognosis for patients with *untreated* WG is very poor [1,8]. Up to 90 percent of patients die within 2 years of presentation, most often due to respiratory or renal failure. Although corticosteroids alone may result in clinical and laboratory improvement in some patients, these responses are usually temporary.

In contrast, *dramatic, long-lasting remissions* can be induced in most patients with the use of cytotoxic agents, particularly cyclophosphamide [2,8-10]. Early institution of therapy is extremely important, since tissue necrosis, once it occurs, cannot be reversed. However, the presence of renal failure severe enough to require dialysis during the *acute phase* of the illness does not necessarily preclude aggressive therapy, since sufficient renal function may return to allow dialysis to be discontinued [11].

Cyclophosphamide is usually initiated orally (1–2 mg/kg/day) when the disease is active but relatively stable. However, patients with more fulminant renal or respiratory involvement should be started on higher doses (4 mg/kg/day for several days). Intermittent intravenous pulse cyclophosphamide (0.5–1.0 gm/m² body surface area) at monthly intervals (as used in lupus nephritis) seems to be less effective than oral therapy in Wegener's granulomatosis.

Corticosteroids, such as prednisone (1 mg/kg/day), are also given simultaneously and are useful in reducing acute inflammation in the eye, skin, and pericardium until cyclophosphamide takes effect (approximately 7–14 days). In addition, intravenous pulses of methylprednisolone (250 mg–1 gm intravenously daily for 3 days, followed by conventional oral doses) may be beneficial in patients with rapidly progressive renal failure. Corticosteroids are continued until the disease is brought under control and are then slowly tapered to alternate-day maintenance therapy.

Cyclophosphamide is continued until there is no evidence of disease activity or toxicity (marrow suppression, infection, or hemorrhagic cystitis) develops. Patients in remission can, at 3 to 4 months, be switched to azathioprine to reduce the incidence of complications [10]. Although azathioprine is generally less effective as initial therapy, it is often sufficient to sustain a cyclophosphamide-induced remission. Cytotoxic therapy must be continued for *at least 1 year* after complete remission has been induced to minimize the risk of relapses. Most relapses in WG are associated with treatment using corticosteroids alone, a reduction in cyclophosphamide dosage, the use of azathioprine in place of cyclophosphamide, or superimposed infection.

Two recent reports suggest a possible, safer alternative to cytotoxic therapy, the antimicrobial combination *trimethoprim-sulfamethoxazole* [12,13]. This regimen has been shown to be effective in inducing and maintaining a remission in a small number of patients, some of whom had become resistant to cyclophosphamide. These findings, which suggest that an infectious process may play a central role in this disorder, clearly need to be confirmed in a larger number of patients.

Patients who develop irreversible, end-stage renal disease may be successfully dialyzed. However, immunosuppressive therapy may still be required if there is continued extrarenal activity. Remission should be achieved before renal transplantation is performed to reduce the likelihood of disease recurrence in the transplanted kidney.

References

1. Black, RM. Vascular diseases of the kidney. In Rose, BD, *Pathophysiology of Renal Disease* (2nd ed). New York: McGraw-Hill, 1987. Pp. 307–310.
2. Fauci, AS, Haynes, BF, Katz, P. The spectrum of vasculitis. Clinical, pathogenic, immunologic, and therapeutic considerations. *Ann Intern Med* 89:660, 1978.
3. Savage, COS, Winearls, CG, Jones, S, Marshall, PD, Lockwood, CM. Prospective study of radioimmunoassay for antibodies against neutrophil cytoplasm in diagnosis of systemic vasculitis. *Lancet* 1:1389, 1987.
4. Case Records of the Massachusetts General Hospital (17-1986). *N Engl J Med* 314:1170, 1986.
5. Woodworth, TG, Abuelo, JG, Austin, HA, III, Esparza, A. Severe glomerulonephritis with late emergence of classic Wegener's granulomatosis. Report of 4 cases and review of the literature. *Medicine* 66:181, 1987.
6. Weiss, MA, Crisman, JD. Segmental necrotizing glomerulonephritis: Diagnostic, prognostic, and therapeutic significance. *Am J Kid Dis* 6:199, 1985.
7. Serra, A, Cameron, JS, Turner, DR, Hartley, B, Ogg, CS, Neild, GH, Williams, DG, Taube, D, Brown, CB, Hicks, JA. Vasculitis affecting the kidney: Presentation, histopathology, and long-term outcome. *Q J Med* 53:181, 1984.
8. Balow, JE. Renal vasculitis. *Kidney Int* 27:954, 1985.
9. Fauci, AS, Haynes, BF, Katz, P, Wolff, SM. Wegener's granulomatosis: Prospective clinical trial and therapeutic experience with eighty-five patients for 21 years. *Ann Intern Med* 98:76, 1983.
10. Pinching, AJ, Lockwood, CM, Pussell, BA, Rees, AJ, Sweeny, P, Evans, DJ, Bowley, N, and Peters, DK. Wegener's granulomatosis: Observations on 18 patients with severe renal disease. *Q J Med* 52:435, 1983.
11. Hind, CRK, Lockwood, CM, Peters, DK, Paraskevakou, H, Evans, DJ, Rees, AJ. Prognosis after immunosuppression of patients with crescentic nephritis requiring dialysis. *Lancet* 1:263, 1983.
12. De Remee, RA, McDonald, TJ, Weiland, LH. Wegener's granulomatosis: Observations on treatment with antimicrobial agents. *Mayo Clin Proc* 60:27, 1985.
13. West, BC, Todd, JR, King, JW. Wegener granulomatosis and trimethoprim-sulfamethoxazole. Complete remission after a twenty-year course. *Ann Intern Med* 106:840, 1987.

40. POLYARTERITIS

Polyarteritis is a disorder associated with inflammatory arterial lesions. Four different forms of polyarteritis, which may or may not be related, have been described: classic polyarteritis nodosa, microscopic polyarteritis, the Churg-Strauss syndrome, and the overlap syndrome [1,2].

Classic Polyarteritis Nodosa

The vasculitis in classic polyarteritis nodosa (PAN) typically affects the small- and medium-sized muscular arteries (Fig. 40-1A). The early inflammatory lesions, which commonly occur at arterial bifurcations, are associated with prominent neutrophilic infiltration and areas of destruction of the vascular wall. Aneurysm formation can develop in the weakened vessel wall, and scarring during the healing phase can lead to a further reduction in the diameter of the vascular lumen (Fig. 40-1B).

The glomerular lesion in PAN is characterized by a focal, segmental necrotizing glomerulonephritis, similar to that seen in Wegener's granulomatosis (see Chap. 39). These changes are primarily ischemic, resulting from vasculitis affecting the small- and medium-sized intrarenal arteries. However, percutaneous renal biopsy may not reveal vasculitis in the extraglomerular vessels (due to sampling error); in this setting, the diag-

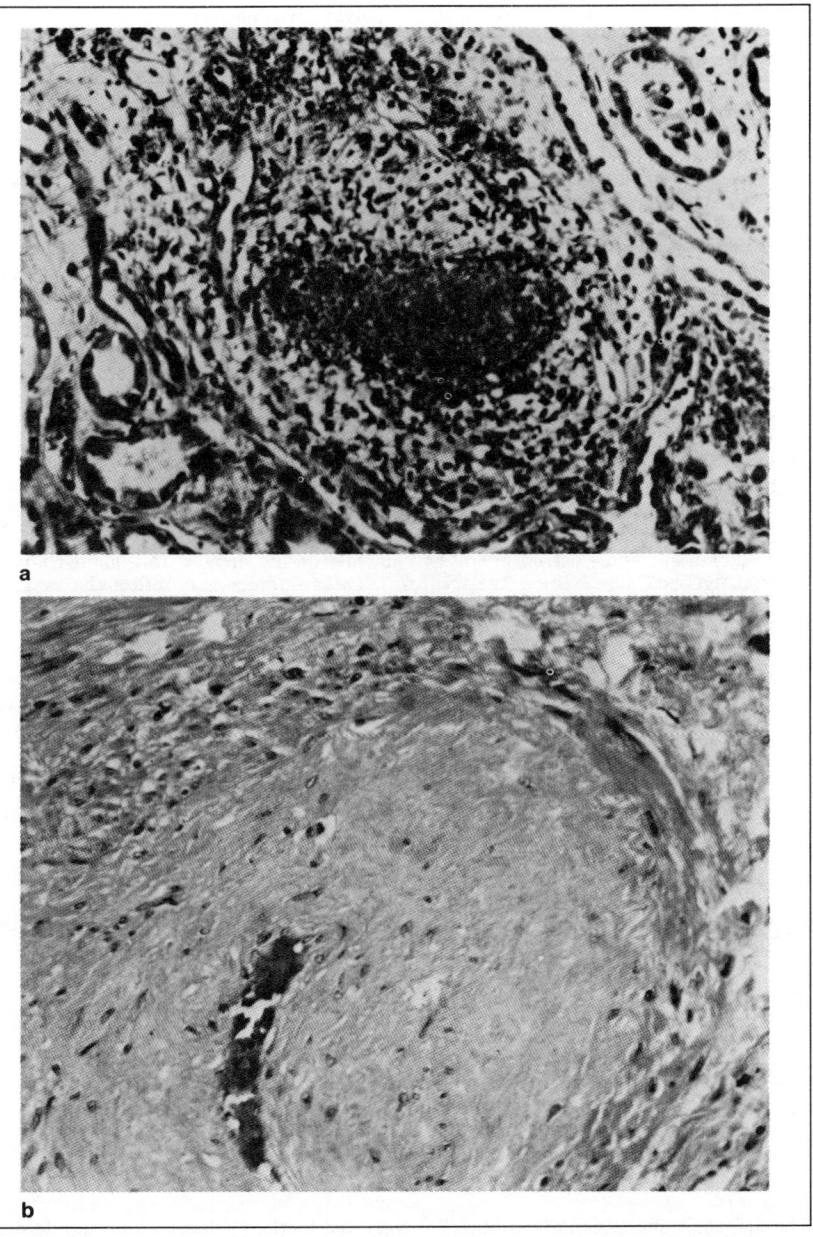

Fig. 40-1. Arterial changes in polyarteritis nodosa. (a) Acute lesion in a medium-sized artery with neutrophilic and mononuclear cell infiltration in the vessel wall. The elastic lamina has been disrupted, and thrombus formation is seen occluding the vascular lumen. (b) A healed lesion reveals a thickened, fibrotic arterial wall, with only a slitlike lumen remaining open. (From Rose, BD. *Pathophysiology of Renal Disease* [2nd ed.]. New York: McGraw-Hill, 1987.)

Table 40-1. Major clinical features of classic polyarteritis nodosa

Organ system	Usual signs and symptoms
Nonspecific symptoms	Fever, anorexia, weight loss, fatigue
Musculoskeletal	Arthralgias, myalgias, arthritis (rare)
Kidney	Abnormal urinary sediment, renal failure, hypertension
Nervous system	Mononeuritis multiplex, cranial neuropathy
Heart	Angina, myocardial infarction, heart failure
Liver	Subclinical to chronic liver disease (only if hepatitis B infection)
Gastrointestinal	Visceral infarction
Skin (uncommon)	Livido reticularis, subcutaneous nodules

nosis is suspected from the necrotizing glomerular injury and the associated systemic findings.

In comparison to other necrotizing glomerular lesions (as seen in lupus nephritis, anti-glomerular basement membrane antibody disease, or bacterial endocarditis), immunofluorescent and electron microscopy usually do not demonstrate glomerular (or arterial) IgG or C3 deposition in PAN [1,2a]. These findings may reflect the rapid removal of immune complexes from the vascular walls or, possibly, a primary role for cellular immunity.

Clinical Presentation
Patients with classic PAN typically present with nonspecific symptoms, including fever, weight loss, arthralgias, and loss of appetite, that presumably reflect the underlying inflammatory process. Other symptoms and signs are dependent on the extent of clinically significant organ involvement (Table 40-1). The finding of an asymmetric polyneuropathy (mononeuritis multiplex) is particularly important because, other than systemic vasculitis, diabetes mellitus is the only systemic disorder that commonly causes this problem.

Renal involvement is observed in most patients at some time during the course of their disease. This is commonly manifested by azotemia and hypertension, the latter being primarily due to ischemic activation of the renin-angiotensin system [3]. The urine sediment is variable in PAN; it may be relatively benign if only the larger vessels are involved, a setting in which there may be glomerular ischemia without much necrosis. However, dysmorphic red blood cells, red cell casts, and mild proteinuria are typically seen when there is prominent glomerular damage [1]. Nephrotic range proteinuria (> 3.5 gm/day), on the other hand is unusual, which probably reflects the secondary nature of the glomerular involvement.

In some patients, an underlying disorder that may have initiated the vasculitis can be identified. In particular, hepatitis B infection may occur in 40 percent of inner-city patients with PAN [4]. Furthermore, a history of intravenous drug abuse (which is more prevalent in this patient population) also may be elicited.

Diagnosis
The diagnosis of classic PAN is initially suggested by the evidence of multisystem involvement. Although the history, physical examination, and laboratory findings may be compatible with this disorder (especially if mononeuritis multiplex is present), a definitive diagnosis can only be made by demonstrating the typical vascular lesions either by angiography or by biopsy of an involved organ. Angiography of the celiac and renal arteries is virtually diagnostic if it demonstrates microaneurysms and irregular, segmental constrictions in the larger vessels, with tapering and occlusion of the smaller intra-

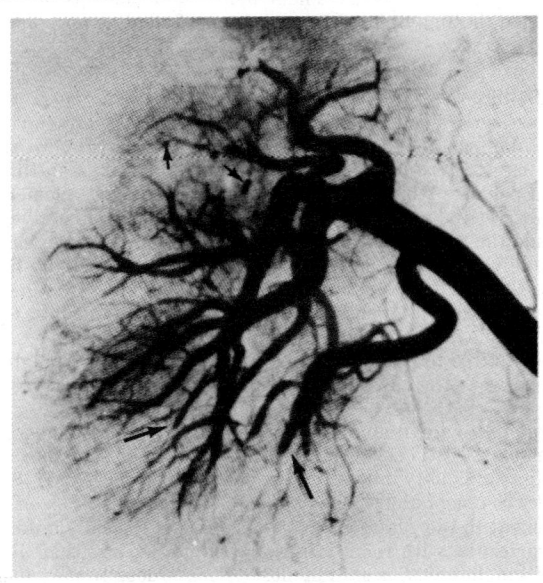

Fig. 40-2. Renal arteriogram in classic polyarteritis nodosa. Both microaneurysms (small arrows) and abrupt cutoff of medium-sized arteries (large arrows) are present, changes which are virtually diagnostic of a large-vessel vasculitis. (From Rose, BD. *Pathophysiology of Renal Disease* [2nd ed.]. New York: McGraw-Hill, 1987.)

renal arteries (Fig. 40-2) [2]. This procedure may be negative, however, in patients in whom only the more distal vessels are involved, as in microscopic polyarteritis.

Renal biopsy is required only if the arteriogram is negative (or cannot be performed) and if no other *easily biopsied* and clinically affected tissue (such as muscle or peripheral nerve) can be identified. As described before, the finding of a segmental, necrotizing glomerulonephritis with negative immunofluorescent staining in a patient with multisystem disease is highly suggestive of systemic vasculitis [1,2a].

Microscopic Polyarteritis

Patients with this variant of polyarteritis exhibit pathologic lesions similar to those observed in classic PAN, but the vessels affected are smaller [1,5]. In the kidney, this is manifested by an arteritis involving the afferent glomerular arterioles and the glomerular capillaries directly. Segmental glomerular necrosis is invariably present, although not all glomeruli may be involved due to the focal nature of the lesion. The glomerular damage is typically more prominent than in classic PAN, where ischemia rather than direct injury is responsible. Immune complexes are not generally detected by immunofluorescent staining or by electron microscopy.

The clinical presentation of patients with microscopic polyarteritis is usually difficult to distinguish from classic PAN. The urinary sediment, however, is more likely to be active due to the direct involvement of glomerular capillaries. Hypertension, which is common in classic PAN, is not usually observed in microscopic polyarteritis; it is unclear why this occurs [1].

Two recent observations suggest that microscopic polyarteritis may be related to Wegener's granulomatosis. First, some patients who present with the renal findings of microscopic polyarteritis later develop classic granulomatous respiratory tract involvement [6]. Second, both disorders (but not classic PAN) seem to be associated with a similar autoantibody directed against a neutrophilic (and perhaps vascular endothelial) cytoplasmic antigen that may represent an epitope of alkaline phosphatase [7].

Churg-Strauss Syndrome

The Churg-Strauss syndrome (or allergic granulomatosis) is characterized by the presence of extravascular granuloma formation, eosinophilic infiltration of arteries and venules, and renal involvement [8]. It may be difficult to distinguish this disorder from other variants of polyarteritis on pathologic examination of the glomeruli. However, a focal or diffuse interstitial nephritis with granulomas and eosinophilic infiltrates may be observed in addition to the characteristic segmental necrotizing glomerular lesions.

The clinical findings in the Churg-Strauss syndrome can usually be distinguished from those of classic PAN. An allergic diathesis is typically the first sign of this disorder, beginning between the ages of 20 and 30. Later, peripheral eosinophilia (often associated with eosinophilic tissue infiltration) is seen, followed by the onset of systemic vasculitis. The time course required to progress from one phase to another is highly variable, but a short interval between the onset of atopy and the development of vasculitis carries a worse prognosis.

Asthmatic symptoms are frequent early findings, particularly during the atopic phase. As systemic vasculitis develops, the lung involvement becomes more prominent with noncavitating pulmonary infiltrates demonstrable on chest x ray [8]. Coronary vasculitis is also very common, and the heart is often the most severely affected organ.

Renal involvement in the Churg-Strauss syndrome is typically milder than in other variants of polyarteritis, with renal failure developing in less than 10 percent of patients. Hypertension, however, is seen in most patients, despite the paucity of clinically severe renal involvement. The reason for this observation is not known.

The clinical findings of an atopic history with asthma and eosinophilia in the presence of multisystem disease should suggest the possibility of the Churg-Strauss syndrome. The diagnosis may be overlooked, however, since all manifestations of the disease may not be present simultaneously. As in other forms of polyarteritis, biopsy of an involved organ is usually necessary to confirm the presence of vasculitis before treatment is initiated.

Overlap Syndrome

Some patients have clinical manifestations that do not allow one variant of polyarteritis to be clearly differentiated from another. Furthermore, skin vasculitis with palpable petechial lesions, similar to those in hypersensitivity vasculitis, also may be present. Patients with these findings are considered to have an "overlap" syndrome but typically have a clinical course and response to treatment similar to classic PAN [9].

Treatment

The outlook for patients with untreated polyarteritis is poor, with the 1- and 5-year survival rates being approximately 50 and 13 percent, respectively [1,2,10]. The prognosis in microscopic polyarteritis may be somewhat better, but long-term survival in this disorder is also limited in the absence of effective therapy.

Treatment with corticosteroids (1 mg/kg/day of prednisone) can substantially improve patient survival in polyarteritis [10,11]. Patients who respond usually do so within the first 3 months of therapy. However, the mortality rate with corticosteroids alone remains high, primarily due to renal failure, cerebral or mesenteric infarction, or cardiac failure. Furthermore, corticosteroid toxicity often occurs in those patients requiring long-term therapy.

In comparison, *long-term remissions* have been induced in classic PAN using cyclophosphamide, even in those patients who do not respond to corticosteroids [1,11,12]. The dosage schedule, possible use of intravenous cyclophosphamide, duration of therapy, and possible conversion to azathioprine after remission has been induced are similar to that described for Wegener's granulomatosis in the preceding chapter and will not be repeated here.

Optimal therapy for classic PAN remains uncertain. Patients with relatively stable disease can be treated initially with corticosteroids alone. Patients who do not respond within 1 month of therapy, who require toxic doses to sustain a remission, or who have more serious disease, as manifested by renal insufficiency or peripheral neuropathy, should be started on both prednisone and cyclophosphamide. Intravenous pulse methylprednisolone (250–1000 mg/day for 3 days) can also be considered as part of the initial regimen in those patients with rapidly progressive renal disease.

It is important to emphasize that improvement in renal function may be seen even in those patients who present with advanced renal failure requiring dialysis [13]. Consequently, severe initial disease does not preclude effective treatment in this disorder. In patients who respond, maintenance therapy should be continued for *1 to 2 years* after remission has been induced to lessen the risk of relapse [1].

Patients with the Churg-Strauss syndrome are more likely to respond to corticosteroids alone. However, cytotoxic therapy has been used in patients with more aggressive disease. Treatment can usually be stopped 1 year after remission, since the vasculitic phase in this disorder usually lasts less than 12 months [8].

Patients with any form of polyarteritis who progress to irreversible end-stage renal disease may be successfully dialyzed. Renal transplantation can be considered in those patients who achieve clinical remission of their extrarenal disease [14]. Cyclophosphamide may, in some patients, have to be substituted for azathioprine (which is frequently given to prevent graft rejection) if the vasculitis recurs.

References

1. Balow, JE. Renal vasculitis. *Kidney Int* 27:954. 1985.
2. Black, RM. Vascular diseases of the kidney. In, Rose, BD, *Pathophysiology of Renal Disease* (2nd ed). New York: McGraw-Hill, 1987. Pp. 300–318.
2a. Weiss, MA, Crissman, JD. Segmental necrotizing glomerulonephritis: Diagnostic, prognostic, and therapeutic significance. *Am J Kid Dis* 6:199, 1985.
3. Stockigt, JR, Topliss, DJ, Hewett, MJ. High-renin hypertension in necrotizing vasculitis. *N Engl J Med* 300:1218, 1979.
4. Shusterman, N, London, WT. Hepatitis B and immune-complex disease. *N Engl J Med* 310:43, 1984.
5. Savage, COS, Winearls, CG, Evans, DJ, Rees, AJ, Lockwood, CM. Microscopic polyarteritis. *Q J Med* 56:467, 1985.
6. Woodworth, TG, Abuelo, JG, Austin, HA, III, Esparaza, A. Severe glomerulonephritis with late emergence of classic Wegener's granulomatosis. Report of 4 cases and review of the literature. *Medicine* 66:181, 1987.
7. Savage, COS, Winearls, CG, Jones, S, Marshall, PD, Lockwood, CM. Prospective study of radioimmunoassay for antibodies versus neutrophil cytoplasm in diagnosis of systemic vasculitis. *Lancet* 1:1389, 1987.
8. Lanham, JG, Elkon, KB, Pusey, CD, Hughes, GR. Systemic vasculitis with asthma and eosinophilia: A clinical approach to the Churg-Strauss syndrome. *Medicine* 63:65. 1984.
9. Leavitt, RY, Fauci, AS. Polyangiitis overlap syndrome. *Am J Med* 81:79. 1986.
10. Frohnert, PP, Sheps, SG. Long-term follow-up study of peri-arteritis nodosa. *Am J Med* 43:8, 1967.
11. Leib, ES, Restivo, Paulus, HE. Immunosuppressive and corticosteroid therapy of polyarteritis nodosa. *Am J Med* 67:941. 1979.
12. Fauci, AS, Katz, P, Haynes, BF, Wolff, SM. Cyclophosphamide therapy of severe systemic necrotizing vasculitis. *N Engl J Med* 301:235, 1979.
13. Hind, CRK, Parakevou, H, Lockwood, CM, Evans, DJ, Peters, DK, Rees, AJ. Prognosis after immunosuppression of patients with crescentic nephritis requiring dialysis. *Lancet* 1:263, 1983.
14. Montalbert, C, Corvallo, A, Broumand, B, Noble, D, Austine, A, Currier, CB, Jr. Successful renal transplantation in polyarteritis nodosa. *Clin Nephrol* 14:206, 1980.

41. HYPERSENSITIVITY VASCULITIS

Hypersensitivity vasculitis is characterized by inflammation of the smaller blood vessels—arterioles, capillaries, and especially postcapillary venules. These changes are especially prominent in the skin, where the blood vessels in the dermis are surrounded by an intense neutrophilic infiltrate, with local hemorrhage and edema. This histologic picture is called a *leukocytoclastic vasculitis* and is manifested by a *palpable* purpuric rash, which is almost always a major clinical sign of this disease.

Hypersensitivity vasculitis is occasionally limited to the skin, but often involves the kidney and other organs. Three major variants of this disorder have been described: Henoch-Schönlein purpura, essential mixed cryoglobulinemia, and serum sickness. Less commonly, skin purpura and renal disease are observed in patients with the "overlap" syndrome of polyarteritis (see Chap. 40) or with urticarial (hypocomplementemic) vasculitis [1,2].

Henoch-Schönlein Purpura

Henoch-Schönlein purpura (HSP) is characterized by the deposition of *IgA-containing* immune complexes at the sites of involvement [1]. Thus, vascular IgA may be found, on immunofluorescent staining, in the purpuric lesions and also occasionally in clinically normal skin [3]. The absence of dermal IgA deposition, however, does not necessarily exclude the diagnosis, since the immune complexes may be removed from the vessel wall in older lesions.

The morphologic changes in the kidney are identical to those observed in IgA nephropathy (see Chap. 32): focal mesangial expansion and cellular proliferation, and, in the more severe cases, diffuse involvement that may include crescent formation and areas of fibrinoid necrosis. These lesions are presumably induced by the mesangial deposition of IgA and complement, which can be detected by immunofluorescent microscopy. True vasculitis is not seen in the kidney, in contrast to the prominent vascular disease in the skin. Why this occurs is not known.

Clinical Manifestations
Henoch-Schönlein purpura most commonly affects children but also can occur in adults [4,5]. The presenting symptoms usually include the characteristic extrarenal triad of abdominal pain, arthritis or arthralgias, and a petechial or purpuric rash. The skin lesions, which are most prominent on the dependent extensor surfaces, are ultimately seen in all patients, although they may not be present on initial examination [4].

Renal involvement is common and is usually evident within a few days to months after the onset of clinical symptoms [5–7]. The urinalysis typically reveals microscopic (or macroscopic) hematuria with red cell and other cellular casts and mild proteinuria. The plasma creatinine concentration is normal or only slightly elevated in most patients at the time of presentation. However, more marked findings, including nephrotic-range proteinuria, hypertension, and renal insufficiency, can be seen in some patients, who may have crescents on renal biopsy.

Diagnosis
The diagnosis of HSP should be considered in any patient with the dermal manifestations of hypersensitivity vasculitis, particularly if abdominal pain and arthritis are also present. Biopsy of involved (or uninvolved) skin may be diagnostic if IgA is detected by immunofluorescent staining in dermal capillaries [3]. (Pathologic examination of the skin without immunofluorescence cannot differentiate this disorder from the other forms of hypersensitivity vasculitis.) Renal biopsy, although generally diagnostic, should be reserved for patients with progressive renal impairment, since HSP is typically a benign, self-limited disorder.

Course and Therapy
Spontaneous resolution of all the clinical manifestations generally occurs in HSP, although recurrent episodes of purpura or glomerulonephritis may be seen [6]. There is

no consistent relationship between recurrent disease and prognosis or between the severity of the glomerulonephritis and the severity of the extrarenal manifestations [7].

The *extent of renal involvement* is usually the most important determinant of the long-term outlook in HSP. The renal prognosis is excellent in most patients who tend to have only focal glomerular involvement and asymptomatic hematuria and proteinuria [8,9]. However, preservation of renal function is less likely in patients who develop acute renal failure, who have nephrotic-range proteinuria, or who have crescents in more than 50 percent of the glomeruli on renal biopsy [7–9]. Less often, progressive renal disease occurs in patients with initially mild renal disease [9].

There is little evidence that conventional therapy with corticosteroids or cyclophosphamide has a beneficial effect on either the skin or renal disease [7,9]. These medications do not appear to reduce the frequency of relapse and do not alter the duration of disease activity. Despite any definitive proof of efficacy, intravenous pulse methylprednisolone (250 mg–1 gm/day for 3 days), cyclophosphamide, or plasmapheresis is usually tried in high-risk patients with crescentic glomerulonephritis and acute renal failure [10,11].

The patient who does not recover normal renal function after the acute episode may ultimately progress on to end-stage renal disease. Successful renal transplantation can be performed, but the disease may recur in the transplanted kidney [12] despite the concurrent administration of immunosuppressive therapy.

Essential Mixed Cryoglobulinemia

Cryoglobulins are antibodies that precipitate in the cold and dissolve on rewarming. The biochemical characteristics that promote cryoprecipitation are not well understood. In essential mixed cryoglobulinemia (EMC), for example, there are usually three components in the circulating cryoprotein complexes: an antigen, an immunoglobulin (usually IgG) directed against the antigen, and a monoclonal IgM rheumatoid factor directed against the immunoglobulin [13]. The inciting antigen cannot usually be identified, although hepatitis B virus and DNA have been found in the cryoprecipitates in isolated cases [14].

The principal pathologic findings in EMC are found in the skin and the kidney. The characteristic changes of a leukocytoclastic vasculitis are seen in the skin. However, IgA is not found in the dermal vessels, in contrast to patients with HSP.

Examination of renal tissue is usually highly suggestive of EMC. Diffuse mesangial and endothelial cell proliferation and basement membrane thickening are generally seen on light microscopy, simulating the appearance of membranoproliferative glomerulonephritis. Of particular importance, however, is the frequent finding of numerous *intraluminal thrombi* composed of precipitated cryoglobulins (Fig. 41-1) [15]. Immunofluorescent staining typically demonstrates granular deposition of IgG, IgM, and C3 in the intraluminal thrombi and along the glomerular basement membrane.

Clinical Presentation

Patients with EMC often present with nonspecific symptoms such as fatigue, lethargy, and arthralgias. Findings more suggestive of this diagnosis are the palpable purpuric rash (mainly affecting the lower extremities), particularly if accompanied by lymphadenopathy, hepatosplenomegaly, peripheral neuropathy, and Raynaud's phenomenon. In addition, hypocomplementemia is often present [15], a finding that is not seen in most other causes of skin purpura, such as HSP and the overlap syndrome of polyarteritis.

Renal involvement, which occurs in about 50 percent of patients with this disorder, always follows the skin lesions [15]. The urinalysis usually reveals mild hematuria and proteinuria, but red cell, white cell, and granular casts may be seen with more severe disease. The plasma creatinine concentration is normal in most patients at the time of presentation.

Liver function tests are often abnormal and may reflect underlying hepatitis B infection in some patients [13]. The hepatic dysfunction also may contribute to the development or persistence of EMC, since the liver is the primary site of removal of cryoglobulins from the plasma [16].

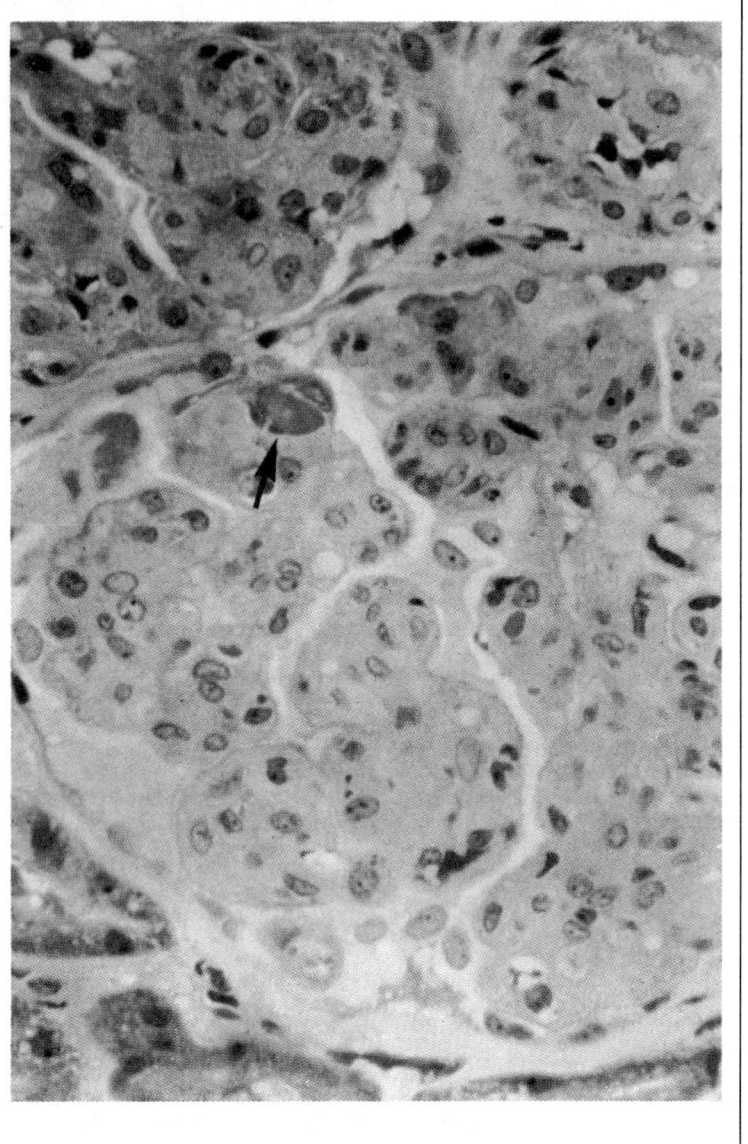

Fig. 41-1. Portion of a glomerulus showing a diffuse proliferative glomerulonephritis with intracapillary thrombus formation (arrow) characteristic of essential mixed cryoglobulinemia. (From Rose, BD. *Pathophysiology of Renal Disease* [2nd ed.]. New York: McGraw-Hill, 1987.)

Diagnosis
The presence of essential mixed cryoglobulinemia should be considered in any patient with a palpable purpuric rash, particularly if accompanied by hypocomplementemia. The diagnosis is then established by the demonstration of a high mixed IgM-IgG (or sometimes IgM-IgA) cryoglobulin titer with a monoclonal component by immunoelectrophoresis [13,15]. Renal biopsy should be reserved for those patients with progressive renal disease or in whom the diagnosis is in doubt.

Course and Treatment
The course of most patients with renal involvement is slowly progressive, with renal insufficiency developing over a period of months to years [13,15]. Neither the cryoglobulin concentration nor the complement levels predicts which patients will ultimately develop end-stage renal disease. Empiric therapy is usually limited to patients with disabling or progressive disease, since the efficacy of specific therapy is uncertain [10]. Patients with fulminant disease (acute renal failure, progressive neuropathy, or distal necrosis requiring amputation) should be treated with plasmapheresis (to remove circulating cryoglobulins and to desaturate reticuloendothelial receptors), prednisone, and cytotoxic agents (such as cyclophosphamide) to limit new antibody formation [17]. It is important that the plasma replacement fluid be warmed prior to infusion to prevent intravascular cryoglobulin precipitation.

Plasmapheresis does not appear to be effective in chronic, slowly progressive disease [15]; some physicians have used prednisone and chlorambucil in this setting with some success [1].

Serum Sickness
Serum sickness is usually caused by medications that probably act as haptens to stimulate an immune response. Many drugs can cause this disorder, but penicillins, sulfonamide derivatives, and phenytoin have been implicated most frequently [18–20]. Certain viral infections (particularly acute hepatitis B infection) also can cause a similar problem [21].

Clinical Presentation
The characteristic presenting picture of serum sickness is a systemic one, with fever, urticaria, arthralgias, lymphadenopathy, and sometimes edema. In most patients, the onset of symptoms is 7 to 10 days after antigen exposure, the time required to produce a sufficient amount of antibody, and subsequently, antigen-antibody complexes. This characteristic time course may be altered with exposure to a previously recognized antigen, as the latent period may be as short as 2 to 7 days. Conversely, a delayed onset and more prolonged course may result from the use of a long-acting drug such as benzathine penicillin [18].

Renal involvement is manifested by an abnormal urinalysis with red blood cells, proteinuria, and cellular casts. Acute renal failure is uncommon but may occur, particularly with prolonged antigen exposure [18]. Renal biopsy in this setting typically reveals an immune complex glomerulonephritis with diffuse cellular proliferation, and deposition of immunoglobulin (mainly IgG) and C3 in the glomerular capillary walls.

Diagnosis and Treatment
The history and physical examination should suggest the presence of serum sickness, particularly if a history of recent antigen exposure (usually a medication) can be elicited. Hypocomplementemia and the presence of circulating hepatitis B surface antigen are also supportive in the appropriate clinical setting.

There is little evidence that immunosuppressive therapy with corticosteroids or cytotoxic agents can prevent the development or alter the course of this disorder. Consequently, therapy in serum sickness should be directed toward identifying and removing the inciting drug or antigen. This should lead to rapid resolution of signs and symptoms within a few days or weeks. A trial of immunosuppressive therapy should be reserved for the infrequent patient with fulminant or progressive organ involvement.

References

1. Black, RM. Vascular diseases of the kidney. In Rose, BD, *Pathophysiology of Renal Disease* (2nd ed). New York: McGraw-Hill, 1987. Pp. 310–317.
2. Shultz, DR, Perez, GO, Volanakis, JE, Pardo, V, Moss, SH. Glomerular disease in two patients with urticarial-cutaneous vasculitis and hypocomplementemia. *Am J Kid Dis* 1:257, 1981.
3. Hene, RJ, Velthuis, P, van de Wiel, A, Klepper, D, Dorhout Mees, EJ, Kater, L. The relevance of IgA deposits in vessel walls of clinically normal skin. *Arch Intern Med* 146:745, 1986.
4. Cameron, JS. Henoch-Schönlein purpura: Clinical presentation. *Contrib Nephrol* 40:246, 1984.
5. Roth, DA, Wilz, DR, Theil, GB. Schönlein-Henoch syndrome in adults. *Q J Med* 55:145, 1985.
6. Koskimies, O, Mir, S, Rapola, J, Vilska, J. Henoch-Schönlein nephritis: Long-term prognosis of unselected patients. *Arch Dis Child* 56:482, 1981.
7. Austin, HA, III, Balow, JE. Henoch-Schönlein nephritis: Long-term prognostic features and the challenge of therapy. *Am J Kid Dis* 2:512, 1983.
8. Meadow, SR. The prognosis of Henoch-Schönlein nephritis. *Clin Nephrol* 9:87, 1978.
9. Counan, R, Winterborn, MH, White, RHR, Heaton, JM, Meadow, SR, Bluet, NH, Swetschin, H, Cameron, JS, Chantler, C. Prognosis of Henoch-Schönlein nephritis in children. *Br Med J* 2:11, 1977.
10. Balow, JE. Renal vasculitis. *Kidney Int* 27:954, 1985.
11. Kauffmann, RH, Houwert, DA. Plasmapheresis in rapidly progressive Henoch-Schönlein glomerulonephritis and the effect on circulating IgA immune complexes. *Clin Nephrol* 16:155, 1981.
12. Baliah, T, Kim, KH, Anthone, S, Montes, M, Andres, GA. Recurrence of Henoch-Schönlein purpura in transplanted kidneys. *Transplantation* 18:343, 1974.
13. Brouet, JC, Clauvel, JP, Danon, F, Klein, M, Seligmann, M. Biologic and clinical significance of cryoglobulins: A report of 86 cases. *Am J Med* 57:775, 1974.
14. Gambles, CN, Rugles, SW. The immunopathogenesis of glomerulonephritis associated with mixed cryoglobulinemia. *N Engl J Med* 299:81, 1978.
15. Gorevic, PD, Kassab, HJ, Levo, Y, Kohn, R, Meltzer, M. Prose, P, Franklin, EC. Mixed cryoglobulinemia: Clinical aspects and long term follow-up of 40 patients. *Am J Med* 69:287, 1980.
16. Levo, Y, Nature of cryoglobulinemia. *Lancet* 1:285, 1984.
17. Ferri, C, Moriconi, L, Gremignai, G, Migliorini, P, Paleologo, G, Fossella, PV, Bombardieri, S. Treatment of the renal involvement in mixed cryoglobulinemia with prolonged plasma exchange. *Nephron* 43:246, 1986.
18. Parker, CW. Allergic reactions in man. *Pharmacol Rev* 34:85, 1982.
19. Mullick, FG, McAllister, HA, Wagner, BM, Fenoglio, JJ, Jr. Drug-related vasculitis: Clinicopathologic correlations in 30 patients. *Hum Pathol* 10:313, 1979.
20. Josephs, SH, Rothman, SF, Buckley, RH. Phenytoin hypersensitivity. *J Allery Clin Immunol* 66:166, 1980.
21. McElgunn, PSJ. Dermatologic manifestations of hepatitis B virus infection. *J Am Acad Dermatol* 8:539, 1983.

42. PROGRESSIVE SYSTEMIC SCLEROSIS

Progressive systemic sclerosis (PSS, scleroderma) is an uncommon multisystem disorder. The skin is typically the most prominent site of involvement but the lungs, gastrointestinal tract, heart, and kidneys are also frequently affected. The renal disease (called scleroderma renal crisis) is of particular importance since, if untreated, it typically progresses to end-stage renal failure and is a major cause of mortality in this condition.

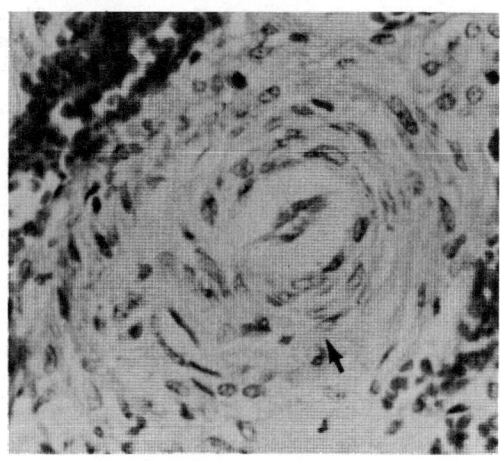

Fig. 42-1. Characteristic renal arterial lesion in progressive systemic sclerosis (PSS), showing concentric onion-skin thickening (arrow) of an interlobular artery, with marked compromise of the vascular lumen. (From Rose, BD. *Pathophysiology of Renal Disease* [2nd ed.]. New York: McGraw-Hill, 1987.)

Pathology

The primary pathologic changes in PSS are seen in the *skin,* where there is a dramatic increase in collagen deposition, and in the *blood vessels.* The renal disease, for example, is associated with obliterative arterial lesions, predominantly affecting the interlobular arteries. These lesions are characterized by concentric, onion-skin thickening that appears to result from proliferation of smooth muscle cells in the media, which then migrate into the intima (Fig. 42-1) [1]. The ensuing narrowing of the vascular lumen can cause ischemic glomerular necrosis and sclerosis and, in some patients, renal cortical infarcts. These vascular changes are not unique to the kidney, as they can often be found in other organs as well.

The histologic abnormalities in PSS may be confused with those observed in polyarteritis, malignant nephrosclerosis, and the hemolytic-uremic syndromes [1]. In comparison to polyarteritis, PSS is not associated with an inflammatory infiltrate in the arterial wall and the elastic membranes are not disrupted. It may not be possible, however, to differentiate the renal pathologic changes in PSS from those in malignant hypertension or the hemolytic-uremic syndromes. Consequently, only the characteristic extrarenal findings of PSS allow the diagnosis to be established.

The above vascular lesions are seen in acute scleroderma nephropathy. In contrast, some patients have evidence of chronic renal disease, manifested clinically by proteinuria and mild renal insufficiency. In this setting, only intimal thickening of the larger renal vessels may be seen. However, the relationships between these findings and PSS is uncertain, since similar changes may be found in patients with atherosclerosis or hypertension. [1].

Pathogenesis

Three theories have been proposed to explain the development of PSS, although the exact pathogenesis remains uncertain [2]. The *vascular* theory hypothesizes that regulatory failure in the microcirculation, leading to arteriolar vasodilation, is the initiating event [3]. The ensuing rise in intracapillary pressure could then damage the vascular endothelium, with the onion-skin changes reflecting cycles of injury and attempted repair. Collagen accumulation, according to this theory, could represent a secondary response to local ischemia. The intracapillary hypertension could also account for the commonly seen edema of the skin and the formation of telangiectases. The observation that the dermal changes in PSS may improve with early aggressive antihypertensive therapy (given for scleroderma renal crisis) is consistent with a central role for microvascular hemodynamics (see the following).

A primary *abnormality in collagen metabolism* has also been proposed, since there is a marked increase in collagen accumulation in the skin and in other organs in this disorder. However, this theory cannot explain many of the other common features of PSS, particularly the development of telangiectases, Raynaud's phenomenon, and edema, all of which may be present before the development of skin fibrosis.

The frequent detection of antinuclear antibodies, some of which are relatively specific for PSS (such as anti-Scl-70; see the following), suggests that the changes in this disorder may be induced by *immunologic injury*. It is possible, however, that these autoantibodies are the result, rather than the cause, of tissue damage.

In summary, the relative roles of these three not mutually exclusive hypotheses are not well defined. Most current data favor the vascular theory, but the event that triggers the microvascular injury remains unknown.

Clinical Presentation

Progressive systemic sclerosis most often affects women between 20 and 50 years of age. The signs and symptoms of the disease are primarily caused either by ischemia from vascular lesions or by an increase in local collagen accumulation.

Early findings suggestive of PSS usually involve the skin, although nonspecific symptoms such as fatigue or musculoskeletal aching also are frequently present. Local or diffuse swelling of the skin is generally the first sign, primarily affecting the hands and face. With time, the skin changes typically become more severe, with progressive induration causing a waxy appearance of the hands and a taut, boardlike appearance of the face. Raynaud's phenomenon is present in as many as 90 percent of patients, and ischemic ulcers may be observed over the fingertips. The early skin findings generally precede clinically evident visceral involvement [2].

The visceral manifestations of PSS depend on the organs affected. Vascular disease and increased collagen deposition in the gastrointestinal tract and lungs, for example, can lead respectively to dysphagia and ulceration or perforation anywhere in the gut, and to dyspnea and cor pulmonale. Renal involvement is also common, affecting 20 to 25 percent of patients.

Scleroderma Renal Crisis

Scleroderma renal crisis is characterized by the sudden onset of acute renal failure, generally with a urine sediment that is normal or that reveals only mild proteinuria with few cells or casts [2,4,5]. These typically benign urinary findings are a reflection of the noninflammatory nature of the vascular disease.

If left untreated, end-stage renal failure usually ensues over a period of 1 to 2 months. Most patients have marked elevations in blood pressure on initial evaluation, which is primarily due to ischemic activation of the renin-angiotensin system. However, the presence of mild hypertension or an elevated plasma renin activity does not necessarily predict which patients with PSS will ultimately develop this complication [4].

Acute scleroderma kidney disease almost always develops within the first 4 years after the onset of the extrarenal manifestations [4]. Most patients present in the cooler months, suggesting a possible role for cold-induced vasospasm.

The pathogenesis of the renal disease is unknown. It has been suggested that a stimulus to renal vasoconstriction (such as heart failure, hypovolemia, or cold exposure) in susceptible patients causes intense renal vasoconstriction. The renal ischemia then increases the release of renin, thereby producing more vasoconstriction and more renal ischemia. The concurrent development of angiotensin-mediated hypertension appears to be a secondary factor in the pathogenesis of scleroderma kidney, since acute renal failure is occasionally observed in the absence of hypertension [1,5].

Diagnosis

The diagnosis of PSS is usually based on the typical dermatologic abnormalities observed on physical examination. Supportive clinical findings include Raynaud's phenomenon, esophageal motility abnormalities, and impaired diffusing capacity on pulmonary function testing.

The findings of acute renal failure in the presence of a relatively normal urinalysis may be diagnostically helpful in those patients without classic extrarenal involvement. This combination is observed in only a few other conditions (see Chap. 16), including prerenal azotemia, urinary tract obstruction, atheroembolic disease, hypercalcemia, myeloma kidney (in which sulfosalicylic acid can be used to screen for urinary light chains), and, less commonly, acute tubular necrosis.

The diagnosis of PSS can be confirmed by skin biopsy. In addition, measurement of antinuclear antibodies also may be helpful in cases where the diagnosis is less apparent. When tested, over 90 percent of patients with PSS have one or more circulating auto-antibodies; some of these antibodies are both relatively specific for this disorder and may correlate with the severity of the disease. For example, anticentromere antibodies may be detected in the serum from patients with limited forms of PSS, such as the CREST syndrome (calcinosis, Raynaud's phenomenon, esophageal motility abnormalities, sclerodactyly, and telangiectasia) [6]. In comparison, approximately 20 percent of patients with diffuse, progressive scleroderma have anti-Scl-70 antibody in their serum; this antibody appears to be directed against the abundant nuclear enzyme, DNA topoisomerase [7].

Treatment

The overall mortality rate in untreated PSS is approximately 65 percent at 7 years [5]. Although some patients have fulminant disease, many patients (such as those with the CREST syndrome) have a more benign and prolonged course, although late progression may occur. Renal failure accounts for about 40 percent of deaths, with the remaining mortality caused by respiratory insufficiency, heart failure, or ischemic gastrointestinal complications (such as visceral perforation) [8].

There is no proved specific therapy for extrarenal PSS. In comparison, the use of antihypertensive drugs in scleroderma renal crisis may dramatically alter the outcome, substantially reducing the incidence of renal failure if begun before irreversible vascular injury has occurred.

The agent of choice in this disorder is a converting enzyme inhibitor, which can specifically reverse the angiotensin II–mediated hypertension in this setting, leading to an improvement in blood pressure in up to 90 percent of patients [9-13]. In addition, early therapy can stabilize or even improve renal function in up to 70 percent of cases [11,12].

The successful treatment of scleroderma renal disease has also been associated with *improvement in the extrarenal manifestations* of PSS in some patients. For example, regression in sclerodermatous skin changes, resolution of a microangiopathic hemolytic anemia if present, and improvement in Raynaud's phenomenon all may be seen [9]. The mechanism by which these changes occur is not well understood; it is possible that they may reflect a concomitant reduction in intracapillary pressures.

The optimal treatment of patients with chronic renal insufficiency without a history of scleroderma renal crisis is uncertain. In most of these patients, a direct link between PSS and renal insufficiency cannot be documented. Therefore, these patients are treated in the same manner as other patients with nonimmunologic progression of renal failure, using strict control of blood pressure (preferably with a converting enzyme inhibitor) and dietary protein restriction, both of which reduce intraglomerular hypertension (see Chap. 56).

Patients who progress to end-stage renal disease may be successfully dialyzed, but unique problems are sometimes observed. Hemodialysis, for example, is likely to be difficult if vascular access is limited by the peripheral vascular disease. This problem can be avoided with continuous ambulatory peritoneal dialysis. However, peritoneal clearances are often reduced in PSS as a result of impaired peritoneal blood flow. Furthermore, peritoneal clearances may change with alterations in the ambient temperature, which are lower during the winter months [14].

Renal transplantation may be performed in patients who are good surgical candidates or who are doing poorly on dialysis. Disease recurrence in the transplant may occur, particularly in those patients who developed end-stage renal failure within 1 year of the clinical onset of the PSS [15]. However, the pathologic findings of scleroderma may be difficult to differentiate from those of chronic transplant rejection, thereby obscuring the true incidence of disease recurrence [1].

References

1. Heptinstall, RH. *Pathology of the Kidney* (3rd ed). Boston: Little, Brown, 1983. Chapter 18.
2. Black, RM. Vascular diseases of the kidney. In Rose, BD, *Pathophysiology of Renal Disease* (2nd ed). New York: McGraw-Hill, 1987. Pp. 318–324.
3. Freis, JF. The microvascular pathogenesis of scleroderma: An hypothesis. *Ann Intern Med* 91:788, 1979.
4. Steen, VD, Medsger, TA, Osial, TA, Ziegler, GL, Shapiro, AP, Rodnan, GP. Factors predicting development of renal involvement in progressive systemic sclerosis. *Am J Med* 76:779, 1984.
5. Cannon, PJ, Hassar, M, Chase, DB, Casarella, WJ, Sommers, SC, LeRoy, EC. The relationship of hypertension and renal failure in scleroderma (progressive systemic sclerosis) to structural and functional abnormalities of the renal cortical circulation. *Medicine.* 53:1, 1974.
6. Kleinsmith, DM, Heinzerling, RH, Burnham, TK. Antinuclear antibodies as immunologic markers for a benign subset and different characteristics of scleroderma. *Arch Dermatol* 118:882, 1982.
7. Shero, JH, Bordwell, B, Rothfield, NF, Earnshaw, WC. High titers of autoantibodies to topoisomerase I (Scl-70) in sera from scleroderma patients. *Science* 231:737, 1986.
8. Follansbee, WP. The cardiovascular manifestations of systemic sclerosis (scleroderma). *Clin Prob Cardio* 11:245, 1986.
9. Lopez-Overjero, JS, Sall, SD, D'Angelo, WA, Cheigh, JS, Stenzel, KH, Laragh, JH. Reversal of vascular and renal crisis of scleroderma by oral angiotensin converting enzyme blockade. *N Engl J Med* 300:1417, 1979.
10. Fries, JF, Wasner, C, Brown, J, Feigenbaum, P. A controlled trial of antihypertensive therapy in systemic sclerosis (scleroderma). *Ann Rheum Dis* 43:407, 1984.
11. Beckett, VL, Donadio, JV, Brennan, LA, Jr, Conn, DL, Chao, EYS, Holley, KE. Use of captopril as early therapy for renal scleroderma: A prospective study. *Mayo Clin Proc* 60:763, 1985.
12. Thurm, RH, Alexander, JC. Captopril in the treatment of scleroderma renal crisis. *Arch Intern Med* 144:733, 1984.
13. Smith, CD, Smith, RD, Korn, JH. Hypertensive crisis in systemic sclerosis: Treatment with the new oral angiotensin converting enzyme inhibitor MK 421 (enalapril) in captopril intolerant patients. *Arth Rheum* 27:826, 1984.
14. Copley, JB, Smith, BJ. Continuous ambulatory peritoneal dialysis in scleroderma *Nephron* 40:353, 1985.
15. Paul, M, Bear, RA, Sugar, L. Renal transplantation in scleroderma. *J Rheumatol* 11:406, 1984.

43. HEMOLYTIC-UREMIC SYNDROMES

The hemolytic-uremic syndromes (HUS) are a group of rare disorders with overlapping clinical findings, typically characterized by a microangiopathic hemolytic anemia, thrombocytopenia, and varying degrees of renal failure. Occlusion of arteries and arterioles by platelet and fibrin thrombi plays a central role in the clinical manifestations of these disorders. The three forms of the HUS—thrombotic thrombocytopenic purpura (TTP), childhood HUS, and adult HUS—differ somewhat in their clinical presentations but have many common features [1].

The histologic changes in the kidney, for example, are similar in each of the forms of the HUS (Fig. 43-1). Patients with acute disease typically have platelet and fibrin

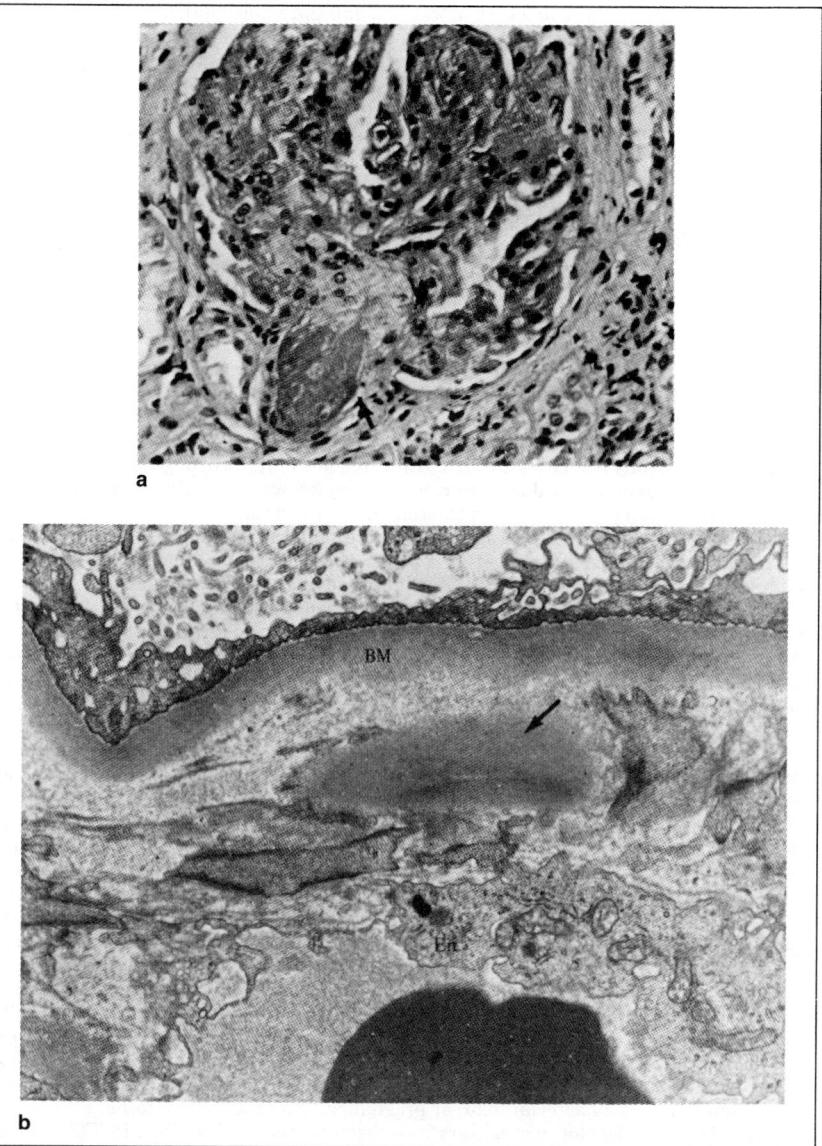

Fig. 43-1. Glomerular abnormalities in the hemolytic-uremic syndrome. (a) Platelet thrombus occluding the afferent arteriole (arrow). (b) Electron microscopy demonstrates widening of the subendothelial space between the glomerular basement membrane (BM) and the endothelial cell (En) in part by the deposition of fibrillar material (arrow), which may represent incompletely polymerized fibrin. (From Rose, BD. *Pathophysiology of Renal Disease* [2nd ed.]. New York: McGraw-Hill, 1987.)

thrombi occluding the small arteries, arterioles, and the glomerular capillaries. In comparison, patients with a more chronic course have prominent obliterative lesions in the interlobular arteries, characterized by concentric, onion-skin thickening, similar to that in scleroderma (see Chap. 42) or malignant hypertension.

Immunofluorescent microscopy usually reveals only fibrin in the arterial and glomerular lesions, with no evidence of immunoglobulin or complement deposition. Electron microscopy shows widening of the subendothelial space in part by fibrillar material that may represent incompletely polymerized fibrin.

Differences in the major site of involvement in the kidney (glomerular versus arterial) appear to be important prognostically [2]. The glomerulus is primarily affected in young children with HUS, a group in which spontaneous recovery is common. In contrast, arterial (in addition to glomerular) lesions are typically observed in adults, a finding associated with more severe hypertension and a lower incidence of spontaneous recovery.

Pathogenesis

The HUS appear to be disorders in which *isolated platelet consumption* is the primary abnormality [1,3]. This is manifested by thrombocytopenia and increased platelet turnover; in comparison, the classic findings of disseminated intravascular coagulation—increased prothrombin and partial thromboplastin times, reduced fibrinogen and factor V levels—are typically absent in the HUS. Elevated levels of fibrin degradation products may be present, presumably due to fibrinolytic breakdown of the fibrin present in the thrombi, rather than by activation of the coagulation system.

The event that triggers platelet aggregation is unknown. Three possible mechanisms have been described: increased levels of a platelet aggregating factor; reduced levels of an inhibitor of platelet aggregation; and primary damage to the vascular endothelium, leading to secondary platelet deposition [1]. The presence of a *platelet aggregating factor* is supported by the observation that normal platelets tend to aggregate when incubated in plasma from patients with TTP [4,5]. Furthermore, the favorable response to plasma exchange in many patients with this disorder may result from the removal of a compound that promotes platelet aggregation. One possible proaggregant in some patients is large factor VIII: von Willebrand factor multimers, the level of which appears to be increased during remission and then falls with acute disease, presumably by consumption in the thrombotic process [1,5]. Other platelet aggregating substances have also been described in selected cases [6].

Alternatively, the intravascular platelet consumption in the HUS could be caused by a *deficiency of a normal inhibitor of platelet aggregation*. The reversal of the disease process occasionally observed in TTP after infusion of fresh-frozen plasma alone is compatible with some deficient factor being replaced [7,8]. Recent studies suggest that the missing factor is, at least in some patients, an *immunoglobulin of the IgG class* [9]. IgG from patients with active HUS lacks this inhibitory activity as does IgG from normal children under the age of 4, the group most likely to develop the childhood HUS [9].

The mechanism of action of this IgG (or other missing inhibitor of platelet aggregation) is currently unknown. It is possible, for example, that these substances normally stimulate the release of prostacyclin from vascular endothelial cells [1] or that they promote the degradation of factor VIII: von Willebrand factor multimers [10]. Thus, their absence would facilitate the formation of platelet thrombi, particularly if some precipitating event (such as a bacterial toxin or pregnancy) has produced endothelial injury.

These defects in platelet aggregation have been primarily described in TTP and in sporadic cases of the adult HUS [1,9,10,10a]. In comparison, *primary endothelial damage* may be the major etiologic factor with drug-induced disease (mitomycin C or cyclosporine) or with classic childhood HUS following an episode of diarrhea [10a,11,12]. In the latter setting, bacterial verotoxins appear to be absorbed from the intestine, leading to endothelial damage and local platelet aggregation [11]. The endothelial injury also may enhance release of the proaggregant factor VIII: von Willebrand factor multimers [11].

Clinical Presentation

Despite their histologic and pathogenetic similarities, the three forms of the HUS have somewhat different clinical characteristics and will therefore be discussed separately.

Thrombotic Thrombocytopenic Purpura

Thrombotic thrombocytopenic purpura is primarily a disease of females between the ages of 10 and 50. It is characterized by the pentad of fever, thrombocytopenia (often with purpura), neurologic abnormalities, a microangiopathic hemolytic anemia, and renal failure [13].

The clinical presentation usually begins with a flulike syndrome that progresses ultimately to purpuric skin lesions and neurologic symptoms. The latter are generally nonlocalizing, such as headaches, mental status abnormalities, seizures, or coma. Less commonly, focal neurologic findings (aphasia or hemiparesis) may be observed.

Abnormal laboratory findings in this syndrome characteristically involve the hematologic and renal systems. A microangiopathic hemolytic anemia with thrombocytopenia is present in virtually all patients at some time in the course of their disease. Other plasma markers of intravascular hemolysis, such as indirect hyperbilirubinemia, low haptoglobin, high plasma lactic dehydrogenase, and moderate reticulocytosis (unless severe renal failure is present) are also common.

The urinalysis is usually abnormal, containing red cells, mild proteinuria, and rarely red cell casts [14]. Mild-to-moderate elevations in the plasma creatinine concentration are most often found, although severe, anuric renal failure may occur [14].

Childhood Hemolytic-Uremic Syndrome

The childhood HUS is a relatively common cause of acute renal failure in children under 4 years of age, but it may also be seen in older children. The observation that certain countries (such as Argentina) and some families have an increased incidence of this disorder suggests a common environmental agent or a genetic predisposition [12].

Childhood HUS typically begins after an episode of bacterial or viral gastroenteritis. This is followed in a few days or weeks by the sudden onset of a bleeding diathesis, usually manifested by petechiae or ecchymoses. Concomitantly, pallor (due to the anemia) and oligoanuria are observed. In more severe cases, neurologic findings may be present, caused by uremia, by electrolyte disturbances (such as hyponatremia), or, as in TTP, by cerebral vascular disease. Hypertension is common and appears to be induced by activation of the renin-angiotensin system by glomerular ischemia.

The laboratory findings in childhood HUS are similar to those observed in TTP. However, the degree of renal failure is characteristically more severe with anuria occurring in up to 50 percent of cases [15]. The urinalysis is frequently only slightly abnormal with minimal proteinuria and few cells or casts, despite the prominent renal function impairment. A somewhat surprising finding in many children is hypocomplementemia; it is unclear how this occurs [16].

Adult Hemolytic-Uremic Syndrome

Adult HUS is another rare disorder; it is often idiopathic, but an underlying condition can sometimes be identified [2]. For example, the adult HUS has been associated with pregnancy, particularly during the postpartum period [17]; estrogen-containing oral contraceptives [18]; mucinous adenocarcinomas of the gastrointestinal tract, pancreas, or prostate [19]; chemotherapy with the mitomycin C [20] or the combination of bleomycin and cisplatin [21]; and the use of cyclosporine [22]. A preceding episode of gastroenteritis, as typically occurs in children, is unusual in adults.

Adult HUS has a clinical presentation similar in many respects to childhood HUS, with thrombocytopenia (and purpura), a microangiopathy, and moderately severe renal failure being the major features. Some patients also develop neurologic symptoms, thereby resulting in a clinical syndrome indistinguishable from TTP. In addition, a cardiomyopathy may be observed in postpartum HUS, a finding that is not generally found in other causes of the HUS [17].

The predominant findings on physical examination are pallor, hypertension, purpura, and if a cardiomyopathy is present, rales and a gallop rhythm. Laboratory findings are similar to TTP; the urinalysis is frequently benign (mild proteinuria), but red cells and red cell casts may be observed in some patients.

Diagnosis

The diagnosis of one of the forms of the HUS is suggested by the classic clinical and laboratory findings and, in some cases, by a known precipitating event. Biopsy of an easily accessible tissue (gingiva or bone marrow) may be diagnostic, if platelet and fibrin thrombi are observed in vessels. However, false-negative biopsies are common, and a more invasive procedure (for example, renal biopsy) may be required in cases where the diagnosis remains unclear, unless precluded by thrombocytopenia [23].

The combination of a microangiopathic hemolytic anemia and acute renal failure can also be seen in patients with disseminated intravascular coagulation (DIC) or systemic vasculitis. When compared to DIC, patients with TTP characteristically have normal coagulation studies other than thrombocytopenia [1,3]. Furthermore, most patients with DIC have an obvious antecedent event (such as sepsis, an obstetrical complication, or hypotension) that appears to have precipitated the disorder.

The HUS can usually be distinguished from systemic vasculitis by the often marked thrombocytopenia and by the absence of musculoskeletal symptoms. Furthermore, neurologic disease in the HUS affects the central nervous system, whereas a peripheral mononeuritis multiplex is typically seen in systemic vasculitis.

Thrombotic thrombocytopenic purpura and the adult HUS are distinguished primarily by the pattern of organ involvement. Neurologic findings are frequently a major problem in patients with TTP, while renal failure tends to be more prominent in adult HUS. However, a common event may cause both disorders, thereby making this distinction less definite. For example, in a study of five patients treated with bleomycin and cisplatin, three presented with the usual features of adult HUS, while the remaining two had symptoms typical of TTP [21].

The diagnosis of childhood HUS can usually be made on the basis of the history, physical examination, and laboratory findings. Tissue biopsy is generally not necessary, since there are very few other disorders affecting this age group that are likely to be confused with the HUS.*

Prognosis

Therapy must be initiated promptly in TTP, since the disease is almost uniformly fatal if untreated, with a 3-month mortality rate of 75 percent [13]. Patients with the *adult HUS* have a lower mortality rate, but the renal prognosis in untreated patients tends to be poor. Recovery may occur within the first few weeks after onset, but it is commonly delayed and usually incomplete. It is estimated that up to 80 percent of adults will ultimately require long-term dialysis or renal transplantation. The outcome appears to be particularly poor in women with postpartum HUS (in part due to the concomitant development of a cardiomyopathy) [17]. In comparison, adult HUS following a diarrheal prodrome or associated with cyclosporine therapy appears to represent a milder form of the disease in which recovery is common.

In contrast, the usual outlook in *childhood HUS* in the United States is good, with a mortality rate presently under 5 percent with supportive care alone (including early peritoneal dialysis and treatment of infection and hypertension) [24]. The hematologic and renal abnormalities generally resolve within 1 to 2 weeks. As described above, glomerular rather than vascular lesions predominate in children, a finding that may explain the better prognosis [2].

There are certain settings, however, where specific therapy may be considered in childhood HUS because more severe disease appears to be present. Relatively bad prognostic signs include no substantial improvement by 1 to 2 weeks after onset, hemorrhage due to severe thrombocytopenia, or central nervous system disease that is not due to uremia or marked hypertension.

---

*Uncommonly, an active urine sediment may be seen in childhood HUS with red blood cells and red cell casts. These urinary findings plus hypertension may suggest the diagnosis of acute glomerulonephritis. Moreover, the presence of hypocomplementemia in some children [16] may raise the possibility of poststreptococcal or membranoproliferative glomerulonephritis. Differentiation from HUS is generally not difficult, however, since neither of these other disorders is associated with the hematologic abnormalities present in the HUS.

Treatment

Therapy in the HUS has been best studied in TTP. Treatment, if effective, can prevent bleeding from thrombocytopenia and can reduce ischemic necrosis induced by the vascular lesions, both of which are major causes of morbidity and mortality in this disorder. In view of the pathogenetic and histopathologic similarities, however, it seems reasonable to consider common therapy in TTP, adult HUS, and fulminant childhood HUS, even though there is at present only anecdotal evidence supporting the efficacy of therapy in the last two disorders [1].

The use of protocols that attempt to replace the missing substance(s) that normally inhibits platelet aggregation or that attempts to remove platelet aggregating factors has dramatically altered the outlook in TTP; in some studies, more than 80 percent of patients undergo long-term remission if therapy is initiated relatively quickly [25].

The increased platelet aggregation and thrombocytopenia can be corrected within 72 hours in some patients by the *infusion of fresh-frozen plasma* [26,27]. This regimen presumably replaces a missing factor that may, for example, stimulate prostacyclin release [1] or promote the degradation of large von Willebrand factor multimers [10]. In other patients, substances that enhance platelet aggregation may be present [1,5,6]; in this setting, their removal by *plasmapheresis* can improve both the symptoms and laboratory parameters [25].

In view of these observations, the following recommendations can be made. Therapy in patients with *stable* TTP without life-threatening signs should be initiated using fresh-frozen plasma (approximately 3 units/day) and antiplatelet agents (such as aspirin and dipyridamole, which are generally ineffective if given alone [28]). If no clinical or laboratory improvement (such as an increased platelet count) is observed within 48 to 72 hours, plasmapheresis (with plasma replacement) should be instituted.

In patients with more aggressive disease, there may not be sufficient time to see if fresh-frozen plasma and antiplatelet agents alone will be effective. As a result, treatment should be initiated with antiplatelet agents and plasmapheresis in this setting*.

Those patients who do not respond to plasma infusion or plasmapheresis may improve if they are treated with gamma globulin infusions or vincristine; the mechanism by which these modalities act is unclear [30–32]. Corticosteroids and splenectomy (both of which have been used in this disorder with only limited success) should be reserved for patients who are refractory to all other therapies.

Two potential complications of treatment in TTP need to be emphasized. First, the use of antiplatelet agents in the presence of thrombocytopenia may cause bleeding in some patients [28]. Second, the infusion of platelets to correct the thrombocytopenia in this disorder has been associated with the acute development or worsening of focal neurologic signs, presumably due to local consumption of the transfused platelets, leading to new or expanded thrombi [33,34]. Therefore, *platelet transfusions should not be given in the absence of severe thrombocytopenia and bleeding.*

In addition to specific therapy, any medications that have been associated with the HUS should be discontinued. For example, spontaneous recovery has been reported in over 50 percent of patients who developed the HUS after treatment with cyclosporine [22]. Reduction in cyclosporine dosage or substitution with an alternative immunosuppressive agent (such as azathioprine) appears to improve the prognosis in this setting.

In summary, plasma infusion and plasmapheresis have dramatically improved the prognosis in TTP (although some patients still die from complications of the disease) [35]. Despite the high incidence of remission, however, careful monitoring is required because relapses may occur in about one-third of patients, often following an episode of infection [35]. These relapses are generally mild and may be manifested only by asymptomatic thrombocytopenia and a microangiopathic hemolytic anemia.

Those patients who develop irreversible renal failure may undergo renal transplantation. There is, however, a risk of recurrent disease in the transplanted kidney. Furthermore, it is uncertain if cyclosporine should be used as an immunosuppressive agent in this setting, since this drug can cause the HUS.

---

*The role of plasmapheresis in drug-induced HUS is uncertain. Preliminary studies in mitomycin C–induced disease suggest that some benefit may be achieved [29].

References

1. Remuzzi, G, HUS and TTP: Variable expression of a single entity. *Kidney Int* 32:292, 1987.
2. Morel-Maroger, L, Kanfer, A, Solez, K, Sraer, JD, Richet, G. Prognostic importance of vascular lesions in acute renal failure with microangiopathic hemolytic anemia (hemolytic-uremic syndrome): Clinicopathologic study in 20 adults. *Kidney Int* 15:548, 1979.
3. Neame, PB, Hirsh, J, Browman, G, Denburg, J, D'Souza, TJ, Gallus, A, Brian, MC. Thrombotic thrombocytopenic purpura: A syndrome of intravascular platelet consumption. *Can Med Assoc J* 144:1108, 1976.
4. Lian, EC-Y. The role of increased platelet aggregation in thrombotic thrombocytopenic purpura. *Sem Thromb Hemostasis* 6:401, 1980.
5. Moake, JL, Rudy, CK, Troll, JH, Weinstein, MJ, Colannino, NM, Azocar, J, Seder, RH, Hong, SL, Deykin, D. Unusually large plasma factor VIII: von Willebrand factor multimers in chronic relapsing thrombotic thrombocytopenic purpura. *N Engl J Med* 307:1432, 1982.
6. Kelton, JG, Moore, J, Santos, A, Sheridan, D. The detection of a platelet-agglutinating factor in TTP. *Ann Intern Med* 101:589, 1984.
7. Byrnes, JJ, Khurana, M. Treatment of Thrombotic thrombocytopenic purpura with plasma. *N Engl J Med* 297:1386, 1977.
8. Lian, EC-Y, Harkness, DR, Byrnes, JJ, Wallach, H, Nunez, R. Presence of a platelet aggregating factor in the plasma of patients with thrombocytopenic purpura (TTP) and its inhibition by normal plasma. *Blood* 53:333, 1979.
9. Lian, EC-Y, Mui, PTK, Siddiqui, FA, Chiu, A, Chiu, LLS. Inhibition of platelet-aggregating activity in thrombotic thrombocytopenic plasma by normal adult immunoglobulin G. *J Clin Invest* 73:548, 1984.
10. Moake, JL, Byrnes, JJ, Troll, JH, Rudy, CK, Hong, SL, Weinstein, JH, Colannino, NM. Effects of fresh frozen plasma and its cryosupernatant fraction on von Willebrand factor multimeric forms in chronic relapsing TTP. *Blood* 65:1232, 1985.
10a. Walters, MDS, Levin, M, Smith, C, et al. Intravascular platelet activation in the hemolytic uremic syndrome. *Kidney Int* 33:107, 1988.
11. Editorial. Unravelling HUS. *Lancet* 2:1437, 1987.
12. Drummond, KN. Hemolytic-uremic syndrome — then and now. *N Engl J Med* 312:116, 1985.
13. Amorosi, EL, Ultmann, JE. Thrombotic thrombocytopenic purpura: Report of 16 cases and review of the literature. *Medicine* 45:139, 1966.
14. Eknoyan, G, Riggs, SA. Renal involvement in patients with thrombotic thrombocytopenic purpura. *Am J Nephrol* 6:117, 1986.
15. Siegler, R, Berry, PL, Hogg, RL. Comparison of the epidemiologic and clinical features of endemic and sporadic forms of hemolytic-uremic syndrome (HUS) in 210 USA children. Report of the Southwest Pediatric Nephrology Study Group (abstract). *Kidney Int* 29:104, 1986.
16. Monnens, L, Molenaar, J, Lambert, PH, Proesmans, W, van Munster, P. The complement system in hemolytic-uremic syndrome in childhood. *Clin Nephrol* 13:168, 1980.
17. Hayslett, JP. Postpartum renal failure. *N Engl J Med* 312:1556, 1985.
18. Hauglustaine, D, van Damme, B, van Renterghem, Y, Michielsen, P. Recurrent hemolytic-uremic syndrome during oral contraception. *Clin Nephrol* 15:148, 1981.
19. Laffay, DL, Tubbs, RR, Valenzuela, MD, Hall, PM, McCormack, LJ. Chronic glomerular microangiopathy and metastatic carcinoma. *Hum Pathol* 10:433, 1979.
20. Valavaara, R, Nordman, E. Renal complications of mitomycin C therapy with special reference to the total dose. *Cancer* 55:47, 1985.
21. Jackson, AM, Rose, BD, Graff, LG, Jacobs, JB, Schwartz, JH, Strauss, GM, Yang, JPS, Rudnick, MR, Elfenbein, IB, Narins, RG. Thrombotic microangiopathy and renal dysfunction associated with antineoplastic chemotherapy. *Ann Intern Med* 104:41, 1984.
22. Wolfe, JA, McCann, RL, Sanfilippo, F. Cyclosporine-associated microangiopathy in renal transplantation: A severe but potentially reversible form of early graft injury. *Transplantation* 41:541, 1986.

23. Goldenfarb, PB, Finch, SC. Thrombotic thrombocytopenic purpura: A ten-year study. *J Am Med Assoc* 226:644, 1973.
24. Dolislager, D, Tune, B. The hemolytic-uremic syndrome: Spectrum of severity and significance of prodrome. *Am J Dis Child* 132:55, 1978.
25. Myers, TJ, Wakem, CJ, Ball, ED, Tremont, SJ. Thrombotic thrombocytopenic purpura: Combined treatment with plasmapheresis and antiplatelet agents. *Ann Intern Med* 92:149, 1980.
26. Byrnes, JJ, Khurana, M. Treatment of thrombotic thrombocytopenic purpura with plasma. *N Engl J Med* 297:1386, 1977.
27. Aster, RH. Plasma therapy for thrombotic thrombocytopenic purpura. *N Engl J Med* 312:985, 1985.
28. Rosove, NH, Ho, WG, Goldfinger, D. Ineffectiveness of aspirin and dipyridamole in the treatment of thrombotic thrombocytopenic purpura. *Ann Intern Med* 96:27, 1982.
29. Cantrell, JE, Phillips, JM, Schein, PS. Cancer-associated hemolytic-uremic syndrome: A complication of mitomycin C chemotherapy. *J Clin Oncol* 3:723, 1984.
30. Sennett, ML, Conrad, ME. Treatment of thrombotic thrombocytopenic purpura. *Arch Intern Med* 146:266, 1986.
31. Gutterman, LA, Stevenson, TD. Treatment of thrombotic thrombocytopenic purpura with vincristine. *J Am Med Assoc* 247:1433, 1982.
32. Wong, P, Itoh, K, Yoshida, S. Treatment of thrombotic thrombocytopenic purpura with intravenous gamma globulin (letter). *N Engl J Med* 314:385, 1986.
33. Harkness, DR, Byrnes, JJ, Lian, E, Williams, WD. Hensley, GT. Hazard of platelet transfusion in thrombotic thrombocytopenic purpura. *J Am Med Assoc.* 246:1931, 1981.
34. Lind, SE. Thrombocytopenic purpura and platelet transfusions (letter). *Ann Intern Med* 106:478, 1987.
35. Rose, M, Eldor, A. High incidence of relapses in thrombotic thrombocytopenic purpura. Clinical study of 35 patients. *Am J Med* 83:437, 1987.

44. THE KIDNEY IN PREGNANCY AND PREECLAMPSIA

Systemic and Renal Hemodynamics

Normal pregnancy is characterized by major changes in blood pressure, sodium balance, and renal function [1,2]. The blood pressure typically falls early in gestation and is often 10 mm Hg below baseline during the second trimester, declining to a mean of 105/60. This decrease in pressure is caused by a reduction in systemic vascular resistance that is in part due to impaired vascular responsiveness to the pressor actions of angiotensin II and norepinephrine [3]. As the pregnancy nears term, these changes become attenuated, and blood pressure returns toward normal.

This reduction in blood pressure is accompanied by the retention of 900 to 1000 meq of sodium and 6 to 8 liters of water [2]. Some of this excess fluid is required to meet the needs of the placenta and the fetus. However, true volume expansion is also present as indicated by elevations in cardiac output and renal perfusion. Several factors may stimulate tubular sodium reabsorption in this setting, including estrogens, aldosterone, and the fall in blood pressure itself.

Renal function is also altered during normal pregnancy. This is manifested by increases in the renal plasma flow and the glomerular filtration rate, resulting both from the elevation in cardiac output and from neurohumoral factors, possibly including enhanced secretion of prolactin [4]. The rise in the glomerular filtration rate begins early in the first trimester and reaches a peak (about 50% above nonpregnant levels) by the beginning of the second trimester [1]. The net effect is a reduction in the plasma creatinine concentration to about 0.4 to 0.5 mg/dl; in comparison, a relatively "normal" plasma creatinine concentration of 0.8 mg/dl at this time is generally indicative of some impairment in renal function. The glomerular filtration rate returns toward baseline during the ninth month of gestation, although it is still well above nonpregnant levels.

Preeclampsia

Preeclampsia is usually characterized by the gradual onset of hypertension, proteinuria, and edema, beginning after the twentieth week of gestation.* It is seen in about 5 to 10 percent of all pregnancies (most often during the last trimester of a first pregnancy) and may progress to a convulsive phase called eclampsia.

Pathogenesis

The placenta is thought to play a central role in the development of preeclampsia, since delivery usually results in the rapid resolution of the clinical manifestations. However, the factors that ultimately lead to placental dysfunction are uncertain.

A primary role for *uterine ischemia* is suggested by the observation that preeclampsia develops primarily in those patients in whom a decrease in placental perfusion would be likely to occur. Primigravidas, for example, may have a less-developed uterine vasculature than multiparous women. The prevalence of preeclampsia is also increased with multiple births or a hydatidiform mole (where metabolic needs may be markedly enhanced, exceeding the placental blood supply) or with underlying vascular diseases, such as diabetes mellitus or hypertension.

Three theories have been proposed to explain the uteroplacental ischemia in preeclampsia: decreased migration of cytotrophoblasts, abnormal prostaglandin metabolism, and activation of the coagulation system [1,5,6].

1. It has been suggested that *decreased migration of cytotrophoblasts* could be the initiating event in the development of the uterine ischemia in preeclampsia [5,6]. In normal pregnancy, cytotrophoblasts grow into the spiral arteries of the uterus; this leads to loss of the musculoelastic tissue in these vessels, thereby resulting in persistent vasodilation. By contrast, the myometrial segments of the uteroplacental arterioles are not invaded in preeclampsia; as a result, these vessels retain their musculoelastic tissue, possibly predisposing them to thromboxane B_2-, norepinephrine-, and angiotensin II–mediated vasoconstriction [5,6]. Why this might occur is not known.

2. *Prostaglandin metabolism* appears to be abnormal during preeclampsia. Normal pregnancy is characterized by increased synthesis of vasodilator prostaglandins; this response helps to preserve uterine perfusion, since inhibition of prostaglandin synthesis by indomethacin causes a concomitant reduction in uterine blood flow [7]. In comparison, preeclampsia may be associated with a relative increase in the production of the vasoconstrictor and platelet aggregator, *thromboxane B_2* [8]. This change could both diminish uterine perfusion and enhance the sensitivity to the pressor effect of infused angiotensin II, the earliest clinical manifestation of preeclampsia (Fig. 44-1) [8]. The possible protective effect of low-dose aspirin in high-risk pregnancies, for example, may be mediated by a preferential inhibition of thromboxane synthesis (see "Prevention").

3. *Activation of the coagulation system,* leading to obliteration of placental vessels by platelets and fibrin, also has been found in preeclampsia [1]. The mechanism by which this might occur is uncertain, although thromboxanes may play a contributory role. Furthermore, ischemic placental degeneration may result in the release of thromboplastins into the systemic circulation, leading to fibrin deposition in the kidney and other organs.

In addition to vascular insufficiency, *immunologic factors* also may be important in at least some cases of preeclampsia. It has been suggested that the production of "blocking antibodies" (antibodies that can block the generation of an immune response against paternal antigens in the fetoplacental unit) is lowest during a first pregnancy. This hypothesis could explain the increased frequency of preeclampsia both in primigravidas and in multiparous women who have a first child with a different father [9].

---

*It should be emphasized that none of these findings in isolation is diagnostic of preeclampsia. Edema, for example, is common in normal pregnancy, partially due to compression of the inferior vena cava by the pregnant uterus.

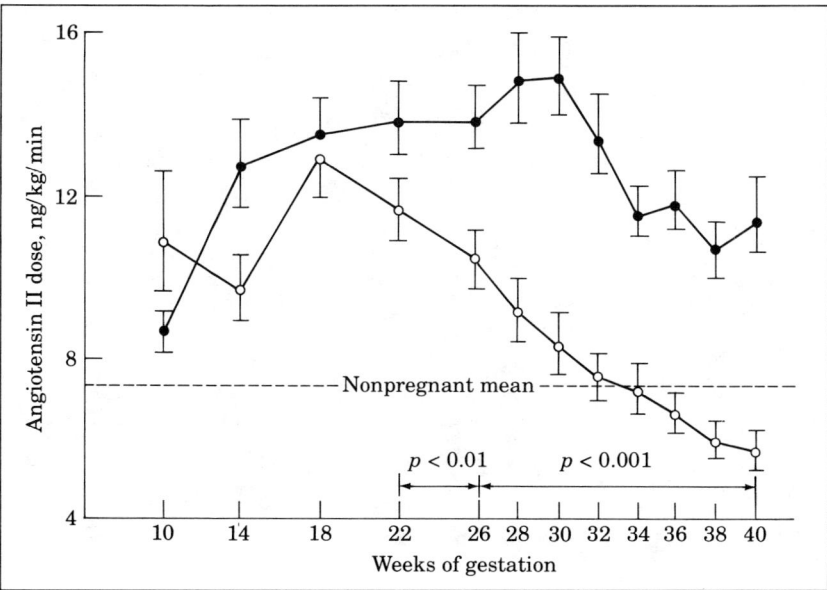

Fig. 44-1. Comparison of the average angiotensin II dose required to raise the diastolic blood pressure by 20 mm Hg in primigravidas. The solid circles represent women who did not develop preeclampsia; a higher dose is required than in nonpregnant women, indicating resistance to the pressor effects of angiotensin II (perhaps due in part to increased prostaglandins). By comparison, women who became preeclamptic (open circles) show a progressive fall in angiotensin II resistance that was significant after the twenty-third week. (From Gant, NF, Daley, GI, Chand, S, Whalley, PJ, MacDonald, PC. *J Clin Invest* 52:2682, 1973, by copyright permission of the American Society for Clinical Investigation.)

Pathology

The principal pathologic changes in the kidney in preeclampsia are seen in the glomeruli (Fig. 44-2). On light microscopy, swelling of endothelial and mesangial cells is observed, resulting in narrowing or obliteration of the glomerular capillary lumens. This characteristic ballooning of endothelial cells (the pathogenesis of which may be related to fibrin deposition) is called *glomerular endotheliosis* [10]. In addition to the increase in cell volume, electron microscopy typically reveals widening of the glomerular basement membrane, in part by fibrillar material that may represent incompletely polymerized fibrin. There is usually no substantial deposition of immunoglobulins or complement on immunofluorescent staining.

In most patients with preeclampsia, the pathologic abnormalities in the kidney begin to resolve shortly after delivery, and glomerular histology typically returns to normal within 2 to 3 weeks. However, rapid resolution does not occur in all cases. There is often extensive glomerular deposition of fibrin and platelets in severe preeclampsia, changes that may be associated with renal cortical necrosis or delayed or incomplete functional recovery. Similar findings may be observed in other organs, including the placenta and liver, and, in patients who progress to eclampsia, the brain and adrenal and pituitary glands.

Clinical Presentation

Preeclampsia is most commonly observed in the third trimester of a first pregnancy, with hypertension usually being the earliest clinical finding [1,11]. Its occurrence during a

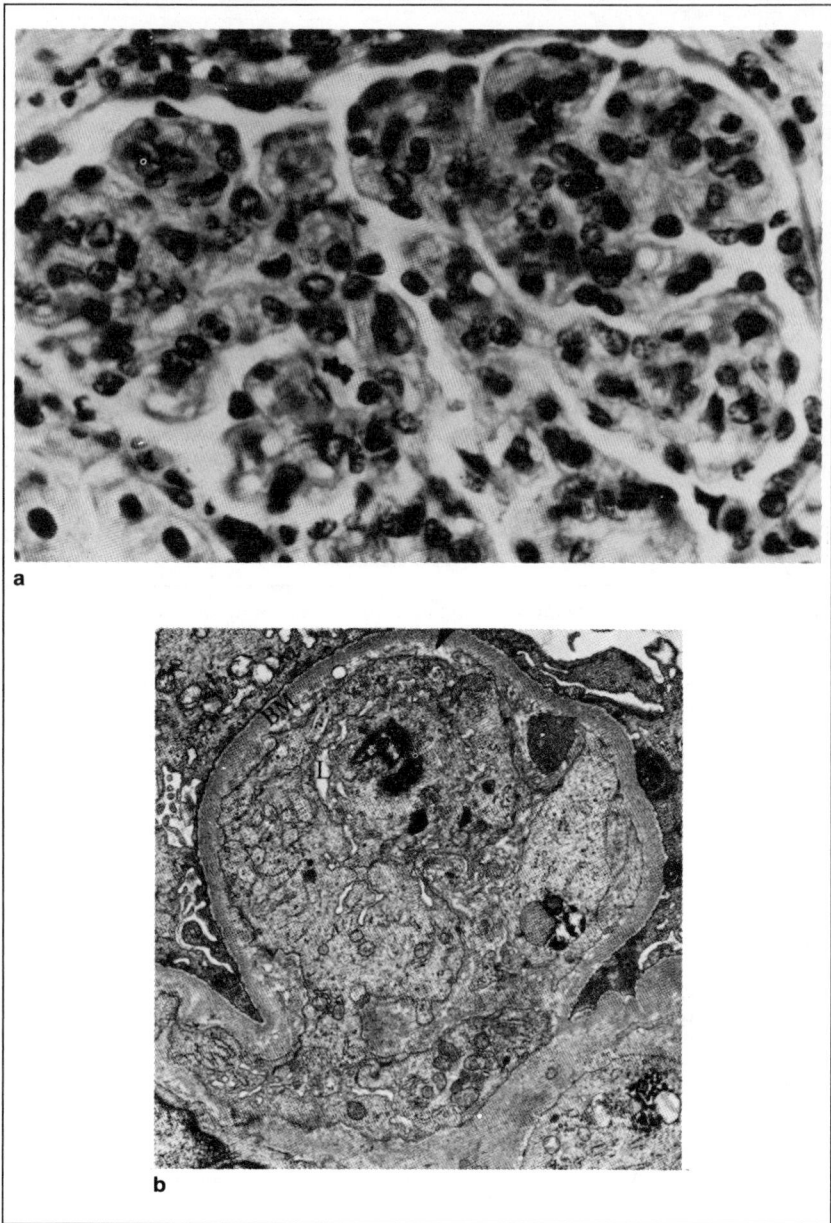

Fig. 44-2. Glomerular endotheliosis in preeclampsia. (a) Light microscopy reveals obliteration of the capillary lumens although cellularity is relatively normal. (b) These changes are better seen on electron microscopy, which shows that marked swelling of the endothelial cell is responsible for virtual loss of the capillary lumen (L). (From Rose, BD. *Pathophysiology of Renal Disease* [2nd ed.]. New York: McGraw-Hill, 1987.)

later pregnancy generally indicates preexistent vascular disease, most often due to hypertension or underlying renal disease.

The blood pressure (which may be labile) gradually begins to increase after the twentieth week of gestation but occasionally as early as 9 to 12 weeks in women who eventually develop preeclampsia [1]. Hypertensive levels (>140/90) are typically reached in the third trimester, often after the thirty-seventh week of gestation.

The degree of hypertension in preeclampsia usually correlates directly with the duration and severity of the disease. Only mild hypertension may be initially present; however, the blood pressure can eventually exceed 180/120 if fetal delivery is delayed.

In addition to hypertension, most patients with preeclampsia have both peripheral edema, which also is commonly seen in normal pregnancy, and proteinuria. Urinary protein excretion increases gradually, often reaching the nephrotic range (>3.5 gm/day). The urine sediment is usually benign, containing only a few red or white cells. Moreover, renal function is generally well maintained with only minor increases in the plasma creatinine concentration (0.2–0.3 mg/dl), unless disseminated intravascular coagulation with renal cortical necrosis develops.

Additional abnormalities may be found in those patients with more severe preeclampsia. Common symptoms and signs include headache, epigastric or right subcostal pain (due to distention of the liver capsule caused by hepatic edema or hemorrhage), visual disturbances, and hyperactive deep tendon reflexes. In some patients, *h*emolysis (with a microangiopathic blood smear), *e*levated *l*iver enzymes, and a *l*ow *p*latelet count (HELLP syndrome) are seen, findings that may reflect hepatic ischemia caused by vascular obstruction [11,12]. Seizures, when they occur, are considered diagnostic of eclampsia.

Diagnosis

The presence of preeclampsia is suggested when hypertension and proteinuria are observed, particularly if developing in the third trimester in a primigravida. An earlier onset or development in a multigravid woman suggests an underlying disorder such as essential hypertension, primary renal disease, diabetes mellitus, or a hydatidiform mole [13,13a]. In one large series, for example, the clinical diagnosis of preeclampsia could be confirmed by postpartum renal biopsy in 85 percent of primigravidas but only 38 percent of multigravidas, most of whom had benign nephrosclerosis or other underlying renal disease [13a].

In general, three issues must be addressed in the diagnosis (and management) of preeclampsia: early diagnosis, distinguishing preeclampsia from other forms of hypertension, and differentiating the renal disease of preeclampsia from other forms of renal disease developing during pregnancy.

EARLY DIAGNOSIS OF PREECLAMPSIA.   The optimal step in early diagnosis is to identify those patients who are at highest risk of developing this disorder. This may be particularly important from a therapeutic standpoint, since close monitoring of the pregnancy can be undertaken and consideration given to the use of prophylactic low-dose aspirin, which may be beneficial in this setting (see the following).

Patients with underlying vascular disease, for example, are predisposed to the development of preeclampsia, presumably due to impaired uteroplacental perfusion. This may explain why preeclampsia is more common in patients with diabetes mellitus or chronic hypertension.

There are also several laboratory abnormalities that vary in their ability to predict which women will subsequently develop this disorder. For example, patients with established preeclampsia frequently have *hyperuricemia* and *hypocalciuria* (due to increased tubular reabsorption of uric acid and calcium, respectively) [14,15]. In isolation, however, these findings are of limited value in early diagnosis, as they may be normal until other, more specific, markers of preeclampsia (such as hypertension) are also present.

The demonstration of increased pressor responsiveness to angiotensin II appears to be the *earliest predictor* of pregnancy-induced hypertension or preeclampsia [16]. Patients prone to develop these problems characteristically demonstrate an increased blood pressure response to infused angiotensin II as early as the twenty-fourth week of gestation (Fig. 44-1). In one large study, for example, the incidence of subsequent hypertension or preeclampsia was 45 percent in positive responders versus less than 5 percent in those with a negative test [16].

The "roll-over" test, which compares the difference in blood pressure between the left lateral recumbent and supine positions, has also been used in an attempt to identify patients who are more likely to develop preeclampsia [17]. This test is performed at 28 weeks, with a positive result defined as an increase in blood pressure (when supine) of 20 mm Hg or more. This exaggerated response to changes in posture may reflect enhanced sensitivity to vasoconstrictors, as exemplified by the response to infused angiotensin II. Although this test is easier to perform than serial angiotensin II infusions, it may be less sensitive and specific.

PREGNANCY-INDUCED HYPERTENSION. Hypertension is considered to be present during pregnancy when the blood pressure is above 140/90, or when there has been more than a 15 mm Hg increase in the diastolic pressure or a 30 mm Hg increase in systolic blood pressure above baseline values. High blood pressure in this setting may be caused by preeclampsia (pregnancy-induced hypertension), an underlying hypertensive tendency, or late or transient gestational hypertension (that resolves after delivery).

In the absence of a past history of hypertension, differentiating between preeclampsia and chronic hypertension may be difficult due to the reduction in pressure typically seen by the second trimester. Consequently, patients with preexistent but undiagnosed essential hypertension may have pressures that fall into the normal range when first seen by the physician. As the blood pressure then rises during the third trimester, factors such as the patient's age, gravid status, degree of protein and calcium excretion, and plasma uric acid concentration all may be helpful in establishing the correct diagnosis (Table 44-1). Calcium excretion below 100 mg/day and a plasma uric acid concentration above 5.5 mg/dl, for example, are suggestive of preeclampsia [14,15].

The onset of *isolated,* mild (and often transient) hypertension during the third trimester is occasionally observed in the absence of concurrent proteinuria. This finding appears to have little adverse effect on the mother or fetus but may be a predictor of future essential hypertension [18].

DISTINGUISHING PRIMARY RENAL DISEASE FROM PREECLAMPSIA. Preeclampsia is the most common form of renal disease occurring during the later stages of pregnancy. It can usually be distinguished easily from other causes of renal disease that occur during pregnancy (Table 44-2); in contrast to preeclampsia, these disorders are often associated with moderate-to-marked reductions in the glomerular filtration rate and with little or no proteinuria.*

It is often difficult to distinguish between severe preeclampsia with disseminated intravascular coagulation (DIC) and the postpartum hemolytic-uremic syndrome (HUS). However, the history and laboratory findings are frequently helpful. The HUS is usually associated with an uncomplicated pregnancy and delivery and with normal coagulation tests (prothrombin time, partial thromboplastin time, and fibrinogen levels), findings that are opposite from those in severe preeclampsia with DIC. This distinction is extremely important from a therapeutic viewpoint, since preeclampsia typically resolves after delivery, whereas plasma infusion or plasmapheresis may be indicated in the postpartum HUS (see Chap. 43).

The exclusion of urinary tract obstruction is another problem that may arise in the pregnant patient with renal failure. Relaxation of ureteral smooth muscle (caused in part by prostaglandins) and pressure on the ureters by the pregnant uterus typically causes some degree of dilatation of the calyceal system in normal gestation. This "functional" hydronephrosis can be detected by renal ultrasound and is, therefore, not diagnostic of urinary tract obstruction in this setting. Rarely, the pregnant uterus may cause sufficient obstruction to produce a reduction in the glomerular filtration rate [20]. Normalization of renal function in the lateral recumbent position and its recurrence when supine should suggest this possibility.

*Acute fatty liver (fatty infiltration of hepatocytes without inflammation or necrosis) is an uncommon complication of pregnancy that is associated with acute renal failure in up to 60 percent of patients. The majority of these patients have evidence of decreased renal perfusion or acute tubular necrosis, although mild preeclampsia may also be present [19].

Table 44-1. Characteristics of preeclampsia and essential hypertension in pregnancy

Finding	Preeclampsia	Essential hypertension
Age	Often < 20	Frequently > 30
Gravida	Usually primigravida	Primigravida or multigravida
History of hypertension	No	May be present
Proteinuria	Present	Usually absent
Plasma uric acid concentration	> 5.5 mg/dl	< 5.5 mg/dl
24-hour urine calcium	< 100 mg/day	> 200 mg/day
Postpartum blood pressure	Normal by 6–12 weeks in most women	Hypertension often persists
Risk of chronic hypertension	Similar to control population in primigravidas	High

Table 44-2. Major causes of renal disease in pregnancy

First half
    Acute tubular necrosis resulting from septic abortion
    Prerenal disease due to hyperemesis gravidarum
Second half
    Preeclampsia
    Renal cortical necrosis or acute tubular necrosis due to abruptio placentae or placenta previa
    Postpartum hemolytic-uremic syndrome
    Urinary tract obstruction

Treatment

Untreated, preeclampsia is associated with an increased incidence of stillbirths, neonatal deaths, and, in patients who progress to severe preeclampsia or eclampsia, maternal mortality primarily due to intracerebral hemorrhage. Definitive therapy is delivery of the fetus and placenta. The only reason to delay delivery in established preeclampsia is evidence of fetal immaturity. In this setting, bed rest in the lateral recumbent position and antihypertensive agents (if the diastolic pressure is above 100–105 mm Hg) can be used until delivery can be safely performed. However, delivery should not be delayed if there are signs that the mother is at risk, including uncontrollable hypertension, visual disturbances, seizures, the HELLP syndrome, or DIC.

In comparison, isolated mild hypertension that develops during the third trimester does not usually necessitate immediate delivery. Although the minimum level of blood pressure elevation that will injure the fetus is unknown, an adverse outcome from mild hypertension is uncommon in patients who do not progress to preeclampsia [21].

The data on therapy of pregnant women with chronic hypertension during pregnancy is also incomplete. A substantial drop in maternal blood pressure with therapy could impair uteroplacental blood flow, thereby compromising fetal survival. On the other hand, a persistent moderate-to-severe elevation in blood pressure could jeopardize both the mother and the fetus.

Despite these problems, a reasonable approach is to institute therapy in women with chronic hypertension if the diastolic blood pressure is above 90 to 95 mm Hg in the first or second trimester or above 100 mm Hg in the third trimester [6,21a,22]. In addition, a diastolic pressure above 105 to 110 mm Hg should always be treated (whether acute or chronic) to reduce the risk of maternal intracerebral hemorrhage.

Once a decision to initiate medical therapy is made, only those antihypertensive agents that appear to be safe during pregnancy should be given: methyldopa, β-blockers, and hydralazine [21a,22]. The problems associated with these medications are relatively minor and include transient neonatal tremors, neonatal bradycardia and hypoglycemia, and lack of hypotensive effect when used alone, respectively. Diuretics are generally avoided, since preeclampsia tends to be associated with a low plasma volume which, if diminished further, can exacerbate the placental ischemia. The safety of calcium channel blockers is also uncertain, although they can effectively reduce the blood pressure toward normal [6,23].

More potent and rapidly acting agents, such as diazoxide, are required in patients with severe hypertension or evidence of central nervous system involvement. An intravenous "mini" bolus of diazoxide (30 mg) can minimize the potential problems of uterine atony (with arrest of labor) and an excessive drop in blood pressure that could jeopardize the fetus [24].

Other medications, such as nitroprusside and converting enzyme inhibitors, are *contraindicated* in pregnancy. Nitroprusside, which can cause cyanide poisoning, and converting enzyme inhibitors, which reduce the generation of angiotensin II, have both caused fetal death in animals [22,25]. Angiotensin II appears to promote uterine vasodilator prostaglandin formation during pregnancy, the inhibition of which leads to uteroplacental ischemia [25].

Prevention

The optimal approach to preeclampsia would be to prevent its occurrence. Preliminary reports suggest that *low-dose aspirin* may minimize the development of preeclampsia in susceptible patients [26,27]. In one recent study, for example, 46 primigravidas predisposed to the development of preeclampsia (as detected by increased sensitivity to infused angiotensin II) were treated with low-dose aspirin (60 mg) or placebo [27]. Preeclampsia, eclampsia, or pregnancy-induced hypertension was observed in 12 of 23 patients treated with placebo but in only 2 of 23 patients treated with aspirin. This beneficial effect may be related to inhibition of thromboxane synthesis, possibly leading to improved uterine perfusion and less platelet aggregation. More clinical trials are needed before this approach to the prevention of preeclampsia can be used on a large scale, however, since at least larger doses of aspirin may have an adverse effect on fetal outcome [28].

Prognosis

Preeclampsia in primigravidas is generally a self-limited disease. There is no increase in the later development of hypertension or renal disease compared with age-matched controls [1,13a]. Furthermore, the risk of developing preeclampsia in a subsequent pregnancy is low (<4%). These general observations, however, may not apply to primigravidas with severe preeclampsia or eclampsia; in this setting, there seems to be an increased incidence of late hypertension and of preeclampsia in subsequent pregnancies [29]. Late hypertension is also more likely with preeclampsia in multigravidas, who often have underlying essential hypertension or renal disease [13a].

Isolated mild hypertension during pregnancy (diastolic blood pressure < 100 mm Hg without proteinuria or renal insufficiency) characteristically has little adverse effect on fetal or maternal outcome. Periodic monitoring is necessary, however, since the risk of late hypertension appears to be increased, especially in patients whose blood pressure has not returned to normal levels by the tenth postpartum day [18,21a].

References

1. Black, RM. Vascular diseases of the kidney. In BD Rose, *Pathophysiology of Renal Disease* (2nd ed). New York: McGraw-Hill, 1987. Pp. 338-348.
2. Lindheimer, MD, Katz, AI. Sodium and diuretics in pregnancy. *N Engl J Med* 288:891, 1973.
3. Gant, NF, Worley, RJ, Everett, R, MacDonald, PC. Control of vascular responsiveness during human pregnancy. *Kidney Int* 18:255, 1980.
4. Conrad, KP, Brinck-Johnsen, T, Adler, RA. Evidence that chronic hyperprolactine-

mia increases renal hemodynamics (abstract). *Clin Res* 34:695A, 1986.
5. Dennis, EJ, McFarland, KF, Hester, JR, LL. The preeclampsia-eclampsia syndrome. In DN Danforth (Ed), *Obstetrics and Gynecology,* (4th ed). New York: Harper and Row, 1982. Pp. 464-465.
6. Redman, CWG. Hypertension in pregnancy: A case discussion. *Kidney Int* 32:151, 1987.
7. Editorial: Prostaglandin synthesis inhibitors in obstetrics and after. *Lancet* 2:185, 1980.
8. Walsh, SW. Preeclampsia: An imbalance in placental thromboxane production. *Am J Obstet Gynecol* 152:335, 1985.
9. Need, JA. Preeclampsia in pregnancies by different fathers: Immunological studies. *Br Med J* 1:548, 1975.
10. Heptinstall, RH. *Pathology of the Kidney* (3rd ed). Boston: Little, Brown, 1983. Chap. 19.
11. Weiner, CP. The clinical spectrum of preeclampsia. *Am J Kid Dis* 9:312, 1987.
12. Weinstein, L. Syndrome of hemolysis, elevated liver enzymes, and low platelet count: A severe consequence of hypertension in pregnancy. *Am J Obstet Gynecol* 142:159, 1982.
13. Ihle, BU, Long, P, Oats, J. Early-onset preeclampsia: Recognition of underlying renal disease. *Br Med J* 294:79, 1987.
13a. Fisher, KA, Luger, A, Spargo, BH, Lindheimer, MD. Hypertension in pregnancy: Clinical-pathological correlations and late prognosis. *Medicine* 60:267, 1981.
14. Fadel, HE, Northrop, G, Misenhimer, HR. Hyperuricemia in pre-eclampsia: A reappraisal. *Am J Obstet Gynecol* 125:640, 1976.
15. Taufield, PA, Ales, KL, Resnick, LM, Druzin, ML, Gertner, JM, Laragh, JH. Hypocalciuria in preeclampsia. *N Engl J Med* 316:715, 1987.
16. Oney, T, Kaulhausen, H. The value of the angiotensin sensitivity test in the early diagnosis of hypertensive disorders in pregnancy. *Am J Obstet Gynecol* 142:17, 1982.
17. Gant, NF, Chand, S, Worley, RJ, Shalley, PJ, Crosby, UD, MacDonald, PC. A clinical test useful for predicting the development of acute hypertension in pregnancy. *Am J Obstet Gynecol* 120:1, 1974.
18. Chesley, LC. *Hypertensive Disorders in Pregnancy* New York: Appleton, Century-Crofts, 1978.
19. Grunfeld, J-P, Pertuiset, N. Acute renal failure in pregnancy: 1987. *Am J Kid Dis* 9:359, 1987.
20. Homans, DC, Blake, GD, Harrington, JT, Cetrulo, CL. Acute renal failure caused by ureteral obstruction by a gravid uterus. *J Am Med Assoc* 246:1230, 1981.
21. Sabai, BM, Abdella, TN, Anderson, GD. Pregnancy outcome in 211 patients with mild chronic hypertension. *Obstet Gynecol* 61:571, 1983.
21a. Lindheimer, MD, Katz, AI. Hypertension in pregnancy. *N Engl J Med* 313:675, 1985.
22. Redman, CWG. The management of hypertension in pregnancy. *Sem Nephrol* 4:270, 1984.
23. Walters, BNJ, Redman, CWG. Treatment of severe pregnancy associated hypertension with the calcium antagonist nifedipine. *Br J Obstet Gynaecol* 91:330, 1984.
24. Dudley, DKL. Minibolus diazoxide in the management of severe hypertension in pregnancy. *Am J Obstet Gynecol* 151:196, 1985.
25. Ferris, TAF, and Weir, EK. Effects of captopril on uterine blood flow and prostaglandin E synthesis in the pregnant rabbit. *J Clin Invest* 71:809, 1983.
26. Wallenburg, HCS, Makovitz, JW, Dekker, GA, Rotmans, P. Low-dose aspirin prevents pregnancy-induced hypertension and pre-eclampsia in angiotensin-sensitive primigravidae. *Lancet* 1:1, 1986.
27. Beaufils, M, Uzan, S, Donsimoni, R, Colau, JC. Prevention of preeclampsia by early anti-platelet therapy. *Lancet* 1:840, 1985.
28. Turner, G, Collins, E. Fetal effects of regular salicylate ingestion in pregnancy. *Lancet* 2:338, 1975.
29. Sibai, BM, El-Nazer, A, Gonzalez-Ruiz, A. Severe preeclampsia-eclampsia in young primigravid women: Subsequent pregnancy outcome and remote prognosis. *Am J Obstet Gynecol* 155:1011, 1986.

45. THROMBOEMBOLIC DISEASES

Thrombus formation or embolization can involve either the renal arterial or venous circulations. This chapter will discuss only the major arterial disorders: renal artery thrombosis, clot emboli, and atheroemboli. Renal vein thrombosis is reviewed separately in Chap. 26, since this problem most commonly occurs in patients with the nephrotic syndrome.

Arterial thromboemboli (or a dissecting aortic aneurysm) can cause either ischemic infarction or ischemic atrophy, depending on the extent of vascular occlusion, the rapidity with which it develops, and whether the vascular lesions are due to clot or to atheroemboli. The renal circulation is particularly susceptible to embolic disease, since the kidneys normally receive about 20 percent of the cardiac output.

Acute Nonatheromatous Occlusion of the Renal Arteries

A variety of conditions can lead to nonatheromatous occlusion of the renal arteries. The primary sources of renal *emboli* are mural thrombi (especially in patients with atrial arrhythmias or a prior myocardial infarction) and vegetations in bacterial endocarditis. Less often, tumor or fat emboli may be observed. In comparison, *thrombosis* of the renal artery is usually superimposed on an underlying atheromatous lesion or follows a traumatic intimal tear [1,2]. It may also rarely occur as a spontaneous finding.

Pathology and Pathogenesis
A wedge-shaped infarct radiating outward from the affected vessel is the classic pathologic change seen in the kidney [1]. The magnitude of the renal injury is dependent on the extent and duration of the vascular occlusion. Irreversible necrosis usually ensues if the renal artery is totally occluded for 2 hours or more [3]. In comparison, total occlusion for a lesser duration may result in acute tubular necrosis rather than infarction. The time course is less predictable if the occlusion is incomplete or if there is adequate collateral flow [2]. In this setting, longer periods of renal ischemia can be tolerated without irreversible renal damage; ischemic atrophy is often seen, a pathologic finding similar to that typically found with atheroemboli.

Clinical Presentation and Diagnosis
The clinical findings in renal arterial occlusion are variable [4]. Patients may be asymptomatic if the occlusion is incomplete, but nausea, vomiting, flank pain, and fever are common in symptomatic patients. Flank or abdominal tenderness are commonly seen on physical examination and a careful search should be undertaken for signs of extrarenal embolization, such as skin lesions or focal neurologic deficits. In addition, an underlying predisposition to arterial embolization, such as atrial fibrillation or a recent myocardial infarction, can often be identified.

Most routine laboratory tests are nondiagnostic. The white blood cell count may be elevated, and the plasma creatinine concentration may increase (particularly in patients with bilateral disease). Gross or microscopic hematuria is observed in only about one-third of patients; its frequent absence may reflect the marked reduction in blood supply to the infarcted area, resulting in the local cessation of glomerular filtration and urine flow [4].

There is, however, one laboratory finding that, in the appropriate clinical setting, is highly suggestive of renal infarction: *a markedly elevated plasma lactate dehydrogenase (LDH) level* (usually > 5 times the upper limit of normal), with little or no elevation of plasma transaminase levels [4,5]. The other conditions in which this enzyme pattern is commonly seen (late myocardial infarction, hemolysis, and renal transplant rejection) can be differentiated from renal infarction on clinical grounds or by measuring urinary LDH excretion. This enzyme is too large to be filtered and urinary LDH is therefore normal in the extrarenal disorders but is elevated in renal infarction and in transplant rejection, conditions where the urinary enzyme is derived from the kidney [6].

A *radioisotope renogram* is the screening procedure of choice to demonstrate a segmental or generalized decrease in renal perfusion. This procedure has the advantage of being noninvasive and may obviate the need for renal arteriography or contrast-enhanced CT scanning. An intravenous pyelogram is generally less sensitive; it often reveals partial or complete nonvisualization of the affected kidney but may be normal in patients with segmental lesions.

Course and Treatment
Irreversible infarction results from complete renal arterial occlusion, unless blood flow is restored within 2 to 3 hours. It is unlikely, therefore, that patients with complete occlusion can be admitted to the hospital, stabilized, and undergo surgical embolectomy (which can result in improved renal function in some patients) in a time frame rapid enough to preserve the affected renal mass. In many patients, however, collateral flow is sufficient to maintain viability for 24 to 48 hours or even later with incomplete occlusion [2].

The optimal therapy of renal infarction is uncertain. Although surgery can restore vascular patency, it appears to be associated with a higher mortality rate and with *no apparent increase in renal functional recovery* when compared to anticoagulation alone [4,7]. Even patients with bilateral embolization and advanced renal failure usually regain a substantial amount of renal function when treated only with anticoagulants [4]. The latter modality may have two beneficial effects: it can decrease the degree of renal infarction by preventing extention of the clot, and it can reduce the incidence of further embolization.

Patients with renal thromboemboli have usually been treated with intravenous heparin followed by warfarin [4,7]. A possibly more effective alternative is to initiate therapy with a thrombolytic agent (such as streptokinase) in an attempt to lyse the occluding blood clot [8]. Local intraarterial infusion, rather than intravenous therapy, can diminish the total dose and therefore reduce the risk of systemic bleeding [9].

Surgery, which is not usually indicated in the initial therapy of this disorder, may be considered in patients with severe renal failure who show no improvement in renal function after 4 to 6 weeks of anticoagulant therapy. In selected patients, late embolectomy has led to improved renal function, indicating that ischemic atrophy can still be reversed.

Other than preventing new emboli, chronic therapy also may require treatment of hypertension. The blood pressure often rises several days after an acute renal infarction and then usually returns to the baseline level after a period of 2 to 3 weeks [10]. In some patients, however, hypertension persists and may be severe. Converting enzyme inhibitors (with diuretics, if necessary) will generally control the blood pressure, since it is generally mediated by the ischemic activation of the renin-angiotensin system.

The prognosis in patients with thromboembolic disease is limited due both to extrarenal embolization (to the brain or intestine) and to the underlying abnormality predisposing to this disorder (such as cardiac disease with mural thrombi). In comparison, patients with traumatic renal artery thrombosis usually have a better prognosis, particularly if renal failure or severe hypertension do not develop [2,11].

Renal Atheroemboli
Renal atheroembolic disease typically occurs in patients with widespread, ulcerated atherosclerotic disease. Clinically important atheroemboli most often result from manipulation of the aorta (or other large arteries) during arteriography, angioplasty, or surgery [11]. They may also be induced by chronic warfarin therapy, in which anticoagulation may interfere with the healing of ulcerated atheromatous plaques [12]. In addition, spontaneous atheroemboli are not uncommon, being demonstrable at autopsy in up to 12 percent of patients over the age of 80 [13]. These atheroemboli, however, are usually clinically silent and not associated with a substantial reduction in renal function.

Pathology and Pathogenesis
Light microscopic examination of renal tissue is often pathognomonic of atheroembolism, revealing fragments of acellular material with biconcave slits (representing dissolved cholesterol crystals) in the medium-sized and small renal arteries (Fig. 45-1). The emboli are nondistensible and irregularly shaped; as a result, they produce incomplete

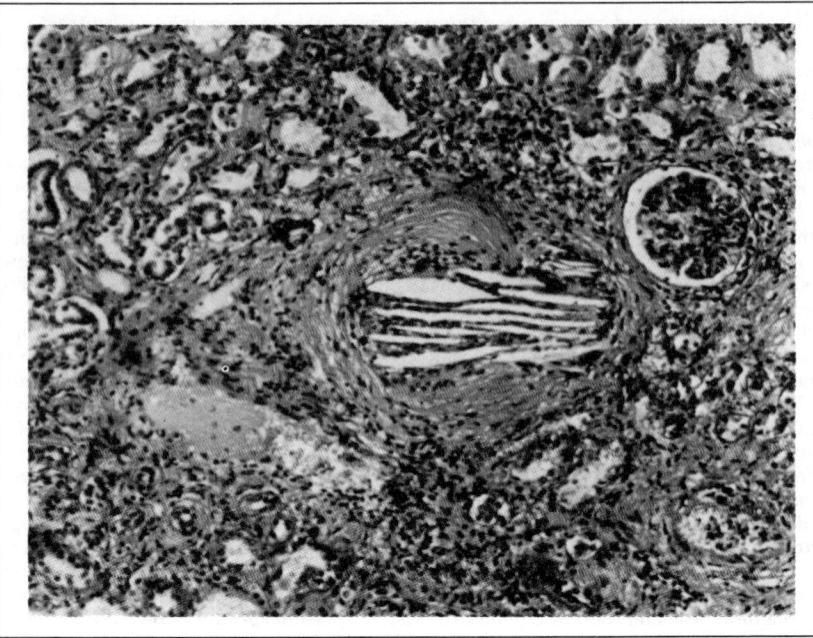

Fig. 45-1. Atheroembolus lodged in a small renal artery with occlusion of the vascular lumen. The biconcave parallel slits (representing cholesterol crystals that have been dissolved during paraffin fixation) are characteristic of this disorder. (From Rose, BD. *Pathophysiology of Renal Disease* [2nd ed.]. New York: McGraw-Hill, 1987.)

occlusion and secondary ischemic atrophy rather than infarction [1]. With time, a foreign-body reaction often ensues, causing intimal proliferation, macrophage infiltration, giant cell formation, and fibrosis with further narrowing of the vascular lumen. Similar emboli are commonly present in other organs as well.

The localization of atheroemboli within the kidney is focal. Consequently, a percutaneous renal biopsy may, by sampling error, miss the characteristic arterial lesions, even in patients with documented atheroemboli in other organs or in the kidney at postmortem examination.

Clinical Presentation
The severe, erosive vascular disease required for atheroemboli is most commonly observed in patients over the age of 50. Since the vascular occlusion is typically incomplete, atheroemboli usually do not produce renal infarction with its characteristic clinical (flank pain) and laboratory (increased lactate dehydrogenase levels) findings [11]. As a result, most patients have *no symptoms referable to the kidneys.*

The history and physical examination may, however, reveal changes due to *extrarenal* atheroemboli. Visual deficits, abdominal pain due to acute pancreatitis or splenic infarction, and myalgias all may be seen. These peripheral emboli also can lead to changes that are detectable on physical examination, including orange plaques in the retinal arterioles, livedo reticularis in the skin of the lower extremities, and areas of gangrene in the toes (in the presence of intact pedal pulses) [12,14,15]. Angiotensin II–mediated hypertension is also frequently present and may be severe [16].

Laboratory findings are nonspecific and include an acute rise in the plasma creatinine concentration shortly after a surgical or radiologic vascular procedure. The urinalysis is typically benign with few cells or casts, consistent with the presence of ischemic atrophy.

However, some patients with renal failure from atheroembolic disease have a more active urinary sediment, with hematuria and cellular (including red cell) casts [17]. In this setting, the presence of glomerulonephritis or systemic vasculitis may be suspected, particularly in patients with concomitant extrarenal manifestations [18,19]. A systemic disease or acute interstitial nephritis may also be suspected from the frequent presence of hypocomplementemia and eosinophilia in this disorder [20,21]. These changes are presumably related to immunologic activation at the exposed surface of the atheroembolus.

Diagnosis
The history and course often suggest the possible presence of atheroemboli. For example, renal failure developing after vascular surgery, arteriography, or angioplasty may be caused by atheroemboli, although acute tubular necrosis (ATN) is probably more common. Evidence of extrarenal embolization, if present, favors the diagnosis of atheroembolic disease in these settings. In addition, the course of these two disorders is typically different. Patients with ATN characteristically have a progressive rise in the plasma creatinine concentration, with renal function then stabilizing and eventually returning spontaneously toward baseline after a variable period of 4 to 21 days. In contrast, patients with atheroemboli usually have an *acute, self-limited* (depending on the degree of embolization) but *irreversible* decline in renal function (since the atheroemboli cannot be lysed or recanalized) [11]. Occasional patients, however, have some improvement in renal function with time, presumably due to resolution of concurrent ATN or the development of collateral flow to ischemic areas [14,22].

The diagnosis may be especially difficult if there is no identifiable precipitating event (as with spontaneous atheroemboli) or if the course of the disease is atypical. For example, subacute progressive renal failure can occur in patients with fibrotic scarring in response to the atheroemboli or with showers of new emboli. In this setting, biopsy of an affected organ (such as skin or kidney) may be necessary. This may be particularly important when extrarenal symptoms, an active urine sediment, or hypocomplementemia or eosinophilia suggest a systemic disorder [18–21]. However, a negative renal biopsy does not necessarily exclude atheroemboli, since affected vessels may be missed.

Treatment and Course
There is no specific treatment for this disorder. In patients at high risk for the development of atheroemboli, procedures such as arteriography should be avoided if other less invasive procedures can provide the same information. Once the disease has occurred, treatment of hypertension (if present) and dietary protein restriction should be considered to slow further hemodynamically mediated glomerular injury (see Chap. 56).

The plasma creatinine concentration often remains stable after the acute episode although, as described before, a progressive decline in renal function can result from scarring of the arterial lesions or new emboli. Patients who develop end-stage renal disease may be successfully dialyzed, but long-term survival is limited by severe, generalized atherosclerosis.

References

1. Heptinstall, RH. *Pathology of the Kidney* (3rd ed). Boston: Little, Brown, 1983. Chap. 21.
2. Cosby, RL, Miller, PD, Schrier, RW. Traumatic renal artery thrombosis. *Am J Med* 81:890, 1986.
3. Hoffman, RM, Stieper, KW, Johnson, RW, Belzer, FO. Renal ischemic tolerance. *Arch Surg* 109:550, 1974.
4. Lessman, RK, Johnson, SR, Coburn, JW, Kaufman, JJ. Renal artery embolism: Clinical features and long-term follow-up of 17 cases. *Ann Intern Med* 89:477, 1978.
5. Winzelberg, GG, Hull, JD, Agar, JWM, Rose, BD, Pletka, PG. Elevation of serum lactate dehydrogenase levels in renal infarction. *J Am Med Assoc* 242:268, 1979.
6. London, RL, Hoffster, P, Perkoff, GT, Pennington, TG. Renal infarction: Elevation of serum and urinary lactate dehydrogenase (LDH). *Arch Intern Med* 121:87, 1968.

7. Moyer, JD, Rao, CN, Wildrich, WC, Olson, CA. Conservative management of renal artery embolus. *J Urol* 109:138, 1973.
8. Steckel, A, Johnston, J, Fraley, DS, Bruns, FJ, Segel, DP, Adler, S. The use of streptokinase to treat renal artery thromboembolism. *Am J Kid Dis* 4:166, 1984.
9. Fisher, CP, Konnak, JW, Cho, KJ, Eckhauser, FE, Stanley, JC. Renal artery embolism: Therapy with intra-arterial streptokinase infusion. *J Urol* 125:402, 1981.
10. Margolin, EG, Merrill, JP, Harrison, JH. Diagnosis of hypertension due to occlusion of the renal artery. *N Engl J Med* 292:1387, 1975.
11. Black, RM. Vascular diseases of the kidney. In BD Rose, *Pathophysiology of Renal Disease* (2nd ed). New York: McGraw-Hill, 1987. Pp. 353-360.
12. Hyman, BT, Landas, SK, Ashwan, RF, Schelper, RL, Robinson, RA. Warfarin-related purple toes syndrome and cholesterol microembolization. *Am J Med* 82:1233, 1987.
13. Sieniewicz, DJ, Moore, S, Moir, FD, McDade, DF. Atheromatous emboli in the kidneys. *Radiology* 92:1231. 1969.
14. McGowan, JA, Greenberg, A. Cholesterol atheroembolic renal disease. Report of 3 cases with emphasis on diagnosis by skin biopsy and extended survival. *Am J Nephrol* 6:135, 1986.
15. Kalter, DC, Rudolph, A, McGavran, M. Livedo reticularis due to multiple cholesterol emboli. *J Am Acad Dermatol* 13:235, 1985.
16. Dalakos, TG, Streeten, DHP, Jones, D, Obeid, A. "Malignant" hypertension resulting from atheromatous embolization predominantly of one kidney. *Am J Med* 57:135, 1974.
17. Clinicopathological Conference. Progressive renal failure with hematuria in a 62-year-old man. *Am J Med* 71:468, 1981.
18. Richards, AM, Eliot, RS, Kanjuh, VI, Bloemendaal, RD, Edwards, JE. Cholesterol embolism: A multiple-system disease masquerading as polyarteritis nodosa. *Am J Cardiol* 15:696, 1965.
19. Case Records of the Massachusetts General Hospital: Case 30-1986. *N Engl J Med* 315:308, 1986.
20. Cosio, FG, Zager, RA, Sharma, HM. Atheroembolic renal disease causes hypocomplementaemia. *Lancet* 2:118, 1985.
21. Bidani, A, Kasinath, BS, Corwin, HL, Schwartz, MM, Lewis, EJ. Eosinophilia in the diagnosis of atheroembolic renal disease (abstract). *Kidney Int* 27:134, 1985.
22. Smith, MC, Ghose, MK, Henry, AR. The clinical spectrum of renal cholesterol embolization. *Am J Med* 71:174, 1981.

VII. TUBULOINTERSTITIAL DISEASES

46. ACUTE DRUG-INDUCED INTERSTITIAL NEPHRITIS: METHICILLIN AND NONSTEROIDAL ANTI-INFLAMMATORY DRUGS

Interstitial nephritis is a disorder that is characterized in its acute stages by a prominent interstitial infiltrate consisting of lymphocytes, monocytes, and, in some patients, neutrophils, eosinophils, or plasma cells. Tubular injury is also commonly present, due primarily to damage induced by the inflammatory cells. With chronic disease, the acute inflammatory changes are largely replaced by interstitial fibrosis and tubular atrophy.

Drugs and infection are the most common causes of interstitial nephritis (Table 46-1) [1,2]. This disorder is also seen less frequently in other settings, including transplant rejection (see Chap. 60), sarcoidosis (see Chap. 53), tumor infiltration of the kidney, systemic lupus erythematosus, Sjögren's syndrome, idiopathic interstitial nephritis, and anti-tubular basement membrane antibody disease, either as a primary disorder or as part of anti-glomerular basement membrane antibody disease [2-8].

This chapter will review two common causes of *acute* drug-induced interstitial nephritis: methicillin (which produces a picture similar to that seen with most of the other drugs in Table 46-1) and nonsteroidal anti-inflammatory drugs (NSAIDs). The major causes of *chronic* drug-induced interstitial nephritis, analgesic abuse and cyclosporine, are discussed separately elsewhere in the book.

The diagnosis of acute interstitial nephritis is usually suspected from the temporal association between drug use and renal disease, the characteristic urinary findings, renal biopsy (if indicated), and at least partial resolution of the disease following discontinuation of the drug. One very helpful urinary abnormality in many but not all patients is the presence of *eosinophils* in the urine sediment. These cells are best identified with Hansel's stain, which is also used to stain eosinophils in bronchial secretions [9]. Eosinophiluria is commonly found in interstitial nephritis but not in most other causes of acute renal failure, including acute tubular necrosis. For unknown reasons, urinary eosinophils may also be seen in rapidly progressive glomerulonephritis [9]. This disorder, however, can usually be distinguished from interstitial nephritis by the presence of red cell casts and the typical lack of a relevant history of drug ingestion.

Methicillin Nephritis

Thymic-derived lymphocytes (T cells) are thought to play a central role in most forms of drug-induced interstitial nephritis, including that due to methicillin. The interstitial filtrate, for example, is usually composed primarily of T cells [10,11]; these cells can then release soluble mediators that can directly produce tubulointerstitial injury and, by chemotaxis, can promote the infiltration of eosinophils [10].

Localization of activated T cells within the kidney probably requires the renal accumulation of the inciting drug or drug-hapten complex. In patients with methicillin nephritis, for example, a methicillin-derived antigen, dimethoxyphenylpenicilloyl (DPO) is deposited along the tubular basement membranes (TBM) [12]. In theory, this antigen could also activate humoral mechanisms. Occasional patients with methicillin nephritis have linear deposition of IgG, DPO, and C3 along the tubular basement membranes and circulating anti-TBM antibodies (which are presumably directed against a DPO-TBM conjugate) [13]. It is not clear, however, whether these antibodies play a primary pathogenetic role or are merely a secondary event induced by initial cell-mediated injury that results in exposure of previously "unseen" TBM antigens.

Clinical Presentation and Diagnosis

Infected patients treated with methicillin usually respond initially with defervescence in fever and improvement in symptoms. After a latent period that generally exceeds 10 days (but may be as short as 3 days), fever recurs, occasionally accompanied by a rash [12,14,15]. At this time, peripheral eosinophilia may be present and the urinalysis typically reveals hematuria (which may be macroscopic), pyuria, eosinophiluria (the absence of which does not exclude the diagnosis), white cell casts, and mild proteinuria. The plasma creatinine concentration is usually elevated at the time of diagnosis; however, the changes in the urine sediment can precede any decline in the glomerular fil-

Table 46-1. Drugs associated with interstitial nephritis*

Strong association	Probable association	Weak association
ACUTE		
Methicillin	Carbenicillin	Phenytoin
Penicillin	Cephalosporins	Tetracycline
Nonsteroidal anti-inflammatory drugs	Oxacillin	Probenecid
	Ampicillin	Captopril
Cimetidine	Sulfonamides	Allopurinol
Cephalothin	Rifampin	Erythromycin
Leukocyte interferon	Thiazides	Chloramphenicol
	Furosemide	Clofibrate
	Phenindione	
CHRONIC		
Analgesic abuse	Lithium	
Cyclosporine		
Nitrosoureas		

*Adapted from Adler, SG, Cohen, AH, Border, WA. *Am J Kid Dis* 5:75, 1985.

tration rate by as much as 1 week [15]. The fractional excretion of sodium is generally elevated but may be below 1 percent in some patients, similar to that seen in prerenal disease [16]. This finding is somewhat surprising, since it might be expected that tubular damage would limit the ability to conserve sodium maximally.

The diagnosis of methicillin nephritis is usually suspected from the history and urinary findings. Although signs of systemic allergy, such as fever, rash, and eosinophilia, may be present, their absence *does not preclude the presence of interstitial nephritis*. The urinalysis, however, usually is very helpful. The triad of hematuria, pyuria, and white cell casts is quite different from the granular and epithelial cell casts characteristically seen in acute tubular necrosis, the other common cause of drug-induced acute renal failure. It has been suggested that, in patients taking multiple drugs, gallium scanning also may be helpful in differentiating between these disorders, being negative in acute tubular necrosis but markedly positive in most cases of acute interstitial nephritis [17].

Another potential difficulty in differential diagnosis arises when methicillin is used to treat bacterial endocarditis. In this disorder, interstitial nephritis must be differentiated from an infection-induced immune complex glomerulonephritis that can produce similar urinary findings. In this setting, the timing of the onset of the renal disease is often helpful. The glomerulonephritis, which may also be associated with red cell casts, is generally present at the time of diagnosis and begins to improve shortly after the institution of appropriate antimicrobial therapy. In comparison, interstitial nephritis is characterized by late onset, well after therapy has been initiated.

Renal biopsy can be performed to confirm the diagnosis of interstitial nephritis. This is often not necessary, however, when the history and urinalysis are highly suggestive.

Treatment
The most important aspect of treatment with any form of drug-induced interstitial nephritis is discontinuation of the drug. Clearing of the urine sediment may occur within several days in patients without renal insufficiency. On the other hand, recovery may take as long as 2 to 4 months in untreated patients with severe acute disease [14]. Furthermore, residual renal insufficiency, as evidenced by a plasma creatinine concentration that is higher than the pretreatment baseline, is not uncommon in the latter setting [14].

The role of corticosteroids is not well defined. In an uncontrolled study of patients with methicillin-induced disease, prednisone appeared to induce a more complete (final plasma creatinine concentration 1.2 mg/dl versus 1.9 mg/dl in untreated patients) and more rapid (9 days versus 54 days) resolution of the renal injury [14]. The initial prednisone dose was 60 mg/day, followed by rapid tapering as a response occurred. Relapses were occasionally seen as the prednisone was discontinued.

These findings suggest that it is probably prudent to institute a trial of prednisone therapy in patients with relatively severe disease (plasma creatinine concentration above 2.5–3.0 mg/dl). In comparison, therapy can probably be safely withheld with milder involvement, since spontaneous recovery is the rule.

Nonsteroidal Anti-Inflammatory Drugs

The interstitial nephritis associated with NSAIDs differs in several important ways from that seen with most other drugs:

1. The latent period may be as long as 18 months in some patients [18].

2. Signs of systemic and local allergy, such as fever, rash, eosinophilia, and eosinophiluria, are usually absent [19].

3. The acute renal failure and active urine sediment is, in most patients, associated with concurrent *nephrotic syndrome* due to minimal change disease* [18,19]. Although the interstitial and glomerular disease usually occur together, some patients have only one or the other [19].

4. The fractional excretion of sodium is typically below 1 percent, perhaps a reflection of the removal of the normally natriuretic effect of renal prostaglandins [19].

Although acute interstitial nephritis can be induced by almost any NSAID, this problem most commonly occurs with the proprionic acid derivatives, particularly *fenoprofen,* which causes approximately 60 percent of cases [19,20]. The mechanism by which these agents produce renal disease is unclear, but T cells again appear to play a primary role, constituting most of the cells in the interstitial infiltrate [20]. These cells could also be responsible for the glomerular injury by the release of a toxic lymphokine [21]. It is possible, for example, that inhibition of the cyclooxygenase pathway facilitates the conversion of arachidonate to leukotrienes, rather than prostaglandins [19]. This change could then promote the activation of helper T cells [22], although it is uncertain why only the kidney would become involved.

The diagnosis of interstitial nephritis due to a NSAID is usually suggested by the triad of drug intake, acute renal failure with hematuria and pyuria (but not red cell casts), and the presence of the nephrotic syndrome. This constellation of findings is so characteristic that a renal biopsy is often not necessary, unless the disease persists long after discontinuation of the drug. This disorder can usually be easily distinguished from other causes of the nephrotic syndrome, such as membranous nephropathy or idiopathic minimal change disease, since both the urine sediment and the plasma creatinine concentration in the latter conditions are relatively normal in most patients at the time of presentation.

Spontaneous recovery to the previous baseline generally occurs within weeks to a few months after the NSAID has been discontinued [18]. There is little evidence that corticosteroids are beneficial in this setting [18].

References

1. Adler, SG, Cohen, AH, Border, WA. Hypersensitivity phenomena and the kidney: Role of drugs and environmental agents. *Am J Kid Dis* 5:75, 1985.

2. Rose, BD. *Pathophysiology of Renal Disease* (2nd ed). New York: McGraw-Hill, 1987. Pp. 389-394.

3. Coggins, CH. Renal failure in lymphoma. *Kidney Int* 17:847, 1980.

*The nephrotic syndrome in acute interstitial nephritis has also been described in isolated cases due to ampicillin, leukocyte interferon, and rifampin [2].

4. Tron, F, Ganeval, D, Droz, D. Immunologically-mediated acute renal failure of non-glomerular origin in the course of SLE. *Am J Med* 67:259, 1979.
5. Winer, RL, Cohen, AH, Sawhney, AS, Gorman, JT. Sjögren's syndrome with immune complex tubulointerstitial disease. *Clin Immunol Immunopathol* 8:494, 1974.
6. Spital, A, Panner, BJ, Sterns, RH. Acute idiopathic tubulointerstitial nephritis: Report of 2 cases and review of the literature. *Am J Kid Dis* 9:71, 1987.
7. Fliger, FD, Wieslander, J, Brentjens, JR, Andres, GA, Butkowski, RJ. Identification of a target antigen in human anti-tubular basement membrane nephritis. *Kidney Int* 31:800, 1987.
8. Andres, G, Brentjens, J, Kohli, R, Anthone, R, Anthone, S, Bliah, T, Montes, M, Mookerjee, BK, Prezyna, A, Sepulveda, M, Venuto, R, Elwood, C. Histology of human tubulointerstitial nephritis associated with antibodies to renal basement membranes. *Kidney Int* 13:480, 1978.
9. Nolan, CR, III, Anger, MS, Kelleher, SP. Eosinophiluria—a new method of detection and definition of the clinical spectrum. *N Engl J Med* 315:1516, 1986.
10. Wilson, CB, Blantz, RC. Nephroimmunopathology and pathophysiology. *Am J Physiol* 248:F319, 1985.
11. Boucher, A, Droz, D, Adafer, E, Noel, L-H. Characterization of mononuclear cell subsets in renal cellular interstitial infiltrates. *Kidney Int* 29:1043, 1986.
12. Baldwin, DS, Levine, BB, McCluskey, RT, Gallo, GR. Renal failure and interstitial nephritis due to penicillin and methicillin. *N Engl J Med* 291:1245, 1968.
13. Border, WA, Lehman, DH, Egan, JD, Sass, HJ, Globe, JE, Wilson, CB. Antitubular basement-membrane antibodies in methicillin-associated interstitial nephritis. *N Engl J Med* 291:381, 1974.
14. Galpin, JE, Shinaberger, JH, Stanley, TM, Blumenkrantz, MJ, Bayer, AS, Friedman, GS, Montgomerie, JZ, Guze, LB, Coburn, JW, Glassock, RJ. Acute interstitial nephritis due to methicillin. *Am J Med* 65:756, 1978.
15. Nolan, CM, Abernathy, RS. Nephropathy associated with methicillin therapy: Prevalence and determinants in patients with staphylococcal bacteremia. *Arch Intern Med* 137:997, 1977.
16. Lins, RL, Verpooten, GA, De Clerck, DS, De Broe, ME. Urinary indices in acute interstitial nephritis. *Clin Nephrol* 26:131, 1986.
17. Linton, AL, Richmond, JM, Clark, WF, Lindsay, RM, Dreidger, AA, Lamki, LM. Gallium scintigraphy in the diagnosis of acute renal failure. *Clin Nephrol* 24:84, 1985.
18. Clive, DM, Stoff, JS. Renal syndromes associated with nonsteroidal antiinflammatory drugs. *N Engl J Med* 310:563, 1984.
19. Abraham, PA, Keane, WF. Glomerular and interstitial disease induced by nonsteroidal anti-inflammatory drugs. *Am J Nephrol* 4:1, 1984.
20. Finkelstein, A, Fraley, DS, Stachura, I, Feldman, HA, Gandy, DR, Bourke, E. Fenoprofen nephropathy: Lipoid nephrosis and interstitial nephritis. A possible T-lymphocyte disorder. *Am J Med* 72:81, 1982.
21. Schnaper, HW, Aune, TM. Steroid-sensitive mechanism of soluble immune response suppressor production in steroid-responsive nephrotic syndrome. *J Clin Invest* 79:257.
22. Goodwin, JS, Atluru, D, Sierakowsky, S, Lianos, EA. Mechanism of action of glucocorticosteroids. Interference of T cell proliferation and interleukin 2 production by hydrocortisone is reversed by leukotriene B_4. *J Clin Invest* 77:1244, 1986.

47. CHRONIC PYELONEPHRITIS AND REFLUX NEPHROPATHY

Chronic pyelonephritis refers to renal injury induced by recurrent or persistent infection of the kidneys. It is seen only in patients who have a major anatomic abnormality in the urinary tract such as obstruction, renal calculi, or most commonly *vesicoureteral reflux in children* [1]. Furthermore, chronic pyelonephritis generally has *no relation to acute pyelonephritis.* The latter disorder typically occurs in women who have a normal urinary tract and is associated with little long-term morbidity.

Pathogenesis

Chronic pyelonephritis is characterized by prominent renal scarring on intravenous pyelography (IVP) (Fig. 47-1). In children, these scars are almost always associated with vesicoureteral reflux [2-4], a congenital defect that results in incompetence of the ureterovesical valve, most often due to a short intramural segment*. Children with gross reflux (reflux back to the renal pelvis with secondary ureteral dilation) are at greatest risk, with the incidence of renal scarring being 60 percent or more [1].

It is thought that the renal damage in chronic pyelonephritis (also called reflux nephropathy) is due to two problems: the reflux of *infected urine* up the ureters and then *into the renal parenchyma* (called intrarenal reflux) (Fig. 47-2) [2-5]. The papillary collecting duct orifices in young children are normally wide open at the upper and lower poles, allowing intrarenal reflux to occur. However, normal renal growth results in spontaneous cessation of intrarenal reflux by the age of 6. This probably explains why *almost all renal scars occur before 6 years of age* [4], since vesicoureteral reflux without intrarenal reflux is unlikely to produce renal injury [5]. Older children may show contraction of old scars but generally do not form new scars.

The importance of infected urine in the genesis of renal scars is suggested from sequential IVP studies in children with vesicoureteral reflux. New scars form only in those children who develop a urinary tract infection [4]. In addition, prevention of infection by the chronic administration of antimicrobials prevents new scar formation and allows normal renal growth to occur, even in the presence of persistent vesicoureteral reflux [6].

Clinical Presentation

The age at which chronic pyelonephritis becomes clinically evident is variable. Many infants or young children present with a symptomatic urinary tract infection. Radiologic evaluation of these children is essential since 30 to 45 percent will have vesicoureteral reflux [2,3].

However, the presence of a urinary tract infection can easily be missed since some infections are asymptomatic and others are associated with relatively nonspecific findings such as fever, failure to thrive, and abdominal distress. In these settings, the presence of chronic pyelonephritis is often discovered incidentally because of the finding of hypertension, anemia, an abnormal urinalysis, or an elevated plasma creatinine concentration on routine examination. Other patients do not seek medical care until they have signs and symptoms of uremia, including weakness, anorexia, pallor, and nocturia.

In comparison to children with vesicoureteral reflux, patients with obstruction or renal stones may present with symptoms related to their underlying disease. Thus, there may be a history of passing stones, episodes of renal colic or gross hematuria, or, with chronically infected struvite stones, persistent back pain.

The urinalysis in chronic pyelonephritis typically reveals pyuria and less frequently white cell casts. Bacteriuria will be found only if the patient is infected or has a struvite stone. Protein excretion is generally less than 1 gm/day, a finding compatible with the primary tubulointerstitial damage in this disorder. However, nephrotic-range proteinuria (but usually without hypoalbuminemia or edema) often occurs in patients with advanced disease. Glomerulosclerosis is found at this time and is thought to reflect hemodynamically mediated injury resulting from the initial nephron loss (see Chap. 56) [1,7].

Diagnosis

Chronic pyelonephritis is a radiologic diagnosis established by the characteristic calyceal blunting and overlying segmental renal scars on IVP (Fig. 47-1). Ureteral dilation also may be present, since these patients generally have marked reflux. These radiologic

*Vesicoureteral reflux and renal scarring can also result from the combination of urinary infection and a flaccid bladder in patients with a spinal cord injury.

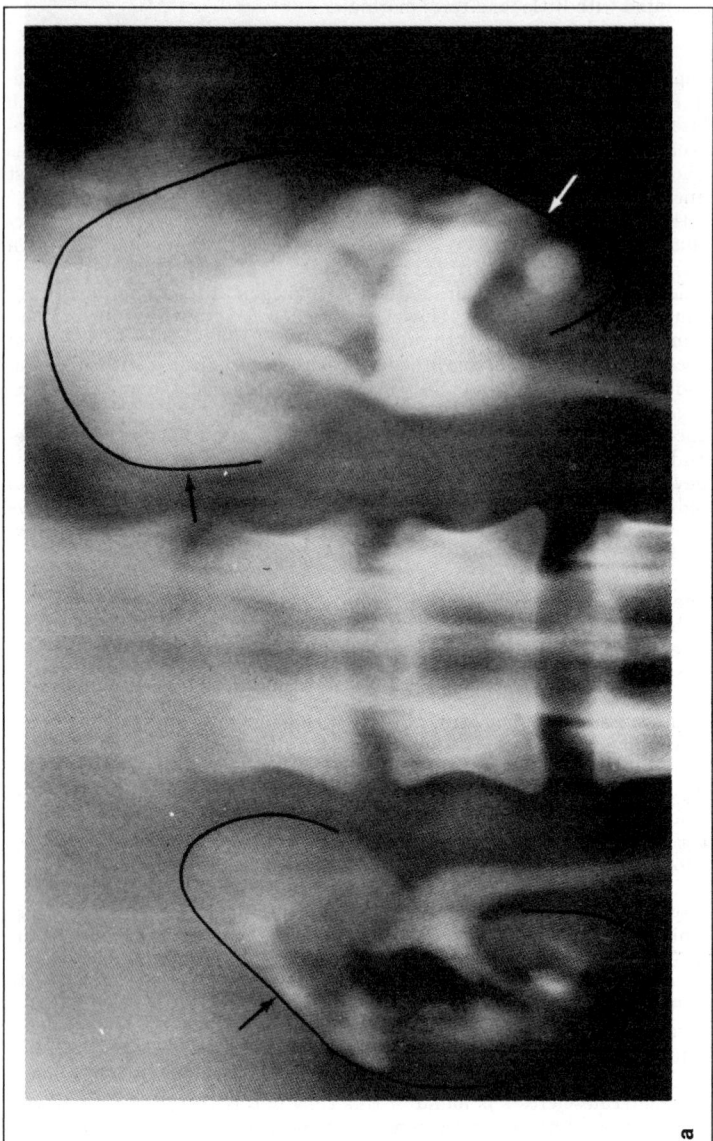

Fig. 47-1. Radiologic changes in chronic pyelonephritis. (a) Intravenous pyelogram demonstrates blunting of the calyces and scarring with loss of parenchyma in both upper poles and the left lower pole (arrows).

a

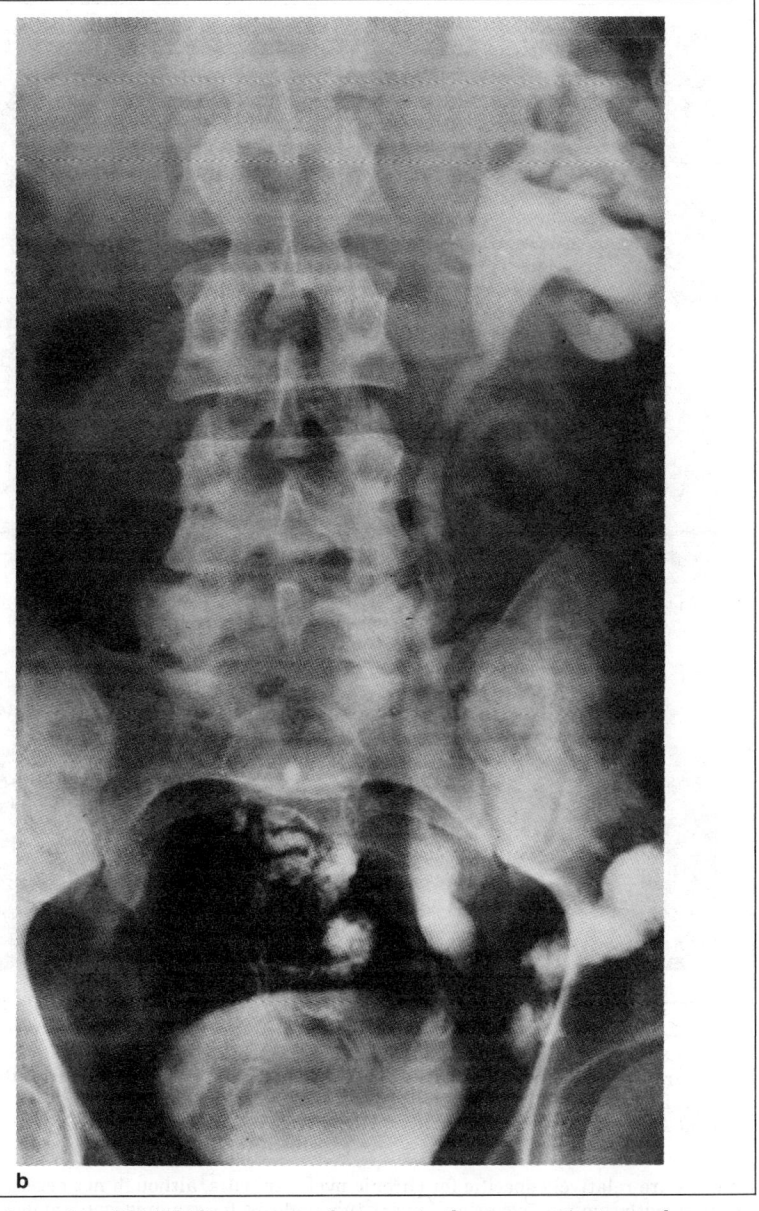

Fig. 47-1 (continued) (b) Voiding cystourethrogram in the same patient reveals gross reflux into the left renal collecting system. Although reflux is not seen on the right, cystoscopy, if performed, often demonstrates changes at the ureteral orifice compatible with previous reflux. (From Rose, BD. *Pathophysiology of Renal Disease* [2nd ed.]. New York: McGraw-Hill, 1987.)

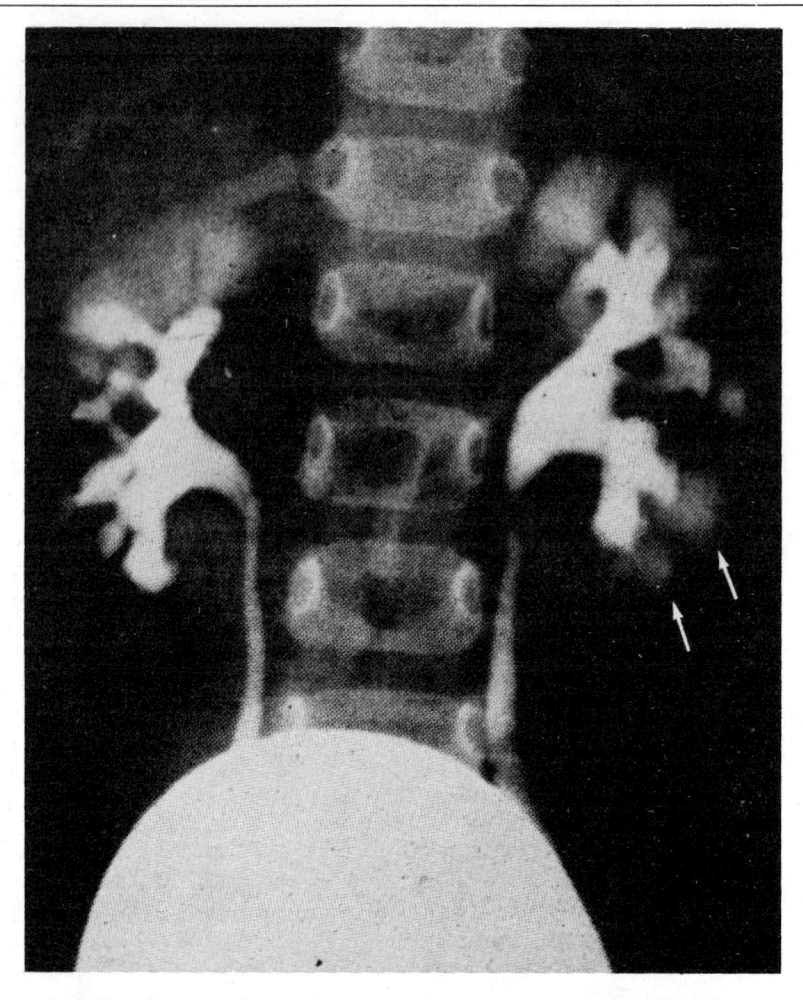

Fig. 47-2. Voiding cystourethrogram in a 4-year-old girl with recurrent urinary tract infections. Gross reflux is seen bilaterally into the renal collecting systems and the renal parenchyma. Arrows indicate the intrarenal reflux in the lower pole of the left kidney. (From Amar, AD. *J Am Med Assoc* 213:293, 1970. Copyright, American Medical Association, 1970.)

findings are relatively specific for chronic pyelonephritis, although not necessarily for infection with common bacteria. Urinary tuberculosis, for example, can produce similar renal changes; it is often accompanied, however, by ureteral strictures and a contracted bladder due to concurrent lower urinary tract involvement. This combination of upper and lower urinary tract scarring is highly suggestive of tuberculous infection [8].

Detection of renal scarring by IVP in a young child should be followed by a voiding cystourethrogram to determine if vesicoureteral reflux is present. In many cases, however, reflux can no longer be demonstrated [6,9]. This is most likely to be seen after puberty, since increased length of the submucosal portion of the terminal ureter during growth usually leads to cessation of reflux.

A somewhat separate issue is the appropriate evaluation of the child with a urinary tract infection, since early treatment of chronic pyelonephritis is essential if end-stage renal disease is to be prevented. Children over the age of 5 to 6 should have a plain film of the abdomen (looking for renal stones) and a renal ultrasound which, if the kidneys are well visualized, should detect substantial renal scarring [10]. No further evaluation is required if scarring appears to be absent, since the loss of intrarenal reflux in these older children [5] largely eliminates the risk of forming new scars [4]. Indications for an IVP include either inadequate visualization of the kidneys or the presence of scarring on ultrasonography.

The sequential work-up of younger children is similar except that a voiding cystourethrogram should be part of the initial radiologic evaluation; these children are still at risk of new scar formation if gross reflux is present.

It may also be reasonable to perform a screening renal ultrasound in *siblings* of children with chronic pyelonephritis. Vesicoureteral reflux occurs with increased frequency within families; in one study, 32 percent of siblings of children with documented reflux also had reflux, often without a history of urinary tract infection [11]. Furthermore, 15 percent of the affected siblings had renal scars.

Course and Treatment

Chronic pyelonephritis is often a progressive disease, accounting for approximately 20 to 30 percent of cases of end-stage renal disease in children. As described before, two factors seem to be most responsible for continued renal damage: *recurrent infection* [4,6] and *hemodynamically mediated glomerulosclerosis* [1,7]. The use of continuous prophylactic antimicrobial therapy with low-dose trimethoprim-sulfamethoxazole or nitrofurantoin has demonstrated the importance of preventing infection [6]. This regimen, when given over a 5- to 10-year period, is associated with normal renal growth and no new scars in over 90 percent of refluxing kidneys and spontaneous disappearance of reflux (due to growth of the intramural portion of the ureter) in 80 percent of cases.

The development of focal glomerulosclerosis is a relatively late occurrence in chronic pyelonephritis, typically occurring when the plasma creatinine concentration is above 2 mg/dl [1,7]. The primary clue suggesting the presence of superimposed glomerular disease is protein excretion in excess of 1.0 to 1.5 gm/day. At this relatively late stage, neither surgical correction of reflux nor continuous antimicrobial therapy (i.e., two modalities that cure the underlying disease) prevents a progressive deterioration in renal function [1,12]. It is presumed that compensatory intraglomerular hypertension, resulting from nephron loss, plays a major role in this secondary glomerular injury (see Chap. 56). Although as yet unproved, therapy aimed at lowering the intraglomerular pressure with a converting enzyme inhibitor or dietary protein restriction, or both, may be most likely to preserve renal function in this setting.

Indications for Surgical Correction of Reflux

The role of surgical correction of vesicoureteral reflux is not well defined [13]. If infection is prevented with antimicrobial therapy, then conservative management is *as effective as surgery* in preventing new scar formation and preserving renal function both in children [6,13,14] and in adults [15]. This is not surprising since intrarenal reflux disappears spontaneously over the age of 5 [5]. Furthermore, vesicoureteral reflux also tends to correct by puberty in most but not all cases [6,9].

Surgery is also not required, if infection can be prevented, in patients with unilateral reflux and scarring. The normal contralateral kidney plus continued growth in the affected kidney result in the maintenance of good renal function [16].

The *major indications for surgery* are (1) the presence of gross reflux and ureteral dilatation in a young child (particularly if under 2 years of age) without marked scarring, since new scars may develop in up to 60 percent of such cases [1]; (2) a child who becomes infected because of incomplete compliance with antimicrobial therapy and shows progressive scarring; and (3) a patient with large staghorn calculi due to an infected struvite stone. Antimicrobial therapy is usually ineffective in the last setting because the bacteria become deeply embedded in the stone. Stone removal is generally the procedure of choice; however, nephrectomy is indicated for control of infection if the affected kidney has little or no residual renal function.

References

1. Cotran, RS. Glomerulosclerosis in reflux nephropathy. *Kidney Int* 21:528, 1982.
2. Shah, KJ, Robins, DG, White, RHR. Renal scarring and vesicoureteric reflux. *Arch Dis Child* 53:210, 1978.
3. Smellie, JM, Normand, IC, Katz, G. Children with urinary infection: Comparison of those with and those without vesicoureteric reflux. *Kidney Int* 20:717, 1981.
4. Smellie, JM, Ransley, PG, Normand, IC, Prescod, N, Edwards, D. Development of new renal scars: A collaborative study. *Br Med J* 290:1957, 1985.
5. Rolleston, GL, Maling, TMJ, Hodson, CJ. Intrarenal reflux and the scarred kidney. *Arch Dis Child* 49:531, 1974.
6. Edwards, D, Normand, ICS, Prescod, N, Smellie, JM. Disappearance of vesicoureteric reflux during long-term prophylaxis of urinary tract infection in children. *Br Med J* 2:285, 1977.
7. Bhathena, DB, Weiss, JH, Holland, NH, McMorrow, RG, Curtis, JJ, Lucas, BA, Luke, RG. Focal and segmental glomerular sclerosis in reflux nephropathy. *Am J Med* 68:886, 1980.
8. Kollins, SA, Hartman, GW, Carr, DT, Sergura, JW, Hattery, RR. Roentgenographic findings in urinary tract tuberculosis. *Am J Roentgenol Rad Ther Nucl Med* 121:487, 1974.
9. Lenaghan, D, Whitaker, JG, Jensen, F, Stephens, FD. The natural history of reflux and long-term effects of reflux on the kidney. *J Urol* 115:728, 1976.
10. Sherwood, T, Whitaker, RH. Initial screening of children with urinary tract infections: Is plain film radiography and ultrasonography enough? *Br Med J* 288:827, 1984.
11. Jerkins, GR, Noe, HN. Familial vesicoureteral reflux: A prospective study. *J Urol* 128:774, 1982.
12. Senkkjian, HO, Stinebaugh, BJ, Mattioli, CA, Suki, WN. Irreversible renal failure following vesicoureteral reflux. *J Am Med Assoc* 241:160, 1979.
13. Birmingham Reflux Study Group. Prospective trial of operative versus non-operative treatment of severe vesicoureteric reflux in children: Five years' observation. *Br Med J* 295:237, 1987.
14. Kincaid-Smith, P. Reflux nephropathy. *Br Med J* 286:2002, 1983.
15. Neves, RJ, Torres, VE, Malek, RS, Svensson, J. Vesicoureteral reflux in the adult. IV. Medical versus surgical management. *J Urol* 132:882, 1984.
16. Claesson, I, Jacobsson, B, Jodal, U, Winberg, J. Compensatory kidney growth in children with urinary tract infection and unilateral renal scarring: An epidemiologic study. *Kidney Int* 20:759, 1981.

48. URIC ACID KIDNEY DISEASE

Uric acid, which is an end product of purine metabolism, can precipitate within the tubules, medullary interstitium, or collecting system, leading to three different types of renal disease: acute uric acid nephropathy, chronic urate nephropathy, and uric acid nephrolithiasis [1]. The settings in which these disorders are likely to occur are determined in part by the chemical characteristics of undissociated uric acid and its urate salt:

$$\text{Urate}^- + \text{H}^+ \rightleftharpoons \text{Uric acid}$$

The relative amounts of these two compounds in the urine (where the pK_a is about 5.35) can be predicted from the Henderson-Hasselbalch equation [2]:

$$pH = 5.35 + \log [\text{urate}^-]/[\text{uric acid}]$$

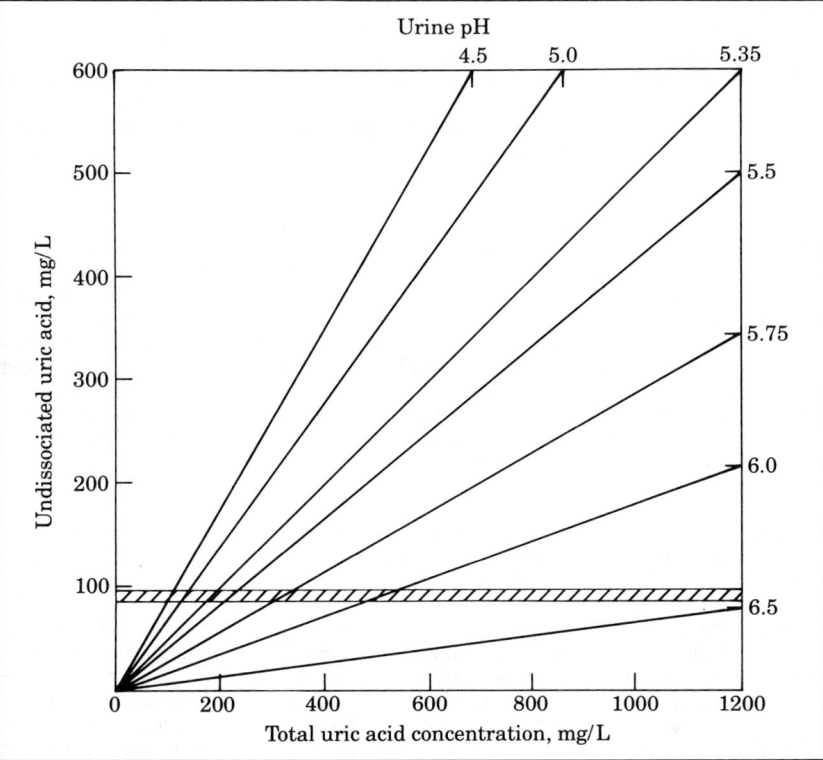

Fig. 48-1. Nomogram depicting the undissociated uric acid concentration at different values of total uric acid concentration (uric acid plus urate) and urine pH. The cross-hatched bar indicates the maximum solubility of undissociated uric acid in urine, which is approximately 100 mg/L. At an acid urine pH of 4.5 to 5.0, there is more uric acid than urate; consequently, the solubility limit for uric acid can be exceeded at a total uric acid concentration under 200 mg/L. In comparison, more than 1200 mg/L remains soluble when the urine pH is 6.5 or above because almost all of the urinary uric acid exists as the much more soluble urate salt. (From Coe, FL. *Kidney Int* 24:392, 1983. Reprinted by permission from Kidney International.)

At the normal arterial pH of 7.40, urate comprises 99 percent of the circulating total uric acid. This relationship changes dramatically in the urine, where acidification to a pH as low as 4.5 to 5.0 converts most of the urate to uric acid. This is important clinically because undissociated uric acid is relatively insoluble in urine (with a solubility of about 100 mg/L) (Fig. 48-1) when compared to the urate salt [2].

Thus, the likelihood of uric acid precipitation within the kidney is dependent on two primary factors: *concentration* (a function of excretion rate and the urine volume) and *pH*. Uric acid excretion is determined by the interplay between four sequential steps: filtration; almost total reabsorption by an anion exchange mechanism (such as urate$^-$/ OH$^-$ exchange) in the early proximal tubule; secretion from the plasma into the lumen by the proximal organic acid secretory pathway; and a variable degree of postsecretory reabsorption, occurring in the late proximal tubule [3].

The highest uric acid concentrations in both the tubules and interstitium occur in the medulla because of the countercurrent mechanism. Within the collecting tubule, the combination of high solute concentration (due to water removal in the presence of antidiuretic hormone) and an acid urine pH favors the intratubular precipitation of undissociated uric acid in susceptible subjects. The result can be acute renal failure or uric acid stone formation. In contrast, *urate* precipitation occurs only in the medullary interstitium where the pH and therefore the urate concentration are relatively high (the latter being due to the diffusion of urate out of the vasa recta capillaries into the interstitium). This can potentially lead to local microtophus formation and chronic interstitial fibrosis.

Acute Uric Acid Nephropathy
Acute uric acid nephropathy is a condition characterized by acute renal failure due to the widespread precipitation of uric acid within the collecting tubules, leading to secondary tubular obstruction. It typically occurs in settings in which there is marked overproduction and subsequent overexcretion of uric acid [4,5]. This is most often seen when there is massive tissue breakdown (and consequent purine release) in lymphomas, leukemias, or polycythemia vera, particularly after chemotherapy or radiation has induced rapid cell lysis [4,5]. Less common causes of this disorder are (1) tissue catabolism due to seizures, ischemia, or the treatment of solid tumors or (2) primary overproduction due to the rare syndrome of hypoxanthine-guanine phosphoribosyltransferase (HGPRTase) deficiency [1,6].

Clinical Presentation
Acute uric acid nephropathy is characterized by the abrupt onset of oliguria or anuria in one of the above settings. There are usually no other symptoms referable to the urinary tract, although flank pain can occur if obstruction develops within the renal pelves or ureters.

Initial laboratory evaluation reveals marked hyperuricemia, with the total plasma uric acid concentration generally exceeding 15 mg/dl [5]. This is in comparison to values below 12 mg/dl in most other forms of acute or chronic renal failure, except for prerenal disease (see the following) [7]. The urinalysis may be normal or show uric acid and urate crystals, findings that are suggestive but not diagnostic of acute uric acid nephropathy.

It is also important to realize that tissue catabolism can lead to the release of a variety of cellular constituents other than purines. As a result, marked elevations can be seen in the plasma concentrations of potassium, urea nitrogen, lactate dehydrogenase, and phosphorus (leading to the formation of calcium phosphate and secondary hypocalcemia). The last problem can induce acute renal failure, due to calcium phosphate rather than urate deposition within the kidney [8].

Diagnosis
The diagnosis of acute uric acid nephropathy is usually suggested by the appropriate history of tissue breakdown plus the presence of marked hyperuricemia. Measurement of the urine uric acid to creatinine ratio on a random urine specimen can, in some patients, help to confirm the presence of overexcretion of uric acid [9]. This value is usually above 1.0 in acute uric acid nephropathy and generally below 0.75 in normals and patients with other forms of acute renal failure.

There are, however, two other settings in which hyperuricemia can accompany acute renal failure. First, trauma or hypotension can lead to ischemic tissue breakdown plus acute tubular necrosis. This diagnosis is suggested by the different urinary findings (granular and epithelial cell casts) and by less marked hyperuricemia (generally below 15 mg/dl).

Second, prerenal disease (as with heart failure treated with diuretics) can produce hyperuricemia due to enhanced proximal reabsorption of sodium and secondarily uric acid. The history, low urine sodium concentration, and low fractional excretion of sodium all distinguish this disorder from acute uric acid nephropathy.

Treatment
Despite the severity of the renal failure, the prognosis for near complete recovery of renal function is excellent if treatment is initiated rapidly [5]. Therapy consists of attempting to wash out the obstructing uric acid crystals with a loop diuretic and fluids,

and of diminishing further uric acid production by the administration of allopurinol. Those patients in whom a diuresis cannot be achieved should be treated with hemodialysis to remove the excess circulating uric acid.

The benefit of urinary alkalinization with acetazolamide and sodium bicarbonate is not certain. Experimental models of acute uric acid nephropathy suggest that hydration alone is as effective as alkalinization in minimizing intratubular precipitation [10]. Furthermore, alkalinization has the potential disadvantage of promoting calcium phosphate deposition in patients with marked hyperphosphatemia.

Prevention
Clearly, prevention is preferable to treating already established disease. Patients about to receive chemotherapy or radiation for lymphoma, leukemia, or other rapidly growing malignancy should be pretreated with allopurinol (in higher-than-normal doses of 600–900 mg/day) plus induction of a diuresis with fluid loading (over 2.5–3.0 liters/day) with or without sodium bicarbonate for urinary alkalinization. Even with optimal prophylactic therapy, however, the degree of cell lysis may be so great that acute renal failure still occurs [5].

Chronic prophylactic therapy with allopurinol may also be indicated in patients who continuously overproduce uric acid and who may be at risk for acute renal failure during periods of dehydration [4,6]. This can occur with polycythemia vera or less commonly with primary gout or HGPRTase deficiency. As a result, 24-hour urine uric acid excretion should be measured in patients with hyperuricemia (even if mild) and one of the aforementioned conditions; allopurinol should probably be administered if excretion exceeds 900 to 1000 mg/day [2,6,11]. An alternate prophylactic regimen consists of maintenance of a high fluid intake plus alkali therapy (with bicarbonate or citrate, for example) to raise the urine pH to 6.5 (Fig. 48-1).

Chronic Urate Nephropathy
Chronic *urate* nephropathy is associated with the deposition of sodium urate crystals within the medulla interstitium. This leads to a secondary inflammatory response (similar to microtophus formation elsewhere) and ultimately interstitial fibrosis, tubular atrophy, and slowly progressive renal failure [4,12].

Patients with urate nephropathy typically have no symptoms referable to the kidney. They tend to have tophaceous gout, an elevated plasma creatinine concentration, and a relatively normal urinalysis [12]. The only laboratory finding suggestive of this disorder is hyperuricemia out of proportion to the degree of renal insufficiency.

Is Chronic Urate Nephropathy a Current Problem?
Recent studies suggest that chronic urate nephropathy is at present a rare problem in the absence of marked hyperuricemia (plasma uric acid concentration >13 mg/dl in men and >10 mg/dl in women) that persists for several decades [13-15]. If these observations are correct, then some other explanation is required for the apparent relationship between hyperuricemia and otherwise unexplained renal failure. One possibility, which has been confirmed in two trials, is that *chronic lead intoxication* plays a primary role in many of these patients [16,17]. Lead both interferes with the excretion of uric acid (perhaps by diminishing tubular secretion) and produces progressive renal damage. The diagnosis of lead intoxication is best established by the demonstration of increased urinary lead excretion after the administration of EDTA (ethylenediaminetetraacetic acid). Treatment of this disorder consists of avoidance of further lead intake (moonshine whiskey and occupational exposure are common current sources) and of removing the excess lead by chelation with EDTA.

Uric Acid Nephrolithiasis
Uric acid stones (which are nonopaque on radiologic examination) occur in approximately 20 percent of patients with primary gout; they also may be seen in occasional patients with other disorders, including polycythemia vera, chronic diarrhea, or the use of a uricosuric agent (such as probenecid or aspirin) [2,18]. As described before, the major factors promoting uric acid precipitation are a high urinary concentration and an acid urine pH. In primary gout, for example, the incidence of stone formation varies with

the rate of uric acid excretion, reaching 40 to 50 percent when excretion exceeds 1000 mg/day [18]. However, stone formation can occur even in gouty patients in whom daily uric acid excretion is normal. In this setting, a persistently acid urine pH (below 5.0–5.5) is present, apparently reflecting a metabolic abnormality associated with gout [18]. As shown in Fig. 48-1, an acid urine markedly increases the likelihood of exceeding the solubility of even normal amounts of uric acid.

The importance of concentration and pH can also be illustrated by patients with chronic diarrhea. In this condition, volume depletion (leading to a fall in urine output and therefore a rise in the uric acid concentration) and metabolic acidosis (leading to an acid urine pH) can promote uric acid nephrolithiasis even though uric acid excretion is in the low-normal range [19].

Therapy is aimed at decreasing the urinary concentration of the relatively insoluble uric acid (Fig. 48-1). This can be achieved by the use of a high fluid-low purine intake plus urinary alkalinization (to a pH of 6.5 for at least part of the day); this regimen can dissolve already existing stones and prevent new stone formation [2,20]. Potassium bicarbonate or citrate (which is metabolized to bicarbonate) is the preferable alkalinizing agent; use of the comparable sodium salt leads to an increase in both sodium and calcium excretion, since the reabsorption of calcium indirectly follows that of sodium [20]. This is clinically important because urinary uric acid can also promote the formation of calcium oxalate stones (see Chap. 54) [2].

Chronic allopurinol therapy can also be used to diminish uric acid excretion. This is particularly indicated in those stone formers who overexcrete uric acid (24-hour excretion >900–1000 mg/day) [2].

References

1. Rose, BD. *Pathophysiology of Renal Disease* (2nd ed). New York: McGraw-Hill, 1987. Pp. 418-425.
2. Coe, FL. Uric acid and calcium oxalate nephrolithiasis. *Kidney Int* 24:392, 1983.
3. Kahn, AM. Weinman, EJ. Urate transport in the proximal tubule: In vivo and vesicle studies. *Am J Physiol* 249:F789, 1985.
4. Emmerson, BT, Row, PG. An evaluation of the pathogenesis of the gouty kidney. *Kidney Int* 8:65, 1975.
5. Kjellstrand, CM, Campbell, DC, von Hartitzch, B, Buselmeier, TJ. Hyperuricemic acute renal failure. *Arch Intern Med* 138:612, 1978.
6. Emmerson, BT, Thompson, L. The spectrum of hypoxanthine-guanine-phosphoribosyltransferase deficiency. *Q J Med* 42:423, 1973.
7. Steele, TH, Rieselbach, RE. The contribution of residual nephrons within the chronically diseased kidney to urate homeostasis in man. *Am J Med* 43:876, 1967.
8. Manballyu, J, Zachee, P, Verbeckmoes, R, Boogaerts, MA. Transient acute renal failure due to tumor-lysis-induced severe phosphate load in a patient with Burkitt's lymphoma. *Clin Nephrol* 22:47, 1984.
9. Wortmann, RL, Fox, IH. Limited value of uric acid to creatinine ratios in estimating uric acid excretion. *Ann Intern Med* 93:822, 1980.
10. Conger, JD, Falk, SA, Guggenheim, SJ, Burke, TJ. A micropuncture study of the early phase of acute urate nephropathy. *J Clin Invest* 58:681, 1976.
11. Liang, MH, Fries, JF. Asymptomatic hyperuricemia: The case for conservative management. *Ann Intern Med* 88:666, 1978.
12. Talbott, JH, Terplan, KL. The kidney in gout. *Medicine* 39:405, 1960.
13. Fessel, WJ. Renal outcomes of gout and hyperuricemia. *Am J Med* 67:74, 1979.
14. Beck, LH. Requiem for gouty nephropathy. *Kidney Int* 30:280, 1986.
15. Campion, EW, Glynn, RJ, DeLabry, LO. Asymptomatic hyperuricemia. Risks and consequences in the Normative Aging Study. *Am J Med* 82:421, 1987.
16. Batuman, V, Maesaka, JK, Haddad, B, Tepper, E, Landy, E, Wedeen, RP. The role of lead in gout nephropathy. *N Engl J Med* 304:520, 1981.

17. Craswell, PW, Price, J, Boyle, PD, Heazlewood, VJ, Baddeley, H, Lloyd, HM, Thomas, BJ, Thomas, BW. Chronic renal failure with gout. *Kidney Int* 26:319, 1984.
18. Yu, Ts-F. Urolithiasis in hyperuricemia and gout. *J Urol* 126:424, 1981.
19. Deren, JJ, Porush, JC, Levitt, MF, Khilvani, MT. Nephrolithiasis as a complication of ulcerative colitis and regional enteritis. *Ann Intern Med* 56:843, 1962.
20. Pak, CYC, Sakhaee, K, Fuller, C. Successful treatment of uric acid nephrolithiasis with potassium citrate. *Kidney Int* 30:422, 1986.

49. ANALGESIC ABUSE NEPHROPATHY AND PAPILLARY NECROSIS

Chronic renal failure associated with excessive consumption of analgesics is a relatively common problem. Its incidence is variable, depending in large part on regional differences in analgesic intake. It is estimated, for example, that analgesic abuse nephropathy (AAN) has been responsible for approximately 1 to 3 percent of cases of end-stage renal disease in the United States as a whole, up to 10 percent in northwestern North Carolina, and 20 percent or more in Australia [1]. Early diagnosis is especially important in this disorder since progressive renal injury can usually be prevented by cessation of analgesic use.

Pathogenesis

The renal damage in AAN is most prominent in the medulla. The earliest changes consist of prominent thickening of the vasa recta capillaries and patchy areas of necrosis of the cells in the loop of Henle and in the medullary interstitium [2]. Similar vascular abnormalities can be found in the renal pelvis and ureter; they are thought to represent an "analgesic microangiopathy" that may reflect primary damage to the vascular endothelial cells [3].

Progression of the vascular lesions leads to enlarging areas of necrosis, beginning in the papilla and extending into the outer medulla. Total papillary necrosis is the eventual result, a change that can be detected by intravenous pyelogram (IVP) if the papilla is sloughed (see the following).

Analgesic nephropathy in humans is usually associated with the ingestion of both phenacetin and aspirin [1,4]. In a prospective 10-year study of women, for example, 12 percent of those with heavy analgesic consumption had a rise in the plasma creatinine concentration versus only 1.4 percent in the control group [5]. In comparison, papillary necrosis leading to renal insufficiency is an unusual problem in patients taking aspirin, phenacetin, or acetaminophen (the major metabolite of phenacetin) alone [1,4,6]. There are occasional patients who develop papillary necrosis after the use of nonsteroidal anti-inflammatory drugs; however, the degree of damage is usually relatively mild in this setting.

Minor abnormalities in renal function, such as decreased concentrating ability or a small reduction in the glomerular filtration rate, can occasionally be detected after cumulative analgesic intake of as little as 1 kg [4]. In contrast, clinically evident renal disease usually requires the ingestion of more than 2 to 3 kg each of phenacetin and aspirin [4]. This will take *5 to 8 years* in a patient using 6 to 8 tablets (or about 1 gm of phenacetin) each day.

The mechanism by which these agents combine to produce renal damage is incompletely understood [7]. Phenacetin is metabolized in the liver to acetaminophen and to N-hydroxylated compounds that may have potent alkylating activity [8]. In addition, metabolism by local hydroperoxidases within the kidney can lead to the production of reactive intermediates that cause tissue damage by lipid peroxidation [7]. These metabolites tend to accumulate in the kidney along the medullary osmotic gradient; as a result, the highest concentrations occur at the papillary tip, the site of the initial pathologic lesions. In comparison to phenacetin, acetaminophen does not appear to form these toxic compounds [8]; this may explain why conventional use of this agent does not seem to lead to papillary injury [1,6].

The potentiating role of aspirin in analgesic nephropathy may be related to two factors. First, aspirin can diminish medullary blood flow by inhibiting the production of vasodilator prostaglandins. The ensuing medullary ischemia could both enhance the toxic effect of phenacetin metabolites and minimize the rate of their removal. Second, aspirin impairs the activity of the hexose monophosphate shunt, thereby lowering the concentration of glutathione, which may normally inactivate the phenacetin metabolites.

Clinical Presentation and Diagnosis

Patients with AAN usually present with fairly characteristic findings (Table 49-1) [4]. Middle-aged women with a chronic history of headache or back pain are most often affected. In many patients, hypertension or an elevated plasma creatinine concentration is discovered on routine examination. Other patients present with symptoms related to analgesic use (such as peptic ulcer disease) or to the renal disease. The latter include flank pain or hematuria, resulting from passage of a sloughed papilla into the renal pelvis or ureter; early symptoms of uremia such as anorexia, fatigue, and weakness; or dysuria and fever due to urinary tract infection, which occurs with increased frequency in AAN.

The urinalysis may be normal or show sterile pyuria, occasionally with mild proteinuria (< 1.5 gm/day). Protein excretion can, however, reach the nephrotic range in patients with advanced disease, presumably due to hemodynamically mediated glomerulosclerosis (see Chap. 56).

The diagnosis of AAN should be considered in any patient (particularly a middle-aged woman) with the combination of chronic renal insufficiency and a relatively normal urinalysis (see Chap. 16). Confirmation of this possibility requires a history of analgesic ingestion. Questioning family and friends may be helpful in this setting, since many patients deny excessive drug use.

An IVP also may be important (Fig. 49-1) [9]. Although papillary necrosis is present on histologic examination in almost all patients, this abnormality can be detected radiologically only if part or all of the papilla has been sloughed*. Partial or complete papillary necrosis can be seen in 25 to 40 percent of patients; the remaining cases usually show small kidneys, occasionally with blunted calyces similar to that found in chronic pyelonephritis.

Course

Continued analgesic ingestion is associated with progressive renal damage, eventually leading to end-stage renal disease. In contrast, renal function often stabilizes or mildly improves in patients who discontinue analgesics [1,11,12]. Even aspirin alone, which is not toxic in patients with normal kidneys, may promote further renal damage in established AAN [11,12]. Propoxyphene and codeine are the only commonly used analgesics that have not been associated with papillary necrosis [4,13].

Progressive renal disease can, however, occur even in those patients in whom analgesic intake is stopped. Secondary, hemodynamically mediated glomerular injury (induced by the initial nephron loss) may play an important role in this setting; as a result,

---

*The radiologic finding of papillary necrosis is not specific for AAN, since this problem can occur in a variety of other disorders including diabetes mellitus, urinary tract obstruction, sickle cell disease, acute pyelonephritis, and renal tuberculosis [10]. The history and appropriate laboratory tests typically allow these conditions to be differentiated from AAN.

Table 49-1. Clinical characteristics of analgesic abuse nephropathy

Primarily affects women in the 30–70-year age range
History of chronic headache or back pain
Ulcerlike symptoms and psychiatric disturbances also common
Hypertension
Urinalysis—sterile pyuria, mild proteinuria, or normal
Intravenous pyelogram
    Papillary necrosis in 25–40%
    Small kidneys in 50–65%
    Normal in 5–15%
Urinary tract infection

it is possible that attempting to lower the intraglomerular pressure with a converting enzyme inhibitor or dietary protein restriction, or both, may have a beneficial long-term effect (see Chap. 56).

In addition to renal disease, AAN also may be complicated by an increased incidence of two other problems: *urinary tract malignancy* and *atherosclerotic vascular disease.* Transitional cell carcinomas of the renal pelvis, ureter, and bladder (which may be multiple and bilateral) and renal cell carcinoma occur in as many as 8 to 10 percent of patients [8,14,15]. In young women (under the age of 50), for example, analgesic abuse is the most common cause of bladder cancer [15]. Furthermore, urothelial atypia has been found in *almost 50 percent* of nephrectomy specimens obtained prior to renal transplantation [14]. It is presumed that the intrarenal accumulation of carcinogenic phenacetin metabolites is responsible for this problem [8]. Similar metabolites do not seem to be formed with acetaminophen alone [8], which does not appear to promote the development of neoplasia [6].

These tumors generally become apparent after 15 to 25 years of analgesic abuse. Most patients are still analgesic users at the time of diagnosis; however, clinically evident disease can occur as late as several years after analgesics have been discontinued and even after renal transplantation has been performed [14].

The major presenting symptom of urinary tract malignancy in AAN is microscopic or gross hematuria. Thus, monitoring the urinalysis is important, looking for the new onset of hematuria. This finding should be investigated with urinary cytology, intravenous pyelography, and, if indicated, cystoscopy with retrograde pyelography. It is also prudent to obtain routine yearly urinary cytology and to consider removing the native kidneys in patients about to receive a renal transplant [14].

Patients with AAN are also more likely to develop atherosclerotic vascular disease (including myocardial infarction and thrombotic stroke), which is often accompanied by premature aging and graying [4]. The mechanism by which this occurs is not well understood. The incidence of other risk factors, such as hypercholesterolemia, smoking, and hypertension, does not appear to be increased when compared to patients with other types of renal disease. It is possible, however, that the analgesic microangiopathy described before [3], which may reflect primary toxic vascular damage, plays an important role in this problem.

Prevention
Optimal therapy of AAN is prevention, by limiting the intake of combination analgesics. The incidence of new cases of this condition, for example, has diminished markedly when phenacetin has been removed from over-the-counter analgesic compounds [1,11]. These compounds have largely been replaced by the use of aspirin, acetaminophen, or ibuprofen, agents that rarely produce papillary necrosis when given alone [1,4,6].

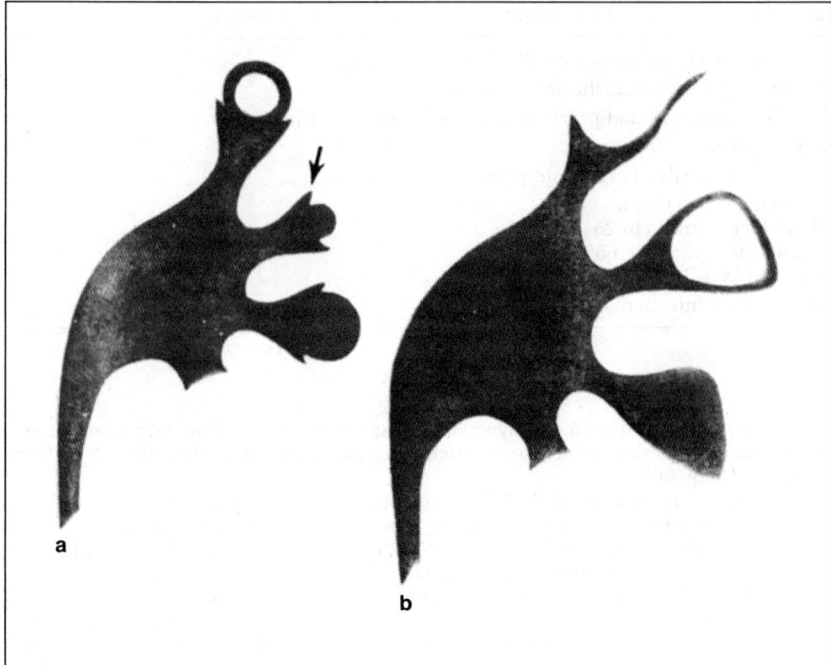

Fig. 49-1. Radiographic findings of renal papillary necrosis in which the papilla has been partially or completely sloughed. (a) Schematization of partial papillary necrosis in which the fornices (arrow) are intact. The three calyces respectively show a medullary ring (the clear area represents a part of the sloughed papilla that has remained in place) and a small and large cavity that are due to partial sloughing of the papilla. (b) The fornices are also lost in complete papillary necrosis, leading to a clubbed appearance. Ring shadow in the middle calyx is again due to a sequestered papilla. (c) Retrograde pyelogram from a patient with analgesic abuse nephropathy. All the calyces are involved with complete papillary necrosis in the lower calyx and partial papillary necrosis in the other calyces, one of which has a medullary ring (arrow). (Adapted from Harrow, BR, Sloane, JA, Liebman, NC, *J Am Med Assoc* 184:445, 1963. By permission of the American Medical Association, copyright, 1963.)

References

1. Buckalew, VM, Jr, Schey, H. Renal disease from habitual antipyretic analgesic consumption: An assessment of the epidemiologic evidence. *Medicine* 65:291, 1986.
2. Gloor, FJ. Changing concepts in pathogenesis and morphology of analgesic nephropathy as seen in Europe. *Kidney Int* 13:27, 1978.
3. Mihatsch, MJ, Hofer, HO, Gudat, F, Knusli, C, Torhorst, J, Zollinger, HU. Capillary sclerosis of the urinary tract and analgesic nephropathy. *Clin Nephrol* 20:285, 1983.
4. Nanra, RS, Stuart-Taylor, JM, deLeon, AH, White, KH. Analgesic nephropathy: Etiology, clinical syndrome, and clinicopathologic correlations in Australia. *Kidney Int* 13:79, 1978.
5. Dubach, VC, Rosner, B, Pfister, EP. Epidemiologic study of abuse of analgesics containing phenacetin. Renal morbidity and mortality (1968-1979). *N Engl J Med* 308:357, 1983.
6. McCredie, M, Stewart, JH. Does paracetamol cause renal papillary necrosis or cancer of the kidney or urinary tract (abstract). *Kidney Int* 30:616, 1986.

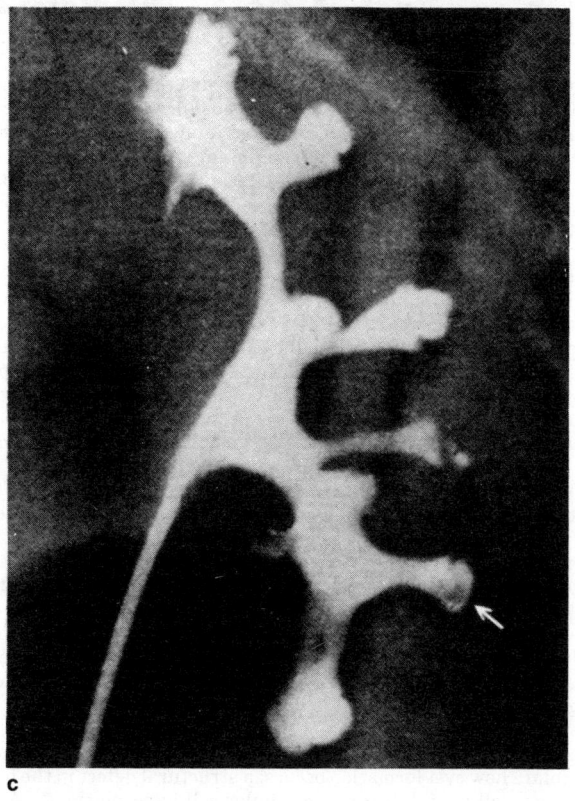

c

Fig. 49-1 (continued)

7. Bach, PH, Hardy, TL. Relevance of animal models to analgesic-associated renal papillary necrosis in humans. *Kidney Int* 28:605, 1985.
8. McCredie, M, Stewart, JH, Carter, JJ, Turner, J, Mahoney, JF. Phenacetin and papillary necrosis: Independent risk factors of renal pelvic cancer, *Kidney Int* 30:81, 1986.
9. Hartman, GW, Torres, VE, Leago, GF, Williamson, B, Jr, Hattery, RR. Analgesic-associated nephropathy. Pathophysiologic and radiological correlation. *J Am Med Assoc* 251:1734, 1984.
10. Eknoyan, G, Qunibi, WY, Grissom, RT, Tuma, SN, Ayus, JC. Renal papillary necrosis: An update. *Medicine* 61:55, 1982.
11. Gault, MH, Wilson, DR. Analgesic nephropathy in Canada: Clinical syndrome, management, and outcome. *Kidney Int* 13:58, 1978.
12. Murray, TG, Goldberg, M. Analgesic-associated nephropathy in the U.S.A.: Epidemiologic, clinical, and pathogenetic features. *Kidney Int* 13:64, 1978.
13. Shelley, JHL. Pharmacologic mechanisms of analgesic nephropathy. *Kidney Int* 13:15, 1978.
14. Blohme, I, Johansson, S. Renal pelvic neoplasms and atypical urothelium in patients with end-stage analgesic nephropathy. *Kidney Int* 20:671, 1981.
15. Piper, JM, Tonascia, J, Matanoski, GM. Heavy phenacetin use and bladder cancer in women aged 20 to 49 years. *N Engl J Med* 313:292, 1985.

50. POLYCYSTIC KIDNEY DISEASE

Adult polycystic kidney disease (PKD) is a common disorder, occurring in approximately 1 out of every 1250 live births [1]. It is also responsible for 10 to 12 percent of cases of end-stage renal disease, a reflection of its almost uniformly progressive course.

Adult PKD is inherited as an autosomal dominant trait, with virtually complete penetrance if the patient lives to 80 years of age [1]. A sporadic form has also been described; it is possible, however, that some of these cases represent familial disease in which affected subjects remain asymptomatic because of delayed expression*.

Pathogenesis

The kidneys in PKD contain multiple cysts of varying size throughout the renal parenchyma. The cysts can develop at any site in the nephron, most often affecting the proximal and collecting tubules [2]. The epithelial cells lining the cysts retain their transport functions; as a result, the composition of the cystic fluid reflects that nephron segment in which they are formed: similar to plasma in the proximal tubule and low sodium–high potassium concentration in the distal nephron [3].

Several studies suggest that only a small proportion of nephrons undergo cyst formation [2,4]. Furthermore, the number of cysts early in the course, when renal function is still relatively normal, is similar to that in azotemic patients [2]. Thus, it is cyst growth, due to an increasing volume of cyst fluid, that is primarily responsible for the development of renal failure by causing compression and eventual atrophy of adjacent noncystic nephrons [2]. The majority of enlarging cysts do not appear to be connected to functioning nephrons [2]. Consequently, cyst growth results from secretion of plasma into the cyst, rather than from glomerular filtration.

Cyst formation, similar to that seen in the kidneys, also occurs in other organs, including the liver, pancreas, and spleen [1]. In addition, structural weakness of the walls of the cerebral arteries can lead to aneurysm formation and intracerebral or subarachnoid bleeding in approximately 10 percent of patients [5].

The biochemical defect in PKD has not been identified, although the abnormal gene has been localized to the short arm of chromosome 16 [6]. Two major theories have been proposed to explain how cyst formation occurs: a structural defect in the basement membrane or abnormal cell growth leading to tubular cell hyperplasia [7]. According to the former hypothesis, weakness of the tubular basement membranes can, even in the presence of normal intratubular pressures, lead to local distention of the tubules and cyst formation. A primary basement membrane abnormality can also explain all of the extrarenal abnormalities that have been seen in this disorder, including cysts in other organs, cerebral aneurysms, colonic diverticula, and aortic regurgitation due to dilatation of the aortic root and annulus [8,9]. Despite the attractiveness of this hypothesis, however, studies in a variety of experimental models reveal no evidence that the tubular basement membranes are structurally weakened [7].

It seems more likely that the primary event in cyst formation is hyperplasia of the tubular epithelial cells, perhaps due to abnormal function of growth factors [7]. Epithelial hyperplasia can be identified within many cysts [2]; furthermore, some patients with PKD develop renal cell carcinoma (which may be bilateral), suggesting the presence of multiple foci of cellular proliferation [10].

Clinical Presentation

Symptoms related to PKD usually do not become apparent until the age of 30 to 50, although the diagnosis may be made earlier in patients who are prospectively evaluated because of a positive family history. Late presentation, however, is not a uniform finding since renal failure occasionally occurs in children of affected parents [11].

The most common initial complaints in PKD are flank pain, vague abdominal discomfort, symptoms of a urinary tract infection, episodic gross hematuria, or the incidental

---

*Infantile and childhood forms of PKD also occur. These rare disorders, which will not be discussed further, are transmitted as an autosomal recessive trait.

discovery of hypertension [1,12]. Hypertension eventually develops in up to 70 percent of patients, generally before the onset of renal failure [13]. Focal compression of the intrarenal arteries by the cysts appears to play at least a contributory role by promoting renin secretion and subsequent sodium and water retention [13].

The initial physical examination may be normal or reveal only hypertension. Palpable kidneys are a relatively late finding, when multiple large cysts lead to an increase in renal size.

The laboratory findings are also variable in PKD. The plasma creatinine concentration is often somewhat elevated at the time of presentation, although advanced renal failure may occasionally be present. The urinalysis may be normal or reveal hematuria, pyuria (if infection is present), or mild proteinuria. An elevation in hemoglobin concentration is another infrequent finding, as about 5 percent of nonazotemic men have a value above 18 gm/dl [14]; a higher-than-expected hemoglobin concentration may also be found in patients with renal insufficiency [12]. Increased production of erythropoietin as cyst compression leads to local ischemia is thought to be responsible for these observations.

Diagnosis

The presence of PKD, which may be suspected from the family history or physical examination, must be confirmed by a radiologic study. Although an intravenous pyelogram may be helpful, this procedure has been replaced by ultrasonography and CT scanning. The former can detect cysts as small as 1.0 to 1.5 cm in diameter; CT scanning is even more sensitive, as cysts with a diameter of 0.5 cm can be seen. Either of these tests is usually diagnostic in patients with established disease, revealing renal enlargement due to bilateral and diffuse cyst formation, with few areas of normal parenchyma being seen between the cysts (Fig. 50-1). Cysts may also be seen in the liver, pancreas, and spleen.

More subtle changes, however, are often present when ultrasonography or CT scanning is used to screen asymptomatic children or siblings of affected patients. The minimal criteria for a positive test are at least one cyst in each kidney with at least one kidney having two or more cysts*; extrarenal cysts, if present, can also be used to establish the diagnosis [6,15]. The likelihood of finding a positive test increases with age, a reflection of the progressive increase in cyst size. Thus, the probability of diagnosing PKD with ultrasonography in the *50 percent of first-degree relatives who will eventually develop the disease* is as high as 30 percent in children (with another 30% having suggestive but not definitive changes) [11] and reaches almost 100 percent by the age of 35 to 40 [15]. Thus, a negative ultrasonogram cannot, with certainty, rule out the diagnosis of PKD under the age of 40 [15]. CT scanning, however, can detect smaller cysts, lowering the age at which a negative study virtually excludes the disease to about 20 to 25.

These difficulties with early radiologic diagnosis may be overcome in the future by using DNA probes in the region adjacent to the PKD gene on chromosome 16 [16]. This technique, which has identified DNA markers that are tightly linked to the PKD gene, may allow greater than 99 percent accuracy in screening even asymptomatic subjects without cysts on radiologic examination.

Prophylactic screening is not usually performed for the presence of a cerebral aneurysm [5]. However, patients with a positive family history of intracerebral bleeding seem to be at greater risk of developing this complication; as a result, CT scanning or magnetic resonance imaging may be helpful in this setting.

Course

PKD is characterized in most patients by a progressive decline in the glomerular filtration rate over a period of many years [12,17]. As described before, this deterioration in kidney function appears to result from cyst formation in a minority of nephrons; increasing size of these cysts then leads to atrophy of adjacent noncystic nephrons [2,4]. End-

---

*These minimal changes alone are not diagnostic of PKD, since similar findings can be seen with multiple simple cysts. Patients with the latter disorder, however, do not have a positive family history of PKD and are generally above the age of 50, a time at which much more advanced radiologic changes would be expected in PKD.

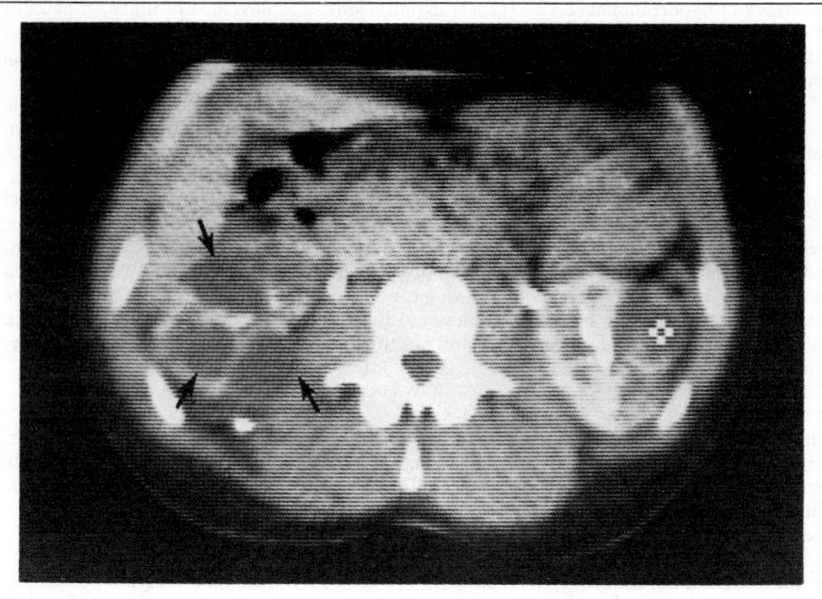

Fig. 50-1. CT scan reveals multiple cysts in each kidney with little visible parenchyma between the cysts. Arrows demonstrate cysts in right kidney. (From Rose, BD. *Pathophysiology of Renal Disease* [2nd ed.]. New York: McGraw-Hill, 1987.)

stage renal disease is unusual before the age of 40 (although it can rarely occur in children [11]) but is seen in approximately 25 percent of patients by age 50 and 75 percent by age 65 [12,17].

In addition to renal failure, PKD can be complicated by a number of other renal and extrarenal problems including gross hematuria and flank pain due to bleeding into a cyst, severe pain resulting from enlargement of a cyst, subarachnoid or intracerebral bleeding, nephrolithiasis, renal cell carcinoma (the presence of which is suggested by hematuria, flank pain, and systemic symptoms such as anorexia and weight loss), and urinary tract infection [1,5,10,12].

Urinary tract infections occur primarily in women; they are generally due to ascending infection from the bladder and may follow urinary tract instrumentation, which should be avoided if possible [12,18]. Either acute pyelonephritis or an infected cyst can occur [18,19]. Treatment is generally begun with conventional antimicrobials that will eradicate parenchymal infection. If, however, the patient does not respond to appropriate therapy, it is likely that an infected cyst is present. Treatment of the latter disorder requires the use of an antimicrobial agent that is both active against the infecting organism and is *able to penetrate the cyst* [19,20]. Ampicillin, cephalosporins, and aminoglycosides, for example, generally do not achieve therapeutic concentrations within the cyst. On the other hand, lipid-soluble agents, such as trimethoprim-sulfamethoxazole and chloramphenicol, are usually able to achieve therapeutic concentrations within the cyst and are therefore more likely to be effective if the organism is sensitive [18-20].

Treatment

There is as yet no proved therapy to slow or prevent progressive renal dysfunction in PKD. There is, however, preliminary evidence that dietary protein restriction may be beneficial, presumably by minimizing hemodynamically mediated glomerular injury (see Chap. 56) [21,22]. It is possible that a similar benefit could be achieved with antihypertensive therapy, preferentially using a converting enzyme inhibitor. Lowering the systemic blood pressure might also have an additional benefit in that it might reduce the risk of cerebral aneurysm rupture.

References

1. Suki, WN. Polycystic kidney disease. *Kidney Int* 22:571, 1982.
2. Grantham, JJ, Geiser, JL, Evan, EP. Cyst formation and growth in autosomal dominant polycystic kidney disease. *Kidney Int* 31:1145, 1987.
3. Huseman, R, Grady, A, Welling, D, Grantham, JJ. Macropuncture study of polycystic disease in adult human kidneys. *Kidney Int* 18:375, 1980.
4. Birenboim, N, Donosco, VS, Huseman, RA, Grantham, JJ. Renal excretion and cyst accumulation of β_2 microglobulin in polycystic kidney disease. *Kidney Int* 31:85, 1987.
5. Levey, AS, Pauker, SG, Kassirer, JP. Occult intracranial aneurysms in polycystic kidney disease. When is cerebral arteriography indicated? *N Engl J Med* 308:986, 1983.
6. Reeders, ST, Breuning, MH, Corney, G, Jeremiah, SJ, Meera Khan, P, Davies, KE, Hopkinson, DA, Pearson, PL, Weatherall, DJ. Two genetic markers closely linked to adult polycystic kidney disease on chromosome 16. *Br Med J* 292:851, 1986.
7. Grantham, JJ, Donoso, VS, Evan, AP, Carone, FA, and Gardner, KD, Jr. Viscoelastic properties of tubule basement membranes in experimental renal cystic disease. *Kidney Int* 32:187, 1987.
8. Scheff, RT, Zuckerman, G, Harter, H, Delmez, J, Koehler, R. Diverticular disease in patients with chronic renal failure due to polycystic kidney disease. *Ann Intern Med* 92:202, 1980.
9. Leier, CV, Baker, PB, Kilman, JW, Wooley, CF. Cardiovascular abnormalities associated with adult polycystic kidney disease. *Ann Intern Med* 100:683, 1984.
10. Kumar, SA, Cedarbaum, AI, Pletka, PG. Renal cell carcinoma in polycystic kidneys: Case report and review of the literature. *J Urol* 124:708, 1980.
11. Sedman, A, Bell, P, Manco-Johnson, M, Schrier, R, Warady, BA, Heard, EO, Butler-Simon, N, Gabow, PA. Autosomal dominant polycystic kidney disease in childhood: A longitudinal study. *Kidney Int* 31:1000, 1987.
12. Milutinovic, J, Fialkow, PJ, Agodoa, LY, Phillips, LA, Rudd, TG, Bryant, JI. Autosomal dominant polycystic kidney disease: Symptoms and clinical findings. *Q J Med* 53:511, 1984.
13. Nash, DA, Jr. Hypertension in polycystic kidney disease without renal failure. *Arch Intern Med* 137:1571, 1977.
14. Gabow, PA, Ikle, DW, Holmes, JH. Polycystic kidney disease: Prospective analysis of nonazotemic patients and family members. *Ann Intern Med* 101:238, 1984.
15. Bear, JC, McManamon, P, Morgan, J, Payne, RH, Lewis, H, Gault, MH, Churchill, DN. Age at clinical onset and at ultrasonographic detection of adult polycystic kidney disease: Data for genetic counselling. *Am J Med Genet* 18:45, 1984.
16. Breuning, MH, Reeders, ST, Brunner, H, et al. Improved early diagnosis of adult polycystic kidney disease with flanking DNA markers. *Lancet* 2:1359, 1987.
17. Churchill, BN, Bear, JC, Morgan, J, Payne, RH, McManamon, PJ, Gault, MH. Prognosis of adult onset polycystic kidney disease reevaluated. *Kidney Int* 26:190, 1981.
18. Schwab, SJ, Bander, SJ, Klahr, S. Renal infection in autosomal dominant polycystic kidney disease. *Am J Med* 82:714, 1987.
19. Sklar, AH, Caruana, RJ, Lammers, JE, Strauser, GD. Renal infections in autosomal dominant polycystic kidney disease. *Am J Kid Dis* 10:81, 1987.
20. Bennett, WM, Elzinga, L, Pulliam, JP, Rashad, AL, Barry, JM. Cyst fluid antibiotic concentrations in autosomal-dominant polycystic kidney disease. *Am J Kid Dis* 6:400, 1985.
21. Oldrizzi, L, Rugiu, C, Valvo, E, Lupo, A, Loschiavo, L, Gammaro, L, Tessitore, N, Fabris, A, Panzetta, G, Maschio, G. Progression of renal failure in patients with renal disease of diverse etiology on protein-restricted diet. *Kidney Int* 27:553, 1985.
22. Rosman, JB, ter Wee, PM, Meiser, S, Piers-Becht, TPhM, Sluiter, WJ, Donker, AbJM. Prospective randomized trial of early dietary protein restriction in chronic renal failure. *Lancet* 2:1291, 1984.

51. MEDULLARY CYSTIC KIDNEY DISEASE, MEDULLARY SPONGE KIDNEY, AND SIMPLE CYSTS

In addition to polycystic kidney disease, there are several other conditions associated with renal cyst formation, including medullary cystic kidney disease, medullary sponge kidney, simple renal cysts, cysts that can undergo malignant transformation (as in the von Hippel-Lindau syndrome and rarely in tuberous sclerosis), and acquired cystic disease in patients with chronic renal failure (see Chap. 58). The clinical characteristics of the first two disorders, in comparison to polycystic kidney disease, are summarized in Table 51-1.

Medullary Cystic Kidney Disease
Medullary cystic kidney disease is a rare disorder in children that is associated with inevitable progression to end-stage renal disease [1,2]. Another condition, familial juvenile nephronophthisis, appears to be histologically and clinically similar to medullary cystic kidney disease except that it becomes clinically evident at a later age [2]. Although they may occur sporadically, these disorders are more commonly inherited usually as an autosomal recessive trait in medullary cystic kidney disease and an autosomal dominant trait in familial juvenile nephronophthisis [2]. In addition, X-linked inheritance has been described in selected cases.

Pathogenesis
Medullary cystic kidney disease is characterized by the presence of multiple cysts, ranging in size from less than 1 mm to 1 cm or more. The cysts arise from intact distal and collecting tubules and are primarily located at the corticomedullary junction and in the medulla. Disease progression is associated with interstitial inflammation and fibrosis, tubular atrophy, and eventual glomerulosclerosis.

The mechanism by which cyst formation occurs is not well understood. It has been suggested that there is a primary defect in the tubular basement membranes, which are initially thin (and perhaps weakened) and later show thickening with a laminated appearance [3]. Furthermore, there tends to be diminished binding of anti-tubular basement membrane antibodies (obtained from a patient with interstitial nephritis), suggesting that a specific basement membrane protein may be missing in this disorder [3]. These *tubular* basement membrane abnormalities are somewhat similar to those seen in the *glomerular* basement membranes in a different disorder, hereditary nephritis. The latter condition, in which a different basement membrane protein appears to be absent, is characterized by initially thin glomerular basement membranes that progress to a laminated appearance and by lack of binding by anti-glomerular basement membrane antibodies obtained from patients with Goodpasture's syndrome (see Chap. 33).

Clinical Presentation
Medullary cystic kidney disease is a slowly progressive condition that produces no symptoms referable to the kidney. As a result, patients typically present with manifestations of advanced renal failure. These include nocturia (due to diminished concentrating ability), anorexia, nausea, and easy fatiguing [1,2]. End-stage renal disease generally occurs before the age of 20 in dominant familial juvenile nephronophthsis and as late as 40 to 50 in autosomal recessive medullary cystic kidney disease [2].

The urinalysis tends to be normal, reflecting the noninflammatory nature of the disease. Abnormal tubular function, however, is common and can lead to early defects in sodium and water reabsorption. The tendency to sodium wasting accounts for the infrequent occurrence of hypertension (even in patients with advanced disease) and for the propensity to develop volume depletion if sodium intake is reduced.

Diagnosis and Treatment
The diagnosis of medullary cystic kidney disease is often made by inference from the clinical presentation and the frequent presence of a positive family history. Obstructive uropathy and chronic pyelonephritis are the other major conditions that can produce

Table 51-1. Clinical characteristics of cystic diseases of the kidney

	Medullary cystic kidney disease	Medullary sponge kidney	Polycystic kidney disease, adult type
Heredity	Variable—autosomal recessive or dominant or not familial	Usually not familial	Autosomal dominant or sporadic
Location of cysts	Primarily at corticomedullary junction	Terminal collecting ducts	Throughout nephron
Flank pain	Absent	Only with complications	Common
Hypertension	Unusual	Unusual	Common
Hematuria	Absent	Only with complications	Frequent
Intravenous pyelography	Small kidneys	Papillary cavities, stones	Large kidneys with cysts
Azotemia after onset	Invariable	Only with complications	Frequent
Age at uremia	20 to 40	Not present	Usually greater than 50

Source: From S. H. Goldman, S. R. Walker, T. C. Merigan, Jr., K. D. Gardner, Jr., and J. M. C. Bull, *N. Engl. J. Med.*, 274:984, 1966. Reprinted by permission from the *New England Journal of Medicine.*

chronic renal failure with a normal urinalysis in this age group. These disorders can be differentiated by ultrasonography: hydronephrosis in urinary obstruction, segmental scarring in chronic pyelonephritis, and multiple small and occasional larger cysts at the corticomedullary junction in medullary cystic kidney disease [4].

There is no known treatment for medullary cystic kidney disease. Patients with this disorder invariably progress to end-stage renal disease, requiring dialysis or transplantation.

Medullary Sponge Kidney
Medullary sponge kidney is a very different disorder from medullary cystic kidney disease. It is characterized by malformation of the terminal collecting ducts with cyst formation [1,5]. These changes are congenital, although there is no evidence for genetic transmission in most patients.

Pathogenesis
Medullary sponge kidney is a disorder affecting the terminal collecting ducts in the pericalyceal region of the renal pyramids. Both small (microscopic) and large cysts may be present. In general, the cysts are diffuse and bilateral; in some patients, however, there is focal involvement of one kidney or of only some calyces.

The factors responsible for these changes are not understood. It is of interest that examination of relatives of patients with medullary cystic kidney disease has in some cases revealed a high incidence of medullary sponge kidney [6]. Furthermore, medullary sponge kidney and polycystic kidney disease have been described in the same patient [7]. These observations suggest that, in at least some patients, medullary sponge kidney may be a *forme fruste* of the other, more serious cystic diseases.

Clinical Presentation and Course
Many patients with medullary sponge kidney are asymptomatic and the diagnosis is never made unless an intravenous pyelogram (IVP) is performed. Symptoms occur only

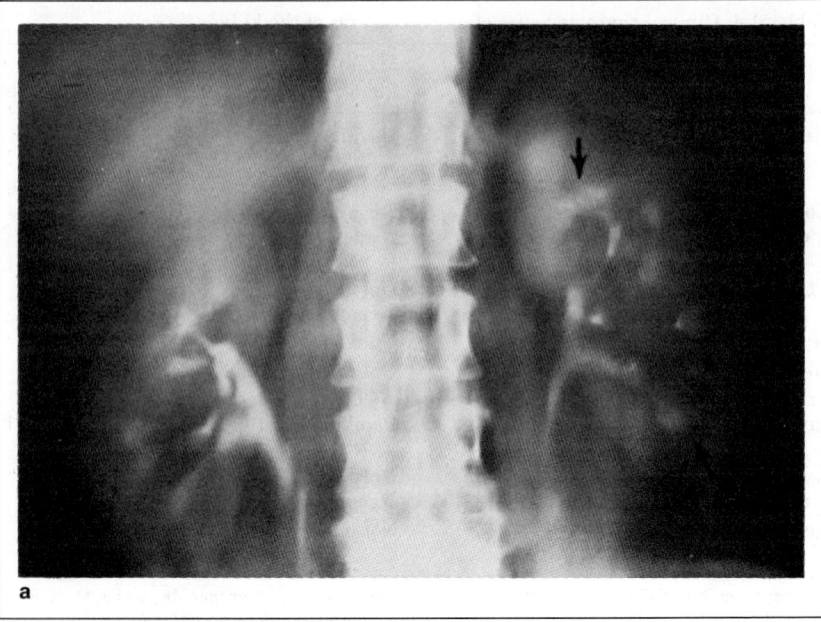

Fig. 51-1. Radiologic findings in medullary sponge kidney. (a) An intravenous
pyelogram shows diffuse involvement of all the calyces, which have a brushlike
appearance radiating out from the calyces (arrows). (b) Calcium stones on
nephrotomography are bunched around the upper and lower calyces of the left kidney
(arrows) in a patient in whom these were the only pyramids that were involved. (From
Rose, BD. *Pathophysiology of Renal Disease* [2nd ed.]. New York: McGraw-Hill, 1987.)

with infection or with the passage of a renal stone, leading to flank pain and hematuria.
Stone formation, originating within the cysts, is relatively common in this disorder.
Most stones are composed of calcium salts that precipitate in part because of stasis
within the abnormal collecting tubules. Hypercalciuria and hyperuricosuria increase
the likelihood of stone formation in this disorder, as they do in patients without underlying renal disease [8].

Medullary sponge kidney is a benign disorder with an excellent long-term prognosis.
The plasma creatinine concentration is usually normal, although it may rise slightly if
passage of a stone leads to unilateral urinary tract obstruction.

Most patients require no specific therapy. Recurrent stone formers, however, may be
treated in an attempt to reduce the frequency of new stones. Possible modalities include
a thiazide diuretic (for hypercalciuria), allopurinol (for hyperuricosuria, which can promote calcium stone formation), or potassium citrate (for hypocitraturia, since urinary
citrate normally inhibits the precipitation of calcium salts) (see Chap. 54) [9,10].

Diagnosis
The diagnosis of medullary sponge kidney is made on an IVP. Opacifications, which
represent the dilated terminal collecting ducts, are seen in the pericalcyeal regions of
some or all of the calyces, leading to the appearance of a brush radiating outward from
the calyx (Fig. 51-1). Calcium stones may also be visible; they are typically small, occur
in clusters, and are found only in the affected calyces.

Simple Renal Cysts
Simple cysts are the most common renal masses. They are most often seen in patients
over the age of 50, up to one-half of whom may have simple cysts (as determined by

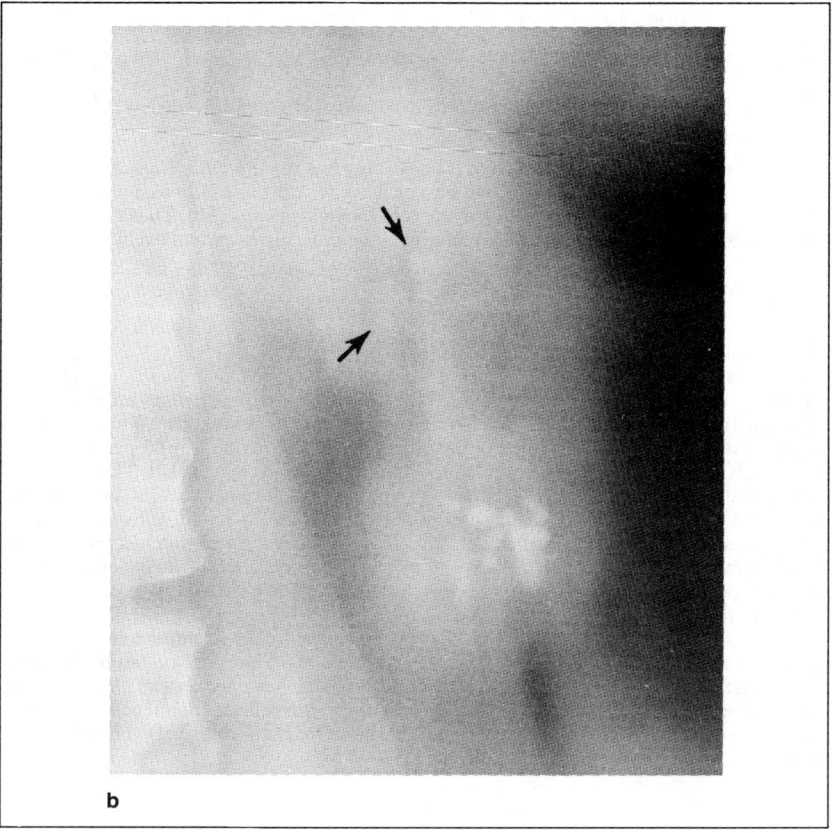

b

Fig. 51-1 (continued)

postmortem examination). These cysts are usually asymptomatic, although they can on occasion lead to flank or abdominal pain [11]. They are usually discovered incidentally on a plain film of the abdomen, IVP, or renal ultrasound. There may be a single cyst or multiple cysts involving both kidneys.

The major concern is distinguishing simple cysts from two more serious conditions: polycystic kidney disease (see Chap. 50) and solid masses, such as a renal cell carcinoma or a renal abscess [11,12]. Ultrasonography and CT scanning are generally able to establish the correct diagnosis in this setting. The criteria favoring a simple cyst on ultrasonography are [12]

1. The mass has sharp margins with smooth walls.
2. There are no echoes (anechoic) within the cyst.
3. There is a strong posterior wall echo, indicating good transmission through the water-filled cyst.

The presence of all three of these findings makes the likelihood of a malignancy extremely small and no further evaluation is required. A CT scan should be performed when there is incomplete renal visualization, calcifications or septae are seen, or if multiple cysts are clustered in a pattern that could mask an underlying carcinoma. A simple cyst is considered to be present on CT scan if [12]

1. The cyst is sharply demarcated from the surrounding parenchyma and has a smooth, thin wall.
2. The fluid within the cyst is homogeneous (like water) with a density of 0 to 20 Hounsfield units.
3. There is no enhancement of the cyst fluid following the administration of radiocontrast media.

The accuracy of ultrasonography and CT scanning has resulted in a dramatic decrease in the necessity for cyst puncture (which can lead to a perirenal hematoma or gross hematuria in up to 4% of cases) [11] or for renal arteriography [12]. These procedures should be considered only if the initial, noninvasive procedures cannot exclude a benign cyst.

Other Cystic Disorders

Cystic lesions can also develop in other uncommon conditions such as the von Hippel-Lindau syndrome and tuberous sclerosis, both of which are inherited as an autosomal dominant trait [1,13]. The von Hippel-Lindau syndrome is characterized primarily by cerebellar and retinal hemangioblastomas. In addition, approximately 65 percent of patients with this disorder develop multiple renal cysts or angiomas [13]. This cyst formation is of particular concern because malignant transformation in at least one of these cysts occurs in as many as one-half of patients [13]. As a result, ultrasonography or CT scanning should be performed periodically to see if cyst formation has occurred or if there is evidence that a preexistent cyst may not be benign. Renal-sparing enucleation is usually performed if a malignancy occurs; nephrectomy is preferably avoided because of the possibility of a carcinoma developing in the other kidney.

Tuberous sclerosis, on the other hand, is characterized by the formation of angiomyolipomas in the skin, brain, kidneys, and other organs [1]. The renal cysts may become quite large; they are often associated with hypertension that may result from compression of adjacent tissue, leading to local ischemia and renin release. Renal cell carcinoma has only been reported in isolated cases and is therefore not a relatively common problem as in the von Hippel-Lindau syndrome [1].

References

1. Welling, LW, Grantham, JJ. Cystic and developmental diseases of the kidney, In BM Brenner and FC Rector, Jr (Eds), *The Kidney* (3rd ed.). Philadelphia: Saunders, 1986.
2. Burke, JR, Inglis, JA, Craswell, PW, Mitchell, KR, Emmerson, BT. Juvenile nephronopthisis and medullary cystic disease -- the same disease. Report of a large family with medullary cystic disease associated with gout and epilepsy. *Clin Nephrol* 18:1, 1982.
3. Cohen, AH, Hoyer, JR. Nephronophthisis: A primary tubular basement membrane defect. *Lab Invest* 55:564, 1986.
4. Rego, JD, Jr, Laing, FC, Jeffrey, RB. Ultrasonographic diagnosis of medullary cystic disease. *J Ultrasound Med* 2:433, 1983.
5. Morris, RC, Jr, Yamauchi, H, Palubinskas, AJ, Howenstine, HJ. Medullary sponge kidney. *Am J Med* 38:883, 1965.
6. Bennett, WB. Kindred coexistence of medullary sponge kidney and medullary cystic disease. *Ann Intern Med* 85:829, 1976.
7. Abreo, K, Steele, TH. Simultaneous medullary sponge and adult onset polycystic kidney disease: The need for accurate diagnosis. *Arch Intern Med* 142:163, 1982.
8. O'Neill, M, Breslau, NA, Pak, CYC. Metabolic evaluation of nephrolithiasis in patients with medullary sponge kidney. *J Am Med Assoc* 245:1233, 1981.
9. Pak, CYC, Peters, P, Hurt, G, Kadesky, M, Fine, M, Reisman, D, Splann, F, Caramela, C, Freeman, A, Britton, F, Sakhaee, K, Breslau, NA. Is selective therapy of recurrent nephrolithiasis possible? *Am J Med* 71:615, 1981.

10. Pak, CYC, Fuller, C. Idiopathic hypocitraturic calcium-oxalate nephrolithiasis successfully treated with potassium citrate. *Ann Intern Med* 104:33, 1986.
11. Clayman, RV, Surya, V, Miller, RP, Reinke, DB, Fraley, EE. Pursuit of the renal mass: Is ultrasound enough? *Am J Med* 77:218, 1984.
12. Bosniak, MA. The current radiologic approach to renal cysts. *Radiology* 158:1, 1986.
13. Malek, RS, Omess, PJ, Benson, RC, Jr, Zincke, H. Renal cell carcinoma in von Hippel-Lindau syndrome. *Am J Med* 82:236, 1987.

52. MYELOMA KIDNEY

Abnormal renal function is common in patients with multiple myeloma. This may be manifested by acute renal failure, by the nephrotic syndrome (due to primary amyloidosis or light-chain deposition disease; see Chap. 31), or by tubular abnormalities such as the Fanconi syndrome [1-3]. This chapter will discuss the major cause of acute renal failure in multiple myeloma: *myeloma kidney*, a disorder in which the urinary excretion of immunoglobulin light chains plays a central role. Hypercalcemia (see Chap. 53), dehydration, and the administration of radiocontrast media (which is usually performed after prior fluid restriction) are other factors that can also contribute to an acute decline in the glomerular filtration rate in this setting [2,4].

The pathologic changes in myeloma kidney are most prominent in the distal and collecting tubules [1,2]. Two primary abnormalities are seen in this condition: intratubular obstruction by glassy, eosinophilic casts; and tubular atrophy and dilatation (Fig. 52-1). Immunofluorescent studies have demonstrated that, in addition to precipitated light chains, the casts contain both other filtered proteins (albumin and gamma globulins) and Tamm-Horsfall mucoprotein, which is normally secreted by the tubular cells in the thick ascending limb of the loop of Henle [5].

Pathogenesis

Myeloma kidney is related to the overproduction of immunoglobulin light chains, which occurs in approximately one-half of patients with this disorder [6]. Light chains have a molecular weight of about 22,000. They are freely filtered across the glomerulus and then largely reabsorbed by the proximal tubular cells. Light-chain excretion is normally less than 30 mg/day. However, marked overproduction and subsequent filtration of these proteins in multiple myeloma overwhelms proximal reabsorptive capacity. As a result, light-chain excretion is increased, ranging from 100 mg/day to more than 20 gm/day.

The mechanism by which light chains lead to renal insufficiency is incompletely understood. Tubular obstruction by the proteinaceous casts is clearly one important factor. However, cast formation is relatively minor in some patients, and renal function has been noted to correlate best with the degree of tubular damage and atrophy [2]. Thus, direct tubular toxicity also may play a major role.

The following sequence has been proposed in which tubular damage and cast formation interact synergistically to produce renal failure. The excess filtered light chains are initially taken up by the proximal tubular cells, where they accumulate and interfere with tubular function, including the reabsorptive capacity for small proteins. As a result, more filtered light chains are delivered distally, promoting the development of occluding tubular casts.

Patients with myeloma kidney generally excrete more than 1 gm of light chains per day [2]. However, some patients excrete much larger quantities without any substantial rise in the plasma creatinine concentration [2,7], indicating that different light chains have variable degrees of nephrotoxicity.

The *isoelectric point* of the monoclonal light chain, for example, may be an important determinant of its potential for inducing renal damage [8]. It has been suggested that those proteins with a relatively high isoelectric point ($pI > 5.8$–6.0) are more likely to be associated with renal failure. These light chains will have a cationic charge at the

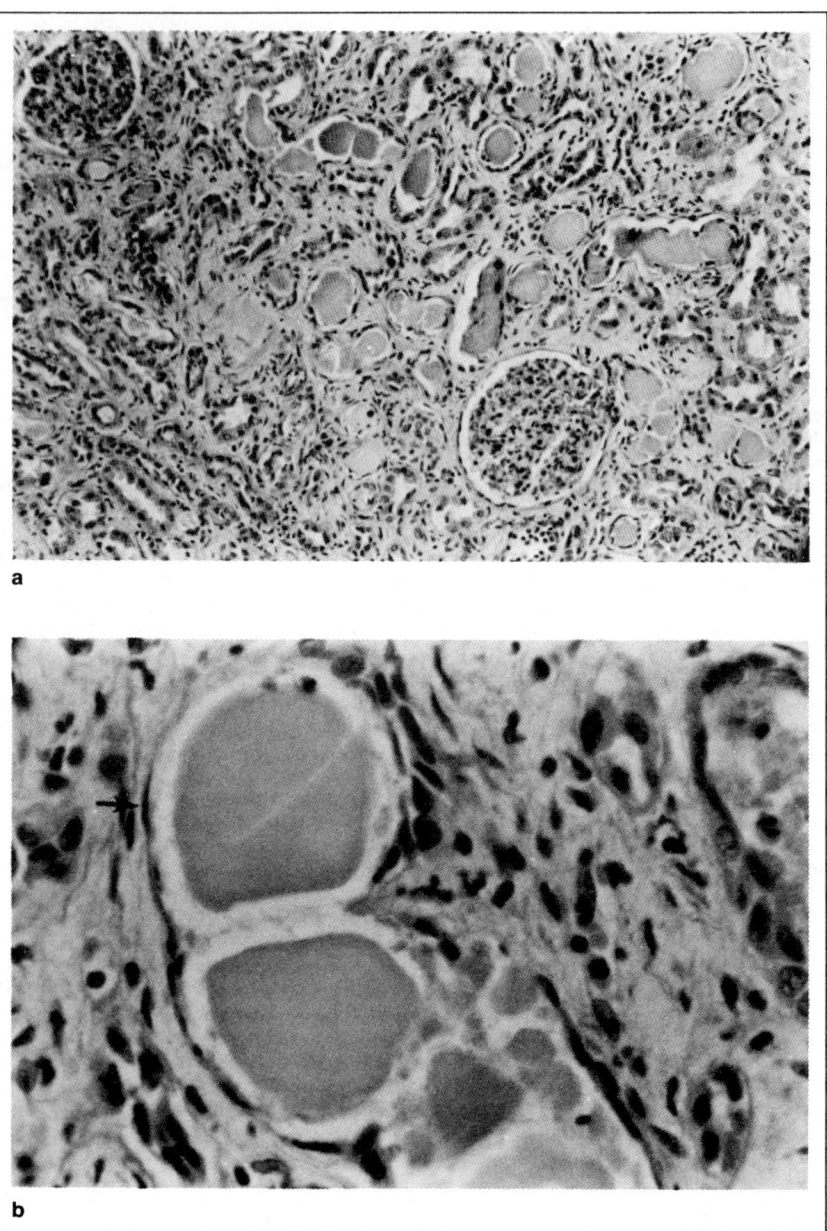

Fig. 52-1. Light microscopy in myeloma kidney demonstrates (a) occlusion of many of the tubules by glassy casts that contain precipitated light chains. Interstitial fibrosis and mononuclear cell infiltration are also present. Higher power (b) shows tubular atrophy with marked flattening of the tubular epithelial cells (arrow). (From Rose, BD. *Pathophysiology of Renal Disease* [2nd ed.]. New York: McGraw-Hill, 1987.)

acid urine pH in the distal nephron. This would allow them to interact with anionic Tamm-Horsfall mucoprotein, thereby forming obstructing casts [5]. Although this interaction may be pathogenetically important, it is not necessarily mediated by charge, since some investigators have been unable to confirm a correlation between nephrotoxicity and the isoelectric point of the excreted light chain [9].

Relation to Amyloidosis and Light-Chain Deposition Disease

Patients who produce excess quantities of monoclonal light chains (and who may or may not have myeloma) can develop two other forms of renal disease: primary amyloidosis and light-chain deposition disease. In these disorders, the light chains are deposited in the tissues (including the glomeruli), but intratubular cast formation is rare [8]. The reasons for this separation are incompletely understood. In both primary amyloidosis and light-chain deposition disease, for example, the light chains must be taken up by macrophages, which then secrete fragments that deposit in the tissues [10]. These fragments may be less nephrotoxic and less likely to promote cast formation than the intact light chains excreted in myeloma kidney.

Clinical Presentation and Diagnosis

Patients with multiple myeloma typically present with systemic symptoms such as weakness, weight loss, and bone pain. The initial laboratory evaluation often reveals anemia, lytic lesions on x ray, and occasionally hypercalcemia.

Renal insufficiency is also found at presentation in about 50 percent of patients [1,2]. The urine sediment is typically benign and albuminuria (as detected by the dipstick that senses only albumin) is mild or absent*. These renal findings are nonspecific; confirmation of the diagnosis requires the demonstration of monoclonal light chains in the urine. This can be done indirectly by testing the urine with sulfosalicylic acid, which senses all urinary proteins. Thus, the constellation of *renal failure, a negative or trace dipstick for protein, and a markedly positive response to sulfosalicylic acid* is highly suggestive of myeloma kidney. A negative sulfosalicylic acid test, however, does not necessarily exclude the diagnosis since this test is not positive unless the concentration of light chains exceeds 1.0 to 1.5 gm/L.

Urinary light chains can be specifically demonstrated by immunoelectrophoresis. It is important to note that only *monoclonal* light chains are suggestive of a plasma cell dyscrasia [6]. The finding of *both* kappa and lambda light chains may be seen with any form of proximal tubular damage (due to many chronic renal diseases) or with a generalized increase in globulin synthesis, as seen in collagen vascular diseases and neoplasms [6].

Course and Treatment

Myeloma kidney is often a progressive disease in which there is a gradual deterioration in renal function. Initial therapy is directed toward those factors that are potentially reversible—hypercalcemia (see Chap. 53), volume depletion, and infection (the last two of which slow flow within the tubules, thereby promoting further cast formation) [2,4]. Thus, saline rehydration and loop diuretics are usually given in an attempt to wash out obstructing casts. Two other modalities also may be effective in selected patients: urinary alkalinization by the administration of sodium bicarbonate (which may decrease the charge interaction between the light chains and Tamm-Horsfall mucoprotein) [11]; and, in refractory acute renal failure, diminishing the circulating light-chain load with plasmapheresis [12]. Using these therapies, even patients who require dialysis due to acutely progressive disease may recover enough renal function to allow dialysis to be discontinued [4].

Once the plasma creatinine concentration is stabilized, therapy is then directed toward treatment of the underlying disease (with prednisone and melphalan) and toward minimization of further cast formation by the maintenance of a high fluid intake (2–3 liters/day). The latter is extremely important because exacerbations of myeloma kidney

---

*Marked albuminuria is usually indicative of concurrent glomerular disease due to amyloidosis or light-chain deposition disease.

commonly occur during periods in which intake is reduced or extrarenal losses are enhanced (due, for example, to diarrhea or vomiting).

References

1. Fang, L-S. Light-chain nephropathy. *Kidney Int* 27:582, 1985.
2. DeFronzo, RA, Cooke, CR, Wright, JR, Humphrey, RL. Renal function in patients with multiple myeloma. *Medicine* 57:151, 1978.
3. Maldonado, JE, Velosa, JA, Kyle, RA, Wagoner, RD, Holley, KE, Salassa, RM. Fanconi syndrome in adults: A manifestation of a latent form of multiple myeloma. *Am J Med* 58:354, 1975.
4. Rota, S, Mougenot, B, Baudouin, B, et al. Multiple myeloma and severe renal failure: A clinicopathologic study of outcome and prognosis in 34 patients. *Medicine* 66:126, 1987.
5. Border, WA, Cohen, AH. Renal biopsy diagnosis of clinically silent multiple myeloma. *Ann Intern Med* 93:43, 1980.
6. Perry, MC, Kyle, RA. The clinical significance of Bence Jones proteinuria. *Mayo Clin Proc* 50:234, 1975.
7. Kyle, RA, Greipp, PR. "Idiopathic" Bence Jones proteinuria: Long-term follow-up in seven patients. *N Engl J Med* 306:564, 1982.
8. Hill, GS, Morel-Maroger, L, Mery, J-P, Brouet, JC, Mignon, F. Renal lesions in multiple myeloma: Their relationship to associated protein abnormalities. *Am J Kid Dis* 2:423, 1983.
9. Smolens, P, Venkatachalam, M, Stein, JH. Myeloma kidney cast nephropathy in a rat model of multiple myeloma. *Kidney Int* 24:192, 1983.
10. Durie, BGM, Persky, B, Soehnlen, BJ, Grogan, TM, Salmon, SE. Amyloid production in human myeloma stem-cell culture, with morphologic evidence of amyloid secretion by associated macrophages *N Engl J Med* 307:1689, 1982.
11. Holland, MD, Galla, JH, Sanders, PW, Luke, RG. Effect of urinary pH and diatrizoate on Bence Jones protein nephrotoxicity in the rat. *Kidney Int* 27:46, 1985.
12. Zucchelli, P, Pasquali, S, Cagnoli, L, Ferrari, G. Controlled plasma exchange trial in acute renal failure due to multiple myeloma. *Kidney Int* 33:1175, 1988.

53. HYPERCALCEMIC AND SARCOID NEPHROPATHY

Hypercalcemia can lead to three major renal problems: nephrolithiasis due to chronic hypercalciuria, polyuria and polydipsia due to nephrogenic diabetes insipidus, and acute and chronic renal failure. The earliest pathologic changes in this condition, which reflect local calcium deposition, are seen in the distal and collecting tubules [1]. Calcification, degeneration, and necrosis of the tubular epithelial cells lead to sloughing and secondarily to intratubular obstruction. More chronic changes include tubular atrophy and interstitial calcification and fibrosis, lesions that are likely to be associated with irreversible renal dysfunction. Calcium deposits also may be found in the blood vessels, glomeruli, and proximal tubules.

The prominent involvement of the collecting tubules probably plays an important role in the acquired resistance to antidiuretic hormone (ADH). ADH-induced generation of cyclic AMP is impaired by hypercalcemia, an effect that may involve the ADH receptor in the cell membrane or the ability of the hormone receptor complex to activate adenyl cyclase [2]. Impaired sodium chloride reabsorption in the loop of Henle also may play a contributory role by interfering with the medullary accumulation of solute, the primary step in the generation of the countercurrent gradient [3].

The pathogenesis of hypercalcemia-induced renal failure appears to be multifactorial. Although the obstructing cellular and calcium casts almost certainly play a role, renal vasoconstriction is also likely to be important. Hypercalcemia directly increases renal vascular tone and lowers the permeability of the glomerular capillary wall, both of which impair the glomerular filtration rate [4]. These vasoconstrictive effects are partially counteracted by the local release of vasodilator prostaglandins [4]. As a result, patients with hypercalcemia are probably at increased risk of developing renal failure when prostaglandin synthesis is impaired by the administration of a nonsteroidal anti-inflammatory drug.

Etiology

Although almost any cause of hypercalcemia can lead to renal dysfunction, the most common are malignancy, primary hyperparathyroidism, and sarcoidosis. In addition to direct osteolysis by bone metastases, it is now clear that humoral factors often play a central role in the tumor-induced increase in bone resorption [5]. Among the substances that have been identified in selected cases are a parathyroid hormonelike peptide; osteoclast activating factors in hematologic malignancies (such as multiple myeloma), which may include tumor necrosis factor and interleukin-1; prostaglandins; and calcitriol (1,25-dihydroxyvitamin D) in some lymphomas [5].

Abnormal vitamin D metabolism also is of primary importance in sarcoidosis. Increased intestinal calcium absorption and subsequent hypercalciuria occur in up to one-half of patients with this disorder [6], with hypercalcemia eventually occurring in 15 to 20 percent of cases. These changes in calcium balance occur only in patients with diffuse sarcoidosis and are due to increased production of calcitriol not by the kidney, but by the *activated mononuclear cells (particularly macrophages)* in the lung and lymph nodes [7,8].

The mechanism by which calcitriol is released by mononuclear cells is unclear; vitamin D has immunomodulatory functions and may therefore be involved in the inflammatory process [9]. This relationship probably also explains the development of hypercalcemia in other granulomatous disorders (such as berylliosis and postsilicon implantation) and in rare cases of lymphoma [5].

Clinical Presentation

Hypercalcemia is most often discovered as an incidental finding on routine examination. On careful questioning, however, many patients have some complaints that may be related to the elevation in the plasma calcium concentration. These include anorexia, nausea, lethargy, constipation, and polyuria and polydipsia.

The physical examination may reveal signs of an underlying malignancy, sarcoidosis or, with chronic elevations in the plasma calcium concentration, calcium deposition along the lateral and medial margins of the cornea (band keratopathy), which is best detected by slit-lamp examination. The laboratory findings, other than hypercalcemia, are nonspecific. Hypokalemia is commonly found, due to increased urinary losses [10]. The mechanism by which this occurs is probably related to defective tubular sodium reabsorption, leading to increased delivery of sodium and water to the potassium-secretory site in the cortical collecting tubule.

The blood urea nitrogen (BUN) and plasma creatinine concentration are often elevated, due both to hypercalcemia and to concomitant volume depletion. The urinalysis is typically normal or near normal, although hematuria can be induced by nephrolithiasis or by hypercalciuria-induced microcalculi [11].

Diagnosis

The presumptive diagnosis of hypercalcemic nephropathy requires only the combination of hypercalcemia and otherwise unexplained renal insufficiency. Plain film of the abdomen in this setting may reveal calcium stones or multiple small parenchymal calcifications (nephrocalcinosis). In addition, hypercalcemia should be excluded (if the plasma calcium concentration has not yet been measured) in any patient with an elevated plasma creatinine concentration and either a normal urinalysis or a known underlying malignancy.

Identifying the cause of hypercalcemia should begin with a careful history, trying to determine if there is excessive vitamin D or calcium intake or symptoms suggestive of an underlying malignancy. In addition, the initial laboratory work-up should include a chest x ray (looking for a malignancy or hilar adenopathy in sarcoidosis), bone scan (looking for a metastatic lesion), protein electrophoresis (looking for a paraprotein, suggestive of multiple myeloma), and measurement of the plasma parathyroid hormone level (in an attempt to distinguish primary hyperparathyroidism from other causes of hypercalcemia in which parathyroid hormone secretion should be appropriately suppressed) [12].

Treatment

Renal function can often be markedly improved by returning the plasma calcium concentration to normal. This improvement is due to reversal of the vasoconstrictive effects of hypercalcemia and to washing out of obstructing tubular casts. Patients with longstanding hypercalcemia, however, may have irreversible tubulointerstitial scarring and persistent renal insufficiency.

Initial therapy of hypercalcemia is directed toward increasing urinary calcium excretion with the combination of a loop diuretic and intravenous saline [13]. The rationale behind this regimen is that calcium is passively reabsorbed in the proximal tubule and the thick ascending limb of the loop of Henle, following gradients established by the reabsorption of sodium and water. Thus, diminishing sodium transport in the proximal tubule (by saline-induced volume expansion) and in the loop of Henle (with a loop diuretic) produces both a natriuresis and a calciuresis. The goal is to maintain the urine output above 2.5 liters/day. It is important to emphasize that producing a diuresis by increasing only water intake will be ineffective; the increase in urine output in this setting is due to an appropriate decrease in the secretion of ADH, thereby lowering water reabsorption in the collecting tubules. Neither sodium nor calcium reabsorption is affected by this regimen.

Corticosteroids also can lower the plasma calcium concentration, particularly in the following conditions: (1) hematologic malignancies in which steroids seem to antagonize the bone resorptive effect of osteoclast-activating factors [5,14]; and (2) sarcoidosis and hypervitaminosis D in which steroids directly diminish intestinal calcium absorption and, in sarcoidosis (and some cases of lymphoma), decrease calcitriol synthesis by the activated macrophages* [16,17]. In contrast, steroid therapy has little effect on the plasma calcium concentration in primary hyperparathyroidism, the other major cause of hypercalcemia.

A variety of other modalities have been used in those patients (usually with an underlying malignancy) who do not respond to saline, a loop diuretic, and corticosteroids [5,13,18]. These include intravenous mithramycin, calcitonin, and, when available, diphosphonates, all of which directly reduce bone resorption. Oral phosphate also may be helpful as chronic therapy, by complexing with intestinal and circulating calcium. The use of intravenous phosphate (which can lead to disseminated calcium phosphate deposition) or hemodialysis to treat severe hypercalcemic crisis is only rarely indicated.

Other Forms of Sarcoid Nephropathy

Sarcoidosis is rarely associated with two noncalcium-related types of renal disease: a granulomatous interstitial nephritis and a variety of glomerular disorders. Renal interstitial granuloma formation (similar to that seen in other tissues) is relatively common in sarcoidosis, although involvement that is severe enough to produce renal insufficiency is unusual. When this does occur, it is generally in the setting of diffuse sarcoidosis [19]. Some patients, however, present with an elevated plasma creatinine concentration with no or only minimal extrarenal manifestations [20].

The laboratory findings of sarcoid interstitial nephritis are nonspecific. The urinalysis is typical of other chronic tubulointerstitial diseases, being normal or revealing only sterile pyuria or mild proteinuria. Renal biopsy reveals normal glomeruli, noncaseating granulomas in the interstitium, tubular damage, and interstitial fibrosis. Corticosteroid therapy tends to restore renal function toward normal, although the recovery may be

---

*Recent evidence suggests that chloroquine and hydroxychloroquine also reduce calcitriol synthesis and reverse hypercalcemia and hypercalciuria in sarcoidosis [15]. The latter drug, which has less retinal toxicity, may be preferable in those patients requiring long-term therapy, since it does not produce the multiple steroid-related side effects.

incomplete [20]. In addition, relapses can occur if therapy is tapered too rapidly and irreversible renal failure can be seen in patients with long-standing disease and marked fibrotic changes in the kidney [20].

A variety of glomerular lesions have also been described in selected patients with sarcoidosis [21]. These include proliferative or crescentic glomerulonephritis, membranous nephropathy, and focal glomerulosclerosis. The urinary findings are similar to those in other patients with these disorders, including proteinuria, which can reach the nephrotic range, hematuria, and red cell and other casts. Corticosteroid therapy again appears to improve renal function [21].

The pathogenesis of the glomerular disease in sarcoidosis is not well understood. It has been proposed that primary tubulointerstitial damage can lead to the exposure or release of previously "unseen" tubular antigens, with subsequent antibody formation and local immune complex deposition.

References

1. Benabe, JE, Martinez-Maldonado, M. Hypercalcemic nephropathy. *Arch Intern Med* 138:777, 1978.
2. Wiesmann, W, Sinha, S, Klahr, S. Effects of ionophore A23187 on baseline and vasopressin-stimulated sodium transport in the toad bladder. *J Clin Invest* 59:418, 1977.
3. Galla, JH, Booker, BB, Luke, RG. Role of the loop segment in the concentrating defect of hypercalcemia. *Kidney Int* 29:977, 1986.
4. Levi, M, Ellis, MA, Berl, T. Control of renal hemodynamics and glomerular filtration rate in chronic hypercalcemia. Role of prostaglandins, renin-angiotensin system and calcium. *J Clin Invest* 71:1624, 1983.
5. Mundy, GR. The hypercalcemia of malignancy. *Kidney Int* 31:142, 1987.
6. Muther, RS, McCarron, DA, Bennett, WM. Renal manifestations of sarcoidosis. *Arch Intern Med* 141:643, 1981.
7. Adams, JS, Sharma, OP, Gacod, MA, Singer, FR. Metabolism of 25-hydroxyvitamin D_3 by cultured pulmonary alveolar macrophages in sarcoidosis. *J Clin Invest* 72:1856, 1983.
8. Mason, RS, Frankel, T, Chan, Y-L, Lissner, D, Posen, S. Vitamin D conversion by sarcoid lymph node homogenate. *Ann Intern Med* 100:59, 1984.
9. Manolagas, SC, Deftos, LJ. The vitamin D endocrine system and the hematolymphopoietic tissue. *Ann Intern Med* 100:144, 1984.
10. Aldinger, KA, Samaan, NA. Hypokalemia with hypercalcemia: Prevalence and significance in treatment. *Ann Intern Med* 87:571, 1977.
11. Stapleton, FB, Roy, S, III, Noe, HN, Jenkins, G. Hypercalciuria in children with hematuria. *N Engl J Med* 310:1345, 1984.
12. Lufkin, EG, Kao, PC, Heath, H, III. Parathyroid hormone radioimmunoassays in the differential diagnosis of hypercalcemia due to primary hyperparathyroidism or malignancy. *Ann Intern Med* 106:559, 1987.
13. Stewart, AF. Therapy of malignancy-associated hypercalcemia: 1983. *Am J Med* 74:475, 1983.
14. Mundy, GR, Rick, ME, Turcotte, R, Kowalski, MA. Pathogenesis of hypercalcemia in lymphosarcoma cell leukemia: Role of an osteoclast activating factor-like substance and a mechanism of action for glucocorticoid therapy. *Am J Med* 65:600, 1978.
15. O'Leary, TJ, Jones, G, Yip, A, Lohnes, D, Cohanim, M, Yendt, ER. The effects of chloroquine on serum 1,25-dihydroxyvitamin D and calcium metabolism in sarcoidosis. *N Engl J Med* 315:727, 1986.
16. Sanders, LM, Winearls, CG, Fraher, LJ, Clemens, TL, Smith, R, O'Riordan, JLH. Studies of the hypercalcemia of sarcoidosis: Effects of steroids and exogenous vitamin D_3 in the circulating concentration of 1,25-dihydroxy vitamin D_3. *Q J Med* 53:165, 1984.
17. Breslau, NA, McGuire, JL, Zerwekh, JE, Frenkel, EP, Pak, CYC. Hypercalcemia associated with increased serum calcitriol levels in three patients with lymphoma. *Ann Intern Med* 100:1, 1984.
18. Harinck, HIJ, Bijvoet, OLM, Plantingh, AST, Body, J-J, Elte, JWF, Sleeboom, HP,

Wildiers, J, Neijt, JP. Role of bone and kidney in tumor-induced hypercalcemia and its treatment with bisphosphonate and sodium chloride. *Am J Med* 82:1133, 1987.

19. Korzets, A, Schneider, M, Taragan, R, Bernheim, J, Bernheim, J. Acute renal failure due to sarcoid granulomatous infiltration of the renal parenchyma. *Am J Kid Dis* 6:250, 1985.

20. Singer, DRJ, Evans, DJ. Renal impairment in sarcoidosis: Granulomatous nephritis as an isolated cause (two case reports and review of the literature). *Clin Nephrol* 26:250, 1986.

21. Goldszer, RC, Galvanek, EG, Lazarus, JM. Glomerulonephritis in a patient with sarcoidosis. Report of a case and review of the literature. *Arch Pathol Lab Med* 105:478, 1981.

54. CALCIUM NEPHROLITHIASIS

Humans excrete relatively large quantities of calcium, uric acid, phosphate, and oxalate in the urine. As a result, stone formation is not an uncommon event. It has been estimated, for example, that 12 percent of men and 5 percent of women will have had at least one symptomatic episode due to a renal stone by the age of 70 [1]. Over 80 percent of these stones contain calcium and, therefore, calcium nephrolithiasis will be the focus of this chapter. Uric acid nephrolithiasis, a less common disorder, is covered in Chap. 48.

As will be seen, calcium stones are most likely to form when one or more factors is present that promotes the precipitation of calcium salts. These include (1) an increase in excretion of calcium or oxalate; (2) an increase in concentration of these substances due to a low urine volume; (3) a reduction in excretion of inhibitors of precipitation, such as citrate; and (4) the presence of uric acid crystals, which can act as a nidus for calcium stone formation [2,3]. The urine pH, which is an important determinant of uric acid (low pH) or struvite (high pH) stone formation, has little role in calcium oxalate precipitation. An elevated urine pH in type 1 (distal) renal tubular acidosis can, however, contribute to the development of calcium phosphate stones (see Chap. 8).

Natural History and Evaluation

The diagnostic evaluation and the approach to therapy are in part determined by the natural history in untreated patients. In a subject who has passed a first calcium stone, the likelihood of forming a second stone is about 15 percent at 1 to 3 years and then gradually increases to 50 percent in men and 30 percent in women by 14 years [1,4]. Thus, many patients have relatively indolent disease, although a small subpopulation will form multiple calculi [2].

It is of interest that the frequency and type of metabolic abnormalities are similar in single and recurrent stone formers [5]. In view of the frequently benign course, however, medical therapy is begun only if there is *metabolically active stone disease,* which is defined as the formation of new stones, an increase in the size of an old stone, or the passage of gravel. Even in this group, therapeutic trials have revealed approximately a 60 percent reduction in stone formation with *placebo* therapy [6,7]. These results suggest that there is often a strong "stone-clinic" effect.

A reasonable approach to a patient with a single calcium stone, therefore, is to increase fluid intake to over 2 liters/day, without further evaluation or specific intervention other than intravenous pyelography to look for an anatomic abnormality, such as medullary sponge kidney. A careful dietary history may be helpful at this time, looking for reversible predisposing factors, such as low fluid intake or the use of vitamin D or large doses of vitamin C, which is in part metabolized to oxalate. Periodic monitoring for new stone formation (by renal ultrasonography or a plain film of the abdomen) should then be performed, initially at yearly intervals.

A complete metabolic work-up is indicated only if there is evidence of active stone disease. This evaluation includes *2 to 3* measurements both of the plasma calcium con-

Table 54-1. Normal limits for daily urine excretion

Substance excreted	Men	Women
Calcium, mg	< 300	< 250
Calcium, mg/kg	< 4	< 4
Uric acid, mg	< 800	< 750
Oxalate, mg	< 50	< 50
Citrate, mg	450–600	650–800

centration and of the 24-hour urinary excretion of calcium, uric acid, sodium, and, to assess the completeness of the collection, creatinine (Table 54-1). These urine collections should be obtained in the outpatient setting when the patient is on his or her regular diet. Citrate is somewhat more difficult to measure and its excretion is usually determined only if neither hypercalciuria nor hyperuricosuria is present in a recurrent stone former. Similarly, oxalate excretion is measured only if there is malabsorption or a suspicion of primary hyperoxaluria (see the following).

Idiopathic Hypercalciuria

Idiopathic hypercalciuria is the most common cause of calcium oxalate stones. As many as 50 to 60 percent of men and 70 to 80 percent of women with calcium stones have urinary calcium excretion rates that are elevated (Table 54-1) [8]; in comparison, only 5 percent of normal subjects are hypercalciuric [8].

Pathogenesis
Idiopathic hypercalciuria appears to be inherited, probably as an autosomal dominant trait, in up to 90 percent of cases [9]. The plasma calcium concentration is normal, and another cause for hypercalciuria (such as sarcoidosis or vitamin D ingestion) cannot be identified.

The increase in urinary calcium excretion in this disorder seems to be due to a mild-to-moderate *rise in the plasma concentration of calcitriol* (1,25-dihydroxyvitamin D_3), the major active form of vitamin D [10,11]. The high calcitriol levels cause an increase in gastrointestinal calcium absorption, which then leads to enhanced urinary calcium excretion [11]. The initial calcium retention also may decrease the release of parathyroid hormone [12]; since this hormone normally stimulates active distal tubular calcium reabsorption [13], a reduction in its rate of secretion can contribute to the hypercalciuria.

Elevated calcitriol levels can also cause hypercalciuria by directly promoting bone resorption [14]. This may be particularly important when these patients are put on a low-calcium diet. In this setting, hypercalciuria persists, coming now from bone rather than increased intestinal absorption. These changes can lead to negative calcium balance and, if prolonged, possibly osteopenia [14]. Restricting dietary calcium also has a second potential disadvantage; by decreasing the formation of insoluble calcium oxalate in the gut, it allows oxalate to remain in a soluble state, leading to increased oxalate absorption. The subsequent rise in urinary oxalate excretion can promote further stone formation [15].

A *high-protein intake* also may play a contributory role in selected patients. The associated acid load, generated from the metabolism of sulfur-containing amino acids such as methionine, can both increase the excretion of calcium (in part by release of calcium from bone during bone buffering of some of the excess hydrogen ions) and reduce the excretion of citrate, a potent inhibitor of crystallization (see the following) [16]. Protein loading also can increase uric acid excretion (due to the metabolism of purines), another factor that can promote calcium stone formation [8]. Thus, avoidance of a high-protein diet may be generally beneficial in all patients with calcium stones.

Diagnosis
The diagnosis of idiopathic hypercalciuria is made when there is an otherwise unexplained increase in urinary calcium excretion in a normocalcemic stone former. Measurement of sodium excretion is important in this setting because calcium reabsorption in the kidney passively follows that of sodium in the proximal tubule and loop of Henle. As a result, hypercalciuria can be obscured if the patient happens to be volume depleted at the time of the collection; this can be detected by a low rate of sodium excretion [17]. On the other hand, a high-sodium intake can contribute to the development of hypercalciuria [17].

In addition, the plasma calcium concentration should be measured on at least two occasions, since many patients with primary hyperparathyroidism have mild, intermittent hypercalcemia [18]. If borderline values are obtained (plasma calcium concentration between 10.1 and 10.5 mg/dl), numerous measurements may be required over a period of time to document the presence of hypercalcemia. This is particulary important in women, since primary hyperparathyroidism is more common in women whereas up to 80 percent of patients with idiopathic hypercalciuria are men [4,18].

Treatment
Reducing urinary calcium excretion is the primary aim of therapy in idiopathic hypercalciuria. Given the potential risks associated with dietary calcium restriction (see before), the treatment of choice is a low-sodium diet plus a thiazide diuretic (Table 54-2). These agents (such as 25–50 mg of hydrochlorothiazide) can diminish calcium excretion by up to 150 mg/day, both by inducing volume depletion (with a secondary rise in proximal calcium reabsorption) and by directly enhancing active calcium transport in the distal tubule (via an unknown mechanism) [19]. The net effect in recurrent stone formers is a 90 percent reduction in new stone disease (although there is also an appreciable improvement with placebo therapy) [2,7,19a].

If hypercalciuria persists, compliance with dietary sodium restriction should be checked (by measuring sodium excretion in a 24-hour collection) and the potassium-sparing diuretic amiloride can be added. Amiloride may have two beneficial effects in this setting: it can reduce calcium excretion further by promoting calcium reabsorption at a more distal site in the cortical collecting tubule [19]; and it can reverse thiazide-induced hypokalemia, thereby increasing the urinary excretion of citrate [20]. Urinary citrate acts as inhibitor of crystallization, probably by forming a *nondissociable but soluble complex* with calcium, which limits the availability of free calcium to combine with oxalate or phosphate.

Citrate excretion should be measured in thiazide-treated patients who continue to form stones, since it may be reduced as part of the primary problem [3] or as a secondary response to hypokalemia. Filtered citrate is normally reabsorbed in the proximal tubule by a sodium-citrate cotransporter. Citrate use within the cells is enhanced by a fall in cell pH, thereby lowering the cell citrate concentration [20]. This creates a more favorable gradient for citrate to enter the cells, leading to a reduction in citrate excretion that can promote stone formation. Thus, citrate excretion is diminished in most forms of metabolic acidosis, a change that contributes to the nephrocalcinosis seen in type 1 (distal) renal tubular acidosis (see Chap. 8).

A similar change in cell pH can occur with hypokalemia. As the plasma potassium concentration falls, cellular potassium moves into the extracellular fluid (to replace the losses); electroneutrality is maintained in this setting by sodium and hydrogen entry into the cells. The ensuing intracellular acidosis can then reduce citrate excretion. This may explain why correcting diuretic-induced hypokalemia with potassium citrate or perhaps amiloride can diminish stone formation [21].

Two points concerning citrate administration deserve emphasis. First, the effect of citrate is indirect. The exogenous citrate is rapidly converted to bicarbonate*, and it is the associated rise in extracellular and presumably intracellular pH that is responsible for the increase in citrate excretion [20,21]. Second, the administration of alkali may also enhance tubular calcium reabsorption, thereby *lowering the rate of calcium excre-*

---

*Bicarbonate administration can produce similar results, although it tends to be somewhat less well tolerated than citrate, due in part to gastric distention from the local formation of carbonic acid.

Table 54-2. Medical therapy of the major causes of active calcium stone disease

Disorder	Preferred therapy
All active stone formers	Maintain fluid intake above 2 liters/day Avoidance of a high-protein diet
Idiopathic hypercalciuria	Thiazide diuretic and low-sodium diet Amiloride Potassium citrate Neutral phosphate Avoid dietary calcium restriction
Primary hyperparathyroidism	Surgery Avoid thiazide diuretic
Hyperuricosuric calcium stones	Low-purine diet Allopurinol Potassium citrate
Hypocitraturia	Potassium citrate
Type 1 renal tubular acidosis (see Chap. 8)	Potassium citrate Thiazide diuretic if also hypercalciuric
Enteric hyperoxaluria	Low-fat, low-oxalate diet, if tolerated Potassium citrate, if metabolic acidosis Calcium carbonate Cholestyramine
Primary hyperoxaluria	Neutral phosphate, magnesium, and pyridoxine
Idiopathic calcium stones	Neutral phosphate

tion [22]. This reverses the tendency of the dietary acid load to enhance calcium loss [16].

Second, *potassium*, rather than sodium, citrate must be given (usually in a dose of 60–80 meq/day). Administration of the sodium salt will produce volume expansion, which will decrease proximal sodium and calcium reabsorption; the ensuing rise in calcium excretion may counterbalance any benefit deriving from the elevation in citrate excretion [22]. In comparison, potassium has no effect on renal calcium handling.

One final modality that may also be effective in refractory patients is the administration of neutral phosphate (such as Neutra-Phos) [16]. This agent acts in part by increasing the urinary excretion of pyrophosphate, an inhibitor of calcium precipitation. It also tends to modestly reduce calcium excretion by binding dietary calcium in the intestinal tract, thereby limiting its absorption. About 2 gm of elemental phosphorus must be provided per day, with diarrhea being a complication in some patients.

Primary Hyperparathyroidism

Patients with primary hyperparathyroidism have both hypercalcemia and hypercalciuria. These effects are due in part to the ability of parathyroid hormone (PTH) to increase calcitriol production, both directly and by inducing hypophosphatemia (through a reduction in the tubular reabsorption of phosphate) [13,23]. Increased intestinal calcium reabsorption as well as PTH and calcitriol stimulated bone resorption then raise the plasma calcium level, leading ultimately to hypercalciuria. The plasma level of calcitriol appears to correlate directly with the development of nephrolithiasis in this disorder [24].

The diagnosis of hyperparathyroidism in a calcium stone former is suggested by the presence of hypercalcemia. As described before, however, the rise in the plasma calcium concentration is often mild and intermittent; thus, multiple measurements may be required to establish that the patient (more often a woman) is really hypercalcemic [18]. PTH levels are typically elevated, in comparison to the suppressed levels in other hypercalcemic states associated with nephrolithiasis, such as sarcoidosis (see Chap. 53), excessive vitamin D intake, and the milk-alkali syndrome.

Optimal treatment of the hypercalcemia and nephrolithiasis requires parathyroid surgery. Thiazide diuretics can reduce urinary calcium excretion in this setting, but worsening hypercalcemia is commonly observed because of the inability to normally suppress PTH release as calcium retention occurs.

Hyperuricosuria-Induced Calcium Stone Disease

Uric acid excretion rates are characteristically higher in men with calcium stone disease than in normal subjects. Increased uric acid production (due to a high intake of purine-rich foods that contain meat rather than grain) appears to be the cause of the hyperuricosuria in most patients [8]. The sulfur-containing amino acids in this diet also impose an acid load, which leads to a reduction in the urine pH below 5.3. As a result there is an increase in the urinary concentration of undissociated uric acid (which is relatively insoluble), thereby favoring the formation of uric acid crystals (see Chap. 48).

These crystals can provide an initial surface on which calcium oxalate can deposit. This process occurs because uric acid and calcium oxalate monohydrate have identical patterns of surface charge spacing, so that one crystal type tends to grow on the surface of the other. As a result, calcium oxalate precipitates out of solution at substantially lower urinary concentrations in the presence of uric acid crystals when compared to normal urine.

The diagnosis of hyperuricosuric calcium oxalate stone formation is made by demonstrating an elevated 24-hour urinary uric acid excretion (Table 54-1) with or without associated hypercalciuria [2,8]. This disorder occurs most frequently in middle-aged men.

Treatment

The frequency of calcium oxalate stones can be reduced by decreasing urinary uric acid excretion or by elevating the urine pH (Table 54-2). Hyperuricosuria can usually be reduced by limiting the quantity of purine-containing foods in the diet [8]. Allopurinol (300 mg/day), which diminishes uric acid synthesis, has been shown to be effective when dietary alterations have failed [2,6]. In one study of 60 recurrent hyperuricosuric calcium stone formers, for example, the incidence of new stone formation was reduced by 63 percent in the placebo group versus 81 percent with allopurinol [6].

Raising the urinary pH to above 6.0 with 60 to 80 meq of potassium citrate per day also can reduce the frequency of stone formation in this disorder [25]. Both conversion of uric acid to the more soluble urate salt and increased urinary excretion of citrate may contribute to this beneficial effect.

Reduced Urinary Crystallization Inhibitors

The urine of normal individuals contains compounds that inhibit the formation of calcium oxalate crystals. In some patients, an abnormality in or lack of these substances appears to increase the tendency toward stone formation. Nephrocalcin, for example, is a glycoprotein inhibitor of calcium oxalate crystal growth that is present in normal urine. It appears to act by adhering to the crystal surface. In recurrent stone formers, however, nephrocalcin structure may be abnormal, a change that might contribute to the disease process [26].

It is more likely that diminished citrate excretion is generally of greater importance [3]. As a group, subjects who form calcium oxalate stones excrete less citrate than normals [3]. In those patients who are hypocitraturic, increasing citrate excretion with potassium citrate (60–80 meq/day) may reduce the frequency of new stone formation [27]. A concurrent fall in urinary calcium, induced by the rise in extracellular pH, also may contribute to this beneficial response [22].

Hyperoxaluria

Increased excretion of oxalate as a cause of calcium oxalate stones occurs in two primary settings, enteric and primary hyperoxaluria.

Enteric Hyperoxaluria

Normal subjects absorb only about 10 percent of dietary oxalate, in part because of the formation of insoluble calcium oxalate salts within the intestinal lumen. This limitation is minimized, however, when the intestinal absorption of fatty acids and bile salts is impaired because of small-bowel injury (as in inflammatory bowel disease), surgical removal, or surgical bypass (as treatment for morbid obesity). These substances can bind to calcium, thereby raising the quantity of free oxalate available for absorption [28]. Perhaps more important, however, exposure of the colon to nonabsorbed bile salts can promote oxalate absorption by increasing intestinal permeability to small molecules [29]. Diarrhea-induced fluid losses may also contribute to stone formation in this setting by lowering the urine output (via volume depletion) and by causing metabolic acidosis, which will lower citrate excretion [20].

A low-fat, low-oxalate diet can reduce the quantity of undigested fatty acids and free oxalate in the colon, thereby reducing oxalate absorption and subsequent excretion. These diets, however, are frequently inadequate nutritionally, since patients with the shortest small bowels are those who tend to have the most severe hyperoxaluria. Consequently, dietary restriction is often unfeasible. Cholestyramine, which binds bile acids and oxalate, may also be effective, but side effects frequently limit its use.

At the least, therapy should consist of treatment of the cause of malabsorption (if possible), maintenance of a high fluid intake, and correction of metabolic acidosis, if present, by potassium citrate. The addition of oral calcium carbonate (1–4 gm/day) also may be beneficial by binding oxalate in the intestinal lumen. Although some of the calcium is absorbed, urinary oxalate excretion falls more than the rise in calcium excretion.

Primary Hyperoxaluria

There are two genetic disorders causing hyperoxaluria-induced stone disease. Both are rare and are characterized by extreme elevations of urinary oxalate excretion (up to 150–300 mg/day) due to enzymatic abnormalities in oxalate metabolism. In addition to nephrolithiasis, renal failure frequently develops in childhood due to massive intrarenal calcium oxalate deposition. Not surprisingly, this disorder (if untreated) recurs in the renal transplant and almost universally leads to loss of the graft [30]. There is, however, evidence that combination therapy can at least partially control this disorder. This includes a high fluid intake, the administration of neutral phosphate and magnesium (both pyrophosphate and magnesium are inhibitors of calcium oxalate precipitation), and the use of pyridoxine that, in some cases, promotes the conversion of glyoxalate to glycine rather than oxalate [30,31]. Potassium citrate can also be added if citrate excretion is reduced.

Idiopathic Calcium Stones

In some recurrent calcium stone formers, no abnormality in calcium, uric acid, citrate, or oxalate excretion can be identified. Optimal therapy in this setting is uncertain. At the least, maintenance of fluid intake above 2 liters/day and, for the reasons described before, avoidance of excess dietary protein should be encouraged in all patients. Medical treatment as outlined in Table 54-2 can be tried if the excretion rate of one of the reactants appears to be in the high-normal range, although the efficacy of such a regimen is unproved. In some patients, for example, calcium excretion is higher and citrate excretion is lower than the mean for normals, even though neither level alone would be considered abnormal [3]. It is possible, therefore, that combination therapy with a thiazide and potassium citrate might be beneficial in this setting. As an alternative, neutral phosphate can be given if no treatable metabolic abnormality is apparent.

References

1. Johnson, CM, Wilson, DM, O'Fallon, WM, et al. Renal stone epidemiology: A 25-year study in Rochester, Minnesota. *Kidney Int* 16:624, 1979.
2. Coe, FL, Parks, JH. Pathophysiology of kidney stones and strategies for treatment. *Hosp Pract* 23(3):145, 1988.
3. Parks, JH, Coe, FL. A urinary calcium-citrate index for the evaluation of nephrolithiasis. *Kidney Int* 30:85, 1986.
4. Coe, FL, Keck, J, Norton, E. The natural history of untreated calcium urolithiasis. *J Am Med Assoc* 238:1519, 1977.

5. Strauss, AL, Coe, FL, Parks, JH. Formation of a single calcium stone of renal origin. *Arch Intern Med* 142:504, 1982.

6. Ettinger, B, Tang, A, Citron, JT, Livermore, B, William, T. Randomized trial of allopurinol in the prevention of calcium oxalate calculi. *N Engl J Med* 315:1386, 1986.

7. Churchill, DN, Taylor, DW. Thiazides for patients with recurrent calcium stones: Still an open question. *J Urol* 133:749, 1985.

8. Coe, FL, Kavalach, AG. Hypercalciuria and hyperuricosuria in patients with calcium nephrolithiasis. *N Engl J Med* 291:1344, 1974.

9. Coe, FL, Parks, HJ, Moore, ES. Familial idiopathic hypercalciuria. *N Engl J Med* 300:337, 1979.

10. Broadus, AE, Insogna, KL, Lang, R, et al. A consideration of the hormonal basis and phosphate leak hypothesis of absorptive hypercalciuria. *J Clin Endocrinol Metab* 58:161, 1984.

11. Broadus, AE, Insogna, KC, Lang, R, Ellison, AF, Dreyer, BE. Evidence for disordered control of 1,25-dihydroxyvitamin D production in absorptive hypercalciuria. *N Engl J Med* 311:73, 1984.

12. Olmer, M, Berland, Y, Argemi, B. Absence of secondary hyperparathyroidism in most patients with renal hypercalciuria. *Kidney Int* 24 (suppl 16):S-175, 1983.

13. Kurokawa, K. Calcium-regulating hormones and the kidney. *Kidney Int* 32:760, 1987.

14. Adams, ND, Gray, RW, Lemann, J, Jr. Cheung, HS. Effects of calcitriol administration on calcium metabolism in healthy men. *Kidney Int* 21:90, 1982.

15. Robertson, WG, Peacock, M. The cause of idiopathic calcium stone disease: Hypercalciuria or hyperoxaluria. *Nephron* 26:105, 1980.

16. Lau, K, Wolf, C, Nussbaum, P, et al. Differing effects of acid versus neutral phosphate therapy of hypercalciuria. *Kidney Int* 16:736, 1979.

17. Muldowney, FP, Freaney, R, Moloney, MF. Importance of dietary sodium in the hypercalciuric syndrome. *Kidney Int* 22:292, 1982.

18. Yendt, ER, Gagne, RJA. Detection of primary hyperparathyroidism, with special reference to its occurrence in hypercalciuric females with normal or borderline serum calcium. *Can Med Assoc J* 98:331, 1968.

19. Costanzo, LS. Localization of diuretic action in microperfused rat distal tubules: Ca and Na transport. *Am J Physiol* 248:F527, 1985.

19a. Ettinger, B, Citrov, JT, Livermore, B, Dolman, LI. Chlorthalidone reduces calcium oxalate calculus recurrence but magnesium hydroxide does not. *J Urol* 139:679, 1988.

20. Simpson, DP. Citrate excretion: A window on renal metabolism. *Am J Physiol* 244:F223, 1983.

21. Pak, CYC, Peterson, R, Sakhaee, K, Fuller, C, Preminger, G, Reisch, J. Correction of hypocitraturia and prevention of stone formation by combined thiazide and potassium citrate therapy in thiazide-unresponsive hypercalciuric nephrolithiasis. *Am J Med* 79:284:1985.

22. Sakhaee, K, Nicar, M, Hill, K, Pak, CYC. Contrasting effects of potassium citrate and sodium citrate therapies on urinary chemistries and crystallization of stone-forming salts. *Kidney Int* 24:348, 1983.

23. Holick, MF. Vitamin D and the kidney. *Kidney Int* 32:912, 1987.

24. Broadus, AE, Horst, RL, Lang, R, Littledike, ET, Rasmussen, H. The importance of circulating 1,25-dihydroxyvitamin D in the pathogenesis of hypercalciuria and renal stone formation in primary hyperparathyroidism. *N Engl J Med* 302:421, 1980.

25. Pak, CYC, Peterson, R. Successful treatment of hyperuricosuric calcium oxalate nephrolithiasis with potassium citrate. *Arch Intern Med* 146:863, 1986.

26. Nakagawa, Y, Ahmed, M, Hall, SL, Deganello, S, Coe, FL. Isolation from human calcium oxalate renal stones of nephrocalcin, a glycoprotein inhibitor of calcium oxalate crystal growth. Evidence that nephrocalcin from patients with calcium oxalate nephrolithiasis is deficient in γ-carboxyglutamic acid. *J Clin Invest* 79:1782, 1987.

27. Pak, CYC, Fuller, C. Idiopathic hypocitraturic calcium-oxalate nephrolithiasis successfully treated with potassium citrate. *Ann Intern Med* 104:33, 1986.

28. Chadwick, VS, Modha, K, Dowling, RH. Mechanism for hyperoxaluria in patients with ileal dysfunction. *N Engl J Med* 289:172, 1973.

29. Kathpalia, SC, Favus, MJ, Coe, FL. Evidence for size and charge permselectivity of rat ascending colon. Effects of ricinoleate and bile salts on oxalic acid and neutral sugar transport. *J Clin Invest* 74:805, 1984.
30. Scheinman, JI, Najarian, JS, Mauer, SM. Successful strategies for renal transplantation in primary oxalosis. *Kidney Int* 25:804, 1984.
31. Yendt, ER, Cohanim, M. Response to a physiologic dose of pyridoxine in type I primary hyperoxaluria. *N Engl J Med* 312:953, 1985.

55. URINARY TRACT OBSTRUCTION

Urinary tract obstruction (UTO) is a relatively common cause of renal disease that may be associated with pain, bleeding, infection, and renal insufficiency. These signs and symptoms can usually be improved by relief of the obstruction. It is therefore essential to recognize those clinical settings in which this potentially reversible disorder is likely to be present.

Etiology and Pathogenesis

Obstruction to urine flow can occur at any site within the urinary tract (Table 55-1). The frequency of these disorders is dependent, in part, on the age and sex of the patient. Most cases in children are due to anatomic abnormalities, such as urethral valves or stricture, meatal stenosis, or stenosis at the ureterovesical or ureteropelvic junction. In contrast, obstructing calculi are most common in young adults, whereas prostatic hypertrophy or carcinoma, retroperitoneal or pelvic neoplasms, and calculi are the major causes in older patients.

In terms of renal function, the major event is an *increase in pressure proximal to the obstruction,* due to continued glomerular filtration [1]. This initially leads to dilatation of the proximal ureter (hydroureter) and the renal pelvis (hydronephrosis). These anatomic changes are important clinically because they can be detected noninvasively by ultrasonography or CT scanning (see the following).

The elevation in pressure is also transmitted back to the proximal tubule. If the obstruction is complete, the increase in intratubular pressure eventually counteracts the gradient favoring fluid movement across the glomerulus and glomerular filtration ceases. With partial obstruction, however, the rise in tubular pressure may lower but will not abolish filtration.

These changes are also associated with secondary arteriolar vasoconstriction, leading to a fall in renal blood flow, a reduction in glomerular capillary pressure, and a further decline in the glomerular filtration rate [1,2]. This alteration is mediated in part by angiotensin II and perhaps thromboxanes [1,3], appearing to be regulated locally by the individual obstructed nephrons [2]. If, for example, single nephrons are obstructed in experimental animals, glomerular hemodynamics remain normal in adjacent nonobstructed nephrons. Thus, the local rise in arteriolar resistance can be seen as an appropriate response since it shifts perfusion away from obstructed, nonfunctioning nephrons.

These experimental results may be applicable to humans. The initially elevated intrapelvic pressure seen with complete obstruction slowly returns to or near normal within 4 weeks, a change that could reflect in part the hemodynamically mediated cessation of glomerular filtration [4]. Despite the fall in intrapelvic pressure, however, hydronephrosis persists, presumably due to increased compliance induced by chronic distention.

The degree of impairment in renal function depends on whether the obstruction is bilateral or unilateral, and on its severity. With unilateral obstruction, for example, there is at most a 50 percent reduction in the glomerular filtration rate. In fact, the change is generally less marked because of compensatory hyperfiltration in the contralateral kidney. In comparison, bilateral disease is associated with a variable decline in glomerular filtration rates, the severity of which is related to the degree of obstruction.

Table 55-1. Major causes of urinary tract obstruction

Level of obstruction	Disease process
Renal pelvis	Calculus
	Sloughed papilla
	Stricture or aberrant vessel at ureteropelvic junction
Ureter	Prostate or bladder carcinoma
	Pelvic carcinoma
	Calculus
	Retroperitoneal lymphoma, carcinoma, or fibrosis
	Accidental surgical ligation
	Edema at ureterovesical junction after retrograde catheterization
	Pregnancy
	Blood clot
	Stricture
Urethra or bladder neck	Benign prostatic hypertrophy
	Carcinoma of the prostate or bladder
	Urethral valves, stricture, or meatal stenosis
	Neurogenic bladder

Tubular function is initially normal with obstruction. As a result, the low rate of urine flow may lead to more efficient sodium reabsorption, with the urinary sodium concentration being below 20 meq/L in acute bilateral obstruction, similar to that in prerenal disease [5]. With time, however, the handling (particularly in the distal nephron) of sodium, potassium, hydrogen, and water becomes impaired, presumably due to persistent exposure to the high intratubular pressure or to ischemia resulting from arteriolar vasoconstriction. Potential clinical manifestations include renal salt wasting, hyperkalemia, renal tubular acidosis (see Chap. 8), and nocturia or polyuria due to the defect in concentrating ability. Thus, partial obstruction may paradoxically be associated with a *rise in urine output.* Oliguria or anuria is not seen unless there is severe bilateral obstruction or chronic partial obstruction has led to end-stage renal disease.

Clinical Presentation

The signs and symptoms produced by UTO are dependent on the site and cause of the obstruction and the rapidity with which it has developed. Pain, usually due to distention of the bladder, collecting system, or renal capsule, is one of the most common presenting signs. However, the degree of discomfort is usually more closely related to the *rate* of distention than to the degree of dilatation. As a result, the pain with acute obstruction (as occurs with renal calculi) is frequently characterized as "excruciating"; in comparison, chronic, partial obstruction (from a retroperitoneal malignancy, for example) may produce no symptoms or only vague abdominal, back, or flank discomfort that may be exacerbated by the increase in urine output following a fluid load.

When pain is present, its location is determined by the *site* of obstruction. Upper ureteral or renal pelvic lesions typically lead to flank pain and tenderness, whereas lower ureteral obstruction causes pain that may radiate to the ipsilateral testicle or labia. A paralytic ileus also may occur, which can in some cases obscure the correct diagnosis.

The physical examination may either be normal or reveal flank tenderness in patients with upper tract obstruction. In comparison, a distended, palpable, and possibly painful bladder is the most common abnormality with bladder neck obstruction. A careful rectal and, in women, pelvic examination should always be performed, since it may disclose a local malignancy or prostatic enlargement.

Routine laboratory findings are generally nondiagnostic. The urinalysis is frequently normal, but hematuria may be observed, particularly with stone disease [6]. Although cystine crystals are diagnostic of cystinuria, other crystals (such as calcium oxalate) may be found normally and are not indicative of stone formation. The urine tends to be isosmotic to plasma, and the urinary sodium concentration exceeds 20 meq/L in patients with prolonged obstruction and chronic renal insufficiency, findings that are typical of any chronic renal disease [5,7].

Complications
Urinary tract obstruction also may be associated with a variety of complications, including infection, hypertension, stone formation, papillary necrosis, and volume depletion.

URINARY TRACT INFECTION.   Urinary stasis behind the obstruction may lead to the development of infection. This is particularly likely with bladder neck obstruction, since this impairs bladder washout, which is the primary natural defense against infection [8]. Infection is less common with upper tract disease (as with a ureteral stone) since there is usually only stasis of sterile urine.

Although urinary tract infections are relatively common (particularly cystitis in females), there are certain findings that suggest the possible presence of an underlying urinary tract abnormality, such as obstruction [9]. These include infection in men or young children of either sex, recurrent or persistent infection in women, and infection with an unusual organism, such as *Pseudomonas*. Eradication of the infection in these settings often requires correction of the anatomic abnormality, such as transurethral resection of the prostate.

HYPERTENSION.   Hypertension in a previously normotensive individual is sometimes observed in UTO and may occur by several mechanisms. Activation of the renin-angiotensin system is usually involved in acute unilateral obstruction, where the elevation in blood pressure is generally reversible [10]. In contrast, volume expansion due to sodium and water retention is usually responsible with bilateral obstruction (or obstruction of a solitary kidney) [11]. The hypertension may persist in this setting if there has been permanent renal damage.

CALCULI AND PAPILLARY NECROSIS.   Stone formation and papillary necrosis may result from, as well as cause, UTO. Calculi are most likely to be observed in patients who become infected with a urease-producing organism, such as *Proteus mirabilis*. The ammonia generated by this process alkalinizes the urine, thereby favoring the formation of magnesium-ammonium-phosphate (struvite) stones. These calculi can expand to fill the entire renal pelvis, forming a "staghorn" calculus that can eventually lead to loss of the kidney, if untreated [12].

Severe obstruction can also cause papillary necrosis. Ischemia may be an important determinant of this problem, as the obstruction-induced rise in hydrostatic pressure in the renal pelvis and medullary interstitium may lead to partial occlusion of the vasa recta capillaries in the renal medulla [13].

VOLUME DEPLETION.   As described before, chronic partial obstruction can produce tubular damage, resulting in impaired sodium and water reabsorption. These defects can lead to nocturia or polyuria but fluid balance is usually well maintained as long as the patient is ingesting a regular diet. However, volume depletion or hypernatremia can occur if intake is reduced because of pain or an intercurrent illness [14].

Diagnosis
Urinary tract obstruction should be suspected if any of the symptoms and signs outlined previously are present. The physician should then inquire about a history or symptoms suggestive of a possible underlying disease such as prostatic enlargement; malignancy; previous abdominal, pelvic, or genitourinary surgery; renal calculi; one of the disorders associated with papillary necrosis (including diabetes mellitus, sickle cell disease, and analgesic abuse nephropathy); or migraine headaches treated with methysergide, a drug that can cause retroperitoneal fibrosis when given for a prolonged period.

It is also important to exclude the presence of obstruction in any patient presenting with otherwise unexplained acute or chronic renal insufficiency, particularly if there is a history of malignancy. The urinary findings are generally nondiagnostic with one exception. Although the urine volume may be reduced in any form of renal disease, *anuria* (output < 50 ml/day) is an unusual finding. Complete bilateral obstruction and shock are the two major causes of this problem, while the hemolytic-uremic syndromes, rapidly progressive glomerulonephritis, and bilateral major vascular occlusion are less commonly responsible. It is important to remember, however, that a *normal or high urine output does not exclude partial obstruction,* since tubular dysfunction can lead to impaired sodium and water reabsorption.

Sequential Evaluation
Bladder catheterization can be performed at the bedside if there is any reason to suspect that bladder neck obstruction may be present. If, for example, prostatic obstruction or a neurogenic bladder is the primary problem, catheterization will lead to a brisk diuresis. Relief of the obstruction may also lead to a reduction in the plasma creatinine concentration in patients who have developed renal failure (see the following).

The rate at which the enlarged bladder should be decompressed has been a source of misunderstanding. Two complications can be induced by the sudden drop in pressure within the bladder: *gross hematuria* (due to sudden expansion of attenuated, compressed bladder-wall veins) and rarely reflex *hypotension.* As a result, it has been suggested that the catheter should be clamped after the initial 500 ml has been removed and the bladder then allowed to drain slowly over many hours. However, the pressure within a tense bladder is extremely sensitive to very small reductions in volume, beginning to fall after the removal of only 5 to 15 ml of urine, and decreasing by about 50 percent after the removal of 100 ml [15]. Consequently, partial or intermittent clamping is not likely to avoid the potential complications of rapid drainage.

Radiographic evaluation to exclude obstruction at the level of the ureters or above is required if bladder catheterization does not induce a diuresis. Most radiographic procedures rely on their ability to detect dilatation of the collecting system (hydronephrosis). It is important to remember, therefore, that *obstruction can occur without dilatation* in three situations:

1. Within 1 to 3 days of obstruction, before the collecting system has had time to dilate
2. When the collecting system is encased by retroperitoneal tumor or fibrosis [16,17]
3. When obstruction is mild, usually causing no impairment in renal function

The radiographic procedure of choice is *renal ultrasonography,* since it is noninvasive and avoids the potentially nephrotoxic and allergic complications of radiocontrast media. In the majority of patients, ultrasound can exclude UTO, diagnose obstruction and its cause, or demonstrate another potential etiology of renal failure (such as polycystic kidney disease). CT scanning should be performed if there is inadequate visualization, if the ultrasound results are equivocal, or if the cause of obstruction cannot be identified.

The combination of a plain film of the abdomen (to detect calculi), ultrasonography, and CT scanning (if needed) will be adequate for diagnostic purposes in over 90 percent of cases [18]. An intravenous pyelogram is necessary only in patients with multiple renal or parapelvic cysts or staghorn calculi (since hydronephrosis may not be detectable by the other modalities in this setting) or when CT scanning cannot identify the level of obstruction.

Rarely, the history is so suggestive (as with unexplained acute renal failure in a patient with known pelvic malignancy) that retrograde or antegrade pyelography is performed to exclude obstruction, even though the other tests are negative [19]. More commonly, these procedures are used to relieve, rather than to diagnose, obstruction.

Treatment
The necessity for and type of therapy required may be quite variable. For example, congenital strictures of the ureteropelvic junction are often asymptomatic unless fluid intake is markedly increased. As a result, surgical correction may not be necessary if renal function is well maintained and there is no evidence of renal parenchymal loss on ultrasonography [20]. Even in symptomatic patients, therapy may be delayed for a period of weeks if it is felt that spontaneous correction may occur and there is neither infection behind the obstruction nor uncontrollable pain. This situation is most commonly seen in patients with a unilateral ureteral calculus. As a general guideline, calculi larger than 10 mm in diameter will not pass spontaneously, those 5 to 10 mm may pass, and

those smaller than 5 mm will usually be excreted [21]. Basket extraction, shock-wave lithotripsy [22], or surgical removal can be used if some intervention is required.

A discussion of the therapeutic alternatives for all of the causes of UTO is beyond the scope of this chapter [20,21]. Nevertheless, some general recommendations can be made for those disorders associated with renal failure, particularly tumors or fibrosis obstructing the ureters or ureterovesical junction.

1. The obstruction can initially be relieved by insertion of a catheter via cystoscopy or antegrade nephrostomy [23,24]. In some cases of ureteral obstruction, a ureteral stent can be left in place; this catheter bypasses the obstruction and drains internally into the bladder. This is usually a temporizing measure, since prolonged use of the stent catheter often leads to infection or occlusion. The stent may, however, be left in place in patients with advanced and refractory disease.

2. An important issue in patients with obstruction due to a malignancy is whether one or both kidneys should be decompressed. The aim of therapy in this setting is to regain the maximum amount of renal function at the minimum risk to the patient. Treatment limited to the less affected side is frequently sufficient to restore adequate renal function, particularly if there is evidence that there will be little functional recovery on the contralateral side (as suggested, for example, by marked parenchymal thinning on ultrasonography).

3. Definitive therapeutic modalities for relief of the obstruction include reinsertion of the ureters into a different area of the bladder, if the disease is limited to the area around the ureteral orifice; creation of a urinary diversion, such as a ureteroileostomy or a Kock ileal pouch (which has a continent nipple valve at the abdominal stoma) [25,26] for severe retroperitoneal or bladder involvement; and freeing the obstructed ureters and moving them into the peritoneum in retroperitoneal fibrosis [27]. Consideration of any urinary diversion procedure should be delayed for at least 2 weeks after relief of the obstruction to ascertain that there is adequate remaining renal function, as evidenced by a fall in the plasma creatinine concentration.

4. Urinary diversion is usually not required for a neurogenic bladder, since clean, intermittent self-catheterization several times a day is effective in most patients [28].

Postobstructive Diuresis

Relief of bilateral urinary tract obstruction is characteristically followed by a brisk diuresis, initially due to urine that has been trapped in the dilated collecting system and, if obstructed, the bladder. The high urine flow may then persist for several days. At least three mechanisms appear to contribute to this *postobstructive diuresis* [29]:

1. Fluid retained during the period of obstruction leads to volume expansion. This can promote sodium excretion when the obstruction is relieved by diminishing the excretion of aldosterone and perhaps increasing that of atrial natriuretic peptide. Other nonspecific natriuretic substances also may be retained and can contribute to the ensuing diuresis [1].

2. Urea that accumulates during the period of obstruction acts as an osmotic diuretic once glomerular filtration is reestablished.

3. Resistance to the action of antidiuretic hormone limits renal concentrating ability, leading to impaired water reabsorption.

In the great majority of cases, volume expansion is the primary driving force for the increase in urine output [30]. Therefore, the diuresis and natriuresis are *appropriate* for the patient's volume status and cease spontaneously when euvolemia is restored. As a result, only *maintenance fluids* are typically required during the postobstructive diuresis; attempting to replace the urine output quantitatively leads to persistent hypervolemia and an output that can exceed 10 liters/day.

In about 5 percent of cases or less, the postobstructive diuresis becomes *inappropriate* [30]. Since it is not possible to identify these patients in advance, all patients should be carefully monitored during the diuretic phase for signs of volume depletion. This problem is usually transient but can persist for weeks or months, presumably due to severe tubular damage.

The usual absence of excessive fluid loss does not mean that tubular function has returned to normal. It is likely that some defect in sodium and water reabsorption persists but is counterbalanced by a persistent moderate decline in the glomerular filtration rate. If, however, the filtration rate rapidly returns to normal, the impairment in tubular function can be unmasked; in this setting, an inappropriate diuresis can occur, even in patients with unilateral obstruction [31].

Prognosis
The return of renal function after bilateral UTO or obstruction in a solitary kidney is variable and is dependent both on the duration and the severity of obstruction. The inconsistent recovery pattern is also affected by the possible presence of preexisting renal disease, infection, nephrolithiasis, hypertension, or papillary necrosis. As a result, there is no predictable relationship in humans between the duration of obstruction and the degree of recovery of renal function. As a rule, complete recovery occurs with uncomplicated acute obstruction (lasting 1–2 weeks). However, irreversible renal damage is seen with prolonged complete or severe partial obstruction, leading to a progressive decline in the degree of recoverable renal function [21,32]. For example, little or no improvement appears to occur after more than 12 weeks of complete obstruction [32].

Radionuclide scanning and ultrasonography have been used in an attempt to predict functional recovery. However, these tests have not been found to be very useful; substantial return of renal function has been described even in patients with total nonvisualization on scanning or marked cortical thinning by ultrasonography, signs that had been thought to be indicative of severe and usually irreversible disease [31,33].

Patients in whom recovery to apparently normal renal function occurs may still have residual renal damage. In a rat model in which unilateral obstruction was induced for only 24 hours, up to 15 percent of nephrons were nonfunctional as late as 60 days after release, a change that was presumed to represent irreversible injury [34]. This was obscured, however, by return of the glomerular filtration rate to normal due to hyperfiltration in the remaining functioning nephrons. If these changes also occur in humans, then there is a potential long-term risk of hemodynamically mediated injury in the remaining nephrons (see Chap. 56). Thus, periodic monitoring of the plasma creatinine concentration is probably prudent.

References

1. Klahr, S. Pathophysiology of obstructive nephropathy. *Kidney Int* 23:414, 1983.
2. Tanner, GA. Effects of kidney tubule obstruction on glomerular filtration in rats. *Am J Physiol* 237:F379, 1979.
3. Klotman, PE, Smith, SR, Volpp, BD, et al. Thromboxane inhibition improves function of hydronephrotic rat kidneys. *Am J Physiol* 250:F282, 1986.
4. Michaelson, G. Percutaneous puncture of the renal pelvis, intrapelvic pressure and the concentrating capacity of the kidney in hydronephrosis. *Acta Med Scand* 559:1, 1974.
5. Hoffman, LM, Suki, WN. Obstructive uropathy mimicking volume depletion. *J Am Med Assoc* 236:2096, 1976.
6. Burkholder, BV, Dotin, LN, Thomason, WB, Beach, OD. Unexplained hematuria: How extensive should the evaluation be? *J Am Med Assoc* 210:1729, 1969.
7. Berlyne, GM. Distal tubular function in chronic hydronephrosis. *Q J Med* 30:339, 1961.
8. Lapides, J. Mechanisms of urinary tract infection. *Urology* 14:217, 1979.
9. Komaroff, AL. Urinalysis and urine culture in women with dysuria. *Ann Intern Med* 104:212, 1986.
10. Weidmann, P, Beretta-Picoli, C, Hirsh, D, Reubi, FC, Massry, SG. Curable hypertension with unilateral hydronephrosis. *Ann Intern Med* 87:437, 1977.
11. Palmer, JM, Zweiman, FG, Assaykeen, TA. Renal hypertension due to hydronephrosis with normal plasma renin activity. *N Engl J Med* 283:1032, 1970.
12. Drach, GW. Urinary lithiasis. In PC Walsh, RF Gittes, AD Perlmutter, TA Stamey (Eds.), *Campell's Urology* (5th ed). Philadelphia: Saunders, 1986.
13. Solez, K, Ponchak, S, Buono, RA, Vernon, N, Finer, PM, Miller, M, Heptinstall, RH.

Inner medullary plasma flow in the kidney with ureteral obstruction. *Am J Physiol* 231:1315, 1976.

14. Landsberg, L. Hypernatremia complicating partial urinary-tract obstruction. *N Engl J Med* 283:746, 1970.

15. Osius, TG, Hynman, F, Jr. Dynamics of acute urinary retention: A manometric, radiographic and clinical study. *J Urol* 90:702, 1963.

16. Rascoff, JH, Golden, RA, Spinowitz, BS, Charytan, C. Nondilated obstructive nephropathy. *Arch Intern Med* 143:696, 1983.

17. Laville, M, Maillet, PJ, Pelle-Francey, D, Finaz de Villaire, J, Traeger, J, Pinet, A. Non-dilated obstructive acute renal failure (abstract). *Kidney Int* 28:694, 1985.

18. Webb, JAW, Reznek, RH, White, SE, Cattell, WR, Fry, IK, Baker, LRI. Can ultrasound and computed tomography replace high-dose urography in patients with impaired renal function. *Q J Med* 53:411, 1984.

19. Griner, PF, Mayewski, RJ, Mushlin, AI, Greenland, P. Selection and interpretation of diagnostic tests and procedures. *Ann Intern Med* 94:553, 1981.

20. Klahr, S, Buerkert, J, Morrison, A. Urinary tract obstruction. In BM Brenner, FC Rector, Jr (Eds.), *The Kidney* 3d ed. Philadelphia: Saunders, 1986.

21. Turka, LA. Urinary tract obstruction. In BD Rose, *Pathophysiology of Renal Disease* 2d ed. New York: McGraw-Hill, 1987.

22. Riehle, RA, Jr, Fair, WAR, Baughan, ED, Jr. Extracorporeal shock-wave lithotripsy for upper urinary tract calculi. *J Am Med Assoc* 255:2043, 1986.

23. Andriole, GL, Bettman, MA, Garnick, MB, Richie, JP. Indwelling double-J ureteral stent for temporary and permanent urinary drainage: Experience with 87 patients. *J Urol* 131:239, 1984.

24. Reznek, RH, Talner, LB. Percutaneous nephrostomy. *Radiol Clin N Am* 22:393, 1984.

25. Hendren, WH, Radopoulos, D. Complications of ileal loop and colon conduit diversion. *Urol Clin N Am* 10:451, 1983.

26. Skinner, DG, Lieskowsky, G, Boyd, SD. Continuing experience with the continent ileal reservoir (Kock pouch) as an alternative to cutaneous urinary diversion: An update. *J Urol* 137:1140, 1987.

27. Lepor, H, Walsh, PC. Idiopathic retroperitoneal fibrosis. *J Urol* 122:1, 1979.

28. Retik, A. Urinary tract disorders in children: New approaches. *Hosp Pract* 19(8):121, 1984.

29. Sophasan, S, Sorrasuchart, S. Factors inducing post-obstructive diuresis in rats. *Nephron* 38:125, 1984.

30. Bishop, MC. Diuresis and renal functional recovery in chronic retention. *Br J Urol* 57:1, 1985.

31. Green, J, Vardy, Y, Munichor, M, Better, OS. Extreme unilateral hydronephrosis with normal glomerular filtration rate: Physiological studies in a case of obstructive uropathy. *J Urol* 136:361, 1986.

32. Better, OS, Arieff, AI, Massry, SG, Kleeman, CR, Maxwell, MH. Studies on renal function after relief of complete unilateral obstruction of three month's duration in man. *Am J Med* 54:234, 1973.

33. McAfee, JG, Singh, A, O'Callaghan, JP. Nuclear imaging supplementary to urography in obstructive uropathy. *Radiology* 137:487, 1980.

34. Bander, SJ, Buerkert, JE, Martin, D, Klahr, S. Long-term effects of 24-hour unilateral obstruction on renal function in the rat. *Kidney Int* 28:614, 1985.

VIII. CHRONIC RENAL FAILURE

56. CAN WE PREVENT RENAL FAILURE?

Eventual progression to renal failure is common in patients with kidney disease once the plasma creatinine concentration (P_{cr}) exceeds 1.5 to 2.0 mg/dl. This may occur even if the underlying disorder is "cured." An example of this phenomenon is seen in chronic pyelonephritis, which is usually due to the combination of urinary tract infection and vesicoureteral reflux. Once there is enough damage to produce renal insufficiency and proteinuria, surgical or spontaneous correction of the reflux and maintenance of sterile urine with chronic antimicrobial therapy do not prevent the ultimate development of renal failure [1].

These findings suggest that, after a certain point, a reduction in the number of functioning nephrons eventually leads to loss of the more normal remaining nephrons. Recent experimental observations suggest that this sequence may result from compensatory changes in intrarenal hemodynamics, particularly a rise in intraglomerular pressure [2]. If this mechanism is also important in humans, then therapy aimed at lowering the intraglomerular pressure may delay or prevent progressive damage in a variety of renal diseases.

Experimental Models
The concept of hemodynamically mediated glomerular injury has been derived from several rat models of renal disease, including the remnant kidney, diabetic nephropathy, and primary hypertension.

Remnant Kidney
The remnant kidney is produced by the surgical removal of a variable portion (up to 85–90%) of the renal mass. In this setting, the remaining renal tissue (or remnant) is initially normal histologically. Within a few months, however, these animals develop progressive renal failure characterized by proteinuria, hypertension, and glomerulosclerosis *in the absence of any known renal disease* [3]. The rate and severity of this process increases in proportion to the amount of renal tissue removed [4].

The major changes that are known to occur in the remnant are structural and hemodynamic hypertrophy. The hemodynamic compensation is characterized in part by an increase in single nephron glomerular filtration rate (GFR). Dilatation of the afferent and to a lesser degree efferent glomerular arterioles is responsible for the rise in filtration by producing an increase in both glomerular plasma flow and hydrostatic pressure [3]. This elevation in the nephron filtration rate has generally been regarded as "adaptive" in that it maximizes the total GFR in the remnant. In the long term, however, the intraglomerular hypertension could lead to progressive glomerular injury and sclerosis.

Proof of this hypothesis has come from therapies aimed at lowering the intraglomerular pressure toward normal. One such modality is dietary protein restriction, since protein intake can substantially affect the GFR. A high-protein diet (or an infusion of amino acids), for example, can increase the GFR by 15 to 20 ml/min or more in humans [5]; this can be considered an appropriate response in that the rise in filtration promotes the excretion of potentially toxic protein metabolites such as urea. The mechanism by which amino acids enhance the GFR is unclear. Somatostatin, which has no important direct effect on the GFR, can abolish the hyperfiltration induced by protein loading; this finding suggests that release of a vasoactive hormone, such as glucagon, may be involved [5,5a]. Alternatively, a high-protein diet may have a direct intrarenal effect [6].

On the other hand, a low-protein diet tends to lower the GFR, primarily by constriction of the afferent glomerular arteriole, thereby reducing the intraglomerular pressure [7,8]. When administered to the rat with a remnant kidney, dietary protein restriction reverses the intraglomerular hypertension and *prevents progressive glomerulosclerosis and renal failure* [3,8].

Antihypertensive therapy represents a second method by which the intraglomerular pressure can be lowered. The administration of the converting enzyme inhibitor (CEI) enalapril to a rat with a remnant kidney returns both the systemic and intraglomerular pressures toward normal and minimizes the degree of glomerular injury (Fig. 56-1) [8,9].

The efficacy of dietary protein restriction and enalapril can be demonstrated even if therapy is begun relatively late in the course, after some glomerular injury has already occurred [8]. Furthermore, these modalities do not necessarily reduce the GFR in this setting, as the fall in glomerular pressure may be counteracted by an increase in glomerular capillary permeability (due, for example, to reversal of angiotensin II–induced mesangial contraction) [8]. These experimental observations seem to correlate with the findings in humans with renal disease in whom these therapies may not produce an acute decline in the GFR.

It should not be assumed, however, that all antihypertensive agents are equally protective. It is important to remember that glomerular pressure is dependent on three factors: the systemic blood pressure, the resistance across the afferent (or preglomerular) arteriole, and the resistance across the efferent (or postglomerular) arteriole. Angiotensin II appears to preferentially constrict the efferent arteriole. Consequently, administration of a CEI will dilate the efferent arteriole, which will tend to directly reduce the glomerular pressure (Fig. 56-2). In comparison, an antihypertensive drug that dilates the afferent arteriole might not lower the glomerular pressure, since the systemic hypotensive response is counterbalanced by more of the pressure being transmitted to the glomerulus. This hemodynamic response appears to occur with the triad of hydrochlorothiazide-reserpine-hydralazine (Fig. 56-2). As a result, this form of antihypertensive therapy is not as effective in protecting the kidney in at least some models of renal disease [9,10]. The relative efficacy of β-blockers and calcium channel blockers remains to be determined.

These findings in the remnant kidney provide a model to explain progressive renal disease in humans. As the disease process damages some nephrons, the other more normal nephrons undergo hypertrophy that is characterized in part by a rise in single nephron GFR and intraglomerular pressure. The latter can then lead to progressive glomerular injury (perhaps by direct mechanical damage to the glomerular basement membrane) in the initially spared nephrons and ultimately renal failure. This sequence could explain the long-term findings that may occur with chronic pyelonephritis (in which progression appears to be inevitable once proteinuria and renal insufficiency are present) [1] or with poststreptococcal glomerulonephritis. Despite apparently complete recovery from the acute episode, some patients who have had poststreptococcal glomerulonephritis develop renal failure 10 to 30 years later that is characterized (as in the remnant) by proteinuria, hypertension, and glomerulosclerosis (similar to that in Fig. 56-1a) [11]. It is possible that some permanent nephron loss occurred during the initial illness. This was at first masked by compensatory hyperfiltration in the less affected glomeruli; however, the associated rise in intraglomerular pressure eventually produced progressive glomerular damage.

Diabetic Nephropathy
A different initiating mechanism appears to be operative in diabetic nephropathy. In both experimental animals and humans with insulin-dependent diabetes mellitus, renal vasodilation occurs as a *primary* event, prior to any nephron loss. Although it is not known how this occurs, the net effect is a GFR that is frequently 25 to 50 percent above normal [12,13] and that, by direct measurement in the rat, is associated with a rise in intraglomerular pressure [12].

In experimental diabetes, both dietary protein restriction and administration of a CEI can reverse the intraglomerular hypertension and *prevent proteinuria and diabetic glomerulosclerosis* even in the absence of good glycemic control (Fig. 56-3) [14,15]. These results suggest that hemodynamic rather than metabolic factors may be of primary importance in diabetic nephropathy. Applicability of these findings to humans is supported by the observations that those patients who develop diabetic nephropathy are more likely to have a higher initial GFR (above 150 ml/min), a higher initial systemic blood pressure (although still within the normal range), and a history of hypertension in one or both parents [16,17]. Hemodynamic factors also may contribute to diabetic retinopathy, since dietary protein restriction prevents increased thickness of the retinal capillary basement membrane in the diabetic rat [17a].

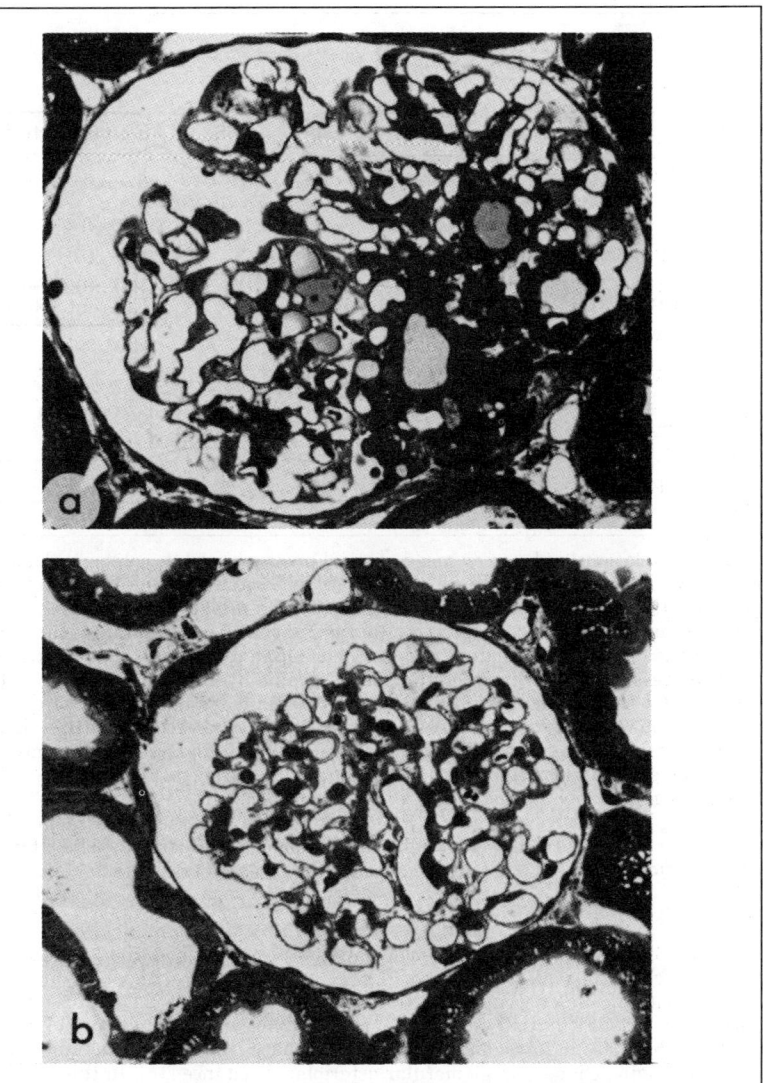

Fig. 56-1. Light microscopy of glomeruli from the remnant kidney of rats 12 weeks after five-sixths nephrectomy. (a) In the control state and after treatment with hydrochlorothiazide-reserpine-hydralazine, approximately 20 to 25 percent of the glomeruli showed areas of capillary collapse and segmental sclerosis as seen in the lower right quadrant. (b) In comparison, almost all of the glomeruli were well preserved in the enalapril-treated rats. (From Anderson, S, Rennke, HG, Brenner, BM. *J Clin Invest* 77:1993, 1986, by copyright permission of the American Society for Clinical Investigation.)

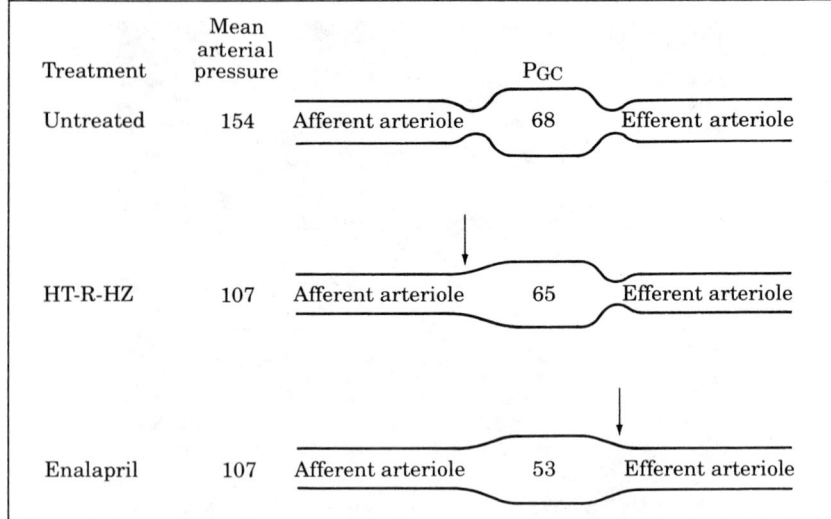

Fig. 56-2. Relationship between mean arterial pressure (middle column), glomerular arteriolar resistance, and glomerular capillary hydrostatic pressure (P_{GC}) in three groups of five-sixths nephrectomized rats. Untreated rats (top column) are hypertensive and have an elevated P_{GC} (normal about 45 mm Hg) that is largely responsible for the compensatory rise in single nephron GFR. Reduction of the mean arterial pressure with hydrochlorothiazide-reserpine-hydralazine (middle panel) is associated with afferent arteriolar dilation, little change in the P_{GC} and no protection against glomerular injury (see Fig. 56-1). In comparison, treatment with enalapril primarily dilates the efferent arteriole, resulting in a fall in P_{GC} and substantial protection against glomerulosclerosis. The afferent arteriole is also partially dilated in this setting, probably due to an autoregulatory response to maintain the GFR by preventing an excessive fall in P_{GC}. (From Anderson, S, Rennke, HG, Brenner, BM. *J Clin Invest* 77:1993, 1986, by copyright permission of the American Society for Clinical Investigation.)

Primary intraglomerular hypertension also may occur early in the course of immune-mediated glomerular diseases. Although the net glomerular permeability is reduced by the immunologic injury (primarily reflecting a decrease in the surface area available for filtration), the GFR initially remains normal. This seemingly appropriate response is mediated by a rise in intraglomerular pressure that is produced by an unknown mechanism involving changes in glomerular arteriolar resistance [18]. In this setting, however, the intraglomerular hypertension could again promote disease progression. It is not surprising, therefore, that both protein restriction and antihypertensive therapy have been shown to ameliorate the degree of glomerular injury in some models of immune-mediated glomerular disease [19,20].

Primary Hypertension
The preceding discussion might suggest that primary hypertension would lead to eventual glomerular damage. It is important to remember, however, that this will occur only if the elevation in pressure is transmitted to the glomeruli. In the spontaneously hypertensive rat (which is thought to resemble essential hypertension in humans), systemic hypertension is associated with renal and afferent arteriolar vasoconstriction in the outer cortex, which contains most of the glomeruli. As a result, in the outer cortical glomeruli, the intraglomerular pressure remains normal [21], there is relatively little glomerulosclerosis [22], and there is no exacerbation of immune-mediated glomerulo-

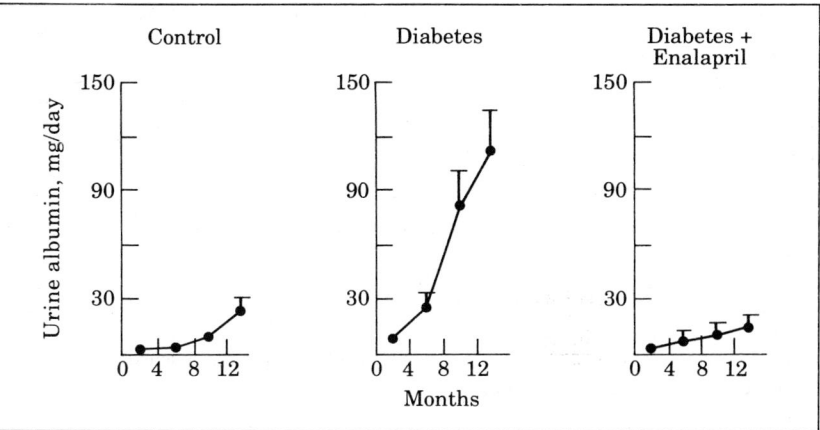

Fig. 56-3. Sequential average daily albumin excretion rates (Ualb. V) in control, untreated diabetic, and enalapril-treated diabetic rats. In contrast to the marked rise in albuminuria with time in the diabetic group, values in the enalapril-treated rats were indistinguishable from control. (From Zatz, R, Dunn, BR, Anderson, S, Rennke, HG, Brenner, BM. *J Clin Invest* 77:1925, 1986, by copyright permission of the American Society for Clinical Investigation.)

nephritis [22a]. Glomerulosclerosis does occur as a late finding in the deep or juxtamedullary glomeruli in which arteriolar resistance and, presumably, intraglomerular pressure, are not as well regulated [22].

These findings may be relevant to patients with essential hypertension, two-thirds of whom have renal vasoconstriction and reduced renal blood flow early in the course of their disease [23]. This could explain why mild-to-moderate hypertension is usually associated with at most only slow progression to renal insufficiency. Furthermore, it could be those patients without early renal vasoconstriction who are at greatest risk of developing glomerular damage.

Hemodynamic Injury in Human Disease

Studies in humans, although necessarily less direct, also support the view that hyperperfused nephrons eventually fail. Table 56-1 lists those disorders in which hemodynamic factors are thought to play an important role. The supporting evidence in chronic pyelonephritis (or reflux nephropathy), poststreptococcal glomerulonephritis, and diabetic nephropathy has been described before and that for the other conditions is presented in the appropriate chapters elsewhere in the book. It is useful, however, to review the renal findings in the human equivalents of the remnant kidney and in aging.

Oligomeganephronia is a rare congenital disease characterized by a marked reduction in nephron number (up to 80%) with compensatory hypertrophy (as exemplified by as much as a fourfold increase in glomerular volume) in those nephrons that are present. Hyperfiltration initially maintains the GFR at an acceptable level but progressive proteinuria, hypertension, and renal failure usually are seen by adolescence [24]. Glomerulosclerosis, similar to that in the rat remnant kidney, is found on histologic examination of the kidney.

The same glomerular changes may be seen with unilateral renal agenesis, a more common disorder that occurs in approximately 1 in every 1000 people [25,26]. The course, however, is less predictable than in oligomeganephronia, presumably because there are more nephrons present and therefore less pronounced intraglomerular hypertension.

The risk of glomerulosclerosis appears to be even less following unilateral nephrectomy [27], a finding that probably reflects a decline in the compensatory response with

Table 56-1. Possible hemodynamically mediated glomerulopathies in humans

Decreased number of functioning nephrons
    Oligomeganephronia
    Unilateral renal agenesis
    Unilateral nephrectomy
"Cured" parenchymal disease causing loss of functioning renal mass
    Poststreptococcal glomerulonephritis
    Chronic pyelonephritis (reflux nephropathy)
    Analgesic abuse nephropathy (with drug cessation)
Primary renal vasodilation
    Diabetes mellitus
    Sickle cell disease
    Obesity
Poorly controlled hypertension (especially with underlying renal disease)
Relative intraglomerular hypertension
    Aging
    Hereditary nephritis

age. This can be appreciated from studies of renal transplant donors. The GFR tends to be unchanged 10 to 15 years after nephrectomy, although there is an increased incidence of proteinuria and hypertension [28,29]. It is possible, however, that more progressive disease will become apparent with longer follow-up.

A decline in renal function is also common with aging. Otherwise healthy adults show a progressive fall in the GFR after the age of 30 to 40; the level in octogenarians is typically about one-half to two-thirds that in young adults [30]. This loss of function is associated with increasing glomerular sclerosis [31] and varies directly with the systemic blood pressure, being most pronounced in hypertensive subjects [32]. These findings suggest that hemodynamic factors may again play an important role. It is possible, for example, that the "normal" glomerular pressures on a typical high-protein American diet are inappropriately high and capable of producing glomerular injury over a period of many years. The observation that glomerulosclerosis also occurs in aging animals and that this change can be diminished by protein restriction [33] are compatible with this hypothesis.

Implications for Therapy
The aforementioned experimental and human studies suggest that reversing intraglomerular hypertension may delay or prevent progressive renal disease. As a result, preliminary (and primarily successful) studies have been conducted evaluating the efficacy of dietary protein restriction and antihypertensive therapy in patients with renal insufficiency of diverse etiologies.

One problem that remains incompletely resolved in these trials has been how to assess changes in the rate of decline in renal function [33a]. Serial measurements of the GFR by inulin or radioisotopic clearance are probably most accurate but are also the most cumbersome to perform. Another widely used method has been to plot the reciprocal of the P_{cr} ($1/P_{cr}$), which should vary directly with the GFR, versus time. (The use and limitations of the P_{cr} are reviewed in Chap. 17.)

In many patients with progressive disease, the GFR declines at a relatively uniform rate. Using serial measurements of $1/P_{cr}$, the slope of the change in the GFR can be calculated both before and after therapy to see if treatment has been of benefit [33a,34]. Figure 56-4 shows sample results from two patients with chronic renal disease who were treated with dietary protein restriction. As can be seen, this form of therapy seemed to prevent further fall in the GFR.

PROTEIN RESTRICTION.   A variety of preliminary studies have suggested a positive effect of protein restriction in up to 75 to 90 percent of cases [34-36]. This occurs in renal

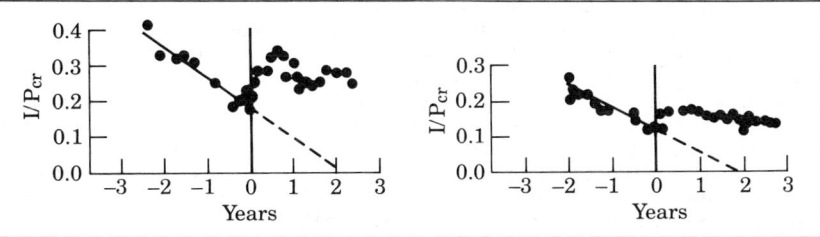

Fig. 56-4. The rate of progression in two patients with chronic renal disease as assessed from the reciprocal of the P_{cr} before and after (vertical bar) the institution of dietary protein restriction. The regression line for pretherapy values is shown as a solid line; the dashed lines represents the expected change if therapy were not successful. Both patients had stabilization of their P_{cr} after limitation of protein intake. (From Mitch, WE, Walser, M, Steinman, TI, Hill, S, Zeger, S, Tungsanga, K. *N Engl J Med* 311:623, 1984. Reprinted by permission from the New England Journal of Medicine.)

diseases of diverse etiology such as chronic glomerulonephritis, chronic pyelonephritis, and polycystic kidney disease. Benefit is less likely if dietary therapy is begun after the P_{cr} is above 8 mg/dl or if the patient has hypertensive nephrosclerosis in which the vascular disease may prevent glomerular hyperfusion [34,35].

These studies, however, cannot be considered to be definitive since they were not prospective, randomized, and double-blinded. Furthermore, use of the reciprocal of the P_{cr} in this setting may be misleading, since lowering dietary protein intake reduces creatinine production and therefore the P_{cr} without change in the GFR; a new steady state may not be achieved for 2 to 3 months [33a]. As a result, a decline in renal function could be masked initially by the diet-induced fall in the P_{cr}. More optimally designed trials are currently being performed that include use of radioisotopic clearances to directly measure the GFR.

Sample daily diets consist of 0.6 gm/kg of high biologic value protein or 20 to 30 gm of protein supplemented with amino acids and their keto analogues. Patient compliance is clearly important if these dietary regimens are to be effective. Assuming that daily intake does not vary widely and that the patient is in a steady state, then nitrogen excretion will be roughly equal to nitrogen intake. The former can be estimated from a 24-hour urine collection [37]:

Urine nitrogen excretion = urine urea nitrogen + nonurea nitrogen

Nonurea nitrogen excretion is roughly constant at about 30 mg/kg of body weight per day. Thus,

Urine nitrogen excretion = urine urea nitrogen + 30 mg/kg

Since each gram of nitrogen is derived from 6.25 gm of protein,

Estimated protein intake = 6.25 (urine urea nitrogen + 30 mg/kg)

If, for example, 24-hour urine urea nitrogen excretion is 7.6 gm in a 70-kg man, then,

Estimated protein intake = 6.25 (7.6 + 2.1) = 60.6 gm

The levels of protein restriction that have been recommended are sufficient to maintain nitrogen balance. However, unsuspected problems may arise with this regimen. For example, limiting dietary protein diminishes the excretion of allopurinol and its active metabolite oxypurinol [38]. Both a fall in the GFR and enhanced tubular reabsorption may contribute to this response, although it is not known how this occurs. The net effect is that the dose of allopurinol should be reduced to minimize toxicity. It is at present unknown if the excretion of other drugs is affected in a similar fashion.

ANTIHYPERTENSIVE THERAPY. Preliminary studies have also been conducted assessing the efficacy of blood pressure reduction. Thus far, these trials have been limited primarily to patients with established diabetic nephropathy and hypertension [39-41]. Both a reduction in the rate of fall in the GFR and a decline in protein excretion have been demonstrated. The issues of CEI versus other forms of antihypertensive therapy and treatment of normotensive patients in an attempt to lower the intraglomerular pressure are currently being addressed. In one preliminary study of patients with renal disease and proteinuria, protein excretion fell by 30 percent with a CEI versus little or no change with other antihypertensive agents [41a]. This finding is compatible with a preferential reduction in intraglomerular pressure with a CEI.

Despite the lack of definitive data at this time, it seems reasonable based on the information presented to consider initiating therapy with a CEI in a patient with slowly progressive renal disease. The aim of treatment should be to reduce the blood pressure to below 130/80 if possible, with serial monitoring of the P_{cr} and the plasma potassium concentration (since a CEI can produce hyperkalemia in patients with renal insufficiency due to a concurrent reduction in the release of aldosterone). Although limiting protein intake may also be beneficial, this modality is more likely to produce problems in patient compliance.

NONSTEROIDAL ANTI-INFLAMMATORY DRUGS. A final form of therapy that may be effective in selected patients is the administration of a nonsteroidal anti-inflammatory drug such as indomethacin or meclofenamate. These agents have been used primarily in patients with the nephrotic syndrome. In many of these patients, there is a 20 to 25 percent decline in the GFR, up to a 75 percent reduction in protein excretion [42-44], a rise in the plasma albumin concentration, and a fall in the plasma cholesterol concentration [43]. These changes could reflect renal vasoconstriction and a fall in intraglomerular pressure produced by the associated decrease in prostaglandin synthesis. It is also possible, if intraglomerular hypertension is ameliorated, that these drugs could slow the rate of progression in those patients who respond [44]. If these findings are confirmed, then renal vasodilation from local prostaglandin synthesis could be a contributing factor to the compensatory glomerular hyperperfusion seen with progressive renal disease.

Alternate Explanations for Progressive Renal Disease

Factors other than intraglomerular hypertension are also likely to contribute to continued tissue injury in chronic renal diseases. These include calcium phosphate deposition, increased local ammonia production, intravascular coagulation, and hyperlipidemia.

The deposition of calcium phosphate in the renal interstitium (due to initial phosphate retention and a subsequent rise in the circulating calcium-phosphate product) may initiate an inflammatory reaction that contributes to tubulointerstitial damage. Increased renal calcium content has been demonstrated in humans relatively early in the course of renal disease, even before the P_{cr} is above 1.5 mg/dl [45]. A potentially deleterious role for these deposits is suggested by the experimental observation that dietary phosphorus restriction is associated with decreased renal calcium deposition and slower disease progression [46]. The applicability of these findings to humans is uncertain, however, since relatively marked phosphorus depletion was induced in these studies [46].

Recent experiments suggest an intriguing role for ammonia in the tubulointerstitial damage that accompanies most forms of chronic renal disease [47]. Nephron loss leads to an increase in a variety of tubular functions, as well as in nephron GFR, in the less affected nephrons. One such adaptive change is a rise in ammonia production in an attempt to excrete the daily acid load. The ensuing local accumulation of ammonia can activate the alternate complement pathway, leading to tubulointerstitial damage and worsening renal function. Lowering the acid load (and therefore the rate of ammonia production) by the administration of sodium bicarbonate minimizes the extent of tubulointerstitial disease and partially preserves renal function in the remnant kidney model [47]. If this finding is confirmed, then alkali therapy might become a standard part of the treatment of chronic renal disease. This is in contrast to the current practice in which the usually mild metabolic acidosis associated with renal insufficiency is frequently not treated.

Endothelial damage, produced either by the primary disease or by secondary intraglomerular hypertension, can activate the coagulation pathways, leading to platelet or fibrin deposition, or both. It is of interest in this regard that antiplatelet agents, such as aspirin and dipyridamole, have been reported to slow the rate of progression in such disparate diseases as membranoproliferative glomerulonephritis and diabetic nephropathy [48,49].

Finally, hyperlipidemia, which can occur in patients with the nephrotic syndrome or diabetes mellitus, also may contribute to secondary glomerular injury [50,51]. For example, studies in a possible rat model of type 2 diabetes have demonstrated that glomerular injury can be minimized by lowering the plasma cholesterol level with different forms of drug therapy [50]. The hyperlipidemia in this setting may produce endothelial injury with a secondary influx of circulating macrophages; this sequence is similar to that seen with the development of atherosclerotic lesions in the larger arteries [51].

Summary
In a variety of slowly progressive renal diseases such as chronic glomerulonephritis, diabetic nephropathy, and polycystic kidney disease, it is at present not possible or, in diabetes mellitus, very difficult to correct the underlying disease. In other conditions such as chronic pyelonephritis, the diagnosis is often not made until there has been substantial renal damage and potentially harmful compensatory hemodynamic mechanisms are already in place. As a result, identification of potentially correctable "secondary" responses offer the greatest hope for delaying or even preventing progression to end-stage renal failure and the requirement for dialysis or transplantation. Trials currently in progress are assessing the effect of reversing intraglomerular hypertension with dietary protein restriction or antihypertensive therapy, preferably beginning with a CEI. Other modalities that may also prove to be effective are use of a nonsteroidal anti-inflammatory drug, limiting net phosphorus intake, alkali therapy to lower ammonia production, the administration of antiplatelet agents, and treatment of associated hyperlipidemia.

References
1. Torres, VE, Velosa, JA, Holley, KE, Kelalis, PP, Stickler, GB, Kurtz, SB. The progression of vesicoureteral reflux. *Ann Intern Med* 92:776, 1980.
2. Brenner, BM. Nephron adaptation to renal injury or ablation. *Am J Physiol* 249:F324, 1985.
3. Hostetter, TH, Olson, JL, Rennke, HG, Venkatachalam, MA, Brenner, BM. Hyperfiltration in remnant nephrons: A potentially adverse response to renal ablation. *Am J Physiol* 241:F85, 1981.
4. Hostetter, TH, Meyer, TW, Rennke, HG, Brenner, BM. Chronic effects of dietary protein in the rat with intact and reduced renal mass. *Kidney Int* 30:509, 1986.
5. Hirschberg, RR, Zipser, RD, Slomowitz, LA, Kopple, ID. Glucagon and prostaglandin are mediators of amino acid-induced rise in renal hemodynamics. *Kidney Int* 33:1147, 1988.
6. Seney, FD, Jr, Persson, AEG, Wright, FS. Modification of tubuloglomerular feedback signal by dietary protein. *Am J Physiol* 252:F83, 1987.
7. Dworkin, LD, Feiner, HD. Glomerular injury in uninephrectomized spontaneously hypertensive rats.A consequence of glomerular capillary hypertension. *J Clin Invest* 77:797, 1986.
8. Meyer, TW, Anderson, SA, Rennke, HG, Brenner, BM. Reversing glomerular hypertension stabilizes established glomerular injury. *Kidney Int* 31:752, 1987.
9. Anderson, S, Rennke, HG, Brenner, BM. Therapeutic advantage of converting enzyme inhibitors in arresting progressive renal disease associated with systemic hypertension in the rat. *J Clin Invest* 77:1993, 1986.
10. Dworkin, LD, Feiner, HD, Randazzo, J. Glomerular hypertension and injury in desoxycorticosterone-salt rats on antihypertensive therapy. *Kidney Int* 31:718, 1987.
11. Baldwin, DS. Chronic glomerulonephritis: Nonimmunologic mechanisms of progressive glomerular damage. *Kidney Int* 21:109, 1982.
12. Hostetter, TH, Troy, JL, Brenner, BM. Glomerular hemodynamics in experimental

diabetes mellitus. *Kidney Int* 19:410, 1981.
13. Mogensen, CE. Diabetes mellitus and the kidney. *Kidney Int* 21:673, 1982.
14. Zatz, R, Meyer, TW, Rennke, HG, Brenner, BM. Predominance of hemodynamic rather than metabolic factors in the pathogenesis of diabetic nephropathy. *Proc Natl Acad Sci (USA)* 82:5963, 1985.
15. Zatz, R, Dunn, BR, Anderson, S, Rennke, HG, Brenner, BM. Prevention of diabetic glomerulopathy by pharmacological amelioration of glomerular capillary hypertension. *J Clin Invest* 77:1925, 1986.
16. Mogensen, CE. Early glomerular hyperfiltration in insulin-dependent diabetics and late nephropathy. *Scand J Clin Lab Invest* 46:201, 1986.
17. Krowlewski, AS, Canessa, M, Warram, JH, et al. Predisposition to hypertension and susceptibility to renal disease in insulin-dependent diabetes mellitus. *N Engl J Med* 318:140, 1988.
17a. Ragalevsky, CA, Sandstrom, DJ, Troy, JL, et al. Prevention of retinal microvascular alterations by dietary protein restriction in long term experimental diabetes mellitus (abstract). *Kidney Int* 31:328, 1987.
18. Kaizu, K, Marsh, D, Zipser, R, Glassock, RJ. Roles of prostaglandins and angiotensin II in experimental glomerulonephritis. *Kidney Int* 28:629, 1985.
19. Neugarten, J, Feiner, HD, Schacht, RG, Baldwin, DS. Amelioration of experimental glomerulonephritis by dietary protein restriction. *Kidney Int* 24:595, 1983.
20. Neugarten, J, Kaminetsky, B, Feiner, H, Schacht, RG, Liu, DT, Baldwin, DS. Nephrotoxic serum nephritis with hypertension: Amelioration by antihypertensive therapy. *Kidney Int* 28:135, 1985.
21. Arendshorst, WJ, Beierwaltes, WH. Renal and nephron hemodynamics in spontaneously hypertensive rats. *Am J Physiol* 236:F246, 1979.
22. Feld, LG, van Liew, JB, Galaske, RG, Boylan, JW. Selectivity of renal injury and progression in the spontaneously hypertensive rat. *Kidney Int* 12:332, 1977.
22a. Stein, HD, Sterzel, RB, Hunt, JD, Pabst, R, Kashgarian, M. No aggravation of the course of experimental glomerulonephritis in spontaneously hypertensive rats. *Am J Pathol* 122:520, 1986.
23. Hollenberg, NK, Borucki, LJ, Adams, DF. The renal vasculature in early essential hypertension. *Medicine* 57:167, 1978.
24. McGraw, M, Poucell, S, Sweet, J, Baumal, R. The significance of focal segmental glomerulosclerosis in oligomeganephronia. *Int J Ped Nephrol* 5:67, 1984.
25. Kiprov, DD, Colvin, RB, McCluskey, RT. Focal and segmental glomerulosclerosis associated with unilateral renal agenesis. *Lab Invest* 46:275, 1982.
26. Gutierrez-Millet, V, Nieto, J, Praga, M, Usera, G, Martinez, MA, Morales, JM. Focal glomerulosclerosis and proteinuria in patients with solitary kidneys. *Arch Intern Med* 146:705, 1986.
27. Zucchelli, P, Cagnoli, L, Lasanova, S, Donini, U, Pasquali, S. Focal glomerulosclerosis in patients with unilateral nephrectomy. *Kidney Int* 24:649, 1983.
28. Watnick, TJ, Jenkins, RR, Rackoff, T, et al. Microalbuminuria and hypertension in long-term renal donors. *Transplantation* 45:59, 1988.
29. Williams, SL, Oler, J, Jorkasky, DK. Long-term renal function in kidney donors: A comparison of donors and their siblings. *Ann Intern Med* 105:1, 1986.
30. Anderson, S, Brenner, BM. Effects of aging on the renal glomerulus. *Am J Med* 80:435, 1986.
31. Kaplan, C, Pasternack, B, Shah, H, Gallo, G. Age-related incidence of sclerotic glomeruli in human kidneys. *Am J Pathol* 80:227, 1975.
32. Lindeman, RD, Tobin, JD, Shock, NW. Association between blood pressure and rate of decline in renal function with age. *Kidney Int* 26:861, 1984.
33. Feldman, DB, McConnell, EE, Knapka, JJ. Growth, kidney disease, and longevity of Syrian hamsters (Mesocricetus auratus) fed varying levels of protein. *Lab Animal Sci* 32:613, 1982.
33a. Mitch, WE. Measuring the rate of progression of renal insufficiency. In WE Mitch (Ed.), *Contemporary Issues in Nephrology. The Progressive Nature of Renal Disease* (Vol. 14). New York: Churchill Livingstone, 1986. Chapter 11.
34. Mitch, WE, Walser, M, Steinman, TI, Hill, S, Zeger, S, Tungsanga, T. The effects of a ketoacid-amino acid supplement to a restricted diet on the progression of chronic

renal failure. *N Engl J Med* 311:623, 1984.
35. El Nahas, AM, Masters-Thomas, A, Brady, SA, Farrington, K, Wilkinson, V, Hilson, AJW, Varghese, Z, Moorhead, JF. Selective effect of low protein diets in chronic renal failure. *Br Med J* 289:1337, 1984.
36. Oldrizzi, L, Rugiu, C, Valvo, E, Lupo, A, Loschiavo, C, Gammaro, L, Tessitore, N, Fabris, A, Panzetta, G, Maschio, G. Progression of renal failure in patients with renal disease of diverse etiology on protein-restricted diet. *Kidney Int* 27:553, 1985.
37. Maroni, BJ, Steinman, TI, Mitch, WE. A method for estimating nitrogen intake of patients with chronic renal failure. *Kidney Int* 27:58, 1985.
38. Berlinger, WG, Park, GD, Spector, R. The effect of dietary protein on the clearance of allopurinol and oxypurinol. *N Engl J Med* 313:771, 1985.
39. Mogensen, CE. Long-term antihypertensive treatment inhibiting progression of diabetic nephropathy. *Br Med J* 285:685, 1982.
40. Parving, H-H, Andersen, AR, Smidt, UM, Homel, E, Mathiessen, ER, Svendsen, PA. Effect of antihypertensive treatment on kidney function in diabetic nephropathy. *Br Med J* 294:1443, 1987.
41. Bjorck, S, Nyberg, G, Mulea, H, Granerus, G, Herlitz, H, Aurell, M. Beneficial effects of angiotensin converting enzyme inhibition on renal function in patients with diabetic nephropathy. *Br Med J* 293:471, 1986.
41a. Heeg, JE, de Jong, PE, van der Hem, GH, de Zeeuw, D. Reduction of proteinuria by angiotensin converting enzyme inhibition. *Kidney Int* 32:78, 1987.
42. Shemesh, O, Ross, JC, Deen, WM, Grant, GW, Myers, BD. Nature of the glomerular capillary injury in human membranous glomerulopathy. *J Clin Invest* 77:868, 1986.
43. Velosa, JA, Torres, VE, Donadio, JV, Jr, Wagoner, RD, Holley, KE, Offord, KP. Treatment of severe nephrotic syndrome with meclofenamate: An uncontrolled pilot study. *Mayo Clin Proc* 60:586, 1985.
44. Velosa, JA, Torres, VE. Benefits and risks of nonsteroidal antiinflammatory drugs in steroid-resistant nephrotic syndrome. *Am J Kid Dis* 8:345, 1986.
45. Gimenez, LF, Solez, K, Walker, WG. Relation between renal calcium content and renal impairment in 246 human renal biopsies. *Kidney Int* 31:93, 1987.
46. Lumbertgul, D, Burke, TJ, Gillum, DM, Alfrey, AC, Harris, DC, Hammond, WS, Schrier, RW. Phosphate depletion arrests progression of chronic renal failure independent of protein intake. *Kidney Int* 29:658, 1986.
47. Nath, KA, Hostetter, MK, Hostetter, TH. Pathophysiology of chronic tubulo-interstitial disease in rats. Interactions of dietary acid load, ammonia, and complement component C3. *J Clin Invest* 76:667, 1985.
48. Donadio, JV, Jr, Anderson, CF, Mitchell, JC, III, Holley, KE, Ilstrup, DM, Fuster, V, Cheesbro, JH. Membranoproliferative glomerulonephritis. A prospective trial of platelet inhibitor therapy. *N Engl J Med* 310:1421, 1984.
49. Donadio, JV, Jr, Ilstrup, DM, Holley, KE, Romero, JC. Platelet inhibitors stabilize diabetic nephropathy: 10-years of prospective study (abstract). *Kidney Int* 31:197, 1987.
50. Kasiske, BL, O'Donnell, MP, Cleary, MP, Keane, WF. Treatment of hyperlipidemia reduces glomerular injury in obese Zucker rats. *Kidney Int* 33:667, 1988.
51. Al-Shebeb, T, Frohlich, J, Magil, AB. Glomerular disease in hypercholesterolemic guinea pigs. A pathogenetic study. *Kidney Int* 33:498, 1988.

57. SIGNS AND SYMPTOMS OF UREMIA

Renal failure may be associated with a variety of signs and symptoms that are collectively referred to as the *uremic state*. There is, however, no predictable correlation between the development of these problems and the severity of the renal disease (as evidenced from the blood urea nitrogen (BUN) and plasma creatinine concentration). For example, pericarditis, anorexia, or neurologic abnormalities (such as confusion or asterixis) may be observed in some patients with a BUN as low as 80 mg/dl. In comparison, other patients may be asymptomatic despite a BUN that is well over 100 mg/dl. This variability is probably related to the fact that neither urea nor creatinine appears to be a major uremic toxin [1].

A complete discussion of all of the complications associated with uremia and their pathogenesis is beyond the scope of this text [1]. This chapter will be limited to three abnormalities that are present at some point in almost all patients with severe renal insufficiency: platelet dysfunction, anemia, and bone disease (renal osteodystrophy).

Platelet Dysfunction

Bleeding complications can occur in both acute and chronic renal failure. This hemorrhagic tendency may have a variety of clinical manifestations, including gastrointestinal or cutaneous bleeding or bleeding from operative sites. It is now clear that this hemostatic defect is primarily related to a *qualitative impairment in platelet function,* as manifested by a *prolonged bleeding time* [2-4]. Although mild thrombocytopenia and nonspecific coagulation abnormalities have also been described, they appear to be of minor clinical importance and are not usually associated with an increased risk of bleeding.

Pathogenesis

Three factors have been proposed to play a pathogenetic role in the defect in platelet function: a circulating toxin that accumulates in uremic plasma, an abnormality in prostaglandin metabolism, and anemia. The contribution of a circulating toxin is supported by the observation that platelet function can be restored toward normal by incubation in normal, rather than uremic, serum [5]. Urea and parathyroid hormone (secondary hyperparathyroidism being almost universally present in these patients; see the following) are among the substances that have been proposed as mediators of this response [2,6]. Their role, however, remains to be proved. Most observers, for example, have been unable to document a relationship between the BUN and the bleeding time in patients with renal insufficiency [4].

Altered prostaglandin metabolism is another factor that could contribute to the impairment in platelet function. A reduction in the platelet synthesis of thromboxane B_2, a potent promoter of platelet aggregation, has been observed in some, but not all, studies [7,8]. Alternatively, the prolonged bleeding time could reflect an endothelial abnormality; uremic vascular tissue has been shown by some observers to release increased amounts of prostacyclin, a change that could diminish platelet adhesion to the vascular wall [9]. How this might occur and its pathogenetic importance are not known.

Finally, anemia may play a central role in the platelet dysfunction. Raising the hematocrit above 27 to 30 percent, either by red cell transfusions or the administration of recombinant human erythropoietin, can frequently normalize the bleeding time (from > 30 minutes in some patients to below 10 minutes) [10,11]. This effect appears to represent a flow-dependent phenomenon. A low hematocrit seems to increase the laminar nature of blood flow, resulting in less platelet-endothelial interaction [2]. Thus, the bleeding time is frequently prolonged even in anemic patients who have normal or near-normal renal function [12].

Treatment

No specific therapy is required in asymptomatic patients. However, attempted correction of the hemostatic defect is indicated in patients who are bleeding or who are being prepared for a surgical procedure, including diagnostic renal biopsy. Several therapeutic modalities are available that can reduce or normalize the bleeding time in this setting (Table 57-1).

Partial or complete correction can often be achieved by *dialysis,* probably due to the removal of some circulating toxin. Both hemodialysis and peritoneal dialysis may be effective [13,14], although the latter may be preferred in patients with active bleeding, since heparin therapy to prevent clotting in the dialyzer is not required. It is important to note, however, that as many as one-third of patients have no improvement in the bleeding time following dialysis [13].

Administration of *cryoprecipitate* is an alternative to dialysis [15]. This modality probably supplies a procoagulant factor that increases platelet aggregation, such as factor

Table 57-1. Correction of a prolonged bleeding time in uremia

Therapy	Dose	Duration of action
Dialysis	1–2 treatments	Variable
Cryoprecipitate	10 units intravenously every 12–24 hours	8–24 hours
dDAVP (desmopressin)	0.3 μg/kg IV over 15–30 minutes in 50 ml of saline	4–8 hours; tachyphylaxis after 1–2 doses limits utility for chronic bleeding
Blood transfusions	Transfuse to raise hematocrit to ≥ 30%	May be prolonged if hematocrit remains elevated
Conjugated estrogen	0.6 mg/kg/day intravenously for 5 days	Peak action at 5–7 days; lasts ≥ 2 weeks

VIII:von Willebrand factor complexes (FVIII:vWF). These multimers appear to act by increasing platelet adhesion to the vascular wall, even though no quantitative or qualitative defect in FVIII:vWF has been identified in uremia [2]. Despite the efficacy of cryoprecipitate, however, the delayed onset of action (12–24 hours) and the risk of transmitting infectious diseases have limited its usefulness.

The simplest and least toxic acute treatment of a prolonged bleeding time in uremia is the intravenous administration of 1-deamino-8-D-arginine *vasopressin* (dDAVP; desmopressin), a long-acting analogue of antidiuretic hormone that lacks pressor activity [16]. The mechanism of action is believed to involve the transient release of endogenous large FVIII:vWF multimers from storage sites, probably in endothelial cells [17]. The improvement in platelet function in this setting is maximal within 1 hour, begins to wane within 4 hours, and is usually gone by 8 hours [16]. Intravenous therapy is preferred; intranasal administration may also be effective [18], but the response is less predictable.

dDAVP is useful only as acute therapy, since rapid tachyphylaxis occurs after the first or second dose. This effect most likely represents depletion of endothelial stores of the FVIII:vWF multimers [2].

Two other modalities can also be used: *transfusions* to raise the hematocrit to 30 percent (see before) [2,10] and the administration of conjugated *estrogens* [19,20]. The latter form of therapy is longer-acting; the peak effect is not usually seen for 5 to 7 days and may persist for 2 weeks or more. The mechanism of action of estrogens in this setting is unclear.

Summary

The treatment of the bleeding uremic patient may require many or all of the above modalities. The preferred acute therapy is intravenous dDAVP plus transfusions to raise the hematocrit above 27 percent. Peritoneal dialysis can also be considered if these agents are unsuccessful, especially if other indications for dialysis are also present (see Chap. 59).

More long-lasting therapy with dialysis, transfusions, dDAVP, estrogens, or a combination of these, can be given to correct a prolonged bleeding time prior to elective surgery or renal biopsy. It is also important to discontinue any medications with antiplatelet activity. Aspirin, for example, may prolong the bleeding time to a greater extent and by mechanisms other than cyclooxygenase inhibition in azotemic patients [21].

Anemia

A normochromic, normocytic anemia is a very common but not universal complication of chronic renal failure. Although there is a large degree of interpatient variability, the hematocrit generally begins to fall when the plasma creatinine concentration is above 2 mg/dl and gets progressively lower as the glomerular filtration rate declines further (Fig. 57-1) [22,23]. By the time that dialysis is required, the hematocrit is typically between 15 and 30 percent, with at least 25 percent of patients requiring intermittent or regular red cell–transfusions [24].

Pathogenesis
The principal cause of anemia in chronic renal failure appears to be decreased secretion of *erythropoietin* (EPO) by the diseased kidneys [24,25]. Human EPO is a glycoprotein hormone made up of 166 amino acids. Experimental studies suggest that EPO is synthesized within the peritubular capillary endothelial cells and released in response to hypoxia [26]. However, the subcellular mechanisms by which the hormone-producing cells recognize altered oxygen availability are unknown.

The normal response to anemia is an increase in EPO production. EPO is then released into the circulation where it stimulates terminal differentiation of erythroid precursors in the bone marrow, increases cellular hemoglobin synthesis, and enhances the effective delivery of new erythrocytes into the circulation.

EPO levels are typically *inappropriately low* for the degree of anemia in chronic renal failure* [22,25]. The importance of this defect has been illustrated by the ability of recombinant human EPO to raise the hematocrit to or near normal levels in many patients being treated with maintenance dialysis [11,24].

A variety of factors other than EPO deficiency may also be important in selected cases [25]. These include

1. Resistance to the effect of EPO by retained uremic toxins [22,27]
2. Mild hemolysis, as evidenced by red cell survival rates that may be 50 percent of normal [28]
3. Bleeding from platelet dysfunction or from blood loss during hemodialysis [29]; the latter problem does not occur with peritoneal dialysis, where blood access is not required [30]
4. Aluminum toxicity, as aluminum interferes with iron uptake by the red cells (see the following) [31]
5. Hyperparathyroidism, either by a direct suppressive effect of parathyroid hormone (PTH) or by marrow fibrosis resulting from renal osteodystrophy [32]
6. Folic acid deficiency due to folate loss during hemodialysis; this appears to be less of a problem with continuous ambulatory peritoneal dialysis (CAPD) [33]
7. Hypersplenism due to silicone released from the dialysis tubing [34]

Diagnosis
Other causes of anemia should be ruled out before ascribing the reduced red cell mass to renal failure. Microcytic and hypochromic indices, for example, suggest either iron deficiency or aluminum intoxication, which are treated by iron replacement or aluminum removal, respectively. A macrocytic anemia, on the other hand, suggests folate or vitamin B_{12} deficiency. Specific therapy for the anemia of renal failure can be initiated once these problems have been excluded or treated.

Treatment
Some patients with chronic renal failure maintain a hematocrit above 30 percent and are asymptomatic. In addition, it is not uncommon for the hematocrit to slowly increase by as much as 5 to 7 percent once dialysis is initiated. It seems likely that the improved erythropoiesis in this setting is due to removal of erythroid inhibitors, although increased EPO production may also occur.

There are, however, a large number of patients with chronic renal failure (some of whom do not yet require dialysis) who have relatively severe anemia that can lead to symptoms such as fatigue, weakness, decreased exercise tolerance, and possibly angina pectoris. It is these patients in whom therapy is indicated.

---

*Much less commonly, a renal cystic disease, such as polycystic kidney disease, can lead to focal areas of ischemia and increased EPO production. The net effect may be a hematocrit that is normal or even elevated, despite the presence of advanced renal failure.

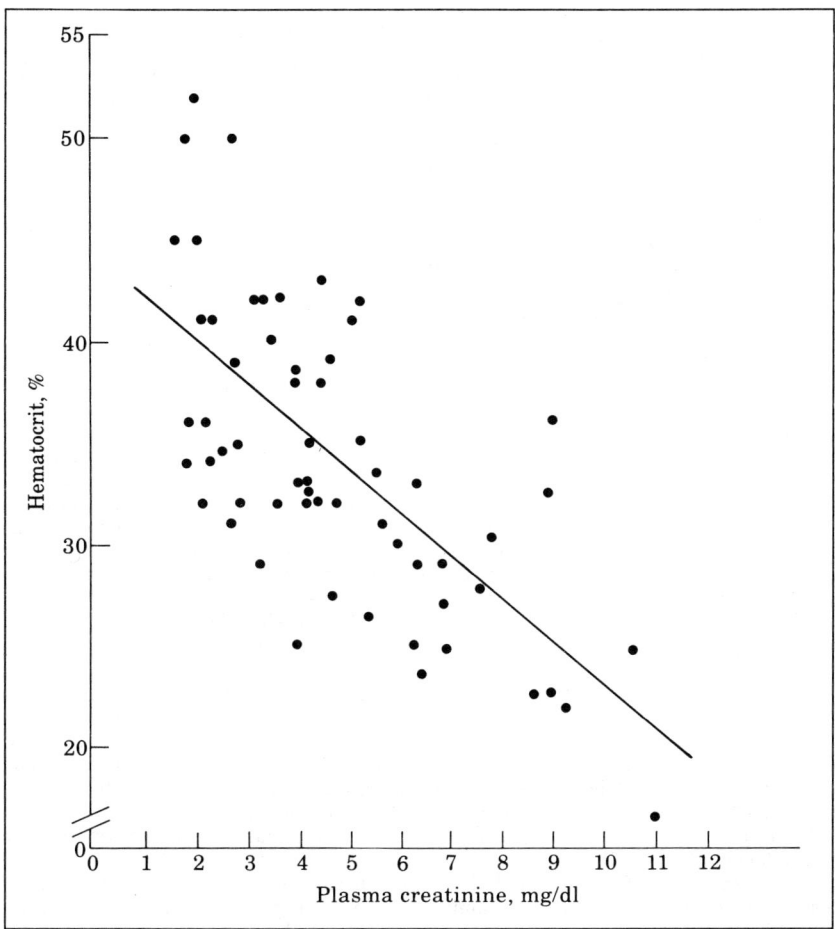

Fig. 57-1. Relationship between the hematocrit and the plasma creatinine concentration in 60 patients with varying degrees of renal insufficiency. There is substantial interpatient variability, however, so that the ability to predict an expected degree of anemia for a given plasma creatinine concentration is limited. (From McGonigle, RJS, Wallin, JD, Shadduck, RK, Fisher, JW. *Kidney Int* 25:437, 1984. Reprinted by permission from Kidney International.)

It seems likely that recombinant human erythropoietin (r-hEPO) will become the *treatment of choice* in this setting [35]. This agent has now been administered in several therapeutic trials to patients with end-stage renal disease undergoing chronic dialysis. There has been, in the majority of cases, a rise in the hematocrit to above 35 percent; this effect usually begins within 1 to 2 weeks and may persist for as long as 6 weeks after treatment has been discontinued [11,24,35]. The drug has generally been given intravenously 3 times per week with each hemodialysis treatment; it can, however, also be administered intraperitoneally in patients on continuous ambulatory peritoneal dialysis (CAPD).

Several complications may develop as a result of r-hEPO administration, most of which are *directly related to correction of the anemia* and to the associated rise in blood viscosity. These include (1) hypertension, due to elimination of anemia-induced peripheral vasodilation and perhaps to increased viscosity; (2) clotting of the arteriovenous fistula used for hemodialysis access, due to correction of the platelet dysfunction and possibly to enhanced viscosity; (3) functional iron deficiency, as a result of the rapid rise in hemoglobin synthesis; and (4) less efficient dialysis, since each ml of blood flowing through the dialyzer now contains less plasma [11,24,36]. The net effect of the last problem may be increments in the BUN, plasma potassium concentration, and the degree of edema [24,36], requiring longer or more efficient dialysis. Increased dietary intake due to the improved sense of well-being also may contribute to these changes [24].

An elevation in the systemic blood pressure may prove to be the most important of these complications. Preliminary results suggest that this problem occurs in almost one-half of patients, occasionally leading to malignant hypertension [36]. If these findings are confirmed, then the end point of r-hEPO therapy may be limited in those patients in whom blood pressure control is a problem. Optimal therapy in this setting may be incomplete correction of the hematocrit to 30 to 35 percent, a level that is high enough to lead to resolution of symptoms without producing a substantial rise in blood pressure.

One last complication, seizures, has been observed in some patients. Although a causal relationship between r-hEPO and neurologic dysfunction has not been proved, a history of seizures is at present a relative contraindication to the use of this agent.

Pending the more widespread availability of r-hEPO, current therapies of uremic anemia include blood transfusions, androgen administration, improved dialysis clearance, and exercise [25,37]. *Packed red cell transfusions* are the most rapid means of improving symptomatic anemia. They are, however, only transiently effective, and their use increases the risk of exposure to hepatitis and other infectious agents. Transfusions also suppress endogenous EPO release and, when given repeatedly, can lead to iron overload and tissue hemosiderosis [25,38]. As a result, transfusions should be used only for symptomatic control, unless the patient is being prepared for renal transplantation (see Chap. 60).

Androgens are the only relatively safe drugs presently available that have the potential for increasing the red cell mass in dialysis patients. When successful (the percentage of patients who will respond is unknown), the hematocrit can be expected to increase by 5 percent or more over a period of months [39,40]. Although there are occasional exceptions, most anephric patients fail to respond, suggesting that androgens act by increasing either the renal release of EPO or its effect on the bone marrow.

Both nandrolone decanoate (1-3 mg/kg/wk, intramuscularly) and fluoxymesterone (0.2–0.5 mg/kg/day, orally) have been successfully used. Side effects are observed in up to 25 percent of patients and include liver and muscle plasma enzyme elevations, cholestasis, hirsutism in women, and priapism in men. Therapy may be discontinued after a maximum response has been obtained, since the elevated hematocrit may persist without maintenance therapy in some patients. Androgen therapy should also be stopped if no response has been observed after 6 months of treatment.

A discussion of the anemia of renal failure would not be complete without emphasizing that some EPO production continues even in scarred, end-stage kidneys. This has been demonstrated by the substantial worsening of anemia that is commonly observed after bilateral nephrectomy. The diseased kidneys also tend to have some urine output, helping to minimize the degree of fluid and electrolyte retention. As a result, bilateral nephrectomy is now rarely performed.

Renal Osteodystrophy

The bone disease that develops in almost all patients with severe chronic renal failure is referred to as renal osteodystrophy [41]. This disorder is often subclinical, its presence being indirectly suggested by abnormal laboratory tests, such as hyperphosphatemia, hypocalcemia, high circulating levels of PTH, and low levels of calcitriol (1,25 dihydroxy-vitamin D_3, the major active metabolite of vitamin D). In some patients, however, renal osteodystrophy is a cause of substantial morbidity. As will be seen, an understanding of the mechanisms involved in the development of this condition is necessary to arrive at a proper approach to diagnosis and therapy.

Pathology
The earliest histologic abnormality (usually found within the first 5 years of renal insufficiency before dialysis has been initiated) is an increase in the amount of unmineralized osteoid that surrounds the mineralized bone surface. This change is believed to reflect secondary hyperparathyroidism, since the bone formation rate is characteristically normal or increased and PTH levels are elevated [41,42].

As the plasma concentration of PTH continues to rise, a more severe form of bone disease, *osteitis fibrosa*, is seen (Table 57-2). Osteoclasts increase in number and size, causing bone resorption and eventual marrow fibrosis [43]. The rate of bone formation often exceeds bone resorption in osteitis fibrosa, leading to an increased bone area in many patients [42]. This rise in bone mass, if severe, can lead to areas of osteosclerosis.

The other major form of uremic bone disease is *osteomalacia*, which is more commonly observed in dialyzed patients with prolonged renal failure. In contrast to osteitis fibrosa, osteomalacia is associated with normal or only mildly elevated PTH levels and a low concentration of calcitriol (Table 57-2). Osteoclasts are reduced in number, fibrosis is absent, and there are prominent areas of uncalcified osteoid, reflecting a low rate of bone formation. It is now clear that *aluminum* plays a major role in this problem; prominent aluminum deposition can usually be detected at the interface between osteoid and mineralized bone (see "Pathogenesis") [44].

Other patients with aluminum deposition have similar findings except that unmineralized osteoid is normal or reduced, not increased. This condition has been called *adynamic or aplastic* bone disease to distinguish it from classic osteomalacia (Table 57-2). Why this occurs is not well understood.

Pathogenesis
The different forms of uremic bone disease are primarily related to the interplay between three factors: secondary hyperparathyroidism, reduced calcitriol production or activity, and the toxic effects of aluminum on normal bone mineralization.

SECONDARY HYPERPARATHYROIDISM AND CALCITRIOL DEFICIENCY. Increased PTH secretion occurs in most patients with advanced renal disease and is the main cause of osteitis fibrosa [41]. The initial event that stimulates PTH release in patients with renal disease is *phosphate retention*, an abnormality caused by the reduction in the glomerular filtration rate and therefore in the filtered phosphate load. The primary role for phosphate in this setting can be illustrated by the observation in experimental animals that restricting phosphate intake (to prevent phosphate retention) can completely prevent the development of secondary hyperparathyroidism [45].

It was initially hypothesized that phosphate retention led to the rise in PTH by combining with circulating calcium, thereby lowering the plasma calcium concentration. However, recent findings suggest that minor elevations in phosphate concentration comparable to those in early renal failure do not decrease the plasma ionized calcium concentration enough to stimulate PTH secretion [41,46]. Consequently, other mechanisms must be involved, the most important of which seems to be a *fall in calcitriol production.*

The synthesis of calcitriol occurs principally in the proximal convoluted tubule by the 1-hydroxylation of 25-hydroxyvitamin D [47]. Secreted calcitriol then acts in the small intestine (where it increases calcium and phosphate absorption) and in bone (where, in concert with PTH, it stimulates bone resorption).

The major physiologic stimuli to calcitriol production are PTH and hypophosphatemia [47]. In normal subjects, for example, calcitriol production rises with dietary phosphate restriction and abruptly declines with phosphate supplementation [48]. Thus, the initial phosphate retention in renal disease plus the associated decrease in functioning renal mass could lower calcitriol levels [49].

Calcitriol deficiency can lead to secondary hyperparathyroidism by two mechanisms: by decreasing the plasma calcium concentration, and, more importantly, by *removing the normal inhibitory effect of calcitriol on the parathyroid gland* [50]. The importance of the latter in humans has been demonstrated by a marked reduction in PTH secretion following the intravenous or intraperitoneal administration of calcitriol to patients on maintenance dialysis [51,52]. In comparison, raising the plasma calcium concentration has a much less pronounced effect.

Table 57-2. Characteristics of different forms of renal osteodystrophy

	Bone formation	Osteoblasts	Osteoclasts	Osteoid	PTH levels*	Aluminum stain
Osteitis fibrosa	Nl-↑	↑	↑	↑	↑↑↑	Variable, usually not present on bone-forming surface
Osteomalacia	↓-0	↓-0	↓-0	↑↑	Nl-sl↑	Prominent at osteoid-bone interface
Adynamic	↓-0	↓-0	↓-0	0 or mild and patchy	Nl-sl↑	Variable, but usually increased

*Calcitriol levels tend to be reduced in each of these disorders.
↑ = increase. ↓ = decrease.

ALUMINUM TOXICITY.   Accumulation of aluminum in bone is a frequent finding in patients requiring chronic dialysis and is often associated with considerable morbidity. Before the use of reverse osmosis for water purification, there was substantial aluminum absorption during hemodialysis in those areas that had a relatively high aluminum content in the local water. Although contamination of the water supply is no longer a problem, *prolonged use of aluminum-containing antacids* as phosphate binders can progressively increase aluminum stores [53,54]. This effect may be exacerbated by enhanced gastrointestinal aluminum absorption in uremia; how this occurs is unknown [55].

In bone, the excess aluminum tends to be deposited at the calcification front, leading to reduced bone turnover and eventual osteomalacia [41,54]. Studies in uremic animals and humans have demonstrated that low PTH and calcitriol levels promote aluminum deposition, an effect that can be reversed by calcitriol replacement [56,57]. These relationships have two important implications. First, some of the aluminum deposition may be a *secondary* event that is promoted by the common reduction in calcitriol synthesis in renal failure (see before) [58]. Second, performing a subtotal parathyroidectomy for osteitis fibrosa can have the deleterious effect of enhancing bone aluminum deposition in patients who also have aluminum-induced osteomalacia [57].

Clinical Manifestations and Diagnosis

In their classic forms, the different types of uremic bone disease have somewhat different clinical features [41]. Advanced osteitis fibrosa, for example, can cause bone pain; proximal muscle weakness; pruritus; spontaneous rupture of tendons; hyperphosphatemia refractory to phosphate binders; and metastatic calcification due to calcium phosphate precipitation out of the plasma, with subsequent deposition in arteries, soft tissues, periarticular areas, and the viscera [1,59,60]. There may also be characteristic radiologic findings, which include skeletal demineralization and subperiosteal resorption that is most prominent in the lateral ends of the clavicles and in the phalanges [60].

It is important to appreciate the role of PTH in this and possible other uremic complications. From the viewpoint of maintenance of the plasma calcium and phosphate concentrations, the increase in PTH secretion is at first *appropriate*. As described before, early renal insufficiency is associated with mild phosphate retention and a small reduction in the plasma calcium concentration, due both to the excess phosphate and to diminished calcitriol production [45,49]. These changes will initially be normalized by PTH, which increases calcium phosphate release from bone and phosphate excretion in the urine.

The "trade-off" for this adaptation, however, is persistent secondary hyperparathyroidism, which can lead to bone disease and can also contribute to a variety of other problems including the platelet dysfunction [6] and disturbed erythropoiesis [32]. Furthermore, the ability of PTH to enhance phosphate excretion (by diminishing proximal tubular resorption) reaches a maximal level when the glomerular filtration rate falls below 20 to 30 ml/min. At this point, further secretion of PTH actually *raises the plasma phosphate concentration,* since its effect on calcium phosphate release from bone is now unopposed [59]. The combination of the near-normal plasma calcium concentration and marked hyperphosphatemia results in a high calcium-phosphate product (over 60–70) that predisposes to metastatic calcification [60].

In comparison, classic uremic osteomalacia is associated with spontaneous fractures, muscle weakness that may be disabling, normal or only slightly elevated plasma PTH levels, and a lesser degree of phosphate retention [1,59]. Dialysis dementia also may occur, a condition probably induced by the deposition of aluminum in brain tissue. Radiologic studies may reveal multiple Looser's zones, rather than subperiosteal resorption.

In the majority of patients, however, there is substantial overlap and these clear clinical distinctions between osteitis fibrosa and aluminum-associated osteomalacia cannot be made. This problem is further complicated by the potential difficulty in interpretation of elevated plasma PTH levels. Hepatic metabolism of PTH leads to the production and, in renal failure, subsequent accumulation of inactive hormone fragments in the plasma [61]. Consequently, high immunoreactivity is not necessarily associated with a comparable level of biologic activity.

Establishing the diagnosis of aluminum-induced bone disease is important if appropriate therapy is to be instituted. Although the gold standard is bone biopsy (of the iliac crest), less invasive procedures have been sought. Random measurement of the plasma aluminum concentration is not sufficiently sensitive; however, the accuracy of this test can be increased by measurement before and after the administrator of the chelator deferoxamine, which can mobilize tissue aluminum stores [62]. The presence of excess aluminum deposition is highly likely if the plasma aluminum concentration rises by more than 500 μg/L and is virtually excluded if the increase is less than 200 μg/L. Intermediate values are considered nondiagnostic and bone biopsy is probably required, particularly in patients who have symptomatic bone disease (characterized by fractures, bone pain, or severe muscle weakness). Bone biopsy is also important if partial parathyroidectomy is being considered, since aluminum deposition in bone increases substantially following parathyroidectomy in patients with concurrent osteomalacia [54,57].

Treatment

GENERAL CONSIDERATIONS.   As described before, phosphate retention plays a central role in uremic bone disease by lowering the plasma calcium concentration and calcitriol production, both of which stimulate the secretion of PTH [45,49-51]. As a result, *correction of hyperphosphatemia* is an essential component of therapy, since it can at least partially reverse these abnormalities [45,49]. This can often be achieved by restricting the intake of inorganic phosphorus to a maximum of 800 mg/day (in a 70-kg adult) plus the administration of phosphate binders. Furthermore, it is not necessary to wait until overt hyperphosphatemia is present. It is probably wise to begin lowering net phosphate intake when the glomerular filtration rate falls below 50 percent of normal, since phosphate retention is already occurring [49].

Phosphate binders are medications that are taken with meals and then combine with dietary phosphorus to diminish its absorption. Aluminum hydroxide–containing antacids (Amphojel, Alternagel, Basaljel, and others)* have been given in this setting in a dose of 15 to 30 ml or more with each meal. The most bothersome acute complication of this therapy is constipation, a problem that may be minimized by using Nephrox (a combination of aluminum hydroxide and mineral oil) or stool softeners. However, the cumulative risk of aluminum toxicity with these agents has led to a search for alternative drugs.

Recent studies suggest that calcium carbonate (in a dose of 2–16 gm/day) has many advantages as a phosphate binder [63]. It reduces aluminum exposure and, by increasing calcium intake, can lead to a rise in the plasma calcium concentration that should suppress PTH secretion. It is important to remember that many foods rich in phosphate are also high in calcium (such as milk and cheese). Thus, phosphorus restriction entails some degree of calcium restriction as well, which can exacerbate the secondary hyperparathyroidism.

Adverse effects, however, may be seen with calcium carbonate, the two most important being hypercalcemia and an inability to correct the hyperphosphatemia. In these settings, aluminum hydroxide can be added to a safe dose of calcium carbonate; this combined regimen will still minimize aluminum exposure.

VITAMIN D REPLACEMENT.   Correction of vitamin D deficiency is another important component of therapy. The exact indications for therapy remain uncertain, since there is evidence that early treatment (when there is only moderate renal insufficiency) will retard or prevent the development of secondary hyperparathyroidism and uremic bone disease. Although this issue remains unresolved, two accepted indications for therapy are persistent hypocalcemia after the plasma phosphate concentration has been normalized, and evidence of marked hyperparathyroidism, since PTH secretion can be directly suppressed by the administration of calcitriol [51,52]. In comparison, uremic osteomalacia is generally refractory to vitamin D, being primarily caused by excess aluminum deposition [41].

---

*Magnesium-containing antacids can also bind dietary phosphorus, but gastrointestinal absorption of magnesium can cause potentially serious hypermagnesemia in renal failure. Consequently, these agents should not be used on a regular basis in azotemic patients.

Table 57-3. Hazards of chronic deferoxamine administration*

Increased susceptibility to *Yersinia* sepsis and to mucomycosis
High-frequency sensorineural hearing loss
Decreased visual acuity
Loss of color vision
Acute mental status changes possibly due to redistribution of aluminum
Hypotension during infusion

*From De Broe, ME, D'Haese, PC, Van de Vyver, FL. Aluminum toxicity. In Daugirdas, JT, Ing, TS (Eds). *Handbook of Dialysis* Boston: Little, Brown, 1988, p. 407.

Calcitriol is probably the vitamin D compound of choice in renal osteodystrophy. In addition to supplying the most active form of the hormone, the short half-life of this medication allows the rapid resolution of hypercalcemia, should this complication occur. The starting oral dose is 0.25–0.5 μg/day, although intravenous (after hemodialysis) or intraperitoneal (with CAPD) administration may be more effective in diminishing PTH release [51,52].

It is essential that an attempt be made to normalize plasma phosphate concentration before institution of calcitriol. This hormone will increase the intestinal absorption of both calcium and phosphate, leading to a rise in their plasma concentrations. If these changes are superimposed on preexisting hyperphosphatemia, the ensuing rise in the calcium-phosphate product can lead to metastatic calcification.

Bone disease can often be stabilized by combined therapy with control of phosphorus intake (by diet or phosphate binders), calcium supplementation, and, when indicated, vitamin D replacement. However, a minority of maintenance dialysis patients remain symptomatic with problems such as recurrent pathologic fractures, muscle pain and weakness, and resistant hyperphosphatemia. In these patients, distinguishing osteitis fibrosa from aluminum-associated osteomalacia is necessary so that appropriate treatment can be instituted [41,54,57].

ALUMINUM REMOVAL. Once aluminum overload has been identified by bone biopsy or the response to deferoxamine infusion, two principal forms of therapy are available. The simplest is to discontinue aluminum-containing antacids, substituting calcium carbonate as the phosphate binder. Using this treatment, plasma aluminum concentrations can be expected to fall and the bone disease may begin to resolve [64]. The excess aluminum is only slowly removed by dialysis, since 80 to 90 percent of circulating aluminum is bound to proteins and is therefore poorly dialyzable.

If this approach is ineffective, chronic administration of deferoxamine can be considered. This agent mobilizes tissue aluminum stores, leading to a marked rise in the plasma aluminum concentration [62]. The aluminum circulates as a relatively small deferoxamine-aluminum complex that can be removed by either peritoneal dialysis or hemodialysis. Successful therapy can, on repeat bone biopsy at 6 months, lead to diminished aluminum staining, an increased rate of bone formation, and evidence of enhanced osteoblast and osteoclast activity [65]. The major limitations in the chronic administration of deferoxamine are its expense and its potentially hazardous, but not completely understood, side effects (Table 57-3). As a result, this form of therapy should currently be used only in patients with severe, refractory disease.

SUBTOTAL PARATHYROIDECTOMY. Patients with predominant osteitis fibrosa who do not respond to phosphate binders and calcitriol may benefit from parathyroidectomy; a portion of one gland is then reimplanted into an accessible area, such as the forearm, in case further surgery is indicated. It is important to remember that aluminum deposition into osteomalacic bone often increases dramatically after parathyroidectomy [54,57]. Consequently, this procedure should be reserved for patients without evidence of aluminum overload, and aluminum-containing antacids should be avoided, if possible, following parathyroid surgery.

References

1. Mujais, SK, Sabatini, S, Kurtzman, NA. Pathophysiology of the uremic syndrome. In BM Brenner, FC Rector, Jr (Eds.), *The Kidney* (3rd ed.). Philadelphia: Saunders, 1986.
2. Woolley, AC. Platelet dysfunction in uremia. *The Kidney* 19:15, 1987.
3. Deykin, D. Uremic bleeding. *Kidney Int* 24:698, 1983.
4. Steiner, RW, Coggins, C, Carvalho, ACA. Bleeding time in uremia: A useful test to assess clinical bleeding. *Am J Hematol* 7:107, 1979.
5. DiMinno, G, Martinez, J, McKean, M, et al. Platelet function in uremia. Multifaceted defect partially corrected by dialysis. *Am J Med* 79:552, 1985.
6. Remuzzi, G, Dodesini, P, Livio, M, et al. Parathyroid hormone inhibits human platelet function. *Lancet* 2:1321, 1981.
7. Remuzzi, G, Benigni, P, Dodesini, A, et al. Reduced platelet thromboxane formation in uremia. Evidence for a functional cyclooxygenase defect. *J Clin Invest* 71:762, 1983.
8. Bloom, A, Greaves, M, Preston, F, et al. Evidence against a platelet cyclooxygenase defect in uremic subjects on chronic hemodialysis. *Br J Haematol* 62:143, 1986.
9. Remuzzi, G, Marchesi, D, Cavenaghi, A, et al. Bleeding in renal failure: A possible role of vascular prostacyclin (PGI_2). *Clin Nephrol* 12:127, 1979.
10. Livio, M, Gotti, E, Marchesi, D, et al. Uremic bleeding: Role of anemia and beneficial effect of red cell transfusion. *Lancet* 2:1013, 1982.
11. Moia, M, Vizzotto, L, Cattaneo, M, et al. Improvement in the haemostatic defect of uraemia after treatment with recombinant human erythropoietin. *Lancet* 2:1227, 1987.
12. Hellem, A, Borchgrevink, C, Ames, S. The role of red cells in hemostasis. The relationship between the hematocrit, bleeding time and platelet adhesiveness. *Br J Haematol* 7:42, 1961.
13. Stewart, JH, Castaldi, PA. Uremic bleeding: A reversible platelet defect corrected by dialysis. *Q J Med* 36:409, 1967.
14. Nenci, G, Berrettini, M, Agnelli, G, et al. The effect of peritoneal dialysis, hemodialysis and kidney transplantation on blood platelet function: Platelet aggregation to ADP and epinephrine. *Nephron* 23:287, 1979.
15. Janson, P, Jubelirer, S, Weinstein, M, et al. Treatment of the bleeding tendency in uremia with cryoprecipitate. *N Engl J Med* 303:1318, 1980.
16. Manucci, PM, Remuzzi, G, Pusineri, F, et al. Deamino-8-D-arginine vasopressin shortens the bleeding time in uremia. *N Engl J Med* 308:8, 1983.
17. Mannucci, PM, Vicente, V, Vianello, L, et al. Controlled trial of desmopressin in liver cirrhosis and other conditions associated with a prolonged bleeding time. *Blood* 67:1148, 1986.
18. Shapiro, M, Kelleher, SP. Intranasal deamino-8-D-arginine vasopressin shortens the bleeding time in uremia. *Am J Nephrol* 4:260, 1984.
19. Liu, Y, Kosfeld, R, Marcum, S. Treatment of uremic bleeding with conjugated estrogen. *Lancet* 2:887, 1984.
20. Livio, M, Manucci, PM, Vigano, G, et al. Conjugated estrogens for the management of bleeding associated with renal failure. *N Engl J Med* 315:731, 1986.
21. Gaspari, F, Vigano, G, Orisio, et al. Aspirin prolongs bleeding time in uremia by a mechanism distinct from platelet cyclooxygenase inhibition. *J Clin Invest* 79:1788, 1987.
22. McGonigle, RJS, Wallin, JD, Shadduck, RK, Fisher, JW. Erythropoietin deficiency and inhibition of erythropoiesis in renal insufficiency. *Kidney Int* 25:437, 1984.
23. Welch, P, Howard A, Gouge, S. The relationship between the degree of anemia and the degree of chronic renal failure (abstract). *Am J Kid Dis* 11:A23, 1988.
24. Eschbach, JW, Egrie, JC, Downing, MR. Correction of the anemia of end-stage renal disease with recombinant human erythropoietin. *N Engl J Med* 316:73, 1987.
25. Eschbach, JW, Adamson, JW. Anemia of end-stage renal disease (ESRD). *Kidney Int* 28:1, 1985.
26. Lacombe, C, Da Silva, J-L, Bruneval, P, et al. Peritubular cells are the site of erythropoietin synthesis in the murine hypoxic kidney. *J Clin Invest* 81:620, 1988.

27. Tadtke, HW, Rege, AB, Lamarche, MB, et al. Identification of spermine as an inhibitor of erythropoiesis in patients with chronic renal failure. *J Clin Invest* 67:1623, 1980.
28. Hocken, AG. Haemolysis in chronic renal failure. *Nephron* 32:28, 1982.
29. Lindsay, RM, Burton, JA, Dargie, HJ, et al. Dialyzer blood loss. *Clin Nephrol* 1:24, 1973.
30. De Paepe, MBJ, Schelstraete, KHG, Ringoir, SMG, et al. Influence of continuous ambulatory peritoneal dialysis on the anemia of end-stage renal disease. *Kidney Int* 23:744, 1983.
31. Short, AIK, Winney, RJ, Robson, JS. Reversible microcytic hypochromic anaemia in dialysis patients due to aluminum intoxication. *Proc Eur Dial Transplant Assoc* 17:226, 1980.
32. Meytes, D, Bogin, E, Ma, A, et al. Effects of parathyroid hormone on erythropoiesis. *J Clin Invest* 67:1263, 1981.
33. Hemmeloff-Andersen, KE. Folic acid status of patients with chronic renal failure maintained by dialysis. *Clin Nephrol* 8:510, 1977.
34. Bommer, J, Ritz, E, Waldherr, R. Silicone-induced splenomegaly. *N Engl J Med* 305:1077, 1981.
35. Eschbach, JW, Adamson, JW. Recombinant human erythropoietin: Implications for nephrology. *Am J Kid Dis* 11:203, 1988.
36. Raine, AEG. Hypertension, blood viscosity and cardiovascular morbidity in renal failure: Implications of erythropoietin therapy. *Lancet 1:97, 1988.*
37. Goldberg, AP, Hagberg, JM, Delmez, JA, et al. Metabolic effects of exercise training in hemodialysis patients. *Kidney Int* 18:754, 1980.
38. Shafer, AI, Cheron, RG, Dluhy, R, et al. Clinical consequences of acquired transfusional iron overload in adults. *N Engl J Med* 304:319, 1981.
39. Hendler, ED, Goffinet, JA, Ross, S, et al. Controlled study of androgen therapy in anemia of patients of maintenance hemodialysis. *N Engl J Med* 291:1046, 1974.
40. Eschbach, JW, Adamson, JW. Anemia of renal disease. In Schrier, RW, Gottschalk, CW (Eds.), *Diseases of the Kidney* (4th ed.). Boston: Little, Brown. 1988, p. 3026.
41. Lee, DBN, Goodman, WG, Coburn, JW. Renal osteodystrophy: Some new questions on an old disorder. *Am J Kid Dis* 11:365, 1988.
42. Sherrard, DJ, Baylink, DJ, Wergedal, JE, et al. Quantitative histological studies on the pathogenesis of uremic bone disease. *J Clin Endocrinol Metab* 39:119, 1974.
43. Kaye, M, Zucher, SW, Leclerc, YG, et al. Osteoclast enlargement in end-stage renal disease. *Kidney Int* 27:574, 1985.
44. Maloney, NA, Ott, SM, Alfrey, AC, et al. Histological quantitation of aluminum in iliac bone from patients with renal failure. *J Lab Clin Med* 99:206, 1982.
45. Slatopolsky, E, Bricker, NS. The role of phosphorus restriction in the prevention of secondary hyperparathyroidism in chronic renal disease. *Kidney Int* 4:141, 1973.
46. Adler, AJ, Ferran, N, Berlyne, GM. Effects of inorganic phosphate on serum ionized calcium concentration in vitro: A reassessment of the "trade off hypothesis." *Kidney Int* 28:932, 1985.
47. Holick, MF. Vitamin D and the kidney. *Kidney Int* 32:912, 1987.
48. Portale, AA, Halloran, BP, Murphy, MM, et al. Oral intake of phosphorus can determine the serum concentration of 1,25-dihydroxyvitamin D by determining its production rate in humans. *J Clin Invest* 77:7, 1986.
49. Llach, F, Massry, SG. On the mechanism of secondary hyperparathyroidism in moderate renal insufficiency. *J Clin Endocrinol Metab* 61:601, 1985.
50. Lopez-Hilker, S, Galceran, T, Chan, Y-L, et al. Hypocalcemia may not be essential for the development of secondary hyperparathyroidism in chronic renal failure. *J Clin Invest* 78:1097, 1986.
51. Slatopolsky, E, Weerts, C, Thielan, T, et al. Marked suppression of secondary hyperparathyroidism by intravenous administration of 1,25-dihydroxycholecalciferol in uremic patients. *J Clin Invest* 74:2136, 1984.
52. Delmez, JA, Dougan, S, Gearing, BK, et al. The effects of intraperitoneal calcitriol on calcium and parathyroid hormone. *Kidney Int* 31:795, 1987.
53. Turner, MW, Ardila, M, Hutchinson, T, et al. Sporadic aluminum osteomalacia: Iden-

tification of patients at risk. *Am J Kid Dis* 11:51, 1988.

54. Slatopolsky, E. The interaction of parathyroid hormone and aluminum in renal osteodystrophy. *Kidney Int* 31:842, 1987.

55. Ittel, TH, Buddington, B, Miller, NL, et al. Enhanced gastrointestinal absorption of aluminum in uremic rats. *Kidney Int* 32:821, 1987.

56. Malluche, HH, Faugere, M-C, Friedler, RM. Calcitriol, parathyroid hormone and accumulation of aluminum in bone in dogs with renal failure. *J Clin Invest* 79:754, 1987.

57. Andress, DL, Ott, SM, Maloney, NA, et al. Effect of parathyroidectomy on bone aluminum accumulation in chronic renal failure. *N Engl J Med* 312:468, 1985.

58. Quarles, LD, Dennis, VW, Gitelman, HJ, et al. Aluminum deposition at the osteoid-bone interface. An epiphenomenon of the osteomalacic state in vitamin D-deficient dogs. *J Clin Invest* 75:1441, 1985.

59. Massry, SG, Coburn, JW, Popovtzer, MD, et al. Secondary hyperparathyroidism in chronic renal failure: The clinical spectrum in uremia, during hemodialysis, and after renal transplantation. *Arch Intern Med* 124:431, 1969.

60. Katz, AI, Hampers, CL, Merill, JP. Secondary hyperparathyroidism and renal osteodystrophy in chronic renal failure: Analysis of 195 patients with observations on the effects of chronic dialysis, kidney transplantation and subtotal parathyroidectomy. *Medicine* 48:333, 1969.

61. Editorial. Measuring the PTH level. *Lancet* 1:94, 1988.

62. Nebeker, HG, Andress, DL, Milliner, DS, et al. Indirect methods for the diagnosis of aluminum bone disease: Plasma aluminum, the desferrioxamine infusion test, and serum iPTH. *Kidney Int* 29 (suppl. 18):S-96, 1986.

63. Slatopolsky, E, Weerts, C, Lopez-Hilker, S, et al. Calcium carbonate as a phosphate binder in patients with chronic renal failure undergoing dialysis. *N Engl J Med* 315:157, 1986.

64. Hercz, G, Andress, DL, Nebeker, HG, et al. Reversal of aluminum-related bone disease after substituting calcium carbonate for aluminum hydroxide. *Am J Kid Dis* 11:70, 1988.

65. Andress, DL, Nebeker, HG, Ott, SM, et al. Bone histologic response to deferoxamine in aluminum-related bone disease. *Kidney Int* 31:1344, 1987.

58. ACQUIRED RENAL CYSTIC DISEASE

In 1977, the development of a unique type of acquired renal cystic disease (ARCD) was reported in hemodialysis patients [1]. Since its initial description, this disorder has been shown to be quite common, having been identified in 25 to 45 percent of patients who have been chronically hemodialyzed for more than 3 years [2,3]. Furthermore, ARCD also may be seen in patients on continuous ambulatory peritoneal dialysis (CAPD) [4,5] as well as those with chronic renal failure not yet requiring dialytic therapy [4,6].

The cysts in ARCD are characteristically small, multiple, and involve both kidneys. They appear to develop from proliferation of both proximal and distal tubular epithelial cells, but the stimulus that initiates cell proliferation is unknown [2,3]. It has been suggested, for example, that cyst formation may be promoted by the higher-than-normal nephron flow rates seen in chronic renal failure (due to the decreased number of functioning nephrons). There is, however, no evidence that the tubular basement membranes in cystic nephrons are structurally weakened, a change that would probably be required if elevated flow rates were to promote the development of cysts [7].

It has also been hypothesized that plasticizers or other substances associated with hemodialysis tubing are the potential toxins that favor cyst formation [3]. However, the observation that patients with chronic renal failure or those treated with CAPD also develop ARCD does not support this theory [4]. Available data suggest that the most important variable in the development of this disorder is the *duration and severity of chronic renal failure.* It seems likely that the compensatory hypertrophy that normally accompanies nephron loss (see Chap. 56) plays a major role in initiating cyst formation.

The importance of this otherwise asymptomatic disease results from the complications that may develop, the most serious of which are *bleeding* and *malignant transformation.* Rupture of an unsupported blood vessel into the cyst may cause local pain or gross hematuria. Less commonly, hemorrhage may extend into the perirenal area, possibly being severe enough to produce hypotension.

However, the most important complication of ARCD is the late development of adenocarcinoma, a change that has been observed in 1 to 4 percent of patients [2,3]. In most cases, this transformation from cyst formation to renal cancer takes place over many (8–10) years, but a shorter interval may be observed [5]. These tumors are occasionally bilateral, a finding that is not unexpected in view of the bilateral nature of ARCD.

As a result of the possibility of malignant degeneration in patients with ARCD, it has been suggested that a *renal ultrasound* be obtained in all patients with end-stage renal disease who have been on chronic dialysis for 1 to 3 years, and if negative, every year thereafter. If ultrasonography reveals ARCD, it is recommended that a CT scan of the kidneys be performed periodically to screen for the development of adenocarcinoma, since the latter modality is more reliable than ultrasonography in detecting solid, intracystic tumors [8].

References

1. Dunnhill, MS, Millard, PR, Oliver, DB. Acquired cystic disease of the kidneys: A hazard of long-term intermittent haemodialysis. *J Clin Pathol* 30:868, 1977.
2. Gardner, KD, Jr, Evan, AP. Cystic kidneys: An enigma evolves. *Am J Kid Dis* 3:403, 1984.
3. Grantham, JJ, Levine, E. Acquired cystic disease: Replacing one kidney disease with another. *Kidney Int* 28:99, 1985.
4. Katz, A, Somobolos, K, Oreopoulos, DG. Acquired cystic disease of the kidney in association with chronic ambulatory peritoneal dialysis. *Am J Kid Dis* 9:426, 1987.
5. Smith, JW, Sallman, AL, Williamson, MR, Lott, CG. Acquired renal cystic disease: Two cases of associated adenocarcinoma and a renal ultrasound survey of a peritoneal dialysis population. *Am J Kid Dis* 10:41, 1987.
6. Narasimhan, N, Golper, TA, Wolfson, M, Rahatzad, M, Bennett, WM. Clinical characteristics and diagnostic considerations in acquired renal cystic disease. *Kidney Int* 30:748, 1986.
7. Grantham, JJ, Donoso, VS, Evan, AP, Carone, FA, and Gardner, KD, Jr. Viscoelastic properties of tubule basement membranes in experimental renal cystic disease. *Kidney Int* 32:187, 1987.
8. Levine, E, Grantham, JJ, Slusher, SL. CT of acquired cystic kidney disease and renal tumors in long-term dialysis patients. *Am J Radiol* 142:125, 1984.

59. DIALYSIS

Loss of renal function results in the accumulation of metabolic waste products and alters the normal homeostatic mechanisms that control water and electrolyte balance. Potential consequences of these abnormalities are the signs and symptoms of uremia. They include fluid accumulation (resulting in hypertension, and peripheral and pulmonary edema), hyperkalemia, pericarditis, and nonlocalizing signs of central nervous system dysfunction (such as confusion, coma, or even seizures).

Using dialysis, the physician can treat these disturbances and improve the quality of life in many patients with chronic, end-stage renal disease. In addition, the fluid, acid-base, and electrolyte problems observed in acute renal failure also can be minimized, thereby sustaining life until the patient's own kidneys recover adequate function. Each of the two types of dialysis, hemodialysis and peritoneal dialysis, are useful in removing fluid, uremic toxins, and potassium.

Hemodialysis

The concept of hemodialysis is simple, but the dialyzers, blood pumps, monitors, dialysate delivery systems, and associated tubing give the appearance of an extraordinarily complex process. Understanding hemodialysis can be made easier by reviewing the basic principles involved.

Blood access from the chronic hemodialysis patient is obtained from an arteriovenous fistula (usually constructed in the nondominant forearm) or, in patients with acute renal failure, from a catheter inserted into a large bore vein, such as the subclavian or femoral vein. Smaller vessels limit the rate of blood flow to the dialysis cartridge, thereby reducing solute clearance.

The most commonly constructed arteriovenous fistula is formed at the level of the wrist by an anastomosis between the radial artery and the cephalic vein. Dialysis needles are inserted into the venous side of the fistula after the vein has developed a larger diameter and a thicker wall, a process requiring 3 to 6 weeks or more. Consequently, the fistula usually cannot be used for dialysis access in the patient with *acute* renal failure. In comparison, a catheter placed into the subclavian or femoral vein can be used immediately.

The technique of hemodialysis requires blood to be pumped from the patient through tubing into a dialysis cartridge or dialyzer (Fig. 59-1). Regardless of the dialyzer used, the principle of dialysis is the same. A semipermeable membrane separates the patient's blood from a constantly replenished volume of dialysis solution (or dialysate). Solutes diffuse across the dialyzer membrane down their concentration gradients. For example, urea diffuses from the patient's blood (high urea concentration) across the membrane into the dialysis solution (which contains no urea). For any given dialyzer, the major determinants of the rate of solute transfer (or dialysis clearance) are the rate of blood and dialysate flow through the dialysis cartridge; the size and permeability of the dialyzer membrane; and the size, charge, and blood concentration of the solute being measured.

In some settings (such as hyperkalemia), it may be necessary to dialyze a specific solute at a relatively faster rate than others by adjusting the concentration of the substance in the dialysis solution. For example, the potassium concentration in most standard dialysis solutions is about 2 meq/L; this empirically determined level allows removal of the potassium that has accumulated between dialysis treatments without producing an excessive reduction in the plasma potassium concentration. By using a 0 or 1 meq/L dialysis bath for part or all of the dialysis treatment, the rate of potassium removal can be appropriately increased in the patient with hyperkalemia.

Standard dialysis solutions also contain sodium (about 140 meq/L), acetate or bicarbonate (35–38 meq/L), calcium (5–6 mg/dl, all of which is ionized), and magnesium (1.0–1.5 mg/dl) but no phosphorus. This results in phosphorus removal but the *net addition* of bicarbonate (or acetate, which is rapidly metabolized to bicarbonate) and calcium, which acts to ameliorate the usually present metabolic acidosis and hypocalcemia.

In addition to solutes, plasma water is also removed during dialysis. This process, called *ultrafiltration,* is driven primarily by the hydrostatic pressure gradient across the dialysis membrane. Thus, raising the transmembrane pressure gradient can lead to an increased rate of fluid removal.* This is particularly useful in those renal failure patients with massive volume overload manifested by pulmonary and peripheral edema.

---

*The transmembrane pressure gradient can be elevated either by increasing the pressure on the blood side of the dialysis membrane or by reducing the pressure on the dialysate side. *Negative pressure,* which is the primary modality currently in use, is generated by creating a vacuum effect on the dialysate side of the membrane. In comparison, *positive pressure* is generated by increasing the rate of blood flow to the dialyzer and by simultaneously increasing the resistance to blood flow back to the patient. The latter is achieved by mechanically constricting the dialysis tubing containing the blood that has already passed through the dialyzer (Fig. 59-1).

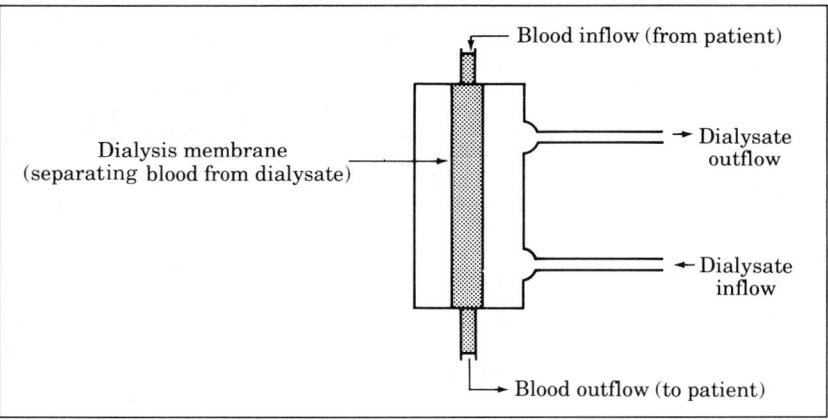

Fig. 59-1. Schematic representation of a hemodialysis cartridge. See text for details.

The risk of inducing hypotension in this setting can be minimized by shutting off the flow of dialysate fluid. This process is called *selective* ultrafiltration [1], since there is no solute diffusion into or out of the dialysate fluid and therefore no osmotic disequilibrium (primarily caused by rapid urea removal) and no excess acetate accumulation, both of which can contribute to a fall in the systemic blood pressure (see the following).

A newer ultrafiltration technique, called *continuous arteriovenous hemofiltration (CAVH),* also has been used for rapid fluid removal in renal failure [2]. During CAVH, blood flow, usually from the femoral artery or vein, is driven by the intravascular pressure (rather than by a mechanical pump) to a hemofilter containing a membrane across which fluid is ultrafiltered. The ultrafiltration rate depends on the pressure generated across the membrane and the permeability characteristics of the hemofilter used.

The blood returning to the patient is subsequently diluted by a fluid replacement system that acts to prevent excessive volume depletion, since more than 1 liter/hour can be removed by CAVH. Despite the often rapid rate of net fluid removal, hypotension is less common than with conventional hemodialysis [3]; the absence of dialysate and solute diffusion probably accounts for this relative protection.

In addition to its use in renal failure, CAVH also may be helpful in selected patients with fluid overload due to refractory congestive heart failure (unresponsive to inotropic drugs, vasodilators, and diuretics) [4]. In this setting, an increase in urine output and an enhanced sensitivity to diuretics often follows the CAVH treatment, although the pathogenesis of these effects is not known. There is, however, a risk of thrombosis if the catheter is left in the femoral artery for a prolonged period. Furthermore, bleeding (from continuous heparinization) or hypotension (if the balance equipment that controls the replacement fluid is inaccurate) may occur [5].

Peritoneal Dialysis

Peritoneal dialysis is an alternative to hemodialysis in patients with acute and chronic renal failure. With this modality, solute and water movement occur across the peritoneal membrane, rather than an external dialyzer. A dialysis cycle in peritoneal dialysis is begun by infusing 1 to 2 liters of dialysis solution into the abdomen, usually through a soft Tenckhoff catheter inserted into the peritoneal cavity. The dialysate stays (or dwells) in the abdomen for a variable period and then is drained out by gravity into a container positioned below the patient. New dialysate is then run in after the drainage is complete.

Solute removal in peritoneal dialysis occurs by diffusion, while water moves down an osmotic gradient into the slightly hyperosmotic dialysate fluid (which normally is a 1.5% [1500 mg/dl] glucose solution). Both the daily clearance of uremic toxins and the rate of fluid removal (ultrafiltration) can be enhanced by increasing the volume of dialysate or the number of dialysis exchanges. Ultrafiltration also can be enhanced by raising the glucose concentration and therefore the osmolality in the dialysate (1.5, 2.5, and 4.25% glucose concentrations are available).

The peritoneal clearance rates of urea and creatinine per unit time are substantially lower than those obtained with hemodialysis (Table 59-1). This difference is primarily due to the higher blood and dialysate flow rates attainable with hemodialysis. However, the decreased efficiency of peritoneal dialysis is usually not clinically important, since it is largely overcome by a longer time of dialysis—24 hours, rather than 3 to 4 hours as with hemodialysis. The two settings in which the increased clearance rate with hemodialysis does become important are in the treatment of drug overdoses or severe hyperkalemia where rapid removal of the offending substance may be life-saving.

Although a hemodialysis clearance of over 100 ml/min for urea and creatinine (Table 59-1) seems to be similar to that with two normally functioning kidneys, it is important to appreciate that the patient is being dialyzed for only 12 of the 168 hours per week so that the net clearance is *less than 8 percent* of normal. Thus, the lowest blood urea nitrogen (BUN) and plasma creatinine concentration may be about 50 mg/dl and 7 mg/dl, respectively, if measured just after a hemodialysis treatment; comparable values in the adequately dialyzed peritoneal dialysis patient are about 80 mg/dl and 10 to 12 mg/dl. These differences are somewhat misleading, however, since the BUN and plasma creatinine concentration *rise between treatments* with hemodialysis but are relatively constant with peritoneal dialysis. The net effect is that uremic symptoms, electrolyte abnormalities, and fluid overload can usually be equally well controlled by both methods.

The technique used for patients with chronic end-stage renal disease is called *continuous ambulatory peritoneal dialysis* (CAPD). Typically, 2 liters of dialysis solution dwell inside the abdominal cavity for about 4 hours, at which time the abdomen is drained and a fresh solution is infused. Most patients perform four exchanges each day (including one overnight) and carry on with their normal activities between exchanges.

CAPD has a variety of advantages that has led to an increase in its popularity:

1. It permits the patient with end-stage renal disease to live a more normal life-style; dialysis can be performed at home, at work, and on vacations where access to hemodialysis may be more difficult.
2. The continuous dialysis allows the ingestion of a relatively normal diet, in comparison to the sodium, potassium, and fluid restrictions between treatments in chronic hemodialysis.
3. Stable blood solute concentrations are maintained with CAPD, in contrast to the wide fluctuations observed with hemodialysis; as a result, CAPD does not lead to symptoms related to osmotic disequilibrium (see the following).
4. Transfusion requirements are reduced in patients on CAPD, in part because there is no blood loss due to partial retention in the dialyzer as occurs with each hemodialysis treatment.

There are, however, disadvantages to CAPD, leading to a net conversion rate to hemodialysis of about 30 to 40 percent. Some patients, for example, are unwilling to make the continuous time commitment of 3 to 4 hours every day to perform the dialysis exchanges. Although now less common, recurrent episodes of peritonitis (see the following) can also lead to discontinuation of CAPD.

Indications for Initiation of Dialysis

The indications for starting dialysis are somewhat controversial. It has been suggested, for example, that dialysis be initiated in acute renal failure when the BUN exceeds 100 mg/dl to forestall the development of uremic complications; there is, however, no proof of benefit from prophylactic dialysis (i.e., dialysis in the absence of fluid overload, hyperkalemia, or uremic signs or symptoms; Table 59-2) [6]. Nevertheless, it may be reasonable to initiate early dialysis (when the BUN is > 100 mg/dl) in a patient with acute tubular necrosis in whom persistent oliguria suggests that resolution of the disease is not imminent (see Chap. 24). In comparison, dialysis is usually withheld from a patient with acute renal failure and a similar BUN if there are no symptoms and if the urine output has begun to increase, a sign that may herald the onset of recovery. Dialysis may

Table 59-1. Comparative clearances (ml/min) for hemodialysis and peritoneal dialysis

	Hemodialysis	Peritoneal dialysis
Urea	120–150	18–27
Creatinine	100–130	14–20

Table 59-2. Indications for acute dialysis in patients with renal failure

Absolute	Relative
Otherwise unexplained altered mental status	Nausea and vomiting
Pericarditis	Persistent, severe hyperkalemia
Persistent, severe circulatory overload	Correction of an abnormal bleeding time before surgery
Ingestions (e.g., methanol, ethylene glycol, aspirin)*	

*See Chap. 5

also be postponed in the asymptomatic patient with contrast-induced acute renal failure, since resolution of this disorder characteristically begins within 5 days.

Similar considerations apply to the patient with chronic renal failure. Uncontrollable fluid overload, pericarditis, peripheral neuropathy, or uremic symptoms (nausea, vomiting, confusion) are indications to initiate dialysis. Asymptomatic patients are usually not dialyzed even if the BUN exceeds 150 mg/dl, since only the blood test will be treated at this point.

Duration of Dialysis
The necessary frequency and duration of hemodialysis treatments are variable. Most patients (whether they have acute or chronic renal failure) are dialyzed for about 3 to 4 hours 3 times a week, a total duration that usually permits maintenance of volume and potassium balance and control of uremic symptoms. However, exceptions do occur. This schedule, for example, is frequently increased in the catabolic, acute renal failure patient who is volume overloaded, but who continues to require intravenous fluids. On the other hand, the use of newer, larger, and more permeable high-flux hemodialysis membranes can shorten the duration of dialysis in most chronic patients, since the rate of solute and fluid removal is enhanced [7].

Most peritoneal dialysis patients respond clinically to 8 liters of dialysis solution daily (four 2-liter exchanges, each with a 4–5-hour dwell time, except for the overnight dialysis). However, patients who are severely catabolic or volume overloaded may transiently require more frequent exchanges. With either hemodialysis or peritoneal dialysis, the *adequacy* of dialysis is most often judged by assessment of the patient's clinical condition.

Hemodialysis Versus Peritoneal Dialysis
Once the decision to initiate dialysis has been made, hemodialysis or peritoneal dialysis must be selected. Since both techniques are effective, the decision of which modality to choose is dependent on additional factors including local availability, the clinical condition of the patient, and patient preference.

Many hospitals do not have the availability of hemodialysis, since the frequency with which this procedure would be used is so low that the cost of maintaining a full-time hemodialysis staff is prohibitive. Most patients with acute renal failure in these institutions can be managed adequately using peritoneal dialysis.

In hospitals where both procedures are available, the condition of the patient is the primary determinant in choosing which modality to use. Hemodialysis, for example, is preferred in the presence of severe, symptomatic hyperkalemia, since potassium removal is more rapid using this procedure. It is also the modality of choice in the patient with multiple abdominal operations, in whom adhesions may limit peritoneal clearances and may increase the risk of bowel perforation during insertion of the peritoneal catheter.

In comparison, peritoneal dialysis is especially useful in patients with vascular instability, where hypotension occurring during hemodialysis (see the following) could be catastrophic, and in patients with active bleeding that can be made worse by heparinization during the hemodialysis treatment.

In patients requiring chronic dialysis, the choice is also based in part on the availability of vascular access and the likelihood of obtaining adequate peritoneal clearances, which may be limited in patients with previous abdominal surgery or with progressive systemic sclerosis (see Chap. 42). The decision in patients without contraindications to either procedure is based on the answers to two questions: (1) Does the patient have the mental capacity and manual dexterity to learn and perform CAPD?; and, if so, (2) What is the patient's choice?

Complications of Dialysis
The problems that develop in patients on dialysis are unique and depend on the type of dialysis being used. As a result, the major complications of these procedures will be discussed separately (Table 59-3), although a complete review of all of the disturbances that can occur is beyond the scope of this discussion.

Hemodialysis
The *disequilibrium syndrome* is a disorder that, in its most severe form, is seen less often today than in the past. Patients typically complain of nonlocalizing neurologic symptoms, such as headache, nausea, and restlessness, which may progress to confusion or even seizures. Symptoms are typically observed toward the end of, or within 12 hours after, the hemodialysis treatment.

The disequilibrium syndrome is believed to be caused primarily by rapid urea removal from the extracellular fluid. This lowers the BUN, but urea clearance from the brain occurs less quickly [8]. The resulting osmotic gradient leads to a shift of fluid from the extracellular fluid into the brain, thereby causing cerebral edema and changes in cerebral function [9]. Minimizing the fall in plasma osmolality by, for example, infusing mannitol, can prevent or reduce the patient's symptoms.

The disequilibrium syndrome most often occurs with the first hemodialysis treatment. At this time, the BUN is at its peak, resulting in a maximum gradient between the plasma and the dialysate fluid and therefore a maximum rate of urea removal by diffusion. Osmotic disequilibrium can be ameliorated or prevented in this setting by limiting the rate and amount of urea removed; this can be achieved by using a smaller dialyzer (with a smaller surface area), lower flow rates, and dialyzing for only 2 to 3 hours during the initial treatments [9].

However, disequilibrium cannot always be completely eliminated, as some chronic hemodialysis patients feel weak and nauseated for several hours after each treatment, symptoms that are probably in part due to osmotic water shifts. This problem is not likely to occur with peritoneal dialysis, since the rate of solute clearance is much less and patients are continually not intermittently dialyzed.

Hypotension occurs in 25 to 50 percent of otherwise uncomplicated hemodialysis treatments [10]. It is frequently caused by excessive fluid removal, may occur more often in patients with uremic autonomic neuropathy, and can usually be corrected by the intravenous administration of saline. However, as described above, relatively large volumes of fluid can be removed without an important fall in blood pressure by selective ultrafiltration or CAVH, in both of which the flow of dialystate is discontinued [1,3]. This finding suggests that solute diffusion can play an important role in the development of hypotension. Two factors may contribute to this relationship: the *fall in plasma osmolality* due to rapid urea loss, which promotes extracellular water movement into the cells; and the transfer of *acetate*, which serves as a source of bicarbonate in the dialysis

Table 59-3. Major complications of hemodialysis and peritoneal dialysis

Hemodialysis
    Disequilibrium syndrome
    Hypotension
    Difficulty with vascular access
    Dyspnea
Peritoneal dialysis
    Peritonitis
    Obesity and hypertriglyceridemia due to glucose absorption from the dialysate
    Protein loss

solution, into the blood stream at a rate that exceeds its ability to be metabolized [10,11]. "Acetate intolerance" appears to be mediated by both a reduction in systemic vascular resistance and a decline in myocardial contractility [10,12]. It appears to occur in about 10 percent of patients who are unable to metabolize acetate rapidly [11] and can be avoided by using a bicarbonate, rather than acetate, containing dialysate [10].

Problems with *vascular access* are also common with both acute and chronic hemodialysis [13,14]. If blood flow is inadequate (due, for example, to stenosis or clotting of an arteriovenous fistula), clearances will be low, requiring more frequent dialysis treatments. Injecting radiocontrast media into the fistula is often used to establish the correct diagnosis. A stenotic lesion may be correctable by angioplasty, whereas fibrinolytic agents or direct removal of the clot may be effective with a thrombotic lesion. The latter modalities may be followed by angioplasty (or surgical revision) if the clot formation were due to stasis induced by an underlying stenosis [14].

In addition to these problems that are superimposed on a previously well functioning fistula, it may be difficult to create a functioning fistula in patients with severe vascular disease due, for example, to diabetes mellitus or scleroderma. In this setting, the use of alternate vascular sites (such as the upper arm or lower extremity), synthetic grafts, or even peritoneal dialysis may be required.

Another complaint that can occur during hemodialysis is transient *dyspnea*. This problem usually occurs within the first 30 minutes of the dialysis treatment and is typically accompanied by neutropenia. It appears that these disturbances result from direct complement activation by the dialysis membrane, with secondary chemotaxis of leukocytes to the pulmonary capillaries and the subsequent formation of leukocyte thrombi [15].

Peritoneal Dialysis and CAPD
The most important complication of peritoneal dialysis is *peritonitis* [16]. Peritonitis may be caused by an infection or leak at the catheter insertion site or by a break in sterile technique; in some cases, however, the initiating event allowing bacteria to enter the peritoneal cavity cannot be ascertained. The clinical manifestations are variable, ranging from asymptomatic infection to severe abdominal pain. Systemic signs, such as fever and hypotension, are less common.

Examination of the peritoneal effluent characteristically reveals cloudy fluid with a white blood cell count of over 100 cells/mm^3 (composed of more than 50% neutrophils). Staphylococcal species are the most frequently isolated organisms, with gram-negative bacteria accounting for another 20 to 25 percent of cases. Fungal infections also may occur but are uncommon.

The initial treatment of peritonitis consists of two to three short dialysis cycles to remove by-products of inflammation and fibrin. Following this, normal 3- to 4-hour dwells are reinstituted, with the addition to the dialysis solution of antimicrobials to treat the local infection (Table 59-4) and heparin (500 units/L) to reduce fibrin formation, which may clog the catheter or sequester bacteria. A systemic loading dose of the antimicrobial is usually administered concomitantly if the patient appears toxic. Pending culture results, the typical patient is empirically placed on an aminoglycoside plus

Table 59-4. Antimicrobial dosage during bacterial peritonitis

Antimicrobial	Intraperitoneal maintenance dose
Vancomycin	25 mg/L
Gentamicin	5 mg/L
Tobramycin	5 mg/L
Amikacin	20 mg/L
Clindamycin	25 mg/L
Cephalothin	250 mg/L
Cefazolin	125 mg/L
Cefuroxime	250 mg/L
Cefotaxime	250 mg/L
Ceftazidime	125 mg/L
Ampicillin	125 mg/L
Oxacillin	125 mg/L
Penicillin G	100,000 U/L
Piperacillin	100 mg/L
Ticarcillin	250 mg/L

*A single parenteral loading dose of the antimicrobial may be given at the time intraperitoneal administration is begun if systemic signs of infection are present.

either oxacillin or vancomycin. Single-agent therapy with a cephalosporin may also be used but some less common organisms will not be covered by this regimen.

Treatment, which can generally be performed on an outpatient basis in CAPD, should be continued for at least 5 days after both resolution of clinical symptoms and clearing of the peritoneal effluent; this usually requires a total of 7 to 10 days of antimicrobial therapy [16]. In contrast to the general efficacy of therapy for bacterial infection, the presence of fungal peritonitis almost always requires *removal of the peritoneal catheter* [16].

It is important to be aware of a common problem seen in many patients who develop peritonitis: loss of ultrafiltration leading to weight gain (often with edema) and often an increase in blood pressure. Fluid retention probably develops in this setting because the mesenteric inflammation leads to dilation of the peritoneal capillaries, arterioles, and venules [17], as well as an increase in the peritoneal lymphatic flow rate [18]. The result is increased systemic absorption of the glucose contained in the infused dialysate, thereby minimizing the osmotic gradient that normally promotes fluid removal. This problem usually resolves as the peritonitis clears.

CAPD also may be associated with metabolic complications, including obesity and hypertriglyceridemia (both of which result from absorption of over one-half of the glucose in the dialysate), and protein loss by diffusion. These problems can be prevented by limiting the dietary intake of carbohydrates and calories while maintaining that of protein. In diabetic patients, the addition of insulin to the dialysate can minimize any elevation in the plasma glucose concentration [19].

References

1. Bergstrom, J. Ultrafiltration without dialysis for removal of fluid and solutes in uremia. *Clin Nephrol* 9:156, 1978.
2. Henderson, LW. Hemofiltration. *The Kidney* 20:25, 1987.
3. Henderson, LW. Heterogeneity of the cardiovascular response to hemofiltration. *Kidney Int* 29:901, 1986.
4. Rimondini, A, Cipolla, CM, Della Bella, P, Grazi, S, Sisillo, E, Susini, G, Guazzi, MD.

Hemofiltration as short-term treatment for refractory congestive heart failure. *Am J Med* 83:43, 1987.

5. Bosch, JP, Saccaggi, A, Glabman, S. Alternatives in extracorporeal uremia therapy. In AR Nissenson, RN Fine, DE Gentile (Eds.), *Clinical Dialysis*. Connecticut: Appleton-Century-Crofts, 1984. Pp. 691–702.
6. Gillum, DM, Kelleher, SP, Dillingham, MA, et al. The role of intensive dialysis in acute renal failure. *Clin Nephrol* 25:249, 1986.
7. Keshaviah, P, Luchmann, D, Ilstrup, K, Collins, A. Technical requirements for rapid high-efficiency therapies. *Artif Org* 10:189, 1986.
8. Todrigo, F, Shideman, J, McHugh, R, Buselmeier, TA, Kjellstand, CM. Osmolarity changes during hemodialysis. *Ann Intern Med* 86:554, 1977.
9. Arieff, AI, Massry, SG, Barrientos, A, Kleeman, CR. Brain water and electrolyte metabolism in uremia. Effects of slow and rapid hemodialysis. *Kidney Int* 4:177, 1973.
10. Henrich, WL. Hemodynamic instability during hemodialysis. *Kidney Int* 30:605, 1986.
11. Vinay, P, Prud'homme, M, Vinet, B, et al. Acetate metabolism and bicarbonate generation during hemodialysis: 10 years of observation. *Kidney Int* 31:1194, 1987.
12. Vincent, JL, Vanherwegham, JL, Degante, JP, Berre, J, Dufaye, P, Kahn, R. Acetate induced myocardial depression during hemodialysis for acute renal failure. *Kidney Int* 22:653, 1982.
13. Palder, SB, Kirkman, RL, Whittemore, MD, Hakim, RM, Lazarus, JM, Tilney, NL. Vascular access for hemodialysis. *Ann Surg* 202:235, 1985.
14. Schwab, SJ, Saeed, M, Sussman, SK, McCann, RL, Stickel, DL. Transluminal angioplasty of venous stenoses in polytetrafluorethylene vascular access grafts. *Kidney Int* 32:395, 1987.
15. Wegmuller, E, Montanson, A, Nydegger, U, Descoeudres, C. Biocompatibility of different hemodialysis membranes: Activation of complement and leukopenia. *Int J Artif Org* 9:85, 1986.
16. Bint, AJ, Finch, RG, Gokal, R, Goldsmith, HF, Junor, B, Oliver, D. Diagnosis and management of peritonitis in continuous ambulatory peritoneal dialysis. *Lancet* 1:845, 1987.
17. Nolph, KD, Miller, FN, Pyle, WK, Sorkin, MI. An hypothesis to explain the ultrafiltration characteristics of peritoneal dialysis. *Kidney Int* 20:543, 1981.
18. Mactier, RA, Khanna, R, Twardowski, ZJ, Nolph, KD. Role of peritoneal cavity lymphatic absorption in peritoneal dialysis. *Kidney Int* 32:165, 1987.
19. Amair, P, Khanna, R, Leibel, B, Perratos, A, Vas, S, Meema, E, Blair, G, Chisolm, L, Vas, M, Zingg, W, Digenis, G, Oreopoulos, D. Continuous ambulatory peritoneal dialysis in diabetics with end-stage renal disease. *N Engl J Med* 306:625, 1982.

60. RENAL TRANSPLANTATION

The first renal transplants in humans were performed in the early 1950s when cadaver kidneys were placed into patients with end-stage renal disease [1]. Some kidneys initially functioned well enough to reverse most of the signs and symptoms of uremia. Within 3 to 5 months, however, all of the transplanted kidneys had failed due to rejection, which represents an immunologic reaction directed against the foreign antigens in the graft.

An inability to prevent rejection limited the use of renal transplantation for the next 10 years, so that by 1960 less than 30 transplants had been performed in the United States. It was not until 1961 that the routine use of prednisone and azathioprine allowed transplantation to become a feasible alternative to dialysis. Since that time, newer, more potent, and in some cases more selective immunosuppressive agents have been developed, and our understanding of the immunologic mechanisms of rejection has been enhanced. Both of these factors have contributed to the generally better patient survival currently seen with living related donor transplants when compared with dialysis [2]. The results are presently not quite so good with cadaveric transplantation where patient survival is essentially the same as that on dialysis [3]. The quality of life, however, is likely to be higher with a well-functioning transplant.

Patient Selection

Many more patients are now being considered for renal transplantation, in part because the age limit is increasing. Patient age between 60 and 65 is not now a preclusion to transplantation, whereas an upper limit of 50 was initially recommended. Occasionally, even older patients may be transplanted if they have a strong desire to undergo this procedure and are otherwise healthy, or if they have been doing poorly on dialysis.

In some cases, concomitant medical problems can preclude transplantation. For example, active infection or malignancy are general contraindications because these conditions can be exacerbated by the immunosuppression induced by antirejection therapy. However, transplantation can usually be safely performed if the patient has been tumor-free for at least 1 to 2 years [4]. Even patients with coronary artery disease can be transplanted, although initial coronary revascularization may be necessary in some cases.

The problem of recurrent disease in the transplant will be discussed. Although this is a common complication, loss of the graft to recurrent disease is unusual; as a result, the cause of the primary renal disease does not generally influence the decision concerning transplantation, although some high-risk patients can be identified.

Tissue Typing for Renal Transplantation

The initial step in matching the donor and recipient is to be certain that the major blood group (ABO) antigens are compatible. This is of critical importance because these antigens are localized on vascular endothelium. A major blood group mismatch typically results in an antibody-mediated "hyperacute" rejection beginning while the recipient is still on the operating room table. Rh antigens appear to be less important, in part because they are confined to circulating red blood cells.

Once it is clear that the blood groups are well matched, histocompatibility typing is initiated. The single genetic complex in mammalian species that codes for the major cell-surface antigens capable of eliciting a rejection response is referred to as the *major histocompatibility complex* (MHC). In humans, these proteins are called human leukocyte antigen (HLA) antigens and are encoded on the short arm of chromosome 6.

The HLA antigens, each of which has many alleles, are divided into two classes on the basis of their tissue distribution, function, and structure [5]. *Class I* antigens (primarily HLA-A -B, and -C) are present on *all nucleated cells* and serve as the primary targets for cytotoxic T lymphocytes when there is incompatibility during renal transplantation [5,6]. Matching for HLA-A and -B* is performed serologically (using sera containing antibodies directed against identified antigens) and is especially important in living related donor transplantation. For example, graft survival at 1 year (before the use of cyclosporine) was *85 to 90* percent for HLA identical siblings who were matched at the A and B loci of each chromosome pair (a four-antigen match); in comparison, graft survival at 1 year fell to *70 to 75* percent if only one chromosome was shared with the donor (a one-haplotype match from a sibling, parent, or child in which two of the four A and B antigens were shared). The results tended to be even worse in a living donor with a four-antigen mismatch (in which neither chromosome was shared); in this setting, 1-year graft survival was similar to that in cadaver transplants, being *45 to 55* percent (prior to cyclosporine) [7].†

Matching for HLA-A and B appears to produce a more modest improvement in cadaveric graft survival, with the difference between the best- and worst-matched groups averaging 15 to 25 percent [8,9]. This difference from living related donor transplantation appears to be related in part to incompatibility at the class II, *HLA-D* region [9,10]. Since

---

*The HLA-C antigens appear to be relatively unimportant determinants of transplant survival.
†The results of cadaveric and living related donor transplantation have improved substantially with the addition of cyclosporine, with 1-year graft survival now being above 75 and 90 percent, respectively [7].

both chromosomes come from the same parents, matching at the A and B loci in a sibling-to-sibling transplant should, in the absence of genetic recombination, lead to concordance for the D antigens. In contrast, a four-antigen A and B match is less likely to guarantee identity at the D locus in an unrelated cadaver donor, due to the large number of possible alleles.

The products of the HLA-D region are referred to as *Class II* antigens. They have a more restricted location than the class I antigens, being found primarily on macrophages, B cells, activated T cells, and to a lesser degree vascular endothelial cells, where they serve as the primary targets for helper T cells during transplant rejection [5]. Compatibility between the HLA-D regions of the donor and recipient (and the likelihood of graft survival) can be determined by the standard mixed lymphocyte culture (MLC). This assay, which takes 5 to 7 days to complete, measures the ability of radiation-inactivated donor lymphocytes to stimulate intact recipient lymphocytes in tissue culture. A proliferative response of recipient cells, as assessed by uptake of radiolabelled thymidine, indicates reaction against foreign HLA antigens (a form of in vitro rejection) and is primarily triggered by the HLA-D region.

Although useful in living related transplants, the MLC response cannot be used prospectively for cadaveric testing because of the length of time required. This obstacle has been overcome in part by serologic typing for loci within the HLA-D region (the best studied being HLA-DR) [5]. HLA-DR incompatibility, by activating helper T cells, seems to be largely responsible for induction of the immune reaction against the graft. This response is directed against class II antigens expressed on the vascular endothelial cells in the peritubular capillaries and glomeruli and on macrophage-like *dendritic cells* in the renal interstitium [5,7,11]. Testing for histocompatibility at the HLA-DR locus has enhanced graft survival in cadaveric transplants, even when cyclosporine has been used [9,12].

Pretransplant Crossmatch
In addition to ABO blood group compatibility and HLA matching, a negative pretransplant crossmatch looking for circulating antibodies against HLA antigens is also required. This test is performed by incubating donor T and B cells with recipient serum in the presence of complement and observing for cytotoxicity (as evidenced by cell lysis) [13]. Antibodies against T cells (directed at HLA-A and B antigens) and possibly against B cells (recognizing HLA-D antigens) generally preclude transplantation to a donor with those antigens, since the rapid deposition of these circulating antibodies in the graft can lead to hyperacute rejection (see the following).

In addition to testing at the time of potential transplantation, routine crossmatching against known HLA antigens is usually performed at *monthly* intervals prior to transplantation. In general, a positive crossmatch against a specific antigen within the preceding 6 months is a contraindication to the use of a graft containing that antigen. However, antibody reactivity often decreases with time, possibly due to the development of anti-idiotypic antibodies that specifically down-regulate the immune response [14,15]. Consequently, transplantation is not contraindicated if a patient with a previously positive crossmatch against a specific antigen has had a negative response for at least 6 months.

Some recipients show reactivity against a large number of HLA antigens, despite having been directly exposed to only a few of these antigens via pregnancy, blood transfusions, a previous transplant, or possibly cross-reacting viral infections. This finding may be due to the fact that antibody responses are, in general, not very specific. Antibody production is not usually limited to one specific "private" HLA antigen (such as HLA-B8). More often, the antibody response is directed against "public" antigens, which are antigens that are common to several HLA gene products.

Pretransplant Blood Transfusions
Before the mid-1970s, pretransplant blood transfusions were avoided unless the patient was symptomatic or had coronary artery disease. The aim of this regimen was to minimize patient sensitization to the foreign HLA antigens on the donor white cells and platelets. It was subsequently demonstrated, however, that transfusions confer a substantial *advantage* in graft survival [16]. For example, in the precyclosporine era, pre-

viously transfused cadaver transplant recipients had 10 to 30 percent better graft survival at 1 to 2 years than recipients who had received no transfusions [16,17]. This benefit is in part dose related, being greatest in patients who had received more than 5 to 10 transfusions [16].

Two hypotheses have been developed to explain these findings. The first suggests that the improved graft survival results from patient selection [18]. Sensitization of the potential recipient by blood transfusions selects out those patients who are highly responsive to a given antigen and who therefore would be more likely to reject a graft containing that antigen. This mechanism may be particularly important in living related donor transplantation in which *donor-specific* transfusions are given. Those patients who become sensitized do not receive a transplant from that donor; the remaining nonresponders have a very high rate of transplant survival [19].

However, experimental studies suggest that third-party blood transfusions have a more important action as an immunosuppressive agent, perhaps by activating suppressor T cells. This is evidenced by improved graft function and fewer severe rejection episodes even in patients who were *not sensitized* by transfusions (and who therefore could not have benefited by selection) [16,19,20].

The future role of transfusions, however, is somewhat in doubt because their beneficial effect may be markedly attenuated by the use of cyclosporine [12,21] and by potential complications. In addition to sensitization of the recipient, they can cause transfusion reactions and transmit infectious agents. It is therefore possible that third-party transfusions will cease to be an integral part of the immunosuppressive regimen over the next decade.

Living Related Donor Evaluation

A potential renal transplant donor must be healthy, free of transmissible disease (HIV infection has been transmitted to the recipient after both living related and cadaveric transplantation [22])*, and psychologically stable. The donor cannot be hypertensive or exhibit any functional or anatomic renal abnormality that would increase the risk of surgery or injury to the remaining kidney.

The donor must be informed about the potential acute and chronic risks of kidney donation, as well as the alternatives available to the recipient. Presently, 1-year cadaveric graft survival rates are approaching those of living related transplants with the use of cyclosporine [24]. However, living related kidneys still function longer (10–15% better 1-year survival [25]) and surgery can be electively planned, thereby limiting the time spent on dialysis and avoiding the complications of organ preservation (such as acute tubular necrosis) that are common with cadaveric transplantation.

The short-term risks to the living related donor are small, since most postoperative complications are minor, with major problems occurring in less than 3 percent of cases [25]. The mortality rate is extremely low, averaging about one death per 1600 transplants [26].

One potential risk that at present remains unanswered is the long-term incidence in the donor of hypertension, proteinuria, and even renal insufficiency due to hemodynamically mediated injury to the remaining kidney (see Chap. 56). While some studies have suggested an increased risk of mild proteinuria and hypertension after 10 to 15 years [27], other reports have not observed a higher incidence in either of these parameters when compared to age-matched, related controls [28]. In the absence of longer follow-up, this controversy remains unresolved; most centers, however, believe that a living related transplant should be encouraged if the potential donor and recipient are well matched.

Renal Transplant Surgery

The native, poorly functioning kidneys are not routinely removed at the time of or prior to transplantation. Exceptions include persistent renal parenchymal infection, ex-

---

*In comparison to other transmissible infectious disorders, cytomegalovirus (CMV) positivity in the donor does not preclude organ donation, since the frequency of latent CMV infection is high in the general population. In this setting, the administration of CMV immune globulin to the recipient in the first few months after transplantation may be effective prophylaxis in patients at risk for primary CMV disease [23].

tremely large kidneys leading to inadequate room for the graft (as in a few patients with polycystic kidney disease), and intractable symptoms such as chronic pain.

The transplanted kidney is placed in the right or left lower quadrant of the abdomen outside the peritoneal cavity. The donor renal artery is anastomosed to the hypogastric artery of the recipient, and the donor ureter is implanted into the urinary bladder. Locating the graft in the lower abdomen has the advantage of easy access in the event of an anatomic problem or if renal transplant biopsy is required to diagnose rejection. While not as protected as the native kidneys, the transplant is unlikely to be injured during routine activities; participation in contact sports (such as tackle football or ice hockey), however, is not recommended.

Immunosuppressive Therapy and Its Complications

The major immunosuppressive drugs used to prevent rejection in renal transplantation are corticosteroids, azathioprine, cyclosporine and, in some centers, antilymphocyte or antithymocyte globulin. Many patients are treated with corticosteroids and cyclosporine alone, although the addition of azathioprine to this regimen has been increasingly used in an attempt to reduce cyclosporine nephrotoxicity (see the following and Chap. 61) [13]. Not surprisingly, major mismatches lead to early rejection as *most grafts are lost within the first 6 to 12 months* [9]. Thereafter, there is a slow attrition rate of less than 5 percent per year, due mostly to chronic rejection (see the following).

Corticosteroids
Corticosteroids are believed to directly impair antigen-driven T-cell proliferation. This effect appears to result from impaired release of interleukin-1 (IL-1) from monocytes [29], thereby blocking IL-1–dependent release of interleukin-2 (IL-2) from antigen activated helper T cells (Fig. 60-1). Since IL-2 is the mitogenic signal for T-cell growth, cell proliferation does not occur [30].

The initial dose of prednisone given to prevent renal transplant rejection is 30 mg/day when cyclosporine is administered concomitantly. Side effects attributable to this drug are well known and include the following: increased susceptibility to infection, easy bruising, acne, cushingoid appearance, excessive weight gain, psychosis, hyperlipidemia, hypertension, coronary atherosclerosis, ischemic necrosis of bone, osteoporosis, myopathy, posterior subcapsular cataracts, de novo insulin-dependent diabetes mellitus, delayed wound healing, and a possible increased risk of neoplasia when used in conjunction with other immunosuppressants. Despite these potential complications, rapid tapering to lower doses and avoidance of prolonged high-dose therapy has substantially reduced the rate and severity of complications associated with corticosteroids.

Azathioprine
Azathioprine is metabolized in the liver to 6-mercaptopurine, which exerts its immunosuppressive and myelosuppressive activity by disrupting normal purine metabolism, thus interfering with DNA synthesis and cell proliferation (Fig. 60-1). It causes preferential reduction in the number of natural killer cells, with lesser effects on suppressor/cytotoxic T cells [31].

The usual dose of azathioprine is 1 to 3 mg/kg/day. The dose must be reduced when allopurinol is used concurrently because allopurinol inhibits xanthine oxidase; in addition to its role in uric acid metabolism, this enzyme is also responsible for the further degradation of 6-mercaptopurine to the less toxic 6-thiouric acid. Failure to make this adjustment can lead to very high azathioprine levels and potentially fatal bone marrow suppression.

The two major side effects that azathioprine shares with corticosteroids are an increased susceptibility to infection (due to neutropenia) and late neoplasia [33]. Less common problems include alopecia, stomatitis, hepatitis (and rarely hepatic venoocclusive disease [32]), and thrombocytopenia. Macrocytic indices (with or without anemia) in the presence of normal folic acid and vitamin B_{12} levels are observed in many patients [33].

Cyclosporine
Cyclosporine is a fungal metabolite that has revolutionized organ transplantation. Since its approval by the Food and Drug Administration in November, 1983, graft survival has

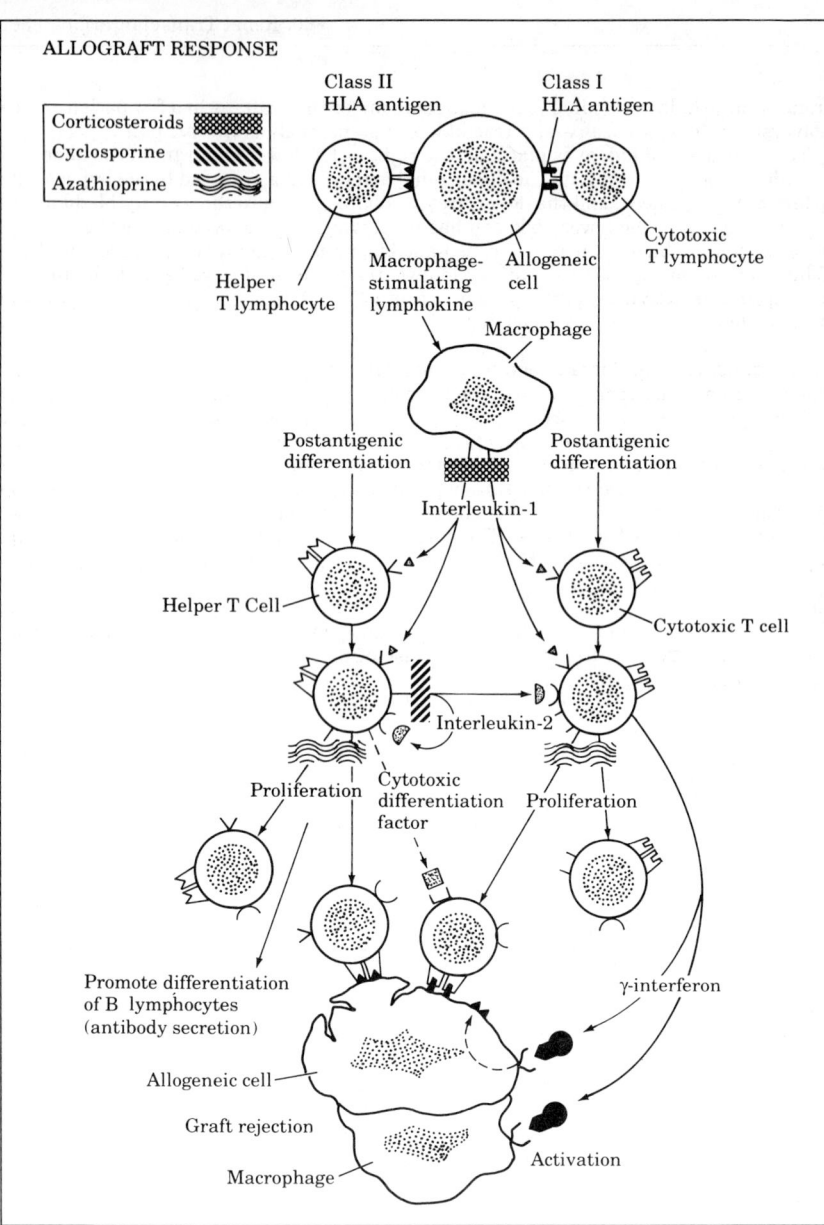

Fig. 60-1. Graft rejection is a complex process that results from the cytodestructive effects of B lymphocytes, helper T cells, cytotoxic T cells, and activated macrophages. Corticosteroids block the production of interleukin-1 (IL-1) by macrophages, thereby inhibiting the IL-1–induced release of interleukin-2 (IL-2) by helper T cells. Cyclosporine, on the other hand, prevents IL-2 production, an action that subsequently impairs the release of the macrophage-activating factor, γ-interferon. Azathioprine has a different mechanism of action, directly impairing cell proliferation. The combined effect of these agents serves to block antigen-driven T cell proliferation and B cell antibody production. (From Strom, TB, Tilney, NL. Immunobiology and immunopharmacology of graft rejection. In RW Schrier, CW Gottschalk (Eds.), *Diseases of the Kidney* (4th ed.). Boston: Little, Brown, 1988. P. 3194).

increased substantially. In several comparative trials, for example, cadaver graft survival rates at 1 year were 50 to 67 percent with corticosteroids and azathioprine versus 73 to 90 percent with corticosteroids and cyclosporine [34,35].

Unlike corticosteroids, cyclosporine does not inhibit the capacity of monocytes to release IL-1. Rather, it blocks IL-2 release from activated helper T lymphocytes via inhibition of messenger RNA (Fig. 60-1) [36,37]. This impairs the subsequent proliferation of helper T cells, antigen-stimulated cytotoxic T cells, and natural and lymphokine-activated killer cells, all of which are dependent on the availability of IL-2 [31,38]. On the other hand, cyclosporine appears to spare suppressor T cells, which may also contribute to its immunosuppressive action [39].

Cyclosporine is lipophilic and is usually administered orally or intravenously. Patients are generally started on 15 to 17 mg/kg/day with the dose decreased over time to 3 to 6 mg/kg/day, depending on the plasma creatinine concentration and blood cyclosporine levels. Cyclosporine levels can be increased by certain drugs, such as cimetidine, erythromycin, diltiazem, and verapamil, although the mechanism of these interactions is uncertain [38,40,41].

In comparison to azathioprine, cyclosporine has little myelosuppressive activity. It is not a panacea, however, since it does have major side effects, the most important of which is nephrotoxicity (see Chap. 61).* The addition of azathioprine to prednisone and cyclosporine or conversion from cyclosporine to azathioprine at 3 to 6 months has been used in an attempt to lower both cyclosporine dosage and subsequent renal injury [42,43]. The long-term efficacy of these regimens remains to be proved. Other adverse reactions to cyclosporine include hypertension, an increased susceptibility to infection and neoplasia, hepatotoxicity, gynecomastia, tremor, seizures, paresthesias, gingival hyperplasia, hypertrichosis, cramps, diarrhea, nausea, vomiting, and flushing [38].

Antilymphocyte and Antithymocyte Globulin
Antilymphocyte (ALG) and antithymocyte (ATG) globulin are produced in horses, goats, or rabbits by immunization with cultured human lymphoblasts (ALG) or thymocytes (ATG). These agents act by coating the surfaces of lymphocytes and causing their sequestration in the liver and spleen.

Side effects include susceptibility to infection and an allergic reaction to the foreign proteins that can lead to fever, chills, phlebitis, thrombocytopenia, leukopenia, serum sickness, and anaphylaxis [44]. These adverse reactions plus the availability of monoclonal antibodies (see the following) have limited the use of these agents to treat rejection, although they are still given for 2 to 3 weeks following transplantation in some centers in an attempt to prevent rejection during this high-risk period [44].

Renal Transplant Rejection
Rejection represents the immunologic response of the recipient against the transplanted kidney. The frequency of this process (which is most common in the first 3 posttransplant months) has been reduced by more potent immunosuppressive agents, but it is still the major cause of graft failure.

Three types of transplant rejection have been identified: hyperacute, acute, and chronic (Table 60-1). Although these disorders vary in their mechanism of tissue injury and time of onset after transplantation, it is not unusual for more than one type of rejection to be present in a given patient.

Hyperacute Rejection
Hyperacute rejection is characterized by the rapid loss of graft function, frequently occurring minutes to several hours after transplantation. In the most severe cases, this process begins during transplant surgery. Microscopic examination of the affected kidney initially reveals neutrophils in the glomerular and vascular walls followed by the widespread formation of platelet and fibrin thrombi, usually leading to total cortical

*Because of its potential for nephrotoxicity, cyclosporine is not typically administered in the immediate posttransplant period until an adequate urine output has been established.

Table 60-1. Types of transplant rejection

Feature	Hyperacute	Acute	Chronic
Onset after transplantation	Usually minutes to hours but may occur later	Usually weeks to months	Months to years
Pathology	Microvascular thrombosis with cortical necrosis; neutrophils in capillaries	Interstitial mononuclear infiltrate, ± necrotizing vasculitis	Arterial and arteriolar intimal thickening
Pathogenesis	Preformed antibodies against HLA antigens in transplant	Both cellular and humoral immunity	Probable combined effects of humoral and cellular immunity
Clinical features	Early loss of graft function	Fever, graft tenderness, hypertension, renal insufficiency	Slowly progressive renal failure, hypertension, and proteinuria
Treatment	Graft nephrectomy	High dose corticosteroids, monoclonal antibodies; less commonly, ALG or ATG	None

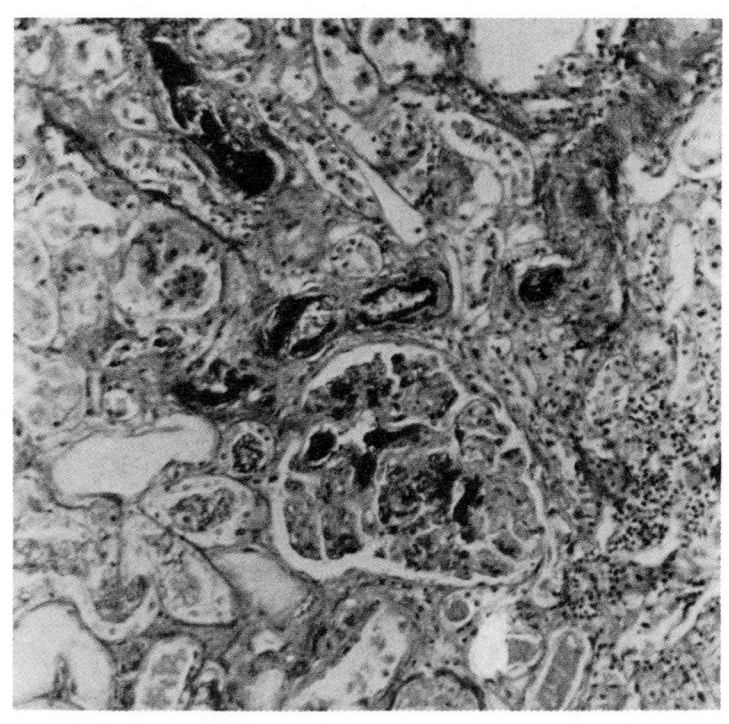

Fig. 60-2. Fibrin thrombi in a glomerulus and in the peritubular capillaries in a patient with hyperacute rejection.

necrosis and irreversible renal failure (Fig. 60-2). There is no effective therapy and transplant nephrectomy is generally required.

Preformed antibodies against donor antigens appear to be responsible for most cases of hyperacute rejection and can be due to ABO incompatibility or to sensitization from transfusions, pregnancy, or a previous transplant. Fortunately, this is now a rare problem because of present crossmatching techniques (see before), which can detect even very low levels of circulating cytotoxic antibodies.

Acute Rejection
Acute rejection is observed in transplant recipients without demonstrable preformed antibodies but with substantial antigenic differences from the donor. It can develop at any time, although most patients have some reaction (which is frequently reversible) within the first 3 posttransplant months. Clinical manifestations of acute rejection include tenderness and enlargement of the graft (although this appears to be less apparent in patients treated with cyclosporine), fever, hypertension, oliguria, and renal insufficiency. The urinary sediment is usually unremarkable, although mononuclear leukocytes (presumably representing cells involved in the rejection response) may be observed in the urinary sediment of some patients.

The primary histologic changes of acute rejection are seen in the interstitium, tubules, and blood vessels (Fig. 60-3). Interstitial infiltration with lymphocytes, lymphoblasts, and plasma cells are the earliest changes and are followed by tubular damage and atrophy. The tubulointerstitial changes in acute rejection are thought to be due to cellular

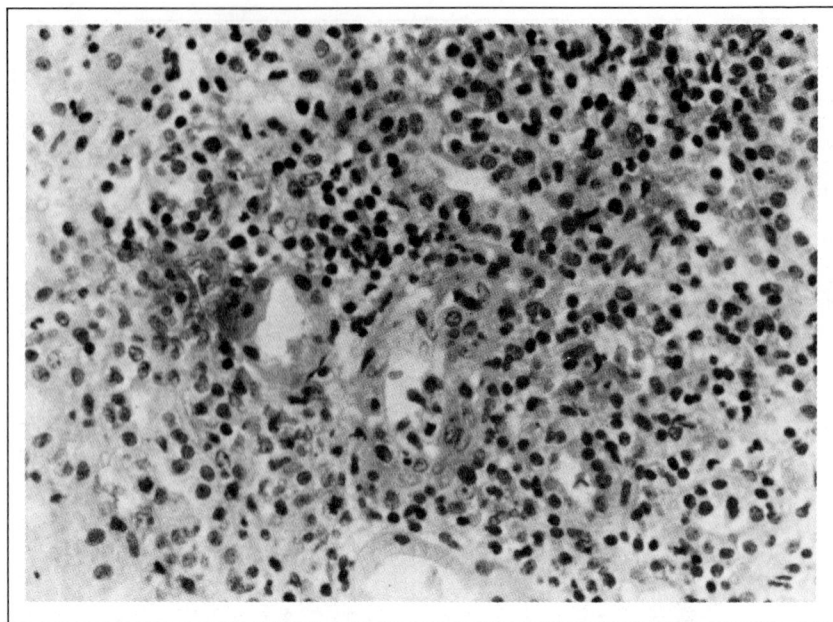

Fig. 60-3. Mononuclear cell infiltrate throughout the interstitium and tubules in acute rejection. Fibrin thrombi similar to those in hyperacute rejection also may be seen at this time.

immunity and may occur in the absence of vascular lesions (with neutrophilic infiltration of vessels and fibrinoid necrosis), which are believed to be caused by humoral mechanisms [13]. Both helper and suppressor/cytotoxic T cells have been identified in these infiltrates, suggesting that collaboration between helper and cytotoxic T cells are important in graft rejection (Fig. 60-1) [45,46].

Treatment of acute rejection first requires the exclusion of other factors that can cause renal insufficiency, such as cyclosporine toxicity or renal transplant obstruction. Ultrasonography and biopsy of the transplant may be required in some cases. With cyclosporine toxicity, for example, tubular injury and focal or diffuse interstitial fibrosis are usually seen (see Chap. 61). These changes are nondiagnostic but are clearly different from the prominent cellular infiltrate of acute rejection.

In the majority of patients, acute rejection responds to treatment with *bolus corticosteroids* (0.25–1.0 gm of intravenous methylprednisolone, given daily for 3–5 days) [13]. A positive response, as evidenced by reduced graft tenderness and a fall in the plasma creatinine concentration, is usually seen within 1 to 3 days. The resolution of fever is nonspecific, however, since high-dose corticosteroid therapy can suppress any febrile response because IL-1 (the release of which is inhibited by these drugs) is an endogenous pyrogen.

Although generally well tolerated, intravenous bolus methylprednisolone has been associated with hypertension, hyperosmolar coma, and rarely fatal ventricular arrhythmias [33]. Consequently, close monitoring is required.

In patients who do not respond to this regimen, *monoclonal OKT3 antibodies* (which have largely replaced ATG and ALG in the treatment of acute rejection) are administered for 10 to 14 days [47,48]. Cyclosporine should be temporarily discontinued during therapy, both to avoid excessive immunosuppression and to reduce nephrotoxicity. By comparison, maintaining prednisone and azathioprine may be beneficial by limiting the host antibody response generated against this foreign protein.

OKT3 antibody (which is administered intravenously over 5 minutes) reacts with the T3 molecule that is present in the cell membrane of all peripheral T cells, where it is required for antigen recognition. The drug appears to act by opsonizing this site, thereby causing the T cells to be removed by the reticuloendothelial system or rendering them incapable of generating an immunologic response. The net effect is that, beginning within minutes after infusion, T3-positive lymphocytes are depleted from the peripheral blood and subsequently from the renal transplant; these changes lead ultimately to reversal of rejection and the restoration of graft function [33,47,48].

OKT3 antibody appears to be effective in up to 90 percent of acute rejection episodes, with improvement beginning within 3 to 5 days after administration [33,47,48].* A variety of side effects may be seen, however, including high fever, chills, dyspnea, chest pain, wheezing, nausea, vomiting, and infection (frequently with cytomegalovirus [49]). Most of these complications occur on the first 2 days of therapy and appear to be related to the release of soluble mediators from the affected T cells [48]. Fatal pulmonary edema (due to a capillary leak syndrome) has also occurred, but appears to be limited to those patients who have mild-to-moderate volume overload before therapy is initiated. As a result, an increased extracellular volume is a contraindication to the use of this agent.

OKT3 antibody should probably be given for only one course, since host antibodies to the foreign protein develop that can lead to loss of effectiveness and possibly to severe adverse reactions during a second course [48]. Consequently, this agent is primarily used for corticosteroid-resistant rejection episodes.

A still experimental alternative to OKT3 antibody (or ATG) is the administration of a monoclonal antibody directed against the IL-2 receptor [50]. This antibody has an important theoretical advantage over OKT3. The latter is directed against all peripheral T cells and therefore induces generalized immunosuppression. In comparison, IL-2 receptors are found *only on activated T cells* and are upregulated by IL-2 itself; as a result, only those cells responding to the graft are removed with the IL-2 receptor antibody, thereby producing specific immunosuppression. Thus, this antibody may prove to be useful either in preventing or in treating acute rejection [50].

Chronic Rejection
In some patients, renal function deteriorates slowly several months to several years after transplantation without signs of acute rejection. Proteinuria, which may reach the nephrotic range, and hypertension commonly accompany the development of renal insufficiency.

The primary histologic changes in chronic rejection are found in the arteries and glomeruli [51]. The interlobular and arcuate arteries are typically the most severely affected, with the characteristic changes being intimal thickening, reduplication of the internal elastic membrane, and narrowing of the vascular lumen similar to that seen in progressive systemic sclerosis (see Chap. 42). The cellular infiltrate typical of acute rejection is usually sparse in chronic rejection and is composed of lymphocytes, plasma cells, and histiocytes. Progressive interstitial fibrosis and tubular atrophy may also occur as a secondary event.

How these changes occur is not well understood but both humoral and cellular immune mechanisms may be involved. Chronic rejection is characteristically unresponsive to modulation of the immunosuppressive regimen and eventually leads to loss of graft function.

Recurrent Disease in the Transplanted Kidney
Although rejection and cyclosporine toxicity are the most common causes of renal insufficiency in the transplant recipient, recurrence of the primary renal disease (or a de novo glomerular disorder, such as membranous nephropathy) may occur [52]. In most cases, the recurrent disease does not appear to have an adverse long-term effect on graft function, but loss of the graft can occur in selected patients (Table 60-2 and the appropriate chapters elsewhere in the book). This is most likely to be seen when the primary disease

*Recurrence of acute rejection at some time after an apparently successful course of OKT3 antibody is not uncommon, occurring in up to 40 to 50 percent of cases.

Table 60-2. Recurrence rates and graft loss from recurrent glomerular disease[a]

Primary disease	Recurrence rate, %	Graft loss, %
Anti-GBM antibody disease	< 5[b]	< 1
Membranoproliferative GN, type II	> 85[c]	10–20
Membranoproliferative GN, type I	15–30[c]	30
Idiopathic RPGN	33	33
IgA nephropathy	50	< 10
Focal glomerulosclerosis	20–30[d]	10–15
Membranous nephropathy	50[c]	0
Lupus nephritis	< 5	< 1
Henoch-Schönlein purpura	0–33	0–25
Systemic vasculitis	Depends on disease activity	Some
Hereditary disorders		
Primary hyperoxaluria	Up to 100	Variable

[a]Adapted from Cameron, JS. *Kidney Int* 23(suppl. 14):24, 1983; and Ward, HJ, Farrer, JH, Rajfer, J, Glassock, RJ, Drumke, A. In Garovoy, MR, Guttman, RD (Eds.), *Renal Transplantation* New York: Churchill Livingstone, 1986. Chap. 11.
[b]Recurrence more likely if circulating anti-GBM antibody is present at the time of transplantation. Thus, the patient is maintained on dialysis, and transplantation is usually delayed 6 to 12 months to allow antibody formation to cease.
[c]Complement levels frequently normal when MPGN recurs in the transplant. In addition, de novo disease, occurring in patients in whom MPGN or membranous nephropathy was not the primary cause of renal failure, is not uncommon and may be related to transplant rejection.
[d]Recurrence rate may be substantially higher in patients with a rapidly progressive course prior to transplantation.

had a rapidly progressive course, causing end-stage renal disease within 1 to 3 years, or when there is a persistent metabolic disorder such as primary hyperoxaluria. With focal glomerulosclerosis, for example, the incidence of recurrent disease is about 50 percent in those with rapid progression versus only 10 to 20 percent in those with a more indolent initial course [53].

Even patients with primary hyperoxaluria, who in the past had almost universal graft loss due to recurrent calcium oxalate deposition within the kidney, can now be successfully transplanted [54]. This has been achieved by the use of combination therapy including neutral phosphate (which leads to increased urinary excretion of pyrophosphate, an inhibitor of calcium oxalate precipitation), magnesium (which binds to urinary oxalate to form the soluble magnesium oxalate salt), and pyridoxine (which can lower the rate of oxalate excretion by promoting the conversion of glyoxalate into glycine, rather than oxalate).

References

1. Hume, DM, Merrill, JP, Miller, BF, Thorn, GW. Experiences with renal homotransplantation in the human: Report of nine cases. *J Clin Invest* 34:327, 1955.
2. Terasaki, PI, Perdue, ST, Saaki, N, et al. Improving success rates of kidney transplantation. *J Am Med Assoc* 250:1065, 1983.
3. Vollmer, WM, Wahl, PW, Blagg, CR. Survival with dialysis and transplantation in patients with end-stage renal disease. *N Engl J Med* 308:1553, 1983.

4. Matas, AJ, Simmons, RL, Buselmeier, TJ, et al. Successful renal transplantation in patients with prior history of malignancy. *Am J Med* 59:791, 1975.
5. Bach, FH, Sachs, DH. Transplantation immunology. *N Engl J Med* 317:489, 1987.
6. Bach, FH, Bach, ML, Sondel, PM. Differential function of major histocompatibility complex antigens in T-lymphocyte activation. *Nature* 259:273, 1976.
7. Morris, PJ. Renal transplantation: Indications, outcome, complications, and results. In RW Schrier, CW Gottschalk (Eds.), *Diseases of the Kidney* (4th ed.). Boston: Little, Brown, 1988. P. 3229.
8. Persijn, GG, Cohen, B, Lansbergen, Q, et al. Effect of HLA-A and HLA-B matching on survival of grafts and recipients after renal transplantation. *N Engl J Med* 307:905, 1982.
9. Festenstein, MB, Doyle, P, Holmes, J. Long-term follow-up in London transplant group recipients of cadaver renal allografts. The influence of HLA matching on transplant outcome. *N Engl J Med* 314:7, 1986.
10. Conti, DJ, Andersen, R, Soper, WD, Wolf, JS. Comparison of clinical response of DR-matched, MLC-compatible cadaver renal allografts and those from HLA-identical related donors. *Transpl Proc* 19:652, 1987.
11. Lechler, RI, Batchelor, JR. Restoration of immunogenicity to passenger cell-depleted kidney allografts by the addition of donor strain dendritic cells. *J Exp Med* 155:31, 1982.
12. Lundgren, G, Albrachtsen, D, Flatmark, A, et al. HLA-matching and pretransplant blood transfusions in cadaveric renal transplantation—A changing picture with cyclosporin. *Lancet* 2:66, 1986.
13. Chan, L, Schrier, RW. New therapeutic protocols in kidney transplantation. *Sem Nephrol* 6:168, 1986.
14. Norman, DJ, Barry, JM, Boehne, C, Wetzstein, P. Natural history of patients who make cytotoxic antibodies following prospective fresh blood transfusions. *Transpl Proc* 17:1072, 1985.
15. Reed, E, Hardy, M, Benvenisty, A. Effect of anti-idiotypic antibodies to HLA on graft survival in renal-allograft recipients. *N Engl J Med* 316:1451, 1987.
16. Opelz, G, Terasaki, PI. Improvement of kidney-graft survival with increased numbers of blood transfusions. *N Engl J Med* 299:799, 1978.
17. D'Apice, AJF, Tah, BD. An elective transfusion policy: Sensitization rates, patient transplantability, and transplant outcome. *Transplantation* 33:191, 1982.
18. MacLeod, AM, Mason, RJ, Shewan, WG, et al. Possible mechanism of action of transfusion effect in renal transplantation. *Lancet* 2:468, 1982.
19. Light, JA, Metz, S, Oddenino, K. Donor-specific transfusion with minimal sensitization. *Transpl Proc* 15:917, 1983.
20. Anderson, CB, Sicard, GA, Etheredge, EE. Pretreatment of renal allograft recipients with azathioprine and donor-specific blood products. *Surgery* 92:315, 1982.
21. Kerman, RH, Flechner, SM, Van Buren, CTA, et al. Immunoregulatory mechanisms in cyclosporine-treated renal allograft recipients. *Transplantation* 43:205, 1987.
22. Prompt, CA, Reis, MM, Grillo, FM, et al. Transmission of AIDS virus at renal transplantation. *Lancet* 2:672, 1985.
23. Snydman, DR, Werner, BG, Heinze-Lacey, B. Use of cytomegalovirus immune globulin to prevent cytomegalovirus disease in renal-transplant recipients. *N Engl J Med* 317:1049, 1987.
24. The Canadian Multicentre Transplant Study Group. A randomized trial of cyclosporine in cadaveric renal transplantation: Analysis at three years. *N Engl J Med* 314:1219, 1986.
25. Weiland, D, Sutherland, DER, Chavers, B, Simmons, RL, Ascher, NL, Najarian, JS. Information on 628 living-related kidney donors at a single institution, with long-term follow-up in 472 cases. *Transpl Proc* 16:5, 1984.
26. Bay, WH, Hevert, LA. The living donor in kidney transplantation. *Ann Intern Med* 106:719, 1987.
27. Watnick, TJ, Jenkins, RR, Rackoff, P, et al. Microalbuminuria and hypertension in long-term renal donors. *Transplantation* 45:59, 1988.
28. Williams, SL, Oler, J, Jorkasky, DK. Long-term renal function in kidney donors: A comparison of donors and their siblings. *Ann Intern Med* 105:1, 1986.

29. Kern, JA, Lamb, RJ, Reed, JC, et al. Dexamethasone inhibition of interleukin 1 beta production by human monocytes. *J Clin Invest* 81:237, 1988.
30. Giles, S, Crabtree, GR, Smith, KA. Gluco-corticoid-induced inhibition of T cell growth factor production. I. The effect on mitogen-induced lymphocyte proliferation. *J Immunol* 123:1624, 1979.
31. Fahey, JL, Sarna, G, Gale, RP, Seeger, R. Immune interventions in disease. *Ann Intern Med* 106:257, 1987.
32. Read, AE, Wiesner, RH, LaBrecque, DR. Hepatic veno-occlusive disease associated with renal transplantation and azathioprine therapy. *Ann Intern Med* 104:651, 1986.
33. Council on Scientific Affairs. Introduction to the management of immunosuppression. *J Am Med Assoc* 257:1781, 1987.
34. Canadian Multicentre Transplant Study Group. A randomized clinical trial of cyclosporine in cadaveric renal transplantation: An analysis at 3 years. *N Engl J Med* 314:1219, 1986.
35. Calne, RY, Thiru, S, McMaster, P, et al. Cyclosporin A in patients receiving renal allografts from cadaver donors. *Lancet* 2:1323, 1978.
36. Dermani-Arab, V, Salehmoghaddam, S, Danovitch, G, Hirji, K, Rezai, A. Mediation of the antiproliferative effect of cyclosporine on human lymphocytes by blockage of interleukin-2 biosynthesis. *Transplantation* 39:439, 1985.
37. Elliott, JF, Lin, Y, Mizel, SB, et al. Induction of interleukin 2 messenger RNA inhibited by cyclosporin A. *Science* 226:1439, 1984.
38. Cohen, DJ, Loertscher, R, Rubin, MF, et al. Cyclosporine: A new immunosuppressive agent for organ transplantation. *Ann Intern Med* 101:667, 1984.
39. Hutchinson, IF, Shadur, CA, Duarte, AJS, Strom, TB, Tilney, NL. Cyclosporine A spares selectively lymphocytes with donor specific suppressor characteristics. *Transplantation* 32:210, 1981.
40. Poochet, JM, Pirson, Y. Cyclosporin-diltiazem interaction. *Lancet* 1:979, 1986.
41. Peterson, JC, Brannigan, J, Pickard, T, Thompson, R. Cyclosporine-verapamil interaction (abstract). *Kidney Int* 33:449, 1988.
42. Lorber, MI, Flechner, SM, Van Buren, CT, Sorensen, K, Kerman, Kahan, BD. Cyclosporine toxicity: The effect of combined therapy using cyclosporine, azathioprine, and prednisone. *Am J Kid Dis* 9:476, 1987.
43. Morris, PJ, Allen, RD, Thompson, JF, Chapman, JR, Ting, A, Dunnhill, MS. Cyclosporin conversion versus conventional immunosuppression: Long-term follow-up and histologic evaluation. *Lancet* 1:586, 1987.
44. Monaco, AP. Antilymphocyte globulin: A clinical transplantation research opportunity. *Am J Kid Dis* 2:67, 1982.
45. Steinmuller, D. Which T cells mediate allograft rejection? *Transplantation* 40:229, 1985.
46. Strom, TB. The cellular and molecular basis of allograft rejection: What do we know? *Transplant Proc* 20:143, 1988.
47. Monoclonal antibodies for kidney allograft rejection. *The Medical Letter* 28:97, 1986.
48. Ortho Multicentre Transplant Study Group. A randomized clinical trial of OKT3 monoclonal antibody for acute rejection of cadaveric renal transplants. *N Engl J Med* 313:337, 1985.
49. Hawkins, R, Burgess, E, Klassen, J. High incidence of cytomegalovirus infections in allograft recipients receiving anti-OKT3 monoclonal antibodies (abstract). *Kidney Int* 33:444, 1988.
50. Soulillou, JP, Peyronnet, P, Le Mauff, B, et al. Prevention of rejection of kidney transplants by monoclonal antibody directed against interleukin 2. *Lancet* 1:1339, 1987.
51. Mathew, ATH, Mathews, DC, Hobbs, JB, Kincaid-Smith, P. Glomerular lesions after renal transplantation. *Am J Med* 59:177, 1975.
52. Cameron, JS. Effect of the recipient's disease on the results of transplantation (other than diabetes mellitus). *Kidney Int* 23 (suppl 14):S-14, 1983.
53. Lewis, EJ. Recurrent focal sclerosis after renal transplantation. *Kidney Int* 22:315, 1982.
54. Scheinman, JI, Najarian, JS, Mauer, SM. Successful strategies for renal transplantation in primary oxalosis. *Kidney Int* 25:804, 1984.

61. CYCLOSPORINE NEPHROTOXICITY

Cyclosporine is presently the most potent immunosuppressive agent used routinely for organ transplantation. Its widespread availability has had a major impact by reducing the frequency and severity of early (first 6 months) renal allograft rejection. As a result, present 1- and 2-year cadaver graft survival rates using this medication have approached (but not equalled) those from living related donors [1]. Cyclosporine has also been used in heart and liver transplantation and with some success in a variety of autoimmune diseases, such as rheumatoid arthritis, uveitis, and insulin-dependent (type 1) diabetes mellitus.

The principal action of cyclosporine appears to result from the preferential inhibition of helper (T4-positive) T-cell activation, thereby blocking interleukin-II (IL-2) production [2]. The net effect is potent immunosuppression, since IL-2 normally has at least two important effects: it permits broad expansion of T cells, including both helper/inducer and suppressor/cytotoxic subsets; and it stimulates production of natural and lymphokine-activated killer cells [3].

Despite the beneficial effects of cyclosporine, its use has often been limited by the development of nephrotoxicity in up to two-thirds of patients [2,4]. The associated decline in renal function is most often mild and reversible. However, recent observations have demonstrated that renal insufficiency increases with time and may be severe and sometimes permanent [4]. Moreover, cyclosporine can also lead to hyperkalemia and hypertension, even in patients who have only a mild reduction in the glomerular filtration rate.

Pathophysiology

Evaluation of the mechanisms underlying cyclosporine nephrotoxicity has been limited, in part, because there is as yet no laboratory model that mimics the changes found in humans.* Furthermore, the pathologic findings in cyclosporine nephropathy, which will be discussed, are nonspecific and, therefore, can be seen with other forms of renal injury.

Certain pathophysiologic effects of cyclosporine are well understood, in particular vasoconstriction. Rat aorta segments contract in response to cyclosporine, an effect blocked by calcium channel blockers [5]. Cyclosporine also increases both afferent and efferent glomerular arteriolar resistances [6]. The reduction in the glomerular filtration rate in this setting can be diminished by converting enzyme inhibition, suggesting that angiotensin II is involved, perhaps by causing an increase in the cell calcium concentration [6]. Abnormal prostanoid metabolism, as evidenced by increased renal production of thromboxane B_2, also may play an important role in this renal vasoconstriction [6a].

The irreversibility of renal dysfunction in some patients may be initiated by these ischemic changes, but direct damage to renal arterioles (and, to a lesser degree, proximal tubules) has also been observed [4,7]. Endothelial damage, for example, could contribute to the association between cyclosporine and renal failure due to the hemolytic-uremic syndrome [4]. In addition, cyclosporine-induced proliferation of interstitial mononuclear cells or fibroblasts may result in the fibrosis often observed in chronic cyclosporine nephrotoxicity (see the following).

Clinical Syndromes of Cyclosporine Nephrotoxicity

Four types of renal failure may be caused by cyclosporine: acute, occurring immediately after renal transplantation; subacute, persisting for months after transplantation but reversing after discontinuation of cyclosporine or a reduction in dosage; chronic (sometimes progressive) irreversible renal failure; and the hemolytic-uremic syndrome (discussed in Chap. 43) [4].

---

*The dog and rat are less susceptible to cyclosporine injury than humans. Furthermore, the mechanisms of toxicity may be different in different species. For example, cyclosporine reduces renal blood flow in humans and rats but stimulates angiotensin II production only in the rat.

Acute Posttransplant Renal Failure
Acute renal failure immediately after renal transplantation is most commonly due to acute tubular necrosis, resulting from a long ischemic time between harvesting the cadaver kidney and transplantation. However, early acute renal failure also has been observed in patients receiving cyclosporine for heart and liver transplants, suggesting drug-mediated disease in at least some cases [4,8].

The pathogenesis of cyclosporine-induced acute renal failure is unknown. However, a low-fractional excretion of sodium and high plasma renin activity in some patients suggests that vasoconstriction and renal ischemia may be the initiating event; ischemic injury could then contribute to the prolonged renal failure that may be observed in this setting [8,9]. As a result, many centers do not initiate cyclosporine until an adequate urine output is established following renal transplantation.

Subacute (Reversible) Renal Failure
The use of cyclosporine has been complicated by a reduction in the glomerular filtration rate with a benign urinalysis in up to 70 percent of patients [4]. This is usually accompanied by a gradual rise in the plasma creatinine concentration over a period of weeks or months after therapy is instituted. However, increased tubular secretion of creatinine may, at first, mask the fall in glomerular filtration by minimizing the rise in the plasma creatinine concentration (see Chap. 17) [10]. The decline in renal function may stabilize, but progressive renal failure is common with prolonged use (see the following) [4,11].

The presence of cyclosporine nephrotoxicity is easily recognized when the drug is given for extrarenal disorders. These include heart, liver, and corneal transplants as well as autoimmune diseases, such as insulin-dependent diabetes mellitus or uveitis [11-13].

In comparison, the diagnosis of cyclosporine nephrotoxicity is more difficult in renal transplantation, since it must be differentiated from allograft rejection. Although a high blood level (> 300–400 μg/L) of cyclosporine may suggest drug-induced nephrotoxicity, a renal biopsy is frequently necessary to distinguish between these disorders.

Pathologically, the kidney in cyclosporine nephropathy initially reveals tubular injury with vacuoles, inclusion bodies, and giant mitochondria in the proximal tubules; focal or diffuse interstitial fibrosis are later findings [4,7,11]. However, these abnormalities in isolation are neither sensitive nor specific enough to be diagnostic. Consequently, the diagnosis of cyclosporine nephrotoxicity is one of exclusion, being made on the basis of impaired renal function in the absence of pathologic evidence of transplant rejection (such as an interstitial lymphocytic infiltrate) or other apparent cause of renal failure.

The response to therapy also may be helpful. With cyclosporine nephrotoxicity, a reduction in drug dosage often leads to a fall in the plasma creatinine concentration within a few days. For example, the plasma creatinine concentration in renal transplant recipients treated with cyclosporine is about 0.6 mg/dl higher than in those treated with azathioprine (for example, 2.1 versus 1.5 mg/dl with relatively well functioning grafts); this difference can usually be reversed by switching from cyclosporine to azathioprine [1].

Chronic (Irreversible) Renal Failure
Early studies in renal transplant recipients suggested that the nephrotoxicity from cyclosporine was generally reversible and that progressive disease, when observed, was usually due to chronic rejection. However, studies in heart transplant recipients receiving cyclosporine have shown that *renal function often declines continually with time, even when lower doses are given* (Fig. 61-1) [13a]. Furthermore, maintenance of normal renal function in this setting is rare after 2 years [11a] with some patients progressing to end-stage renal disease [11,11a,13a]. Irreversible renal failure has also been reported in patients treated with cyclosporine for uveitis [13] or the prevention of corneal transplant rejection [12], most of whom received a relatively high dose of greater than 7.5 to 10.0 mg/kg/day.

The pathologic findings in these patients may be nonspecific. They include evidence of irreversibility, such as focal or diffuse interstitial fibrosis, microcalcifications, and tubular atrophy, along with focal and segmental glomerular sclerosis [4]. However, most

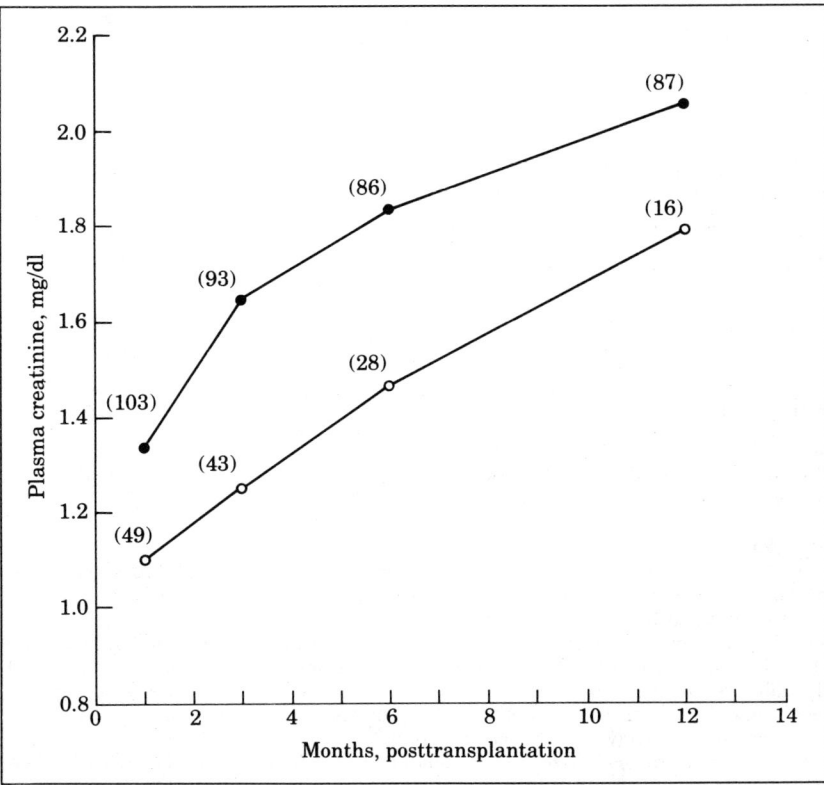

Fig. 61-1. Mean plasma creatinine concentration during the first year following heart transplantation in patients treated with cyclosporine in either high (approximately 7 mg/kg, solid circles) or low (4 mg/kg, open circles) doses. Although the plasma creatinine concentration is initially lower with reduced dosage, the same progressive rise with time is seen in both treatment groups. The numbers in parentheses refer to the number of patients treated at each point in time. (From BD Myers. *Kidney Int* 30:964, 1986. Reprinted by permission from Kidney International.)

patients also have a prominent obliterative arteriopathy that is highly suggestive of cyclosporine nephropathy [13a].

In an attempt to avoid or limit nephrotoxicity, many centers now use triple therapy with prednisone, azathioprine, and cyclosporine, a regimen that may allow lower doses of cyclosporine to be administered [14]. Alternatively, some transplant centers use cyclosporine and prednisone in the early posttransplant period but then substitute azathioprine for cyclosporine at 3 to 6 months. The latter protocol has reduced the degree of renal impairment in most patients but has also been associated with a higher frequency of renal transplant rejection in some [15,16], but not all [17] studies. The timing of this change in therapy may be important; use of cyclosporine for more than 1 year may be associated with progressive renal injury, even after cyclosporine has been discontinued [13a].

Another possible alternative, which has been evaluated in experimental animals, is interfering with the increase in renal thromboxane synthesis by giving cyclosporine in fish oil containing eicosapentaenoic acid [6a]. This regimen partially reverses the de-

Table 61-1. Causes of posttransplant hypertension*

Immunosuppressive therapy
  Corticosteroids
  Cyclosporine
Renal insufficiency
  Chronic transplant rejection
  Recurrent disease developing in the renal transplant
Potentially surgically correctable disorders
  Allograft renal artery stenosis
  Hypertension caused by native kidneys
Other speculative etiologies
  Recurrent essential hypertension
  De novo essential hypertension from donor kidney

*Adapted from RG Luke. *Kidney Int* 31:1024, 1987. Reprinted by permission from Kidney International.

cline in the glomerular filtration rate and minimizes the degree of tubular injury. Its applicability to humans remains to be established.

Hyperkalemia

Serum potassium concentrations are characteristically higher in patients receiving cyclosporine and prednisone (Cy-P) than in those on conventional immunosuppressive therapy with azathioprine and prednisone (Aza-P) [18]. Hyperkalemia is often associated with a normal anion gap metabolic acidosis but normal urinary acidification (urine pH < 5.5), findings suggestive of aldosterone resistance or deficiency (see Chap. 11). Hypoaldosteronism has been documented in some cases [19] but, in others, aldosterone secretion has apparently been normal [20]. A direct tubular defect limiting potassium secretion may be involved in the latter setting.

It is important to emphasize that incidence and severity of hyperkalemia are likely to be enhanced when potassium handling is already impaired. This problem may be seen in cyclosporine-treated patients who have underlying renal insufficiency or who are concomitantly taking β-adrenergic blockers, converting enzyme inhibitors, nonsteroidal anti-inflammatory drugs, or potassium-sparing diuretics (see Chap. 11).

Hypertension

The major causes of hypertension following renal transplantation are listed in Table 61-1, with chronic transplant rejection probably being most common [21]. However, the frequency of hypertension in patients receiving Cy-P appears to be substantially higher than in those treated with Aza-P (67 versus 45%), suggesting that cyclosporine may directly raise the blood pressure [22]. This hypothesis is supported by an increased frequency of hypertension in cyclosporine-treated recipients of bone marrow and heart transplants [23,24].

The pathogenesis of cyclosporine-associated hypertension is unclear, but renal insufficiency with secondary volume expansion may be important. Vasoconstriction due to a direct vascular effect [6] or to drug-induced inhibition of endothelial prostacyclin synthesis [25] also may play a contributory role. In comparison, the renin-angiotensin and sympathetic nervous systems do not seem to be involved.

Cyclosporine-associated hypertension is a relatively late finding, perhaps because its presence is masked by fewer rejection episodes than seen with conventional immunosuppressive agents [4]. In a recent study of 200 patients, for example, there was no difference in the frequency of hypertension in patients treated with Cy-P or Aza-P at 1 and 6 months following transplantation [26]. By 1 to 2 years, however, the level of blood pressure (or the need for antihypertensive therapy) was substantially greater in patients receiving cyclosporine.

Cyclosporine-induced hypertension may respond to a reduction in drug dosage, if indicated. Alternatively, conventional antihypertensive therapy should be instituted if the diastolic blood pressure remains above 90 to 95 mm Hg. Diuretic-induced hypokalemia is less of a problem in this setting than in normals, probably due to the cyclosporine-induced defect in potassium excretion. On the other hand, hyperkalemia may become more prominent if a converting enzyme inhibitor is used, due to the associated reduction in the release of aldosterone (which is normally stimulated by angiotensin II). As a result, the plasma potassium concentration should be monitored carefully when a converting enzyme inhibitor is added to cyclosporine.

References

1. Canadian Multicentre Transplant Study Group. A randomized clinical trial of cyclosporine in cadaveric renal transplantation: An analysis at 3 years. *N Engl J Med* 314:1219, 1986.
2. Cohen, DJ, Loertscher, R, Rubin, MF, Tilney, NL, Carpenter, CB, Strom, TG. Cyclosporine: a new immunosuppressive agent for organ transplantation. *Ann Intern Med* 101:667, 1984.
3. Fahey, JL, Sarna, G, Gale, RP, Seeger, R. Immune interventions in disease. *Ann Intern Med* 106:257, 1987.
4. Myers, BD. Cyclosporine nephrotoxicity. *Kidney Int* 30:964, 1986.
5. Xue, H, Bukoski, RD, McCarron, DA, Bennett, WM. Induction of contraction of isolated rat aorta by cyclosporine. *Transplantation* 43:715, 1987.
6. Barros, EJG, Boim, MA, Ajzen H, Ramos OL, Schor, N. Glomerular hemodynamics and hormonal participation on cyclosporine nephrotoxicity. *Kidney Int* 32:19, 1987.
6a. Elzinga, L, Kelley, VE, Houghton, DC, Bennett, WM. Modification of experimental nephrotoxicity with fish oil as the vehicle for cyclosporine. *Transplantation* 43:271, 1987.
7. Humes, HD, Jackson, NM, O'Connor, RP, Hunt, DA, and White, MD. Pathogenetic mechanisms of nephrotoxicity: Insights into cyclosporine nephrotoxicity. *Transplant Proc* 17 (suppl 1):51, 1985.
8. Powell-Jackson, PR, Young, B, Calne, RY, Williams, R. Nephrotoxicity of parenterally administered cyclosporine after orthotopic liver transplantation. *Transplantation* 36:505, 1983.
9. Canadian Multicentre Transplant Group. A randomized clinical trial of cyclosporine in cadaveric renal transplantation. *N Engl J Med* 309:809, 1983.
10. Ross, EA, Wilkinson, A, Hawkins, RA, Danovitch, GM. The plasma creatinine concentration is not an accurate reflection of the glomerular filtration rate in stable renal transplant patients receiving cyclosporine. *Am J Kid Dis* 10:113, 1987.
11. Myers, BD, Ross, J, Newton, K. Luetscher, J, Perlroth, M. Cyclosporine-associated chronic nephropathy. *N Engl J Med* 311:699, 1984.
11a. Greenberg, JW, Engel, ME, Thompson, ME, et al. Early and late forms of cyclosporine nephrotoxicity: Studies in cardiac transplant recipients. *Am J Kid Dis* 9:12, 1987.
12. Nahman, NS, Jr, Cosia, FG, Olkin, SK, Mendell, JR, Sharma, HM. Cyclosporine nephrotoxicity without major organ transplantation. *Ann Intern Med* 106:400, 1987.
13. Palestine, AG, Austin, HA, Balow, JE, Antonovych, TT, Sabnis, SG, Preuss, HG, Nussenblatt. Renal histopathologic alterations in patients treated with cyclosporine for uveitis. *N Engl J Med* 314:1293, 1986.
13a. Myers, BD, Sibley, R, Newton, L, et al. The long-term course of cyclosporine-associated chronic nephropathy. *Kidney Int* 33:590, 1988.
14. Lorber, MI, Flechner, SM, Van Buren, CT, Sorensen, K, Kerman, Kahan, BD. Cyclosporine toxicity: The effect of combined therapy using cyclosporine, azathioprine, and prednisone. *Am J Kid Dis* 9:476, 1987.
15. Flechner, SM, Van Buren, CT, Jarowenko, M. The fate of patients converted from cyclosporine to azathioprine to improve renal function. *Transplant Proc* 17:1227, 1985.
16. Morris, PJ, Allen, RD, Thompson, JF, Chapman, JR, Ting, A, Dunnhill, MS. Cyclosporin conversion versus conventional immunosuppression: Long-term follow-up and histologic evaluation. *Lancet* 1:586, 1987.
17. Hoitsma, AJ, van Lier, HJJ, Wetzels, JFM, Berden, JHM, Berden, JHM, Koene, RAP.

Cyclosporin treatment with conversion after three months versus conventional immunosuppression in renal allograft recipients. *Lancet* 1:584, 1987.

18. European Multicentre Trial. Cyclosporine A as sole immunosuppressive agent in recipients of kidney allografts from cadaver donors. *Lancet* 2:57, 1982.

19. Adu, D, Michael, J, Turney, J. Hyperkalemia in cyclosporine-treated renal allograft recipients. *Lancet* 2:370, 1983.

20. Bantle, JP, Nath, KA, Sutherland, DER, Najarian, JS, Ferris, TF. Effect of cyclosporine in the renin-angiotensin system and potassium excretion in renal transplant recipients. *Arch Intern Med* 145:505, 1985.

21. Luke, RG. Hypertension in renal transplant recipients. *Kidney Int* 31:1024, 1987.

22. Hamilton, DV, Carmichael, DJS, Evans, DB. Hypertension in renal transplant recipients on cyclosporin A and corticosteroids and azathioprine. *Transplant Proc* 14:597, 1982.

23. Barrett, AJ, Kendra, JR. Cyclosporine A as prophylaxis against graft-versus-host disease in 36 patients. *Br Med J* 285:162, 1982.

24. Bellet, M, Cabrol, C, Sassano, F, et al. Systemic hypertension after cardiac transplantation: Effect of cyclosporine on the renin angiotensin aldosterone system. *Am J Cardiol* 56:927, 1985.

25. Neild, GH, Ivory, K, Williams, DG. Glomerular thrombi and infarction in rabbits with serum sickness following cyclosporine therapy. *Transplant Proc* 15:2782, 1982.

26. Jarowenko, MV, Flechner, SM, Van Buren, CAT, et al. Influence of cyclosporine on posttransplant blood pressure response. *Am J Kid Dis* 10:98, 1987.

INDEX

INDEX

☑ I accept your invitation to become a subscriber to <u>Medical Rounds</u>. Enter my subscription as I've indicated below, with this understanding: I may cancel my subscription at <u>any</u> time and receive a <u>complete</u> refund for **all** unmailed issues.

I'd like to pay by: (Prepayment is Required)
☐ Check or cash (payable to Medical Rounds in U.S. funds only)   ☐ MasterCard   ☐ VISA   ☐ Amex

Card number _____

Expires On _____

Signature _____
(Signature required to process credit card orders)

Name _____

Address _____

City, State, Zip _____

	Individual	Resident	Institution
U.S. & Possessions	$45.00	$22.00	$55.00
Canada & Foreign	$56.00	$29.00	$69.00
Special 3-Year Rate		$39.00	

NO STAMP OR ADDRESSING NEEDED. MAIL THIS ENVELOPE WITH YOUR PAYMENT OR CHARGE CARD INFORMATION TODAY. Prepayment required.

Y8IN01

New
in
1988!

The All-in-One Diagnostic and Therapeutic Tool for Staff Physicians and Residents

Medical Rounds

A new journal from Little, Brown — Publishers of the SPIRAL® Manual Series

4072

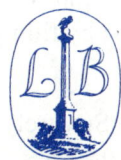

Inaugural Year Offer — Money-Back Guarantee
If You Are Not Completely Satisfied

Rush! New Journal Order!

Dear Physician:

How often have you wished, on rounds or in clinic, for really good, current reviews on common diseases or clinical syndromes?

Now you'll find those reviews in *Medical Rounds*, a uniquely useful new journal from Little, Brown, edited by Faith T. Fitzgerald, M.D., of the University of California at Davis.

The inaugural issue came out in February 1988 to rave reviews. And six times a year *Medical Rounds* will publish comprehensive, cohesive, and current reviews of important topics in internal medicine and its allied specialties. Reviews that are peer reviewed, extensively referenced, and authoritative. The reviews you've wished for.

Pressed for time? Let *Medical Rounds* spare you hours of researching, photocopying, and compiling the articles and information you may need to confirm a patient's differential diagnosis. Or, turn to *Medical Rounds* for consultation on your clinical management strategy.

Preparing for rounds? The information in *Medical Rounds* is more clinically useful than many research articles.

Working on a talk or a student review? *Medical Rounds* provides access to information that is far more current than any textbook.

Need a current and authoritative review of a common disease or syndrome? *Medical Rounds* is more focused on your teaching and learning needs than any other resource available.

Don't miss another issue of this exciting new journal. Reserve your copy of the next issue by filling in and returning this subscription form today.

Sincerely,

Joel H. Baron
Publisher

*P.S.   Remember, your subscription is completely risk-free. If for any reason **Medical Rounds** does not meet your expectations within 30 days after you receive your first issue, we will send your money back. No questions.*